Cancer Pain Management: Principles and Practice

Cancer Pain Management: Principles and Practice

Winston C.V. Parris, M.D., F.A.C.P.M.
Professor of Anesthesiology and Director of Pain Control Center, Vanderbilt
University Medical Center; Attending Anesthesiologist, Vanderbilt University
Hospital, Nashville, Tennessee

Forewords by
Henry W. Foster, Jr., M.D.
Professor of Obstetrics and Gynecology, Meharry Medical College, Nashville,
Tennessee; Senior Advisor to President Clinton on Teenage Pregnancy Reduction and
Youth Issues

and

Ronald Melzack, Ph.D., F.R.S.C.
Professor of Psychology, McGill University, Montreal, Quebec, Canada

Butterworth–Heinemann
Boston   Oxford   Johannesburg   Melbourne   New Delhi   Singapore

Copyright © 1997 by Butterworth–Heinemann

 A member of the Reed Elsevier group

Library of Congress Cataloging-in-Publication Data

Cancer pain management : principles and practice / [edited by] Winston
   C.V. Parris ; forewords by Henry W. Foster, Jr., Ronald Melzack.
      p.   cm.
   Includes bibliographical references and index.
   ISBN 0-7506-9491-2 (alk. paper)
   1. Cancer pain—Treatment. 2. Cancer—Palliative treatment.
  I. Parris, Winston C. V.
   [DNLM: 1. Pain, Intractable—therapy. 2. Neoplasms—therapy. WL
704 C215 1996]
RC262.C291192 1996
616.99'406—dc20
DNLM/DLC
for Library of Congress   96-28928
                                     CIP

British Library Cataloguing-in-Publication Data
A catalogue record for this book is available from the British Library.

The publisher offers special discounts on bulk orders of this book.
For information, please contact:

Manager of Special Sales
Butterworth–Heinemann
313 Washington Street
Newton, MA 02158–1626
Tel: 617-928-2500
Fax: 617-928-2620

For information on all medical publications available, contact our World Wide Web
home page at: http://www.bh.com/med

10 9 8 7 6 5 4 3 2 1

Printed in the United States of America

To the ladies who have filled my life with love, purpose, and happiness: my late wife, Shirley V. Parris, my late mother, Julia A. Parris, and my daughter, Sharon P.J. Parris

Contents

Contributing Authors

Robert C. Adler, D.M.D., M.S.
Lecturer in Head and Orofacial Pain, UCLA School of Dentistry; Staff Surgeon, Department of Surgery, Century City Hospital, Los Angeles, California

C. W. Allwood, M.D., B.A., M.B.Ch.B., F.C., M.Med.
Acting Head of Department of Psychiatry, Witwatersrand University School of Health Sciences; Principal Specialist in Psychiatry, Tara Hospital, Johannesburg, South Africa

Jeff M. Arthur, M.D., D.A.B.A
Assistant Professor of Anesthesiology, Texas Tech Health Science Center and University Medical Center, Lubbock, Texas

Marshall D. Bedder, M.D., F.R.C.P.(C)
Medical Director, Advanced Pain Management Group, Inc., Providence St. Vincent Hospital and Medical Center, Portland, Oregon

Serge Blond, M.D.
Neurosurgeon, C.H.R.U. Hospital of Salengzo, Lille, France

Bennett Blumenkopf, M.D.
Associate Professor of Neurosurgery, Vanderbilt University School of Medicine; Attending Neurosurgeon, Vanderbilt University Medical Center, Nashville, Tennessee

William S. Breitbart, M.D.
Associate Professor of Psychiatry, Cornell University Medical College, New York, New York

Reverend Jeanne Maguire Brenneis, M.Div., S.T.M.
Director, Bioethics Center and Chaplain, Hospice of Northern Virginia, Falls Church, Virginia

Daniel B. Carr, M.D., F.A.B.P.M.
Saltonstall Professor of Pain Research, Departments of Anesthesia and Medicine, Tufts University School of Medicine; Medical Director, Pain Management Program, Department of Anesthesia, New England Medical Center, Boston, Massachusetts

Sonja W. Chandler, Pharm.D., M.S.
Pharmacy Pain Specialist, Department of Pharmacoeconomics, University of Texas M.D. Anderson Cancer Center, Houston, Texas

Joachim Chrubasik, M.D., P.R.I.V., D.O.Z.
Professor and Head of the Pain Unit and Ambulatory Anesthesia Pain Service, Pain Clinic, University of Heidelberg, Germany

Sigrun Chrubasik, M.D.
Department of Internal Medicine I, University of Heidelberg, Germany

Dipankar Das Gupta, D.A., M.D., M.M.A.M.S.
Professor in Anesthesia, University of Bombay; Consultant Anesthesiologist, Pain Clinic and Intensive Care Unit, Tata Memorial Hospital, Bombay, Maharashtra, India

Denise L. Dunlap, B.S.
Public Relations Coordinator, Department of Development and Community Relations, Alive Hospice, Inc., Nashville, Tennessee

John M. Flexner, M.D.
Professor of Medicine, Vanderbilt University School of Medicine, Nashville, Tennessee

John P. Greer, M.D.
Associate Professor of Medicine and Pediatrics, Vanderbilt University School of Medicine, Nashville, Tennessee

Michele Holevar, M.D., F.A.C.S.
Assistant Professor of Surgery, University of Illinois College of Medicine, Chicago; Associate Director of Trauma, Department of Surgery, Christ Hospital and Medical Center, Oak Lawn, Illinois

Allen H. Hord, M.D.
Assistant Professor of Anesthesiology and Orthopedics and Director, Division of Pain Medicine, Emory University School of Medicine; Director, Center for Pain Medicine, Department of Anesthesiology, Emory University Hospital, Atlanta, Georgia

Jeffrey D. Hord, M.D.
Assistant Professor of Pediatrics, University of Pittsburgh School of Medicine; Assistant Professor of Pediatrics, Division of Hematology and Oncology, Children's Hospital of Pittsburgh, Pittsburgh, Pennsylvania

Gordon Irving, M.B., B.S., M.Sc., M.Med., F.F.A.
Associate Professor of Anesthesiology and Medical Director, Center for Pain Medicine, University of Texas Health Science Center at Houston; Associate Professor of Anesthesiology, Hermann Hospital, Houston, Texas

Ada Jacox, R.N., Ph.D.
Associate Dean for Research, College of Nursing, Wayne State University; Director, Center for Health Research, Department of Nursing, Detroit Medical Center, Detroit, Michigan

Subhash Jain, M.D.
Associate Professor of Anesthesiology, Cornell University Medical College; Director, Pain Management, Departments of Anesthesiology and Critical Care Medicine, Memorial Sloan-Kettering Cancer Center, New York, New York

Piotr K. Janicki, M.D., Ph.D., D.Sci.
Research Associate Professor of Anesthesiology, Vanderbilt University School of Medicine, Nashville, Tennessee

Benjamin W. Johnson, Jr., M.D.
Assistant Professor of Anesthesiology, Vanderbilt University School of Medicine; Assistant Director, Vanderbilt Pain Control Center, Department of Anesthesiology, Vanderbilt University Medical Center, Nashville, Tennessee

Reverend Benjamin W. Johnson, Sr.
Past Instructor, Moody Bible Institute; Pastor Emeritus of Christ Community Church, Chicago, Illinois

Robert F. Kaiko, Ph.D.
Former Adjunct Assistant Professor of Pharmacology, Cornell Graduate School of Medical Sciences; Former Assistant Member, Analgesic Studies Section, Memorial Sloan-Kettering Cancer Center, New York, New York

Sri Kantha, M.D.
Medical Director, Meadowlands Pain Management Center, Meadowlands Hospital Medical Center, Seacaucus, New Jersey

Steven P. Key, M.D.
Chief Surgery Resident, Vanderbilt University Hospital, Nashville, Tennessee

M.V.L. Kothari
Attending Anesthesiologist, University of Bombay, Bombay, India

Elliot S. Krames, M.D.
Medical Director, Pacific Pain Treatment Centers, San Francisco, California

Daniel Le Bars, D.Sci., D.V.M.
Research Director, INSERM, Paris, France

V. Levin, B.Sc., M.B.Ch.B., F.F.Rad.(T)
Head of Radiation Oncology, University of Witwatersrand; Chief Specialist, Department of Radiation Oncology, Johannesburg Hospital, Johannesburg, South Africa

Janice M. Livengood, Ph.D., H.S.P.
Clinical Psychologist and Assistant Professor of Anesthesiology, Vanderbilt Pain Control Center and Vanderbilt University Hospital, Nashville, Tennessee

Paolo L. Manfredi, M.D.
Clinical Fellow in Neuro-Oncology, Section of Pain Symptom Management, University of Texas M.D. Anderson Cancer Center, Houston, Texas

Anne Marie McKenzie, M.D.
Assistant Professor of Anesthesiology, Emory University Hospital; Chief, Grady Pain Clinic, Department of Anesthesiology, Grady Memorial Hospital, Atlanta, Georgia

Emma Lee Ann Meffert, R.N., M.A., M.S., M.S.N.
Adult Acute Program, Poplar Springs Hospital, Petersburg, Virginia

Lopa A. Mehta
Attending Anesthesiologist, University of Bombay, Bombay, India

George A. Mensah, M.D., F.A.C.P., F.A.C.C.
Associate Professor of Medicine and Director, Medical Specialties Practice Site, Ambulatory Care Center, Medical College of Georgia, Augusta, Georgia

Jacques Meynadier, M.D.
Chief, Department of Anesthesiology, Intensive Care and Pain Treatment, Centre Oscar Lambret, Lille, France

Stephanie M. Mouton, M.D.
Assistant Professor of Anesthesiology, Vanderbilt University Medical Center, Nashville, Tennessee

Subir Nag, M.D.
Professor of Radiology and Chief of Brachytherapy, Ohio State University College of Medicine, Columbus, Ohio

Tsutom Oyama, M.D.
Professor Emeritus of Anesthesiology, University of Hirosaki School of Medicine, Hirosaki, Aomori-Ken, Japan

James C. Pace, R.N., D.S.N., M.Div.
Associate Professor of Nursing, Department of Adult Health, Emory University School of Medicine and NHW School of Nursing, Altanta, Georgia

Winston C. V. Parris, M.D., F.A.C.P.M.
Professor of Anesthesiology and Director of Pain Control Center, Vanderbilt University Medical Center; Attending Anesthesiologist, Vanderbilt University Hospital, Nashville, Tennessee

Steven D. Passik, Ph.D.
Assistant Professor of Psychology in Psychiatry, Cornell University Medical College, Bronx, New York; Assistant Attending Psychologist, Department of Psychiatry, Memorial Sloan-Kettering Cancer Center, New York, New York

Richard B. Patt, M.D.
Associate Professor of Anesthesiology and Neuro-Oncology, Director, Anesthesia Pain Services, and Deputy Chief, Pain and Symptom Management Section, University of Texas M.D. Anderson Cancer Center, Houston, Texas

David K. Payne, Ph.D.
Post-Doctoral Fellow in Psychiatry, Memorial Sloan-Kettering Cancer Center, New York, New York

Joan M. Payne, R.D., L.D.N.
Clinical Dietitian, Nutrition Services, Vanderbilt University Medical Center, Nashville, Tennessee

Richard Payne, M.D.
Associate Professor of Medicine, Department of Neuro-Oncology, Section of Pain and Symptom Management, University of Texas Medical School at Houston; Chief, Section of Pain and Symptom Management, Department of Neuro-Oncology, University of Texas M.D. Anderson Cancer Center, Houston, Texas

Gabor B. Racz, M.D., Ch.B., D.A.B.P.M.
Professor and Chairman of Anesthesiology, Texas Tech University Health Sciences Center; Attending Anesthesiologist and Director of Institute for Pain Management, Department of Anesthesiology, Texas Tech University Health Sciences Center and University Medical Center, Lubbock, Texas

Hugh Raftery, M.B., B.Ch., F.F.A.R.C.S.I.
Past President, World Society of Pain Clinicians, The Pain Society GB & I and The Irish Pain Society; Retired Consultant, Pain Relief Clinic, Beaumont Hospital, and Member of Board of Directors, St. Frances Hospital, Dublin, Ireland

P. Prithvi Raj, M.D., F.A.C.P.M.
Academic Director of Pain Medicine, UCLA Pain Medicine Center; Clinical Professor of Anesthesiology, UCLA School of Medicine, Los Angeles, California

Gail E. Rasmussen, M.D.
Assistant Professor, Division of Pediatric Critical Care and Anesthesia, Vanderbilt University Medical Center; Attending Physician, Departments of Anesthesiology and Pediatrics, Vanderbilt University Hospital, Nashville, Tennessee

William O. Richards, M.D.
Associate Professor of Surgery, Vanderbilt University School of Medicine, Nashville, Tennessee

E. Shipton, M.B.Ch.B., D.A., F.F.A., M.Med., M.D.
Head, Chief Specialist and Full Professor of Anesthesiology and Pain Management, and Subdean, Hillbrow Hospital, University of Witwatersrand, Johannesburg, South Africa

Gülen Tangören, M.D., F.A.C.A.
Staff Anesthesiologist, Sibley Memorial Hospital, Washington, District of Columbia

Joseph D. Tobias, M.D.
Associate Professor of Anesthesiology and Pediatrics, The University of Missouri; Director, Pediatric Critical Care/Anesthesia, The University of Missouri, Columbia, Missouri

Susan Utley, R.N., M.S.N., O.C.N.
Clinical Associate, Vanderbilt University School of Nursing; Clinical Nurse Specialist and Case Manager in Oncology, Office of Case Management, Vanderbilt University Medical Center, Nashville, Tennessee

Patricia M. Way, R.N., M.N., A.N.P.
Advance Practice Registered Nurse, Division of Bone Marrow Transplantation, University of Utah Health Science Center, Salt Lake City, Utah

Sharon M. Weinstein, M.D.
Assistant Professor of Medicine and Assistant Attending Neurologist, Department of Neuro-Oncology, University of Texas M.D. Anderson Cancer Center, Houston, Texas

Nancy Wells, D.N.Sc., R.N.
Research Assistant Professor, Vanderbilt University School of Nursing; Director of Nursing Research, Patient Care Services, Vanderbilt University Medical Center, Nashville, Tennessee

Jean-Claude Willer, M.D.
Professor of Physiology and Chief, Department of Clinical Neurophysiology, Medical School of Medicine, Pitie Salpetrier, Paris, France

Steven N. Wolff, M.D.
Associate Professor of Medicine, Vanderbilt University School of Medicine; Director, Bone Marrow Transplant Program, Vanderbilt University Hospital, Nashville, Tennessee

Debra Wujcik, R.N, M.S.N., A.O.C.N.
Adjunct Instructor, Vanderbilt University School of Nursing; Clinical Director, Affiliate Network, Vanderbilt Cancer Center, Nashville, Tennessee

Richard M. Zaner, Ph.D.
Ann Geddes Stahlman Professor of Medical Ethics and Director, Clinical Ethics Consultation Service, Department of Medicine and Center for Clinical Research Ethics, Vanderbilt University Medical Center, Nashville, Tennessee

Foreword I

This text, *Cancer Pain Management: Principles and Practice*, constitutes a milestone. It is devoted exclusively to the vagaries of pain caused by cancer. Although pain is the oldest affliction of humankind, it continues to represent the single most frequent reason that medical care is sought. Unremitting pain and a high-quality life are incompatible. Our ability to obtund pain in a scientific sense began only in the nineteenth century with the application of general anesthesia. Hence, it is both appropriate and understandable that the training background of the author of this text and many of his contributors is the field of anesthesiology.

The timeliness of this text is reinforced by the fact that the undertreatment of cancer pain is widespread. This circumstance is frustrating for practitioners and creates indescribable suffering for patients with cancer and their loved ones. Those who ascribe to the tenets of this text can mitigate the problem of cancer pain.

This book has a comprehensive character; this is how it must be, given that pain crosscuts all other medical disciplines. The author and his contributors have taken on an enormous challenge in producing this text on this subject. Confronted with this challenge, they have dutifully gone forth and have produced a quality product.

Forty-eight chapters are included, and there are 61 different contributors including the author. The book has a smooth flow; it commences with a historical background of cancer pain and mechanisms of its etiology. Most appropriately, the epidemiology of pain, in adults and children, is then presented. Existing and new approaches to pain control in cancer patients are discussed, including the topics of controlled-release opioids, intrathecal and epidural opiates, nerve block therapy, implantable technologies for pain, neuraxial analgesic blockade, stereotactic techniques, intraventricular morphine, invasive techniques, and neurolytic procedures.

Included in this text is an enlightened segment devoted to the psychosocial needs of cancer patients. Also discussed is the role of nonphysician providers of care and the provision of care in nonhospital settings. Hence, the role of nurses, social workers, nutritionists, and others is presented. Additionally, the hospice movement and support groups are addressed. The text's closing chapters reveal much about the sensitivity and character of the author and his contributors. Chapters are included that address spirituality and suffering, ethical issues, and governmental guidelines for cancer pain management.

Because cancer and its associated pain affects all medical disciplines, the writing of this text was complex; however, Dr. Winston C. V. Parris and his contributors engaged this challenge undaunted and have produced a significant and quality product for inclusion in the medical literature. All health care providers who manage pain in patients with cancer should be grateful for this fine effort.

Henry W. Foster, Jr.

Foreword II

Few problems are more challenging than the relief of pain in people with cancer. Cancer is rarely painful at its onset or during its early phases. However, patients with metastatic cancer usually develop pain that increases in severity, depending on the site, until it becomes relentless suffering. In addition, some patients develop severe pain directly or indirectly as a result of therapy. The late John J. Bonica estimated that moderate to severe pain is experienced by about 40% of patients with intermediate stages of the disease, and by 60–80% of patients with advanced cancer.

A substantial proportion of cancer patients obtain satisfactory relief of their pain by the judicious use of opiates. Increasingly, physicians have come to believe that a person's final weeks should be as free of pain as possible, and provide drugs such as morphine whenever they are requested by the patient. New delivery systems have evolved in recent decades, such as slow-release morphine capsules, self-administration pumps, and subcutaneous reservoirs that deliver a steady supply of morphine. Many of these techniques are the outcome of slowly evolving changes in our attitudes toward the use of narcotics for cancer patients. Hospices and palliative care services have become increasingly available so that terminally ill patients can live the remainder of their days free of pain and other distressing symptoms.

About 80–90% of cancer patients can achieve freedom from pain and a high quality of life by the appropriate use of opiates, sometimes in combination with other medications such as nonsteroidal anti-inflammatory drugs or tricyclic antidepressants. This is best accomplished in a hospice or a palliative care service in a hospital, but careful observation and regulation of dosages by any health care provider (or team of them) can generally maintain pain at levels that are at least tolerable.

Sometimes, however, cancer pain appears irregularly, so that opiates are inappropriate. At other times, the pain is massive and opiates are just not sufficiently effective. Pain may periodically break through the prevailing level of relief obtained with opiates to produce minutes or hours of hell one or more times a day. These breakthrough pains, because they strike unexpectedly at severe intensity, may present the greatest problem to health care professionals.

An armamentarium of treatments is required to manage cancer pain. Fortunately, Dr. Parris provides us here with excellent chapters describing the multitude of techniques that are available. He has invited contributions from experts in the field, and this single, focused volume provides all the techniques that may be needed to manage cancer pain in its myriad forms. The chapters describe the techniques for managing cancer pain by anesthesiologic, pharmacologic, psychiatric, surgical, and many other procedures. The strengths and weaknesses of the procedures for different kinds of pain are discussed honestly so that the reader can make intelligent, informed decisions. In addition to technical procedures to stop pain, Dr. Parris has invited contributions from outstanding professionals who deal with such important problems as suicide, drug abuse, government regulatory agencies, and ethical issues.

What shines through all the contributions to this volume is the compassion for those who suffer. This compassion and caring for one's fellow human beings is a shining personal characteristic of Dr. Parris, and it has provided a beacon for his contributors. Their concern, above all, is to present their specialized knowledge to help suffering patients.

This is an outstanding book that provides guidelines, techniques, and sensitive, balanced discussions of the complex, challenging problems presented by the suffering of cancer patients. Dr. Parris has made a very valuable contribution by enlisting the help of highly knowledgeable authorities who share their experience with the readers of this book. The relief of pain and suffering is a noble goal in life. This book enables health professionals everywhere to achieve that goal.

Ronald Melzack

Preface

Cancer remains one of those diseases that has always had and still has the implications of a death sentence. Traditionally, the word *cancer* has ominous intonations for two reasons: first, most cancer patients die sooner rather than later, and second, many cancer patients are known to suffer a great deal of pain before and during death. Great strides have been made in treating cancer and, indeed, almost everyone knows someone who has had cancer and is still alive. Moreover, it is encouraging to note that more people are becoming familiar with patients who have had cancer and its associated pain and whose pain has been satisfactorily controlled. Cancer pain management, though far from optimal, is improving largely due to the efforts of the late John Bonica, who sounded the alarm locally, nationally, and internationally that cancer pain was inadequately managed. It would be naive to state that Bonica's admonitions have been heeded; in fact, this is very far from reality. There are many reasons for this shortfall. A major reason is the lack of enthusiasm and/or conviction on the part of medical and nursing educators to introduce pain medicine in general and cancer pain management in particular into the curricula of medical and nursing undergraduate programs and postgraduate residency training programs. At most major medical institutions in the United States today, it is unfortunate that little or no time is allocated to pain medicine. Thus, it is not surprising that the inadequate management of cancer patients in pain is largely due to a deficiency in the fund of knowledge of most health care providers regarding cancer pain. The major objective of this text is to attempt to disseminate information on cancer pain and its management. It is also my hope that discussion of some of the controversial issues trigger the interest of both the informed and the relatively uninformed readers to seek more knowledge on cancer pain and its nuances.

No effort was spared in trying to introduce a multidisciplinary flavor to this text. Experts were invited from many disciplines, countries, and perspectives to collectively create a work that would be as varied as it is interesting and as clear as it broad. To achieve these goals, the authors were selected not only for their expertise on a particular subject but also for their overall commitment and enthusiasm to improving standards of cancer pain management.

A review of the basic sciences, the pathophysiology of cancer pain, and the clinical examination of cancer pain patients provides a good starting point for evaluating and treating cancer pain patients. Several authors have contributed to these areas and have expressed their viewpoints with conviction and clarity, so as to prepare a would-be therapist for the complex task of managing pain in a cancer patient. Thus, I hope we have been successful in stimulating the reader to add to his or her knowledge if possible and to seek more information regarding the diverse and multiple subtleties of cancer pain management.

Physicians and other health care professionals have a noble profession. It is noble and indeed a privilege to have the knowledge and the capacity to treat fellow human beings who are afflicted with various disease processes. It is even more satisfying, yet humbling, to treat patients who have cancer pain. If that treatment is successful, most cancer patients become very grateful. The expression of that gratitude can be rewarding to the recipient: physician, nurse, or other health care provider. As health care reform and the implications of managed competition become apparent, it is clear that the personal touch in medicine is diminished and the interactions between patients and physicians may become more impersonal. The management of cancer pain remains one of those areas in medicine where that nostalgic feeling of being of service may still be experienced. Perhaps it is appropriate to share a small but significant experience with the reader.

As you may have observed, this text is dedicated to the three ladies (my wife, my mother, and my daughter) who have most influenced my life. One of them is my late wife, Shirley Parris, to whom I am eternally grateful for her love and support over the past 25 years and especially during the preparation of this text. During the early phases of preparation, Shirley became gravely ill with cancer and developed a cancer-related pain syndrome (herpes zoster) that produced such excruciating pain one Sunday morning that I felt obligated to do something to to ease her suffering as quickly as possible. I performed a nerve block for Shirley at home, and an expression that I shall never forget shortly after performing that procedure for her was that of a faint smile emerging through streams of quiet tears that had been evoked by the excruciating pain. This faint smile was followed by a softly spoken "Thank you." The memory of that smile and the period around that event represents a moment in my professional life I shall treasure and never forget. Although we were not able to cure Shirley of her cancer, we were able to control the pain most of the time, and it is gratifying to note that she died peacefully and without pain. Although I had been privileged to experience this emotion with several patients over the past 20 years, it was a rare opportunity and privilege to have been able to be of service to a loved one. It is that similar feeling of being of service to the cancer pain patient that I hope most of my colleagues may experience as they practice their noble acts of healing, caring, and cancer pain management.

I am sure there are a few readers who would be familiar with most of the issues discussed in this text. To those readers I suggest that you move straight to Chapter 39 and read "Spirituality and Suffering," by Reverend Jeanne Brenneis. The contents of this chapter are critical to the principles surrounding cancer pain management and to issues of terminal illness and its sequelae. This chapter is informative, inspiring, and extraordinarily profound. Further, it is rewarding to learn of the accounts of two professionals—a physician and a pastor—who both had cancer and pain associated with their cancer and its treatment, and to learn of their perspectives of cancer pain. Their experiences are truly stimulating.

This text also addresses issues dealing with the history of cancer pain, the epidemiology of cancer pain in children and adults, and the assessment of cancer pain. A review of the basic mechanisms of cancer pain is also included. The different modalities for treating the cancer pain patient including medical, surgical, radiotherapeutic, neurosurgical, and other interventional techniques are described in some detail in this work. The importance of morphine as the gold standard in cancer pain management along with different methods of opioid administration and the diverse delivery systems are also discussed. A full chapter is devoted to the role of controlled-release opioids in cancer pain management. Nerve block therapy has a relatively small but distinct place in the management of those patients (approximately 5–10%) who do not satisfactorily respond to conventional pharmacologic management of cancer pain. Most of the nerve blocks used in treating the cancer pain patient are discussed. The use of implantable devices, infusion devices, neuraxial analgesic blockade, and stereotactic techniques for managing cancer pain are also reviewed in detail.

The medical, pharmacologic, and psychological management of cancer pain patients are also examined fully, and the different cancer-related pain syndromes are discussed along with appropriate therapeutic regimens. Most patients with terminal cancer develop nutritional problems either as a result of the progression of disease or as a result of the therapy for the cancer or both. Thus, the biochemical and practical considerations of nutrition are also discussed. In spite of the relative success in treating cancer patients, there is a great deal of dissatisfaction as a result of treatment since the patient's quality of life may not be acceptable either as a result of the cancer or as a result of the treatment for cancer, or both. Thus, the chapter on the quality of life of cancer pain patients represents an important contribution as one assesses efficacy of cancer pain therapies.

The recently released Cancer Pain Guideline by the Agency for Health Care Policy and Research represents an important step in educating physicians and other health care providers in the fundamentals of cancer pain management. Dr. Carr and his colleagues have done a superb job of encapsulating essentials of the guidelines in Chapter 43. As treatments become more aggressive, invasive, and expensive while, simultaneously, fewer funds are available for research and treating patients, a consideration of the ethical issues of cancer pain management has assumed paramount importance. The roles of the nurse and support groups in cancer pain management, not only for the patient but also for the family, have not received much prominence in the past. It is hoped that the information shared in these chapters may give the reader a global perspective on the complex issues relating to cancer pain management. The discussion of some of the unique perspectives of cancer pain management in Japan, India, and South Africa gives the text a little international flavor and lets the reader perceive that different countries deal with their unique problems in different ways, but at the same time, the overall principles of cancer pain management remain the same.

As the cancer pain patient continues to receive treatment, some of those therapeutic modalities may inevitably fail, and the patient and family will soon have to face the issues of dying and death. To effectively address those issues, the practical and philosophical approaches of the hospice movement are very informative in updating the reader on what is available and what should not be denied patients in that seemingly "hopeless hour." In fact, effectively administered hospice care may be most rewarding not only to patients but also to the family. I can truly testify to the tremendous comfort and support that the Hospice Group of Nashville brought to my family and me. It would have been so much more difficult in those closing weeks to have dealt with the issues of death without their support and invaluable assistance. To them and to hospice groups around the world, society owes a great debt of gratitude.

Thus, I am grateful to all the contributing authors for their expertise, contribution, and unselfish dedication. I hope that we have collectively produced a text that would truly represent a significant contribution to the field of medicine in general and to cancer pain management in particular.

I am grateful to the staff of Butterworth-Heinemann and more especially to the Director of Medical Publishing, Susan Pioli, for their general assistance. Susan's patience and cooperative interactions with me have been instrumental in my continuing to complete this work when at times I felt I would abandon it. The vacuum created by the loss of a mother and wife in less than 6 months may seriously impair one's productivity and motivation. The support and consideration of Susan and her team are largely responsible for the timely completion of this work.

I am very grateful to my administrative assistant Louise Efejuku and my secretary Cathryn Ellen for their loyalty, dedication, and hard work during the preparation of this text. The long hours and the unselfish administration of the many unheralded tasks that were necessary in the preparation of this text make their contribution totally invaluable. The typing of manuscripts and correspondence with the publisher and authors were just some of the many laborious duties they performed on behalf of this work.

I also thank Dr. Ronald Melzack for his contribution. As a noted scholar and superb researcher, and indeed a sincere friend, I am truly honored to have his participation in this work. I am truly honored to have Dr. Henry Foster, Senior Advisor to President Clinton on Teenage Pregnancy Reduction and Youth Issues, contribute to this work. His unique perspective on cancer pain management is indeed valuable and highly appreciated.

I honor my late parents, Edward and Julia Parris, for instilling in me those values that have served me well during good times and bad times, and also during the preparation of this work. My late wife Shirley has been the driving force behind me and a tower of support as I planned the outline of this text. Shirley's input, advice, caring, support, friendship, and most especially her love were an irreplaceable source of strength and energy to me and will continue to remain so. My children, Wayne, Wendell, and Sharon have been wonderful in supporting me in dealing with the different crises we faced, and I am truly thankful to the Lord for blessing my life with them. They have been sources of comfort during the closing phases of the preparation of this text, and I am truly proud of them and grateful for their love and support.

To the reader, I hope that you will find this work useful by virtue of its variety, scope, and depth, and I hope that you find it useful in your day-to-day clinical practice.

Winston C. V. Parris

Cancer Pain Management:
Principles and Practice

Chapter 1
Historical Perspectives

Anne Marie McKenzie and Winston C. V. Parris

As an experience, pain cannot be viewed as simply a nociceptive phenomenon because it usually involves the emotions and is tempered by the environment in which it occurs. The concept of pain, its source, and its therapy have undergone several philosophical changes. It is only recently that pain has evolved from a philosophical, almost mystical concept to one based on a scientific foundation. In some instances, religious or superstitious sentiment has altered the view toward pain therapy—e.g., it was once believed that because pain was sent from the gods it was something to be endured rather than eliminated. The Stoics thought that to endure pain silently was a form of dignity. Gout was once a painful condition associated with a life of luxury.[1] Today, analgesia is sometimes withheld in emergency rooms when pain is seen as a warning signal, e.g., suspicion of an acute abdomen. In the case of the patient with cancer, acute onset of back pain may be a sign of metastatic disease. Despite the constantly evolving nature of the study of pain, there are many instances, particularly in the case of chronic pain, where effective therapy is still far from ideal. Even today, most patients with advanced cancer experience a significant amount of pain during the course of their disease, in spite of the new technology that continues to be developed.[2] In addition, there are organizations dedicated to the study of pain, both in the United States and throughout the world, and currently very effective pharmacologic regimens are available to treat patients with cancer pain.

Ancient Cultures

Pain is usually thought of as either originating from an injury or as being due to an abnormal process or growth involving an internal organ, bone, or nerve. In ancient civilizations, external pain, e.g., those injuries sustained in warfare, was not viewed with any special attention; however, pain from disease was mystical and filled with superstition.[3, 4] The tribal concept of pain came from the notion that it was the result of an "intrusion" from outside the body.[3–5] These "intruders" were thought to be evil spirits sent by the gods as a form of punishment. Medicine men or the shaman were required to treat the resulting pain syndrome.[4–7] The spirits were thought to enter the body via several different pathways, and the course of therapy was often determined based on the pathway entered by the spirit. In New Guinea, it was believed that the port of entry for evil spirits was via an arrow or spear, which subsequently produced spontaneous pain. In Egypt, the left nostril was a particularly appealing entry site.[3] The papyri of Ebers and Berlin document that treatment involved expulsion of the offending spirit by sneezing, sweating, vomiting, and urination and even trephination for the treatment of headaches.[3, 4, 5, 7] Sometimes the shaman would suck the evil spirit from the painful wound and neutralize it with his special powers.[4, 5, 7] The analgesic regimen used by the Egyptians included placing electric fish from the Nile over wounds for the treatment of pain—similarly to the way a transcutaneous electrical nerve stimulation unit is used today.[7] The word *pain* is derived from

1

the Latin word *poena,* which means punishment; the word *patient* is derived from the Latin word *patior,* which means to endure suffering or pain.[7, 8] Sacrifices were offered to appease the gods who were seen as the dispensers of punishment in the form of pain.

The treatment of pain in children has also been described in ancient documents. Some of the pediatric pain remedies included having children wear amulets and drink various concoctions. These remedies were often specific for the problem requiring therapy—e.g., children were made to wear amulets filled with a dead man's tooth (Omnibonus Ferrarius, 1577) as a treatment for teething pain.[9] There have also been descriptions of the use of opioids to treat pain in children. The papyrus of Ebers, an Egyptian manuscript that contains a wide variety of pharmacologic information, describes the use of opium for pediatric pain.[3, 9] Despite this history of specific attention to pediatric pain, children remain to this day chronically undertreated. In 1977, Eland demonstrated that only 50% of children (aged 4–8) with postoperative pain were given analgesics. Moreover, the percentage of untreated pediatric patients with cancer pain was even higher. This was mainly due to the erroneous assumption that children were less sensitive to pain, and that the central nervous system was relatively underdeveloped in neonates. It has been recognized only recently that neonates can indeed feel pain, despite their immature nervous systems.[9]

Effect of Religion on Pain Concepts

The concept of pain as a form of punishment from superior beings or as a consequence of sin is not unique to ancient tribal cultures. This concept has also been depicted in early Christian literature.[5] Following her fall from grace, Eve was told by God that she would endure pain during childbirth: "I will greatly multiply your pain in childbearing; in pain you shall bring forth children, yet your desire shall be for your husband, and he shall rule over you" (Gen. 3:16). Consequently, the early Protestant church thought that pain during childbirth was something meant to be endured by women and thus the church opposed the use of analgesia to relieve this pain. In 1847, James Simpson introduced painless childbirth by using chloroform. However, it was not until Queen Victoria was given chloroform for

analgesia during the delivery of her eighth child, Prince Leopold, that painless childbirth was accepted by the church.[10] Epidural analgesia has made childbirth much less painful today, but there are still many countries in which this technique is not readily available. Even the use of surgical anesthesia was questioned. Pope Pius XII in the late nineteenth century had to give his approval before anesthesia could be used for surgical procedures: "The patient, desirous of avoiding or relieving pain, may, without any disquietude of conscience, use the means discovered by science which in themselves are not immoral."[6] The biblical character Job endured pain and suffering as described in the Old Testament:

> Man is also chastened with pain on his bed, and with unceasing complaint in his bones; so that his life loathes bread, and his soul favorite food. His flesh wastes away from sight, and his bones which were not seen stick out. Then his soul draws near to the pit, and his life to those who bring death (Job 33:19–22).

Job was considered a faithful servant by God, and was not guilty of any wrongdoing. He was described as a man who was "blameless and upright, one who feared God and turned away from evil . . ." (Job 1:1) and yet it was God who suggested to Satan: "have you considered my servant Job?" (Job 1:8). Job's friends assumed that there was some great sin in his life for which he was being punished by God. After all, "no harm befalls the righteous" (Prov. 12:21).

In the fifth century, St. Augustine wrote, "All diseases of Christians are to be ascribed to demons, chiefly do they torment the fresh baptized, yea even the guiltless newborn infant," implying that even the innocent infants did not escape the work of demons.[9] Many people in the first century Catholic church were persecuted and suffered ruthless persecution because of their belief in Christ. They often identified their suffering with Christ's suffering on the cross. Based on these beliefs, many present-day cancer pain patients with strong Christian beliefs view pain and suffering as part of their journey toward eternal salvation.

Ancient Approaches to Pain

During the time of the ancient Greeks, the heart and not the brain was considered the center of all sensation.[3, 4, 7, 11, 12] Medicine was considered more of a philosophical pursuit rather than a scientific pursuit. Hippocrates was the first to distinguish between medicine and philosophy. He thought pain was due to an imbalance of the four humors that controlled bodily function (blood, phlegm, yellow bile, and black bile).[4] This imbalance was referred to as *dyscrasia*.[4, 5] The *Hippocratic Collection*, which includes some 60 treatises written between 430–380 B.C., has sections that deal with the treatment of pain.[1, 7] These treatises were not thought to have a single author, but rather to be a collection of schools of thought.[1, 5] The School of Cos (including *The Nature of Man, Air, Water and Places, Prognostics, Epidemics I and III*) was more concerned with prognosis and the School of Cnidus (including *Disease II* and *Internal Ailments*) was more interested in diagnosis.[1] The *Collection* was also an attempt to use the diagnostic skills of the physician without downplaying the importance of verbal interaction and communication with the patient. The patient's description of his symptoms was very important. There has been reference to the *Hippocratic Collection* detailing therapy that treated opposites, but with regard to pain therapy there was some reference to likeminded treatments and remedies—e.g., treating pain with pain as described in *Epidemics V*.[1] The concept of preemptive analgesia dates back as far as the early 1900s to George Washington Crile (1864–1943). His anoci-association theory proposed that postsurgical pain could be alleviated by preventing the impulses from reaching the spinal cord. This could be accomplished by administering anesthesia prior to and during the surgical procedure.[13] Anaxagoras (500–428 B.C.) thought that pain was involved at some level in all sensations, and that this perception was located in the brain.[5] Pythagoras (566–497 B.C.), a Greek philosopher who traveled extensively through the Mediterranean and India, saw pain and suffering as necessary components of self-control.[4] Plato (427–347 B.C.) thought of pain as a sensation as well as a passion. He saw both the liver and heart as centers for experiencing pain. In Plato's theory, the brain was the processing center for distinguishing the perceived sensations.[5] He thought pain and pleasure were intimately linked, with distorted pleasure turning to pain, then being pleasurable again when the proper environment was attained.[5] Alcmaeon, a student of Pythagoras, thought that the brain was the center of all sensation and reason. He developed a theory that included a nervous system network of ducts and vessels carrying sensation through sensory organs to the brain.[3–5] The five senses that he described include taste, touch, smell, hearing, and vision.[5] Although all of these scholars hypothesized that the brain was the important organ for processing sensory information, their theories did not gain much success because they were counteracted by the more popular notion that the heart was the center of sensation. This school of thought was endorsed by Aristotle (384–322 B.C.), philosopher and son of a physician, who termed the heart the *sensorium commune*—being the seat of intelligence as well as the source of sensation.[3–5] He expressed this in *De Amina*, where he said, "Sensations are pleasant when their sensible extremes such as acid and sweet are brought in to their proper ratio, whilst in excess they are painful and destructive."[4, 14] He continued with the notion of five separate senses expressed earlier by Alcmaeon. Aristotle thought that the brain's role was secondary to the heart in that its purpose was to cool blood coming from the heart. It was also useful in inducing sleep.[1] This concept has permeated our language even today with expressions such as "heartache," "heart throb," and "breaking my heart."[5] Pain, according to Aristotle, was essential to the body and was caused by increased sensitivity to all sensations, particularly touch.[4] This Aristotelian concept dominated theories of sensation for several years and heavily influenced the scientific thought process of medicine. In ancient Egypt, the brain was totally ignored as a vital organ and was not even preserved in the embalming process.[3] The Egyptians thought that the *metu*, a network of vessels, carried life to the heart, which they also regarded as the center of all sensation.[4, 5]

The Greek ideology soon became widespread as their culture and practices spread across the Mediterranean Basin. Alexandria soon became known as a city that housed scholars and as a source for intellectual pursuits. It is in this environment that Herophilus (330–250 B.C.) and Erasistratus (310–250 B.C.) explored the anatomy of the nervous system.[1, 3] Herophilus both experimented on live criminals and did postmortem examinations on them. According to Celsus:

> As pain and illness may invade our inner organs, they cannot determine any way of restoring them to integrity without knowing their structure. It is therefore necessary to open up cadavers to scrutinize their viscera and en-

trails; and Herophilus and Erasistratus have gone even further as they have opened up live criminals which kings conveyed to them from the dungeons so they might capture in the raw what nature had kept hidden from them… .[1]

In his neuroanatomy study, Herophilus established that the cerebellum was important in controlling voluntary movement and described seven pairs of cranial nerves.[1] Erasistratus also found anatomic evidence that the brain was part of the central nervous system and delineated two kinds of nerves (sensory and motor). He described sensory nerves as hollow nerves in the meninges and the motor nerves as being in the cerebrum and cerebellum.[1] Galen (130–201 A.D.), a physician from Pergamon, is noted for combining the anatomic basis for medicine with philosophy.[3] He studied in both Greece and Alexandria before becoming a court physician to the emperor, Marcus Aurelius, in Rome. While there, Galen performed anatomic dissections on the nervous systems of newborn pigs. It is from evidence gathered from these dissections that he developed a brain centered complex theory of sensation.[1, 3, 4, 6, 7] He concluded that pain was important in understanding the organization of the nervous system and that pain was a symptom of underlying pathology. He expanded on the work of Erasistratus and Herophilus and established a category for painful nerves, which included three types of nerves: those pertaining to movement ("hard" nerves), sensation ("soft" nerves), and relaying messages of pain.[6] The pain nerves had the lowest sensibility.[3, 6] This concept also met with opposition due to the still prevailing thought that the heart was the center of all sensation. In *De Locis Affectis*, Galen emphasized the diagnostic value of pain in identifying organ or internal disease. He has been credited with many of the descriptive terms currently used for pain symptoms—e.g., "pulsific" (throbbing) and "pungitive" (lancinating). He did not, however, include the sensation of numbness as a specific type of pain.[1] His dissections also gave him insight into the tactile senses and let him emphasize pain as both a symptom and a part of the disease process. Galen thought that pain was under the larger umbrella of perception, and that perception was a combination of a receiving organ, a connecting passageway, and a processing center.[1] He saw pain as a warning of important internal and external changes. Interestingly, he developed a medication, *theriac*, which contained among its contents viper's flesh and opium.[10]

Plato, in *Timaeus*, wrote that the heart and liver were the centers for sensation.[4] He thought there was a three-part spirit, in which the liver and heart were pain centers and the brain was the site of discrimination for the concepts that resulted in these sensations.[4, 5]

Celsus, a first century medical writer, thought of pain as valuable only in terms of providing a diagnosis or as a predictor of prognosis with no positive qualities. In his eight books, he defined several different kinds of pains—each with a different significance. As the presence of pain was, by definition, associated with some form of pathology, measures were to be taken to treat the cause of the pain. He had detailed instructions for analgesic regimens based on the symptoms, e.g., pleuritic chest pain was treated with blood letting if acute, and topical vinegar and mustard application if chronic.[1] In 529 A.D., the Greek Academy was closed by Justinian due to its "perverse pagan teachings." As a result, many of the teachers fled to Persia.[3] A school of medicine was started in Jundishapur and texts were translated into Arabic.[3] Many of the writings were translated in Baghdad by Hunayn ibn Ishaq, a Nestorian Christian.[15] Arabic medicine began to enter Europe in the eleventh century and was influenced by physicians and philosophers such as Avicenna (980–1036 A.D.).

Avicenna, an Arabic physician, thought that all internal senses were within the cerebral ventricles. His theory of pain was based on the four temperaments (heat, cold, moistness, and dryness), which each organ contained to varying degrees. A disturbance in the composition of these temperaments resulted in pain.[6] He also described the anesthetic properties of opium, and his treatise *Canon Medicinae* described the use of herbane and mandrake to relieve pain. He also wrote *Poem Medicinae*, which was an abbreviated version of *Canon Medicinae*.[11] *Canon Medicinae* was widely used, and remained an authoritative medical text in Europe for six centuries.[3, 4, 6, 10, 16] During the time between the fall of Rome and the start of the Renaissance, the influence of Christianity was apparent in the scientific community. The painful crucifixion of Christ was seen as a method of salvation and redemption.[3] It was not until between 1800 and 1850 that pain developed into a scientific concept composed of anatomy and physiology—without its prior associated religious connotation.

Pain and Art

Depictions of therapy for pain have been seen since the Egyptian hieroglyphics.[7] Homer used medical pain descriptors in the *Iliad* and *Odyssey*.[1] He used different words to describe different types of suffering as well as to describe varying types of pain—e.g., a distinction was made between the pains of childbirth and pains sustained following injury by a sword. He also had separate descriptors for persistent and intermittent symptoms. The god of healing was Peon or Apollo and was known to administer "remedies."[1] Helen of Troy was said to have treated her pain with a "drug" that was in her wine.[1]

Leonardo da Vinci (1452–1519), in his famous painting of a man with two faces, depicted artistically the relationship between pain and pleasure, similar to the concepts expressed by Plato.[4, 6] Da Vinci was both a scientist and artist who, after anatomic dissections, concluded that the *sensorium commune* was in the third ventricle, with sensation conducted to the brain via the spinal cord.[4, 6]

In ancient China, the Yin Yang theory (Yin being negative and Yang positive) of two opposing forces prevailed, with pain being caused by an imbalance of these forces. Yin was the force of conservation and Yang of dissipation.[3] The earliest medical text in China, *The Yellow Emperor's Classic of Internal Medicine*, included descriptions of acupuncture for treatment. Acupuncture was described as correcting the imbalance of the opposing forces and is still used to treat painful conditions today. The Chinese used the willow plant (which contains salicylic acid) to treat arthritis.[10] Nonsteroidal anti-inflammatory drugs are a mainstay of treatment for arthritis today.

Use of Medications for Pain Relief

Since the times of ancient civilization, medications have been used to relieve pain. The Babylonians in 2250 B.C. used herbs for pain relief.[12] There have been artifacts from ancient Egypt, Babylon, and Persia that describe various treatments for pain.

Similarly, the *Rig-Veda*, one of the oldest sacred books of India (ca. 4000 B.C.), described pain remedies.[3] Analgesics are referred to in Greek mythology. Aesculapius, the Greek god of medicine, had a herbal analgesic called nepenthe.[12]

As noted previously, mandrake and wine have both been described as being used for pain relief. The apostle Paul advised his disciple, Timothy, to drink some wine for his "frequent ailments" (1 Tim. 5:23). Hippocratic doctors are recorded as using medications such as mandrake, herbane, night shade, and poppies. Hippocratic medicine was practical in nature, with pain being the result of a perturbation of the natural equilibrium of a healthy body. The Hippocratic sense is illustrated in the statement "first do no harm."[3] During the seventeenth century there was some controversy regarding the liberal therapeutic use of opium. Sydenham, who is known for creating laudanum (an analgesic that contained opium), strongly favored the use of opium as a key ingredient for analgesics. He stated, "So necessary an instrument is opium in the hand of a skillful man that medicine would be a cripple without it; and whoever understands it well, will do more with it alone than he could well hope to do from any single medicine."[17] Morphine was isolated from opium by Frederick Serturner, an apothecary's assistant, in Prussia in 1803 and he published his findings in *Principium Somniferum*.[10, 16] This new isolate did not have a significant impact until 1817, when he renamed the drug "morphine," after Morpheus, the Greek god of dreams.[16] The discovery of hypodermic needles in 1853 expanded the use of morphine.[10] Crawford Long gave the first ether anesthetic in 1842. This discovery, which led to the ability to conduct painless surgery, was not recognized until 1846 when William Morton gave the first public demonstration. This revolutionized the field of surgery, allowing previously impossible procedures to be performed. Interestingly, chloroform, nitrous oxide, and ether had all been discovered as substances by 1831 but were used only for recreational purposes.

Alternative methods to pharmacologic therapy for the treatment of pain syndromes have been gaining popularity. Psychological therapy, including biofeedback and hypnosis, is a useful adjunct to pharmacologic therapy for the cancer patient. Acupuncture has been used in some select circumstances with varying success.

Pain Theories

By the nineteenth century, knowledge of anatomy and physiology had developed to the point where more sophisticated theories regarding the sensation and perception of pain were beginning to evolve. In 1826, Johannes Muller proposed a theory that sensory receptor stimulation transmitted pain signals centrally. This paved the way for two other theories: the specificity and intensive theories.[6] The specificity theory was developed in 1858 by Schiff who discovered that pain and touch were independent sensations with different pathways. Erb in 1874 proposed the intensive theory that any stimulus, if intense enough, could produce pain.[6, 8] Nafe in 1934 suggested that cutaneous sensation was characterized by specific patterns of nervous impulses rather than individual routes.[18] Livingston in 1943 tried to explain the summation phenomenon of pain syndromes in terms of specific neural mechanisms. Weddell and Sinclair in 1955 elaborated on the work of Nafe with the development of the pattern theory, which suggested that all fiber endings are alike, with the exception of those innervating hair cells, creating a pattern based on stimulation of nonspecific receptors.[18] Melzack and Wall in 1965 developed the gate control theory of pain that proposed that a central modulator affected large and small nerve fiber input and thus affected pain perception.[18] Although this theory has since undergone multiple revisions, it is still used to help describe pain syndromes.

Hospice Movement

The concept of hospice dates back to Fabiola, a Roman matron during the reign of Emperor Julian the Apostate.[19] She had a place for sick and healthy travelers and also cared for the dying. Hospice is a medieval term representing a welcome place of rest for pilgrims to the Holy Land.[19–21] Hospitals in general began as Christian institutions and, in medieval times, hospitals and hospices were interchangeable. During the eleventh century, there were many monastery-based hospices. St. Vincent de Paul, a seventeenth-century Catholic priest, founded the Sisters of Charity in Paris for the poor, sick, and dying. This influenced Fliedner, a Protestant pastor, to found Kaiserwerth 100 years later.[19–21] Nuns from the Sisters of Charity and Kaiserwerth accompanied Florence Nightingale in the Crimea. In 1902 the Irish Sisters of Charity founded St. Joseph's Hospice, which was to be staffed by Cicely Saunders 50 years later. Cicely Saunders was the first full-time hospice medical officer. She was the founder and medical director of St. Christopher's Hospice in England. Her training began as a nurse and after being injured in the war, she became a medical social worker. She later developed a keen interest in terminal cancer patients and trained to become a physician. She spoke of the importance of taking the patient at his or her word, scheduling dosing of opioids versus as needed dosing, and frequent pain assessment to adequately manage the patient's pain.[19, 21, 22] She sought to convince the medical community that it was totally unnecessary for cancer patients to die in pain.[19–21] Saunders is now considered the mother of palliative care,[19–21, 23] and many of her views are still being taught in medicine and nursing schools today.

Invasive Techniques for the Management of Cancer Pain

As technology advanced in the management of pain, new ways to deliver opioids were developed. Opiate receptors were identified in the brain in 1973, and in 1976 Yaksh demonstrated naloxone reversible analgesia in rats with intrathecal morphine.[24, 25] Two years later, Wang and Behar treated intractable cancer pain using intrathecal and epidural opioids.[26, 27] Since then, continuous infusions of epidural and intrathecal opioids have been successfully used to treat cancer pain, particularly in patients unable to tolerate other routes of opioid delivery.

Neurolysis is another form of analgesia typically reserved for cancer pain patients. Numerous drugs have been used for neurolysis in the past, including silver nitrate, chloroform, glycerin, ricin, and ammonium salts. Phenol and alcohol are the most commonly used agents. Hauck in 1906 used alcohol to treat neuralgias; however, Dogliotti in 1931 was the first to use intrathecal alcohol to treat pain. Phenol, isolated in 1834, was first used as a neurolytic agent in rabbits by Doppler in 1925 in Germany. In 1926 he reported analgesia in 12 patients using a topical application of 7% aqueous solution on femoral arteries in the treatment of peripheral vascular disease.[28] It was not until the late 1950s that phenol became more commonly used for the treatment of chronic pain. Intrathecal phenol neurolysis was first described by Maher in 1955 and success rates of up to 80% have been described. Reports of epidural injections of phenol are sparse. Alcohol has also been used for neurolysis, particularly in the management of pain due to pancreatic cancer, where alcohol celiac plexus blockade is often performed with good success rates.[29] There have been reports of multiple injection techniques over several days using epidural alcohol for intractable cancer pain. Complications of neuraxial neurolysis include bowel and bladder dysfunction, persistent numbness and weakness, and paresthesias. Because their duration of analgesia averages 3–9 months, these procedures are most commonly performed on patients with limited life expectancy, who often have lost their bowel and bladder function.[28]

Surgical techniques have been used in the treatment of cancer pain. Abe and Bennett in 1888 performed the first sensory rhizotomy for chronic pain.[30, 31] In 1905 Spiller, a neurologist, discovered the significance of the anterior spinothalamic tracts in pain, after noting loss of pain and temperature sensation in a patient who had masses compressing the anterior spinal cord. In 1911 he convinced Martin, a neurosurgeon, to perform the first cordotomy for pain relief in a cancer patient.[30, 31] Cordotomy involves the section of the lateral spinothalamic tracts carrying contralateral pain and temperature fibers.[30] The first percutaneous cordotomy was performed by Mullan in 1963.[32] Although cordotomy was helpful for unilateral pain syndromes, midline myelotomy was introduced to treat intractable midline or bilateral pain. Armour performed the first midline myelotomy (division of the spinothalamic decussating fibers) in 1927.[33]

Modern Concepts of Cancer Pain Management

The undertreatment of pain in general, and cancer pain in particular, is receiving greater recognition. The American Pain Society recently published standards for both acute and cancer pain. The Agency for Health Care Policy and Research (AHCPR) published their first set of guidelines on medical care dealing with acute postoperative pain

in March 1994.[34] Their guidelines indicated that at least 50% of postoperative pain patients are undertreated.[34] Fifty percent of patients with cancer and 75% of those with advanced malignant disease will likely experience moderate-to-severe pain.[35, 36] There are multiple barriers to adequate pain management—both patient and physician related. Some of these barriers have originated from the worthwhile fight against illicit drugs. Unfortunately, the result is that patients who need opioids for legitimate pain control may have difficulty obtaining them.[35] There are sometimes inconsistencies in local regulatory agencies with respect to cancer pain management. In a recent survey of state medical board members, 14% thought that prescribing opioids for an extended period to patients with cancer pain was a lawful but generally unacceptable medical practice and should thus be discouraged.[35] Five percent thought that this practice was a probable violation of both federal and state controlled substances laws that warranted investigation.[35] Cancer pain initiatives are volunteer, grass roots, multidisciplinary state level organizations dedicated to overcoming myths and barriers regarding the effective management of cancer pain. The first initiative was organized in Wisconsin in 1986 in response to the realization of a general lack of education about cancer pain and opioids, which was having a negative impact on patient care. This realization came when Congress tried to introduce a bill to legalize heroin (Diamorphine), which has been illegal in the United States since 1924.[37] This measure was opposed because heroin is just a prodrug and gets broken down to morphine.[37, 38] The American Cancer Society (ACS) listed cancer pain as one of their national priorities for the first time in 1993 and has publicly supported state cancer pain initiatives since then. The American Society for Clinical Oncology (ASCO) has developed a curriculum for oncology fellows for training in cancer pain as part of their fellowship. This curriculum was introduced in an attempt to address the lack of formal education regarding pain management offered to most house officers. The Oncology Nursing Society has recently released position papers on cancer pain education and research, with specific guidelines for nurses.[39]

Cancer pain issues are making their way into the media. A landmark legal case in 1991 in North Carolina awarded a large financial sum because of failure to treat a patient's pain. A man with metastatic cancer was sent to a nursing home and once there, was weaned off the narcotics for his pain. He subsequently died a very painful death and his family was awarded $15 million in compensation for the pain and suffering that he endured. There are now societies devoted to advancing knowledge in the area of pain medicine, e.g., the American Pain Society (APS) and the International Association for the Study of Pain (IASP). The APS has recently published a set of standards for the treatment of acute and chronic cancer pain. The multifactorial nature of cancer pain is also being recognized and multidisciplinary pain centers are now gaining acceptance. There have been several surveys of physicians, nurses, and medical students regarding their knowledge and treatment of pain. There is still misunderstanding in the medical community as well as in the lay public with regard to the difference among opioid dependence, tolerance, and addiction. It is clear that education in pain medicine has been underrepresented in most medical and nursing institutions, judging by the scant number of pages devoted to pain in textbooks as well as by the relative paucity of pain lectures.[36] A review of nine American textbooks and monographs on cancer management published prior to 1982 showed that only 17 of 9,300 pages discussed treatment of cancer pain symptoms. This leaves little data for residents to rely on and consequently results in the chronic undertreatment of pain.[40] Despite the fact that there have been advocates for improved pain management for several years, statistics show that pain is still not being well controlled worldwide.

Bonica noted that there was no published epidemiologic data on pain as late as the 1970s. Until then, there was also no data on the psychosocial effects of cancer pain on the patients and their families. There has been a great paucity of pharmacokinetic data on analgesics in cancer patients until recently.[40, 41] This deficiency prompted Bonica to formulate data based on rough estimates and extrapolations from both the United States and worldwide. It is from this data that we know that 50% of all cancer patients and 75% of patients with advanced disease will experience a significant amount of pain. The World Health Organization (WHO) has established a cancer pain relief program to study cancer pain. In 1982, the three-step analgesic ladder, a validated, easy-to-follow, inexpensive guide to cancer pain relief was developed. The analgesic ladder is an algorithm for treating cancer pain, starting from nonopioid analgesics and progressing to strong opioids as the pain increases in severity. It has been shown that more than 75% of patients with cancer pain can be effectively managed using this technique.[42] In order for this strategy to be effective, the WHO has stated that the country must integrate the information into a national policy and implement methods to transfer the information to the community level.[43] Also new is the realization that cancer pain is not a single isolated entity unto itself, but that it has multiple etiologies that may or may not be directly related to the cancer itself.[13, 44, 45] Some pain syndromes may be more responsive to opioids than others—e.g., neuropathic pain may be less responsive to opioids than somatic pain. This fact has resulted in the awareness that treatment must be directed toward the perceived etiology of the pain once it is discovered. Pain does not occur in a vacuum; the psychosocial manifestations of pain must be treated as well as any possible side effects to the treatment. With regards to cancer pain, this is generally stressed in all fields of medicine, but particularly in the field of pain medicine.

References

1. Rey R. Antiquity. In History of Pain. Paris: Éditions la Découverte, XIII, 1993;19.
2. Bonica JJ. Cancer Pain. In JJ Bonica (ed), The Management of Pain. Philadelphia and London: Lea & Febiger, 1990;400.
3. Todd EM. Pain: Historical Perspectives. In GM Aronoff (ed), Evaluation and Treatment of Chronic Pain. Baltimore: Urban and Schwarzenberg, 1985;1.
4. Procacci P, Maresca M. Pain Concept in Western Civilization: A Historical Review. In C Benedetti, et al (eds), Advances in Pain Research and Therapy (Vol. 7). Recent Advances in the Management of Pain. New York: Raven, 1984:1.
5. Procacci P, Maresca M. Evolution of the Concept of Pain. In Sicuteri (ed), Advances in Pain Research and Therapy (Vol. 20). New York: Raven, 1984:1.
6. Jaros JA. The concept of pain. Crit Care Nurs Clin North Am 1991;1:1.
7. Warfield C. A history of pain relief. Hosp Prac 1988; 7:121.
8. Caton D. The secularization of pain. Anesthesiology 1985;62:93.
9. Unruh AM. Voices from the past: Ancient views of pain in childhood. Clin J Pain 1992;8:247.
10. Raja PP. Pain relief: Fact or fancy? Reg Anesth 1990;15:157.

11. Donovan MI. An historical view of pain management. How we got to where we are! Cancer Nurs 1989;12:257.

12. Bonica JJ. History of Pain Concepts and Therapies. In JJ Bonica (ed), The Management of Pain. Philadelphia and London: Lea & Febiger, 1990;2.

13. Katz J. George Washington Crile, anoci-association, and pre-emptive analgesia. Pain 1993;53:243.

14. Aristotelis Ethica Nichomachae. Editit et commentario continuo enstruxit. G. Ramsauer. Lipsiae, in aedibus B. G. Teubneri, 1878.

15. Rey R. The Middle Ages and Pain: A World to Investigate. In History of Pain. Paris: Éditions la Découverte, XIII, 1993;55.

16. Raj PP. History of Pain Management. In PP Raj (ed), Practical Management of Pain. New York: Year Book, 1986;3.

17. Rey R. Pain in the Classical Age. In History of Pain. Paris: Éditions la Découverte, XIII, 1993.

18. Melzack R, Wall PD. Pain mechanisms: A new theory. Science 1965;150:971.

19. Craven J, Wald FS. Hospice care for dying patients. Am J Nurs 1975;75:1816.

20. Allan N. Hospice to hospital in the near east: An instance of continuity and change in late antiquity. Bull Hist Med 1990;64:446.

21. Campbell L. History of the hospice movement. Cancer Nurs 1986;9:333.

22. Saunders C. The last stages of life. Am J Nurs 1965;65:70.

23. Austin C, Cody CP, Eyres PJ, et al. Hospice home care pain management: Four critical variables. Cancer Nurs 1986;9:58.

24. Yaksh TL, Rudy TA. Analgesia mediated by a direct spinal action of narcotics. Science 1976;192:1357.

25. Jacquet YF, Lajtha A. Morphine action at central nervous system sites in rat: Analgesia or hyperalgesia depending on site and dose. Science 1973;182:490.

26. Wang JK, Nauss LA, Thomas JE. Pain relief by intrathecally applied morphine in man. Anesthesiology 1979;50:149.

27. Behar M, Magora F, Olshwang D, et al. Epidural morphine in treatment of pain. Lancet 1979;i:527.

28. Wood KM. The use of phenol as a neurolytic agent: A review. Pain 1978;5:205.

29. Korevaar WC. Transcatheter thoracic epidural neurolysis using ethyl alcohol. Anesthesiology 1988;69:989.

30. Sundaresan N, DiGiaanfo GV, Hughes JO. Neurosurgery in the treatment of cancer pain. Cancer 1989;63:2365.

31. White JC, Sweet WH. Introduction. In Pain and the Neurosurgeon: A Forty Year Experience. Springfield, IL: Charles C. Thomas, 1969;3.

32. Mullan S, Harper PV, Hekmatpanah J, et al. Percutaneous interruption of spinal pain tracts by means of a strontium 90 needle. J Neurosurg 1963;20:931.

33. Armour D. Surgery of the spinal cord and its membranes. Lancet 1927;ii:691.

34. Acute Pain Management in Adults: Operative Procedures. U.S. Department of Health and Human Services. Agency for Health Care Policy and Research, 1992.

35. Joranson D, Cleeland CS, Weissman DE, Gilson AM. Opioids for chronic cancer and noncancer pain: A survey of state medical board members. Fed Bull June 1992;15.

36. Bonica JJ. Treatment of Cancer Pain: Current Status and Future Needs. In Sicuteri (ed), Advances in Pain Research and Therapy (Vol. 9). New York: Raven, 1985;589.

37. Lasagna L. Heroin: A medical "me too." N Engl J Med 1981;304:1539.

38. Kaiko RF, Wallenstein SL, Rogers AG, et al. Analgesic and mood effects of heroin and morphine in cancer patients with postoperative pain. N Engl J Med 1981;304:1501.

39. Spross JA, McGuire DB, Schmitt RM. Oncology Nursing Society position paper on cancer pain. Oncol Nurs Forum 1991;17:595, 751, 943.

40. Bonica JJ. Cancer pain: A major national health problem. Cancer Nurs J 1978;4:313.

41. Baines M, Kirkham SR. Cancer Pain. In PD Wall, R Melzack (eds), Textbook of Pain. New York: Churchill Livingstone, 1989;590.

42. Ventafridda V, Tamburini M, DeConno F, et al. A validation study of the WHO method for cancer pain relief. Cancer 1987;59:851.

43. Teoh N, Stjernsward J. WHO Cancer Pain Relief Program—Ten Years On. IASP Newsletter July/August 1992;5.

44. Abram SE. Advances in chronic pain management since gate control. Reg Anesth 1993;18:66.

45. Sharfman WH, Walsh TD. Has the analgesia efficacy of neurolytic celiac plexus block been demonstrated in pancreatic cancer pain? Pain 1990;41:267.

Chapter 2

Epidemiology of Cancer in Children

Jeffrey D. Hord and John P. Greer

Few risk factors have been identified for neoplasms in children. Epidemiologic studies are severely limited by the relative rarity of childhood cancer; only 2% of malignancies in Western industrialized nations occur in children.[1] It is extremely difficult for a single institution to perform childhood cancer epidemiologic studies owing to the small sample size. To overcome this problem, epidemiologic data from a large number of institutions are aggregated and analyzed by organizations such as the Children's Cancer Group and the Pediatric Oncology Group.

The biological behavior of a malignancy may differ, depending on the histologic subtype, but it is often impossible to study individual subtypes owing to the extremely small sample size. Other problems with pediatric oncology epidemiologic studies include the gathering of data from subjective sources (parents) and the need to consider both prenatal and postnatal factors.[2]

A significant amount of epidemiologic data regarding cancer in the United States comes from the population-based Surveillance, Epidemiology, and End Results (SEER) program based within the National Cancer Institute. The SEER program monitors nine geographic regions scattered throughout the country that are thought to be representative subsets of the U.S. population based on demographic and epidemiologic criteria. The SEER program's database encompasses 9.6% of the U.S. population.[3]

Incidence and Mortality

Cancer is second only to accidents as the leading cause of death among children aged 1–14 years in the United States (Figure 2-1). Approximately 7,800 children are diagnosed with cancer annually[4] and 1,700 children will die during that same period due to cancer.[5] This corresponds to an incidence of 142 per 1 million in white children less than 15 years of age and an incidence of 124 per 1 million in black children of the same age. The cure rate for all malignant neoplasms in pediatrics is approaching 70%.[3]

The types of cancer that occur in children are different from those found in adults and vary with age during childhood (Figure 2-2). For example, neuroblastoma is the most common malignancy in infants and acute lymphoblastic leukemia (ALL) is most common in older children. The ratio of solid tumors to leukemia declines from 5 to 1 in infants to 2 to 1 in children aged 1–14 years.[6]

Studies performed by the International Agency for Research on Cancer demonstrate markedly different incidence rates of cancer in children less than 15 years of age among various countries (Figure 2-3). The highest reported incidence is in Nigeria (Ibadan) at 155.6 per 1 million and the lowest is in Fiji (Indian) at 39.7 per 1 million.[7] Differences among incidence rates may be related to environmental and genetic variables, but the varying quality of medical care throughout the world and the diffi-

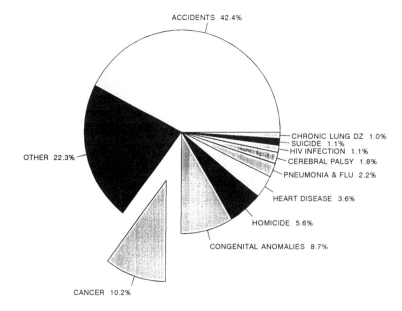

Figure 2-1. Causes of death in children aged 1–14 years in the United States. (Adapted from National Center for Health Statistics: Vital Statistics of the United States, 1989. Washington, DC: Public Health Service, 1992.)

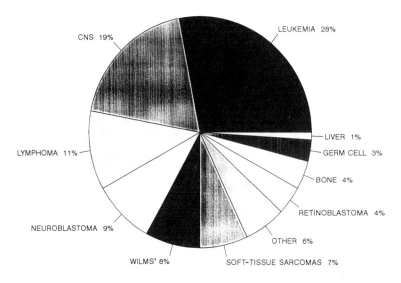

Figure 2-2. Distribution of types of cancer found in US children aged 1–15 years. (Adapted from LL Robison. General Principles of the Epidemiology of Childhood Cancer. In PA Pizzo, DG Poplack [eds], Principles and Practice of Pediatric Oncology. Philadelphia: Lippincott, 1993;3.)

culty in maintaining thorough population-based registries in developing countries may adversely affect the accuracy of the study results.

Recent information from the SEER registry indicates that despite an increase of 7.6% in the incidence rate of childhood malignancies from 1973–1989 in the United States, the overall cancer mortality in children has decreased by 38.9%. The most significant increase in incidence occurred in the two most frequent childhood neoplasms: central nervous system (CNS) tumors (an increase of 28.6%) and ALL (23.7%). During the same period, the mortality for five childhood malignancies decreased by more than 50%: soft tissue sarcomas, Hodgkin's lymphomas, ALL, non-Hodgkin's lymphomas, and malignant bone tumors (Figure 2-4). After the first 5 years of life, the incidence of cancer in childhood increases with age. The incidence of malignancy in children

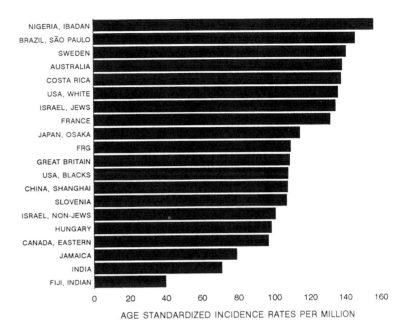

Figure 2-3. Incidence of cancer in children less than 15 years old in selected areas of the world. Rates are age standardized and expressed as per million of the population. (Adapted from LL Robison. General Principles of the Epidemiology of Childhood Cancer. In PA Pizzo, DG Poplack [eds], Principles and Practice of Pediatric Oncology. Philadelphia: Lippincott, 1993;3.)

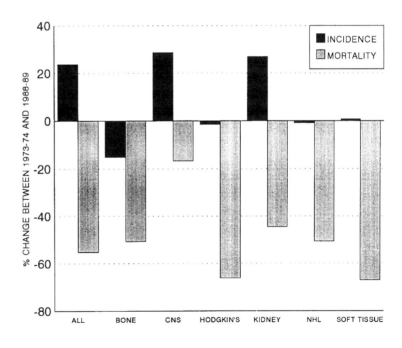

Figure 2-4. Percent change in incidence and mortality rates from 1973–1974 and 1988–1989 in the major types of childhood neoplasms in the United States. (ALL = acute lymphoblastic leukemia; NHL = non-Hodgkin's lymphoma.) (Graph constructed using SEER data from BA Miller, LAG Ries, BF Hankey, CL Kosary, et al. [eds], Cancer Statistics Review: 1973–1989, National Cancer Institute. NIH Pub. No. 92-2789, 1992.)

younger than 5 years of age is greater than for children aged 5–14 years old, regardless of sex or race.[3]

From 1974–1976 to 1983–1988, the 5-year relative survival rate for all pediatric neoplasms increased from 55.3–67.5%. The largest increases in survival occurred in non-Hodgkin's lymphoma (44.1–69.0%), ALL (52.5–72.3%), and acute nonlymphoblastic leukemia (ANLL) patients (14.3–30.3%) (Figure 2-5). These improvements in survival are most certainly related to improved therapeutic modalities and supportive care. The survival curve for all childhood malignancies combined reaches a plateau 8–10 years postdiagnosis.[3]

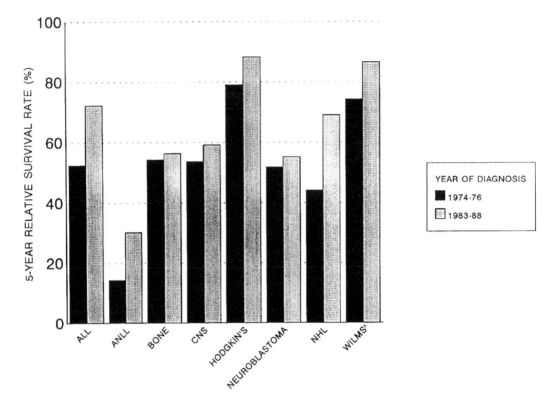

Figure 2-5. A comparison of the 5-year relative survival rate of patients diagnosed with major types of childhood neoplasms in the United States from 1974–1976 to patients diagnosed from 1983–1988. (ALL = acute lymphoblastic leukemia; ANLL = acute nonlymphoblastic leukemia; NHL = non-Hodgkin's lymphoma.) (Graph constructed using SEER data from BA Miller, LAG Ries, BF Hankey, CL Kosary, et al. [eds], Cancer Statistics Review: 1973–1989, National Cancer Institute. NIH Pub. No. 92-2789, 1992.)

Cancer in Infancy

Only 0.05% of all malignancies occur in children younger than 1 year old.[6] In this population, the development of malignant disease is most likely influenced by prezygotic or intrauterine factors[8] and all the steps of carcinogenesis must occur during the time between conception and diagnosis. Embryonal tumors such as retinoblastoma, Wilms' tumor, and hepatoblastoma are relatively more frequent in infants,[6] whereas stage IV-S neuroblastoma occurs exclusively in infants.[9] The majority of bilateral retinoblastomas present during infancy.[10] The bladder, prostate, and vagina are involved twice as often in cancer in infants as in older children.[11]

Germ cell tumors diagnosed in the first year of life, particularly before the age of 6 months, are usually benign. Mesoblastic nephromas, rhabdoid sarcomas, and botryoid tumors are rare outside infancy, whereas bone tumors are rare during infancy.[6] A study conducted by the International Agency for Research on Cancer demonstrated a greater than 12-fold difference between the highest incidence rate of neoplasms in infants throughout the world (Japanese children) and the lowest (African-American children in New York). The reason for this difference is not readily apparent, although genetic factors may play a role. The incidence rates of CNS tumors, neuroblastoma, retinoblastoma, and germ cell tumors appear to be the most variable.[7]

Risk Factors

Environmental Factors

Ionizing Radiation

Exposure to ionizing radiation has been found to induce human cancers. This association is well described in survivors of nuclear bombing and in people exposed to radiation for medical and occupational reasons.[12, 13] The latency period between exposure to radiation and the development of neoplasia varies. An increase in the incidence of leukemia was seen in Japanese children following exposure to atomic bombing, with the peak incidence 4–6 years postexposure. The excess of leukemia began declining 10 years after the bombing; however, it had not disappeared greater than 20 years postdetonation.[14]

In a Children's Cancer Group study, 43 second neoplasms were identified in a cohort of 9,720 children diagnosed with ALL from June 1972 to August 1988. Thirty-two of the 43 second neoplasms appeared in a previously irradiated field. There were 24 CNS tumors and all occurred in patients previously treated with cranial irradiation. No plateau in the incidence of second neoplasms was evident 15 years postradiotherapy.[15] The dose is the major determinant for radiation-induced carcinogenesis, whereas other factors include the type of radiation, fraction size, dose rate, amount of tissue exposed, and age at which exposed.[14] An excess risk of cancer has not been directly measured for a dose of less than 10 rad in adults.[16]

An inverse relationship appears to exist between age and the susceptibility to the harmful effects of ionizing radiation. The potential for developing acute leukemia, thyroid cancer, and breast cancer was greater in those atomic bomb survivors who were exposed at a young age.[12, 14] There is an association between in utero exposure to ionizing radiation and an excess of cancers.[17] Not only is in utero exposure harmful, preconceptual paternal germ cell exposure may also lead to mutations in sperm that may have a carcinogenic effect on subsequent offspring. A case-control study by Gardner et al. examined the excess of childhood leukemia and lymphomas near the Sellafield nuclear plant and found an association between the development of leukemia and non-Hodgkin's lymphoma and preconceptual paternal exposure to penetrating radiation.[18]

Ultraviolet Radiation

Ultraviolet radiation from the sun is known to cause cancer in adults.[19] The incidence and mortality in the white population from skin cancers other than malignant melanoma are inversely related to the distance of the population from the equator. Skin cancer is virtually absent in the pediatric age group, except in children with a genetic disorder predisposing them to the development of cancer, such as xeroderma pigmentosum,[20] dysplastic nevus syndrome,[21] or albinism.[22] Without a genetic predisposition, the cumulative dose of ultraviolet radiation from sunlight does not appear to reach the critical level needed for carcinogenesis during childhood.

Electromagnetic Fields

Recent literature has described reports of an association between environmental exposures to electromagnetic fields from electrical power lines and pediatric malignancies such as leukemia, CNS tumors, and neuroblastoma.[23–26] This association has not withstood critical review to this point and further study is needed.[27, 28]

Chemicals and Drugs

Exposure to a variety of chemicals during childhood may lead to the development of various neoplasms later in life. Although adults may be exposed in the work setting, children are most often exposed to contaminants in the air, soil, and food.[29, 30] Mesotheliomas have developed in adults who lived near asbestos mines during their childhood.[31] The relationship between parental occupation and various pediatric malignancies has been explored but no strong association has been found.

Although alkylating agents are effective for several pediatric disorders including many malignancies, it is well recognized that certain ones (cyclophosphamide, melphalan, nitrosurea) have a leukemogenic potential.[32–35] Topoisomerase II inhibitors such as teniposide and etoposide have also been associated with secondary leukemias.[35] In one study, 21 of 734 ALL patients treated with topoisomerase II inhibitors developed ANLL within 8 years.[36]

Drugs such as hormones and immunosuppressants used for nonmalignant processes have also been linked to the development of cancer.[12, 37–39] One of the best examples of transplacental chemical carcinogenesis is the effect of diethylstilbestrol (DES) on the developing fetus. During the 1940s and 1950s, DES was prescribed to many women to prevent miscarriages. Since the first reports by Herbst and Scully in 1970,[40] it has become evident that young women exposed in utero to DES are at increased risk for developing clear cell carcinoma of the vagina during early adulthood.[41] Cancer has not been reported in male children exposed in utero to DES but there is an increased incidence of oligospermia, epididymal cysts, hypoplastic testes, and microphallus.[42]

Infectious Agents

A relationship appears to exist between certain viruses and the development of cancer, although it has been difficult to document. Epstein-Barr virus (EBV) DNA is present within 95% of African Burkitt's lymphoma tumors but in only 20% of sporadic Burkitt's tumors.[43–45] EBV may cause chronic B-cell stimulation and be critical to the development of African Burkitt's lymphoma.[46] There are also reports of an association between EBV and nasopharyngeal carcinoma,[47] peripheral T-cell lymphoma,[48–51] Hodgkin's disease,[52, 53] and Ki-1 lymphoma.[53]

Chronic hepatitis B infection increases the risk of developing hepatocellular carcinoma later in life[54]; a similar relationship exists between human papillomavirus infection and cervical cancer.[55] There is an increase in the susceptibility to develop Kaposi's sarcoma, non-Hodgkin's B-cell lymphoma, and CNS lymphoma in adults infected with the human immunodeficiency virus (HIV). This increase in susceptibility appears to be multifactorial with the primary factor being a defect in immune surveillance.[56] The relationship between HIV and childhood neoplasms is still being investigated.

The human T-cell lymphotropic virus type I (HTLV-1), a retrovirus endemic to Japan, the Caribbean, and regions of central Africa, can be transmitted by the transfer of infected T lymphocytes via breast milk, semen, or blood products. HTLV-1 has been directly associated with the development of adult T-cell leukemia and lymphoma (ATLL), which typically has an aggressive course. B-cell lymphomas are more common than T-cell lymphomas in most of the world, but T-cell lymphomas are more common in areas with a high frequency of HTLV-1 infections. Although HTLV-1 infection may occur during infancy, the virus may remain latent for an extended period. The direct association between HTLV-1 and human malignancy is based on the following evidence: (1) the areas of

Japan with the highest incidence of ATLL correspond to the areas with the highest prevalence of HTLV-1 infection; (2) individuals with ATLL have antibodies against HTLV-1; (3) HTLV-1 DNA has been isolated from ATLL neoplastic cells; and (4) HTLV-1 immortalizes human T cells.[57]

Genetic Factors

A number of genetic disorders predispose children to the development of cancer. These disorders may consist of a single gene defect, the absence or addition of an entire chromosome, or the interaction of many genes with environmental factors. Malignancies with a genetic origin often have the following features: (1) early age at diagnosis, (2) multifocal lesions within one organ, (3) bilateral lesions in paired organs, (4) development of multiple primary cancers, and (5) association with birth defects.[16, 58]

Twin studies are often helpful in discovering the genetic basis for a disease process. One such study demonstrated that when one twin develops leukemia as an infant, the other twin has nearly a 100% chance of also developing leukemia. The risk decreases after 1 year of age and continues to decline until the age of 6 years when it becomes the same as the risk of other family members. In a karyotyping study performed by Chaganti et al., leukemic blasts from a set of 15-month-old identical twins were found to have identical cytogenetic abnormalities, providing strong evidence that both populations of blasts originated in a single cell. Owing to the early onset of leukemia in these children, it is hypothesized that one twin developed leukemia in utero and the leukemic blasts were transferred to the other twin through placental vessels.[58, 59]

The classic example of an association between a chromosome defect and a malignancy is that of trisomy 21 (Down's syndrome) and leukemia. Children with Down's syndrome have a 10- to 20-fold greater risk of developing leukemia during the first decade of life, with a peak incidence 3 years earlier than that in the general population.[60]

There are more than 200 single gene defects with neoplastic tendencies.[61] Approximately one-third of these are associated with childhood cancer.[16] Some of the more common single gene disorders associated with pediatric malignancies include Wiskott-Aldrich syndrome,[62] ataxia-telangiectasia,[62] Beckwith-Wiedemann syndrome,[63] Fanconi's anemia,[64] and hereditary retinoblastoma.[65]

Retinoblastoma and Knudson's Hypothesis

Much of what is known about the relationship between genetics and cancer was discovered through the study of retinoblastoma. Approximately 30–40% of retinoblastoma cases are transmitted in an autosomal dominant pattern with 90% penetrance.[66] The familial form is characterized by bilateral disease and an early age of onset, with approximately half of the cases diagnosed before 1 year of age.[58, 67, 68] Based on his epidemiologic study of retinoblastoma, Knudson proposed a two-mutation hypothesis of carcinogenesis. This hypothesis states that all retinoblastomas arise from mutations in both alleles of a gene that suppresses tumor development. Patients with the hereditary form of retinoblastoma inherit one mutation and develop the second as the result of some environmental influence. Patients with the sporadic form acquire both mutations following conception.[68]

Knudson's hypothesis was confirmed with the identification of chromosome 13q14 deletions in retinoblastoma. The normal allele at this locus acts to suppress cancer development (tumor suppressor gene) when present in one or two copies. In the hereditary form, patients are born with one normal retinoblastoma gene, but its normal function is lost early in life through point mutation or mitotic recombination.[69] Tumor suppressor genes may also be critical to the development of Wilms' tumor in patients with Miller's syndrome.[70]

Abnormalities in Embryogenesis and Cancer

Sacrococcygeal teratomas may be associated with malformations of the lower spine. Persistence of fetal rest tissues in Rathke's pouch predisposes to the development of craniopharyngioma and remnants of such tissue in brachial cleft cysts or thyroglossal duct cysts predispose to the development of various carcinomas.[71] Abnormal embryogenesis is also responsible for the development of extragonadal germ cell tumors.

The risk of malignancy is approximately 35 times greater than normal in maldescended testes. The more severe the maldescent, the greater the risk of malignancy. In a patient with unilateral cryptorchidism, neoplasia can occur within the normally descended testis or the maldescended testis. Orchiopexy is recommended at 12–18 months of age to reduce the incidence of cancer.[58, 72]

Li-Fraumeni Syndrome

Bottomley in 1967 was one of the first to describe the familial aggregation of cancer.[73] He described a large family with 400 members spanning five generations who had an excess of cancer.[74] Beginning in 1969, Li and Fraumeni described several families with a high frequency of diverse neoplasms.[75, 76] They recognized the high incidence of cancer in relatives of childhood soft tissue sarcoma patients. The malignancies that occurred in excess in these relatives included childhood soft tissue sarcomas, early onset breast cancer, brain tumors, and leukemias. These families have been followed for more than 20 years and there continues to be an excess of cancer.[77] This hereditary cancer syndrome has been labeled the Li-Fraumeni syndrome. Recently, germline mutations in the p53 tumor suppressor gene have been identified in several Li-Fraumeni families.[78–80]

Other familial cancer syndromes include polyposis coli, multiple endocrine neoplasia types I and II, dysplastic nevi syndrome, nevoid basal cell carcinoma, hereditary retinoblastoma, and familial Wilms' tumor. Hereditary cancer syndromes should be suspected when the cancer occurs (1) in more than two generations, (2) in siblings, (3) at an unusual age for the type of tumor, or (4) in association with other genetic disorders or birth defects.[16]

Epidemiology of Selected Pediatric Neoplasms

Acute Lymphoblastic Leukemia

ALL is the most common malignancy in pediatric populations, with the frequency increasing rapidly after birth, peaking before 5 years of age, and declining thereafter.[81] The highest incidence rates of childhood ALL occurs in U.S. whites and in Europe; the lowest rates are found in U.S. blacks, the Middle East, and Africa.[1, 7] Comparative surveys in Africa indicate that ALL is more likely to occur in urban areas within the upper socioeconomic groups. This suggests that conditions associated with higher standards of living may predispose one to ALL.[82, 83] The frequency of T-cell ALL is relatively constant throughout the world. As discussed earlier, certain immunodeficiencies such as agammaglobulinemia and severe combined immunodeficiency predispose to the development of ALL[84] as does Down's syndrome.[60]

Acute Nonlymphoblastic Leukemia

Approximately 20% of all children younger than 15 years old who develop acute leukemia will develop ANLL.[85] There is no particular age at which the frequency of ANLL peaks, but most infants younger than 4 weeks of age with congenital leukemia have ANLL.[86, 87] The highest incidence rates are in Japan and New Zealand, whereas the lowest are in the United States and Europe.[7] The most common subtype of ANLL is acute myelocytic leukemia.[85]

Exposure to ionizing radiation,[14] alkylating agents,[32–35] and topoisomerase II inhibitors [35, 36] all predispose to the development of ANLL. Chromosomal breakage syndromes such as ataxia-telangiectasia, Bloom's syndrome, and Fanconi's anemia are associated with ANLL.[84]

Hodgkin's Lymphoma

The highest incidence rates of Hodgkin's lymphoma are in industrialized Western countries.[7] In the United States, Hodgkin's disease is rare in children younger than 5 years old but the frequency increases thereafter. There is a bimodal distribution with the first peak at 15–34 years of age and the second peak at greater than 50 years of age.[88] Better socioeconomic development is associated with a lower frequency of Hodgkin's disease among children, a higher frequency among young adults, and histologic subtypes with a better prognosis. The role that socioeconomic status plays in the development of Hodgkin's disease is not well defined.[16]

An infectious etiology has been postulated for Hodgkin's lymphoma, with EBV as a possible cause. The EBV genome has been found in Reed-Sternberg cells.[89] There have been more than 100 cases of Hodgkin's disease reported with familial aggregations,[90] thus raising the suspicion of human-to-human transmission or of an inherited genetic defect. One theory that combines several of the previously discussed ideas states that people in higher socioeconomic classes are more likely to become infected with EBV later in life, and that this, in combination with a genetic predisposition, leads to the development of Hodgkin's disease.

Non-Hodgkin's Lymphoma

Non-Hodgkin's lymphoma occurs 1.5 times more often than Hodgkin's disease. Like Hodgkin's disease, non-Hodgkin's lymphoma occurs rarely in children younger than 5 years old but the incidence increases thereafter. The male-to-female ratio in non-Hodgkin's lymphoma is nearly 3 to 1 and the incidence in U.S. white children is nearly twice that found in U.S. black children.[7, 91] The incidence of non-Hodgkin's lymphoma appears to be increasing throughout the world. This increase is probably related to both the expanding number of immunodeficient patients and to environmental factors such as exposure to pesticides,[92] solvents,[93] and hair dyes.[94]

Infectious agents play a role in the pathogenesis of some non-Hodgkin's lymphoma. EBV DNA has been isolated in 95% of African Burkitt's lymphoma,[43–45] and the retrovirus HTLV-1 has been isolated from the neoplastic cells of patients with ATLL.[95, 96] Epidemiologic studies of tropical Africa, where both malaria and Burkitt's lymphoma are endemic, indicate that malaria acts as a cofactor in the development of Burkitt's lymphoma. All children in these areas are infected by malaria before the age of 4 years, and in areas where antimalaria programs have been introduced, the incidence of the tumor has reportedly declined. Chronic malarial infection appears to suppress T-cell function, leading to uncontrolled EBV replication and lymphomagenesis.[97, 98] Similarly, the increased risk of developing B-cell lymphomas in immunodeficient patients with depressed T-cell immunity is related to EBV infection.[99]

Central Nervous System Tumors

Tumors of the CNS make up approximately 20% of neoplasms in patients younger than 14 years of age.[81] The highest incidence of CNS neoplasms occurs in U.S. whites, Denmark, and Sweden, whereas the lowest rates are found in Asia and Africa.[7] The four most common types of CNS neoplasms in children are astrocytomas, glioblastomas, medulloblastomas, and ependymomas, with 60% located infratentorially. Children with neurofibromatosis, tuberous sclerosis, and nevoid basal cell carcinoma are at increased risk for developing malignant neural tumors.[16, 100] Patients who have received cranial irradiation are also at increased risk for CNS neoplasms.[15]

Neuroblastoma

Neuroblastoma is the third most common solid malignancy in children after CNS tumors and lymphomas and the most common malignancy in infants.[6, 7] The highest incidence of neuroblastoma is in North America, Europe, Israel, and Australia, while the lowest incidence is in Africa and Central and South America.[7] Fifty percent of all cases are diagnosed in children younger than 2 years old, whereas 90% are diagnosed before 10 years of age.[81, 101] This tumor most frequently arises from the adrenal medulla and the sympathetic nervous tissue in the chest and pelvis. The male-to-female ratio is 1.3 to 1.0.[16] The presence of nonrandom deletions of chromosome 1p in 70% of neuroblastoma tumors raises the suspicion that a tumor suppressor gene may play a role in the development of this malignancy.[102]

One study found adrenal neuroblastoma in situ incidentally in 1 of every 40 infants younger than 3 months old dying of causes other than cancer and in nearly all fetuses 10–30 weeks' gestation.[103] Neonatal screening for neuroblastoma measuring urinary vanillylmandelic acid and homovanillic acid in Japan and Quebec, Canada has detected mostly early stage disease and has not affected overall mortality.[104, 105] The early disease detected by screening appears to be destined for spontaneous differentiation and resolution.

Wilms' Tumor

The incidence of Wilms' tumor in U.S. white children younger than 15 years of age is estimated at 9 per 1 million and the incidence among U.S. black children is about 25% greater.[7] Approximately 75% of all cases are diagnosed before the age of 5 years.[61] Throughout the world, the incidence among male and female subjects is equal. In Asia, the overall rate is less, a greater proportion of cases are diagnosed within the first year of life, and the male-to-female ratio is 1 to 4.[106]

Epidemiologic studies performed by the National Wilms' Tumor Study failed to confirm many of the previously reported associations between Wilms' tumor and maternal exposure during pregnancy to cigarettes, caffeine, oral contraceptives, and hair dyes.[107] A number of reports have suggested an association between the development of Wilms' tumor and paternal occupational exposure to hydrocarbons and lead, but further study is needed.[108–110]

Associations exist between Wilms' tumor and sporadic aniridia, anomalies of the male urogenital system, hemihypertrophy, hamartomas of the skin, Bloom's syndrome, and the Beckwith-Wiedemann syndrome. Approximately 15% of patients with Wilms' tumor have an associated congenital anomaly.[16, 111–113] Patients with bilateral Wilms' tumor are more likely to have hypospadias or cryptorchidism, whereas those with multifocal disease (either unilateral or bilateral) have a higher incidence of hemihypertrophy and Beckwith-Wiedemann syndrome. There is not an elevated incidence of congenital anomalies in the familial form of Wilms' tumor.[106]

The gene for the Beckwith-Wiedemann syndrome has been located on chromosome 11p15 and a consistent deletion of chromosome 11p13 has been identified in patients with the aniridia–Wilms' syndrome. Each of these sites is suspected to contain a Wilms' tumor gene.[16, 114] It has been suggested that genomic imprinting plays a role in Wilms' tumorigenesis. An imprinted gene is a gene that is expressed differently depending on whether it is of maternal or paternal origin. Based on Knudson's two-hit hypothesis of carcinogenesis, the first hit necessary for the development of Wilms' tumor could be the inactivation of one allele of a Wilms' tumor gene due to genomic imprinting.[115]

Sarcomas

Malignant bone tumors account for only 4% of all neoplasms in children. The two most common types, osteosarcoma and Ewing's sarcoma, occur most often during adolescence, suggesting an association with rapid bone growth.[7, 16] Osteosarcomas make up 60% of malignant bone tumors in U.S. children, and the highest incidence rates worldwide are found in Spain and U.S. Hispanics, whereas the lowest rates are in Asia.[7, 81] External beam irradiation and bone-seeking radionuclides are known to induce osteosarcomas.[116] Survivors of bilateral (hereditary) retinoblastomas develop secondary osteosarcoma at a significantly greater rate than the general population.[117] Molecular studies indicate that deletions of the retinoblastoma gene (chromosome 13q) are critical to the development of hereditary retinoblastoma and secondary osteosarcoma.[118]

Ewing's sarcoma accounts for 30% of bony neoplasms in U.S. children and occurs most often in U.S. whites, New Zealanders, Australians, and Europeans but rarely in blacks, Japanese, and Chinese.[7, 81] There is an association between Ewing's sarcoma and a translocation between chromosomes 11 and 22.[119]

Approximately 50% of the soft tissue sarcomas in U.S. children are rhabdomyosarcomas.[16] There is a bimodal age distribution for rhabdomyosarcoma, with peaks at 2–5 years of age and again at 13–18 years of age.[76, 120] The first peak is created by head, neck, and genitourinary rhabdomyosarcomas, whereas the second peak exists due to primaries of the extremities, trunk, and paratesticular regions.[121] Soft tissue sarcomas are part of several familial cancer syndromes and also occur at a greater than expected frequency in patients with neurofibromatosis.[122, 123]

Summary

Despite improvements in therapy and increases in survival, cancer remains the second leading cause of death in children. Epidemiologic investigations have been limited by the relative rarity of childhood neoplasms. However, the epidemiology of childhood cancer is becoming better characterized owing to the efforts of large multi-institutional cancer groups.

A great deal has been learned about genetics and cancer from studying childhood malignancies. Knudson's two-mutation hypothesis of carcinogenesis was formulated based on epidemiologic studies of retinoblastoma. From epidemiologic studies, Li and Fraumeni identified a familial cancer syndrome. Others have since found that the p53 tumor suppressor gene is abnormal in this syndrome and have started to characterize this gene's role in increasing susceptibility to the development of diverse cancers.

Based on epidemiologic data, associations have been identified between certain childhood infections and the development of cancer either as a child or an adult. Strong relationships exist between Epstein-Barr virus and Burkitt's lymphoma, hepatitis B and hepatocellular carcinoma, and HTLV-1 and adult T-cell leukemia and lymphoma. Ironically, the major source of carcinogenic environmental exposures is the treatment modalities used in cancer therapy. Ionizing radiation, immunosuppressants, and certain chemotherapeutic agents are known to increase the risk of developing a second malignancy.

Much remains to be discovered regarding the epidemiology of childhood cancer. Long-term follow-up of survivors of childhood cancer will continue to yield information regarding the pathogenesis of neoplasia and the impact of current therapy on future generations. As more is learned about the molecular biology of childhood malignancies, screening tests will likely become available to determine which children are at greatest risk for developing cancer, and gene therapy may be able to prevent the development of these diseases.

References

1. Robison LL. General Principles of the Epidemiology of Childhood Cancer. In PA Pizzo, DG Poplack (eds), Principles and Practice of Pediatric Oncology. Philadelphia: Lippincott, 1993;3.
2. Bunin GR, Meadows AT. Epidemiology and Wilms tumor: Approaches and methods. Med Pediatr Oncol 1993;21:169.
3. Miller BA, Ries LAG, Hankey BF, et al. (eds), Cancer Statistics Review: 1973–1989, National Cancer Institute, NIH Pub. No. 92-2789, 1992.
4. American Cancer Society. Cancer Facts and Figures, 1992.
5. National Center for Health Statistics: Vital Statistics of the United States, 1989. Washington, DC: Public Health Service, 1992.
6. Birch JM, Blair V. The epidemiology of infant cancers. Br J Cancer 1992;66(Suppl. XVIII):S2.
7. Parkins DM, Stiller CA, Draper GJ, et al. (eds), International Incidence of Childhood Cancer, International Agency for Research on Cancer. IARC Publ. No. 87, 1988.

8. Miller RW. Prenatal Origins of Cancer in Man: Epidemiologic Evidence. In L Tomatis, U Mohr (eds), Transplacental Carcinogenesis. Lyon, France: International Agency for Research for Cancer, 1973,175.

9. Evans AE, Chatten J, D'Angio GJ, et al. A review of 17 IV-S neuroblastoma patients at the Children's Hospital of Philadelphia. Cancer 1980;45:833.

10. Sanders BM, Draper GJ, Kingston JE. Retinoblastoma in Great Britain 1969–1980: Incidence, treatment and survival. Br J Ophthalmol 1988;72:576.

11. Ragab AH, Heyn R, Tefft M, et al. Infants younger than 1 year of age with rhabdomyosarcoma. Cancer 1986; 58:2606.

12. Boice JD, Fraumeni JF Jr. (eds). Radiation Carcinogenesis. New York: Raven, 1984.

13. Kohn HI, Fry RJM. Radiation carcinogenesis. N Engl J Med 1984;301:504.

14. Committee on the Biological Effects of Ionizing Radiations. The Effects on Populations of Exposure to Low Levels of Ionizing Radiation. Washington, DC: National Academy Press, 1980.

15. Neglia JP, Meadows AT, Robison LL, et al. Second neoplasms after acute lymphoblastic leukemia in childhood. N Engl J Med 1991;325:1330.

16. Li FP. Epidemiology of Cancer in Childhood. In DG Nathan, FA Oski (eds), Hematology of Infancy and Childhood. Philadelphia: Saunders, 1993;30:1102.

17. Yoshimoto Y, Kato H, Schull WJ. Risk of cancer among children exposed in utero to A-bomb radiations 1950–1984. Lancet 1988;2:665.

18. Gardner MJ, Snee MP, Hall AJ, et al. Results of case-control study of leukaemia and lymphoma among young people near Sellafield nuclear plant in West Cumbria. Br Med J 1990;300:423.

19. Scotto J, Fraumeni JF Jr. Skin (Other Than Melanoma). In D Schottenfeld, JF Fraumeni Jr. (eds), Cancer Epidemiology and Prevention. Philadelphia: Saunders, 1982;996.

20. Cleaver JE. Defective repair replication of DNA in xeroderma pigmentosum. Nature 1968;218:652.

21. Perara MIR, Um KI, Greene MH, et al. Hereditary dysplastic nevus syndrome: Lymphoid cell ultraviolet hypermutability in association with increased melanoma susceptibility. Cancer Res 1986;46:1005.

22. Okoro AN. Albinism in Nigeria: A clinical and social study. Br J Dermatol 1975;92:485.

23. Savitz DA, Kaune WT. Childhood cancer in relation to a modified residential wire code. Environ Health Perspect 1993;101:76.

24. Howe GR, Burch DJ, Chiarelli AM, et al. An exploratory case-control study of brain tumors in children. Cancer Res 1989;49:4349.

25. Spitz MR, Johnson CC. Neuroblastoma and paternal occupation. Am J Epidemiol 1985;121:924.

26. Laval G, Tuyns AJ. Environmental factors in childhood leukaemia. Br J Ind Med 1988;45:843.

27. Jackson JD. Are the stray 60-Hz electromagnetic fields associated with the distribution and use of electric power a significant cause of cancer? Proc Natl Acad Sci U S A 1992;89:3508.

28. Ware BJ, Cole P. Selection bias from differential residential mobility as an explanation for association of wire codes with childhood cancer. J Clin Epidemiol 1993;46:545.

29. Miller RW. Environmental causes of cancer in childhood. Adv Pediatr 1978;25:97.

30. Janerich DT, Burnett WS, Feck G, et al. Cancer incidence in the Love Canal area. Science 1981;212:1404.

31. Anderson HA, Lilis R, Daum SM, et al. Household contact asbestos neoplastic risk. Ann NY Acad Sci 1976;271:311.

32. Greene MH, Boice JD, Greer BE, et al. Acute nonlymphocytic leukemia after therapy with alkylating agents for ovarian cancer. N Engl J Med 1982;307:1416.

33. Boice JD, Greene MH, Kille JY Jr., et al. Leukemia and preleukemia after adjuvant treatment of gastrointestinal cancer with Semustine (methyl-CCNU). N Engl J Med 1983;309:1079.

34. Pui CH, Behm FG, Raimondi SC, et al. Secondary acute myeloid leukemia in children treated for acute lymphoid leukemia. N Engl J Med 1989;321:136.

35. Hawkins MM, Wilson LM, Stovall MA, et al. Epipodophyllotoxins, alkylating agents, and radiation and risk of secondary leukaemia after childhood cancer. Br Med J 1992;304:951.

36. Pui CH, Ribeiro RC, Hancock ML, et al. Acute myeloid leukemia in children treated with epipodophyllotoxins for acute lymphoblastic leukemia. N Engl J Med 1991;325:1682.

37. Chilvers C, McPherson K, Peto J, et al. Oral contraceptive use and breast cancer risk in young women. Lancet 1989;1:973.

38. Hoover R, Fraumeni JF Jr. Risk of cancer in renal-transplant recipients. Lancet 1973;2:55.

39. Cutler BS, Forbes AP, Ingersal FM, Scully RE. Endometrial carcinoma after stilbestrol therapy in gonadal dysgenesis. N Engl J Med 1972;287:628.

40. Herbst AL, Scully RE. Adenocarcinoma of the vagina in adolescence: A report of 7 cases including 6 clear-cell carcinomas (so-called mesonephromas). Cancer 1970;25:745.

41. Lanier AP, Noller KL. Cancer and stilbestrol: A follow-up of 1,719 persons exposed to estrogens in utero and born 1943–1959. Mayo Clin Proc 1973;48:793.

42. Gill WB, Schumacher GFB, Bibbo M, et al. Association of diethylstilbestrol exposure *in utero* with cryptorchidism, testicular hypoplasia and semen abnormalities. J Urol 1979;122:36.

43. Magrath IT. The Pathogenesis of Burkitt's Lymphoma. In G Klein, G Van de Woude (eds), Recent Adv Cancer Res 1990;55:133.

44. de-The G. Epidemiology of Epstein-Barr Virus and Associated Disease in Man. In B Roizman (ed), The Herpes Virus (Vol. 1). New York: Plenum, 1982;25.

45. Okano M, Thiele GM, Davis JR, et al. EBV and human diseases: Recent advances in diagnosis. Clin Microbiol Rev 1988;1:300.

46. Sullivan JL. Epstein-Barr virus and lymphoproliferative disorders. Semin Hematol 1988;25:269.

47. Zur Hausen H, Schulte-Holthausen H, Kleim H, et al. EBV-DNA in biopsies of Burkitt's tumor and anaplastic carcinoma of the nasopharynx. Nature 1970;228:1056.

48. Cheng AL, Ih-Jen S, Yao-Chung C, et al. Characteristic clinicopathologic features of Epstein-Barr virus-associated peripheral T-cell lymphoma. Cancer 1993; 72:909.

49. Jones JF, Shurin S, Abramowsky C, et al. T-cell lymphomas containing Epstein-Barr viral DNA in patients with chronic Epstein-Barr virus infection. N Engl J Med 1988;318:733.

50. Su IJ, Lin KH, Chen CJ, et al. Epstein-Barr virus associated peripheral T-cell lymphoma of activated CD8 phenotype. Cancer 1990;66:2557.

51. Su IJ, Hsieh HC, Lin KH, et al. Aggressive peripheral T-cell lymphomas containing Epstein-Barr viral DNA: A clinicopathologic and molecular analysis. Blood 1991;77:799.

52. Pallesen G, Hamilton-Dutoit SJ, Rowe M, Young LS. Expression of Epstein-Barr virus (EBV) latent gene products in tumor cells of Hodgkin's disease. Lancet 1991;337:320.

53. Anagnostopoulos I, Herbst H, Niedobitek G, Stein H. Demonstration of monoclonal EBV genomes in Hodgkin's disease and Ki-1 positive anaplastic large cell lymphoma by combined Southern blot and in situ hybridization. Blood 1989;74:810.

54. Arthur MJP, Hall AJ, Wright R. Hepatitis B, hepatocellular carcinoma, and strategies for prevention. Lancet 1984;1:607.

55. Henderson BE. Establishment of an association between a virus and a human cancer. J Natl Cancer Inst 1989;81:320.

56. Safai B, Diaz B, Schwartz J. Malignant neoplasms associated with human immunodeficiency virus infection. CA Cancer J Clin 1992;42:74.

57. Takatsuki K, Yamaguchi K, Hattori T. Adult T-Cell Leukemia and Lymphoma. In RC Gallo, F Wong-Stall (eds), Retrovirus Biology and Human Disease. New York: Dekker, 1990;147.

58. Mulvihill JJ. Childhood Cancer, the Environment, and Heredity. In PA Pizzo, DG Poplack (eds), Principles and Practice of Pediatric Oncology. Philadelphia: Lippincott, 1993;11.

59. Chaganti RSK, Miller DR, Meyers PA, German J. Cytogenetic evidence of the intrauterine origin of acute leukemia in monozygotic twins. N Engl J Med 1979;300:1032.

60. Fong C, Brodeur GM. Down's syndrome and leukemia: Epidemiology, genetics, cytogenetics and mechanisms of leukemogenesis. Cancer Genet Cytogenet 1987; 28:55.

61. Mulvihill JJ. Genetic Repertory of Human Neoplasia. In JJ Mulvihill, RW Miller (eds), Genetics of Human Cancer. New York: Raven, 1977;137.

62. Filipovich AH, Spector BD, Kersey J. Immunodeficiency in humans as a risk factor in the development of malignancy. Prev Med 1980;9:252.

63. Sotelo-Avila C, Gooch WM III. Neoplasms Associated with the Beckwith-Wiedemann Syndrome. In HS Rosenberg, RP Bolande (eds), Perspectives in Pediatric Pathology (Vol. 3). Chicago: Year Book, 1976;255.

64. Auerbach A, Allen R. Leukemia and preleukemia in Fanconi's anemia patients: A review of the literature and report of the International Fanconi's Anemia Registry. Cancer Genet Cytogenet 1991;51:1.

65. Knudson AG Jr. Hereditary cancer, oncogenes, and antioncogenes. Cancer Res 1985;45:1437.

66. Draper GJ, Sanders BM, Brownbill PA, Hawkins MM. Patterns of risk of hereditary retinoblastoma and application to genetic counseling. Br J Cancer 1992;66:211.

67. Hethcote HW, Knudson AG Jr. Model for the incidence of embryonal cancers: Applications to retinoblastoma. Proc Natl Acad Sci U S A 1978;75:2453.

68. Knudson AG Jr. Mutation and cancer: Statistical study of retinoblastoma. Proc Natl Acad Sci U S A 1971;68:820.

69. Johnson MP, Ramsay N, Cervenka J, Wang N. Retinoblastoma and its association with a deletion in chromosome 13: A survey using high-resolution chromosome techniques. Cancer Genet Cytogenet 1982;6:29.

70. Francke U, Holmes LB, Atkins L, Riccardi VM. Aniridia-Wilms tumor association: Evidence for specific deletion of 11p13. Cytogenet Cell Genet 1979;24:185.

71. Bolande RP. Developmental pathology. Am J Pathol 1979;94:627.

72. Martin DC. Malignancy in the cryptorchid testis. Urol Clin North Am 1982;9:371.

73. Bottomley RH, Condit PT, Chanes RE. Cytogenetic studies in familial malignancy. Clin Res 1967;15:334.

74. Bottomley RH, Trainer AL, Condit PT. Chromosome studies in a "cancer family." Cancer 1971;28:519.

75. Li FP, Fraumeni JF Jr. Soft-tissue sarcomas, breast cancer, and other neoplasms: A familial syndrome? Ann Intern Med 1969;71:747.

76. Li FP, Fraumeni JF Jr. Rhabdomyosarcoma in children: Epidemiologic study and identification of a familial cancer syndrome. J Natl Cancer Inst 1969;43:1365.

77. Li FP, Fraumeni JF Jr, Mulvihill JJ, et al. A cancer family syndrome in twenty-four kindreds. Cancer Res 1988;48:5358.

78. Malkin D, Li FP, Strong LC, et al. Germ line p53 mutations in a familial syndrome of breast cancer, sarcomas, and other neoplasms. Science 1990;250:1233.

79. Strong LC, Williams WR, Tainsky MA. The Li-Fraumeni syndrome: From clinical epidemiology to molecular genetics. Am J Epidemiol 1992;135:190.

80. Srivastava S, Zou Z, Pirollo K, et al. Germ-line transmission of a mutated p53 gene in a cancer-prone family with Li-Fraumeni syndrome. Nature 1990;348:747.

81. Young JL Jr, Ries LG. Cancer incidence, survival, and mortality for children younger than age 15 years. Cancer 1986;58:598.

82. McWhirter WR. The relationship of incidence of childhood lymphoblastic leukemia to social class. Br J Cancer 1982;46:640.

83. Greaves MF. Collaborative group study of the epidemiology of acute lymphoblastic leukemia subtypes: Background and first report. Leuk Res 1985;9:715.

84. Sullivan AK. Classification, pathogenesis, and etiology of neoplastic diseases of the hematopoietic system. In GR Lee, TC Bithell, J Foerster, et al. (eds), Wintrobe's Clinical Hematology. Philadelphia: Lea & Febiger, 1993;2:1725.

85. Choi SI, Simone JV. Acute nonlymphocytic leukemia in 171 children. Med Pediatr Oncol 1976;2:119.

86. Grier HE, Weinstein HJ. Acute nonlymphocytic leukemia. Pediatr Clin North Am 1985;32:653.

87. Pierce MI. Leukemia in the newborn infant. J Pediatr 1959;54:691.

88. Spitz MR, Sider JG. Ethnic patterns of Hodgkin's disease incidence among children and adolescents in the United States, 1973–1982. J Natl Cancer Inst 1986;76:235.

89. Weiss LM, Movahed LA. Detection of Epstein-Barr viral genomes in Reed-Sternberg cells of Hodgkin's disease. N Engl J Med 1989;320:502.

90. Grufferman S, Cole P, Smith PG, Lukes RJ. Hodgkin's disease in siblings. N Engl J Med 1977;296:248.

91. Link MP. Non-Hodgkin's lymphoma in children. Pediatr Clin North Am 1985;32:699.

92. Zahm SH, Blair A. Pesticides and non-Hodgkin's lymphoma. Cancer Res 1992;52:5485.

93. Pearce N, Bethwaite P. Increasing incidence of non-Hodgkin's lymphoma: Occupational and environmental factors. Cancer Res 1992;52:5496.

94. Cantor KP, Blair A, Everett G. Hair dye use and risk of leukemia and lymphoma. Am J Public Health 1988;78:570.

95. Poiesz BJ, Ruscetti FW, Gazdar AF, et al. Detection and isolation of type C retrovirus particles from fresh and cultured lymphocytes of a patient with cutaneous T-cell lymphoma. Proc Natl Acad Sci U S A 1980;77:7415.

96. Hinuma Y, Nagata K, Hanaoka M, et al. Adult T-cell leukemia: Antigen in an adult T-cell leukemia cell line and detection of antibodies to the antigen in human sera. Proc Natl Acad Sci U S A 1981;78:6476.

97. Biggar RJ, Gardiner C, Lennette ET, et al. Malaria, sex, and place of residence as factors in antibody response to Epstein-Barr virus in Ghana, West Africa. Lancet 1981;2:115.

98. de-The G, Geser A, Day NE, et al. Epidemiological evidence for causal relationship between Epstein-Barr virus and Burkitt's lymphoma from Ugandan prospective study. Nature 1978;274:756.

99. Rabkin CS, Devesa SS, Zahm SH, Gail MH. Increasing incidence of non-Hodgkin's lymphoma. Semin Hematol 1993;30:286.

100. Horton WA. Genetics of Central Nervous System Tumors. In D Bergsma (ed), Birth Defects: Original Article Series (Vol. 12). National Foundation March of Dimes 1976;91.

101. Miller RW, Fraumeni JF Jr., Hill JA. Neuroblastoma: Epidemiologic approach to its origin. Am J Dis Child 1968;115:253.

102. Gilbert F, Feder M, Balaban G, et al. Human neuroblastomas and abnormalities of chromosome 1 and 17. Cancer Res 1984;44:5444.

103. Turkel SB, Itabashi HH. The natural history of neuroblastic cells in the fetal adrenal gland. Am J Pathol 1974;76:225.

104. Sawada T, Sugimoto T, Tanaka T, et al. Number and cure rate of neuroblastoma cases detected by the mass screening program in Japan: Future aspects. Med Pediatr Oncol 1987;15:14.

105. Woods WG, Tuchman M, Bernstein ML, et al. Screening for neuroblastoma in North America: 2-year results from the Quebec Project. Am J Pediatr Hematol Oncol 1992;14:312.

106. Breslow N, Olshan A, Beckwith JB, Green DM. Epidemiology of Wilms tumor. Med Pediatr Oncol 1993;21:172.

107. Olshan AF, Breslow NE, Falletta JM, et al. Risk factors for Wilms tumor. Cancer 1993;72:938.

108. Hakulinen T, Salonen T, Teppo L. Cancer in the offspring of fathers in hydrocarbon-related occupations. Br J Prev Soc Med 1976;30:138.

109. Hemminki K, Saloniemi I, Salonen T, et al. Childhood cancer and parental occupation in Finland. J Epidemiol Community Health 1981;35:11.

110. Kantor AF, McCrea Curnen MG, Meigs W, Flannery JT. Occupations of fathers of patients with Wilms' tumor. J Epidemiol Community Health 1979;33:253.

111. Miller RW, Fraumeni JF Jr., Manning MD. Association of Wilms' tumor with aniridia, hemihypertrophy and other congenital malformations. N Engl J Med 1964;270:922.

112. Beckwith JB. Macroglossia, Omphalocele, Adrenal Cytomegaly, Gigantism and Hyperplastic Visceromegaly. In D Bergsma, VA McKusick, JG Hall, CI Scott (eds), BD:OAS (Vol. 5). New York: Stratton Intercon, 1969;188.

113. Wiedemann HR. Complexe malformatif famial avec hernie ombilicale et macroglossie: un syndrome nouveau? J Genet Hum 1964;13:223.

114. Pritchard-Jones K, Fleming S. The candidate Wilms' tumor gene is involved in genitourinary development. Nature 1990;346:194.

115. Wilkins RJ. Genomic imprinting and carcinogenesis. Lancet 1988;1:329.

116. Strong LC, Herson J. Risk of radiation-related subsequent malignant tumors in survivors of Ewing's sarcoma. J Natl Cancer Inst 1979;62:1401.

117. Draper GJ, Sanders BM, Kingston JE. Second primary neoplasms in patients with retinoblastoma. Br J Cancer 1986;53:661.

118. Hansen MF, Koufos A, Gallie BL, et al. Osteosarcoma and retinoblastoma: A shared chromosomal mechanism revealing recessive predisposition. Proc Natl Acad Sci U S A 1985;82:6216.

119. Turc-Carel C, Aurias A, Mugneret F, et al. Chromosomes in Ewing's sarcoma. I. An evaluation of 85 cases and remarkable consistency of t(11;22)(q24;q12). Cancer Genet Cytogenet 1988;32:229.

120. Lacey SR, Jewett TC Jr, Karp MP, et al. Advances in the treatment of rhabdomyosarcoma. Semin Surg Oncol 1986;2:139.

121. Hays DM. Rhabdomyosarcoma and Other Soft Tissue Sarcomas. In DM Hays (ed), Pediatric Surgical Oncology. Orlando, FL: Grune & Stratton, 1986;87.

122. Li FP. Cancer families: Human models of susceptibility to neoplasia. Cancer Res 1988;48:5381.

123. Blatt J, Jaffe J, Deutsch M, Adkins JC. Neurofibromatosis and childhood tumors. Cancer 1986; 57:1225.

Chapter 3

Epidemiology: The Distribution and Determination of Adult Cancer

Steven N. Wolff

Cancer in adults has a major impact on the health care system. This substantial burden is due to a high prevalence, requiring extensive resources for prevention, diagnosis, treatment, and management of disease-specific sequelae. The extent of a disease process is described by the field of epidemiology, which also elaborates on related matters such as distribution, determination, association, prevention, and treatment.

Epidemiology is a complex field with a variety of measures, data sources, and analytical methods. Epidemiology brings into perspective the importance of a disease and interventions such as pain management. This chapter introduces some of these topics and focuses on the changing incidence of various cancers in the adult population. Physicians caring for the cancer patient will therefore gain a better global knowledge of the distribution of the diseases for which they are asked to intervene.

Epidemiologic Measures

The occurrence of a disease in a population is described by classic epidemiologic terms. Cancer, like other common diseases, is studied by measures of incidence, prevalence, mortality, and case fatality.[1] These describe the natural history of a disease and evaluate the effects of treatment.

Prevalence is the total number of affected individuals at one specific time. Incidence is the number of individuals developing the specified process over 1 year. Mortality, similar to incidence, quantitates the number of disease-specific deaths over 1 year. Case fatality is the number of disease-specific deaths in 1 year divided by the incidence of the disease over the same period. All of these measures are recorded for a theoretic population of 100,000. Prevalence is influenced by incidence (accumulation) and by mortality (elimination). These measures help evaluate questions such as are more cancers developing? Are more cancers being diagnosed? Are therapies improving survival? Will more patients need palliation for complications of cancer?

Epidemiology can evaluate phenomena of cause and association. These are of paramount importance because we all wish to reduce the risk of developing various cancers. Etiologic hypotheses are defined by case-control or cohort studies using analytical methods such as regression and survival analyses.

Cohort studies define populations and follow them for the occurrence of a disease. These populations can be prospective or historic and can be chosen to have a particular exposure or therapeutic intervention. Comparison of the outcome of the various populations is used to test the hypothesis. The classic cohort study is the interventional trial.

Case-control studies identify populations with a disease and then evaluate similar populations (case control) but without the disease. These populations are then compared for the putative etiologic factors.

All of these methods have various strengths and weaknesses. Case-control studies are easier and less expensive to perform but are limited to the disease process creating the case controls. Cohort studies can be used to test many hypotheses but are more difficult, lengthy, and expensive to perform.

Cohort and case-control studies express the likelihood of a disease in comparative populations by a ratio called *relative risk*. A better measure may be absolute risk expressing risk over time, which takes into consideration patient age and competing morbidity from other conditions.[2] A ratio of 20 times is relative risk and a risk of 25% of developing cancer over the next 20 years is an absolute risk.

Although these epidemiologic measures are simple to conceptualize, accurate determination is more complex because of limitations of population data. Even when data are readily available, they may not be reliable or may fail to adequately describe subtle nuances required for analysis. For example, although attainable, death certificates do not accurately record precise information. In this sense, epidemiology has many intrinsic limitations because vast populations exist without accurate prospective and detailed databases. The obvious solution to inadequate retrospective population data is prospective information. However, prospective detailed data repositories are costly to initiate and maintain.

Table 3-1. U.S. Mortality in 1989

Rank	Cause of Death	Death Rate[*]	Percent of Total
1	Heart disease	232	34.1
2	Cancer	171	23.1
3	Cerebrovascular accident	44	6.8
4	Accidents	35	4.4
5	Chronic obstructive pulmonary disease	28	3.9
6	Pneumonia	23	3.6
7	Diabetes	16	2.2
8	Suicide	11	1.4
9	Cirrhosis	10	1.2
10	Homicide	9	1.1
11	Artery diseases	8	1.1
12	HIV infection	7	1.0
13	Nephritis	7	1.0
14	Atherosclerosis	6	0.9
15	Septicemia	6	0.9
	All others	96	13.3

[*]Age-adjusted to the 1970 standard population (per 100,000).

Etiologic Inferences

Epidemiology studies are used to evaluate causative or associative hypotheses. If detected, such relationships could lead to interventions avoiding detrimental and encouraging beneficial behavior.[3, 4] Many agents are associated with an increase in the risk of developing cancer.[5, 6] These include ultraviolet and ionizing radiation, parasites, viruses, and many manufactured substances such as alcohol,[7] tobacco,[8–10] environmental pollutants, medications (chemotherapy), chemicals, diets,[11–14] and hormones.[15] Recent advances in oncogenes and tumor suppressor genes substantiate the genetic susceptibility of cancer.[16,17]

Tobacco is a major cause of cancers such as lung, larynx, pharynx, esophagus, mouth, breast, bladder, pancreas, kidney, stomach, cervix, and leukemia. Considering the rapid and substantial increase in the incidence and mortality of lung cancer, smoking must be considered a major public health dilemma.

Cancer Registries

Many independent hospital, community, and state databases have been organized into large-scale national databases. The National Cancer Institute began the Surveillance, Epidemiology, and End Results (SEER) program in 1973, collecting data from cancer registries representing 10% of the total U.S. population. The National Cancer Data Base (NCDB) is a joint project of the American Cancer Society and the Commission of Cancer of the American College of Surgeons.[18] The NCDB requests information from more than 2,000 hospitals and all known cancer registries. At last estimate, the NCDB contained information from 37% of the total expected cancer population of this country. These databases represent the most proficient collections of cancer population information and are frequently used to generate national cancer statistics.

Cancer Statistics

Cancer is the second leading cause of U.S. mortality as shown in Table 3-1.[19] Table 3-2 describes the incidence and mortality of various cancers using data from the SEER program applied to the 1993 census.[19] This table separately reports male and female subjects (although their trends are similar). Mortality trends over the past six decades for common sites of cancer are shown in Figures 3-1 and 3-2.[19] It is ap-

Table 3-2. Estimated Cancer Incidence* and Mortality by Site and Sex in 1993

Site	Male (Incidence/ Mortality)	Female (Incidence/ Mortality)
Melanoma	3%/2%	3%/1%
Oral	3%/2%	2%/1%
Lung	17%/34%	12%/22%
Breast	—	32%/18%
Pancreas	2%/4%	2%/5%
Stomach	3%/3%	—
Colon and rectum	13%/10%	13%/11%
Ovary	—	4%/5%
Prostate	28%/13%	—
Uterus	—	8%/4%
Urinary	9%/5%	4%/3%
Leukemia and lymphoma	8%/8%	6%/8%
All other sites	14%/19%	14%/22%

*Excluding basal and squamous skin cancers and carcinoma in situ.

parent from these figures that there is a marked increase of lung cancer mortality for men and women and a decrease in uterine, stomach, and colorectal mortality. The increasing lung cancer mortality is of most concern in women in whom it has eclipsed carcinoma of the breast to become the most common cause of female cancer mortality. These trends reflect the various environmental changes and specifically the increase in smoking incidence preceding the increase in lung cancer incidence.

Although a crude measure, the comparison of incidence to mortality relates to the success of therapeutic interventions. For example, lung cancer has greater mortality than incidence, indicating ineffective therapy. On the other hand, breast and prostate cancers have relatively lower mortality, suggesting relatively effective overall therapeutic results. The stage or extent of disease at diagnosis also contributes to survival rates. Cancers that are seldom diagnosed at an early stage in their history (e.g., ovary and pancreas) have poor survival rates. Can-

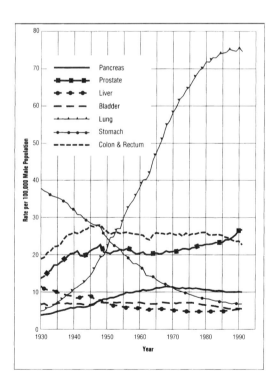

Figure 3-1. Cancer mortality trends among the U.S. male population from 1930–1987. (Reprinted with permission from CC Boring, TS Squires, T Tong. Cancer statistics, 1993. CA Cancer J Clin 1993;1:16.)

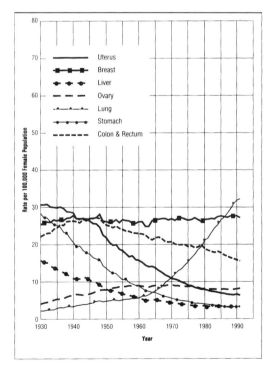

Figure 3-2. Cancer mortality trends among the U.S. female population from 1930–1987. (Reprinted with permission from CC Boring, TS Squires, T Tong. Cancer statistics, 1993. CA Cancer J Clin 1993;1:16.)

Table 3-3. Mortality Ranked for Cancer Sites for Men by Age Groups in 1989

Rank	< 15 Years	15–34 Years	35–54 Years	55–74 Years	75+ Years
1	Leukemia	Leukemia	Lung	Lung	Lung
2	Brain and CNS	Lymphoma	Colorectal	Colorectal	Prostate
3	Endocrine	Brain and CNS	Lymphoma	Prostate	Colorectal
4	Lymphoma	Skin	Brain and CNS	Pancreas	Pancreas
5	Sarcoma	Hodgkin's disease	Skin	Esophagus	Bladder

CNS = central nervous system.

Table 3-4. Mortality Ranked for Cancer Sites for Women by Age Groups in 1989

Rank	< 15 Years	15–34 Years	35–54 Years	55–74 Years	75+ Years
1	Leukemia	Breast	Breast	Lung	Colorectal
2	Brain and CNS	Leukemia	Lung	Breast	Lung
3	Endocrine	Uterus	Uterus	Colorectal	Breast
4	Sarcoma	Brain and CNS	Colorectal	Ovary	Pancreas
5	Bone	Skin	Ovary	Pancreas	Lymphoma

CNS = central nervous system.

Table 3-5.   Average Age-Adjusted Annual Incidence per 100,000 of Selected Cancers (1975–1985)

Site	White	Black	Hispanic	Native American	Chinese	Japanese	Filipino	Hawaiian
All sites	404	490	266	185	293	304	242	399
Esophagus	5	18	3	2	6	6	55	15
Stomach	12	21	21	26	15	39	10	40
Colon	40	41	18	8	34	42	24	26
Lung	82	120	32	14	61	48	40	108
Prostate	77	123	72	46	33	46	47	60
Breast	92	76	51	26	59	57	46	105
Cervix	9	20	17	20	11	6	11	15
Uterus	27	15	11	5	18	18	11	28
Pancreas	11	17	12	9	9	10	8	11
Lymphoma	4	3	3	1	1	1	2	1
Leukemia	14	11	8	6	8	7	9	10
Myeloma	5	10	3	3	3	3	5	6
Bladder	30	15	11	4	14	13	6	11
Testis	4	1	3	2	2	1	1	3

cers that are detected by effective screening programs before dissemination (e.g., breast, cervix, and prostate) lend themselves to better outcomes.

Mortality is even more informative when categorized by age as shown in Tables 3-3 and 3-4.[19] For men, leukemia is prominent up to the ages of 35–54 when lung cancer becomes the leading cause of cancer mortality; for women, leukemia is foremost up to the ages of 15–34 when breast cancer becomes the prominent cause of death. Similar to men, lung cancer assumes mortality leadership beginning at ages 55–74 in women.

The influence of race on cancer incidence and mortality is shown in Tables 3-5 and 3-6.[1] Table 3-5 summarizes the age-adjusted annual incidence of selected cancers by various racial and ethnic groups.

Table 3-6. Five-Year Survival Percentages for Cancer Sites Categorized by Race (1983–1988)*

Site	White (%)	Black (%)
All sites	54	38
Oral and pharynx	54	32
Colon	59	48
Rectum	57	46
Lung	13	11
Larynx	67	53
Cervix	68	55
Breast	79	62
Prostate	78	63
Urinary	79	59
Lymphoma	52	43
Multiple myeloma	26	29
Hodgkin's lymphoma	78	74
Leukemia	38	29
Uterine	84	54

*Standard error of the survival rate is from 5–10%.

This table shows large variations and initiates etiologic speculations such as genetic susceptibility interacting with local environment. Epidemiologic studies on population migrations evaluate the influence of genetic susceptibility and environmental agents. These classic studies suggest that the incidence of many cancers is dependent on environmental influences. These studies support aggressive health care policies for cancer prevention and screening in high-risk groups.

Mortality as well as incidence varies among race and ethnic groups. Table 3-6 summarizes 5-year survival rates categorized by race. As illustrated, blacks have inferior survival rates when compared with whites. These results may be directly related to the disease or indirectly related to the inadequacy of disease management.

The effect of newer and, it is hoped, more effective cancer intervention is demonstrated by the change of mortality over time. Table 3-7 shows in detail the 5-year survival rate for selected sites of cancer for U.S. whites from 1967–1987.[1] The trends in this table demonstrate overall improvement from 39–52%. In general, the rate of improvement was greatest from 1960–1976.

One of the important cancers under recent heavy scientific and political scrutiny is female carcinoma of the breast. Subsequent to 1977, breast cancer incidence rates increased slowly.[20] After 1982, the incidence sharply increased until 1987, whereafter the rates have slightly declined. Coincident with the increase in incidence was improvement in the 3- and 5-year survival rates. This overall phenomenon may be related to improved early detection by self-examination and mammography screening pro-

Table 3-7. Five-Year Relative Survival Percentages for U.S. Whites (1976–1987)

Site	1960–1963 (%)	1970–1973 (%)	1974–1976 (%)	1977–1980 (%)	1981–1987 (%)
All Sites	39	43	50	50	52
Oral	45	43	54	55	54
Esophagus	4	44	5	6	9
Colon	43	49	50	53	58
Pancreas	1	2	3	2	3
Larynx	53	62	66	67	68
Lung	8	10	12	13	13
Breast	63	68	75	75	78
Ovary	32	36	36	38	38
Prostate	50	63	67	72	76
Testis	63	72	78	88	93
Bladder	53	61	74	76	79
Hodgkin's lymphoma	40	67	71	73	77
Lymphoma	31	41	47	48	51
Leukemia	14	22	34	36	36
Cervix	58	64	69	68	68
Uterine	73	81	89	86	84
Myeloma	12	19	24	25	26

grams.[21] Diagnosing breast cancer at an earlier stage can lead to improved survival.

Summary

Due to improved health care, the median age range of the U.S. population is increasing. Formerly untreatable diseases now have more effective management and treatment. Patients with cancer may anticipate more effective care, resulting in a higher cure rate with a prolonged survival with active cancer. Taken together, these two processes will increase the prevalence of patients developing cancer sequelae. Pain as a late manifestation of cancer will thus demand more response from the health care community. Considering the many forms of cancer that can cause pain, there will be significantly more demands on physicians managing pain control.

References

1. Fraumeni JF, Hoover RN, Devesa SS, Linlen LJ. Epidemiology of Cancer. In VT DeVita Jr., S Hellman, SA Rosenberg (eds), Cancer Principles and Practice of Oncology. Philadelphia: Lippincott, 1993;150.
2. Dupont WD. Converting relative risks to absolute risks: A graphical approach. Stat Med 1989;8:641.
3. Vanio H, Wilbourn J. Cancer etiology: Agents causally associated with human cancer. Pharmacol Toxicol 1993;72(Suppl 1):4.
4. Goodman GE. Chemoprophylaxis strategies in high-risk groups with an emphasis on lung cancer. Chest 1993;103(Suppl 1):60S.
5. Mansfield CM. A review of the etiology of breast cancer. J Natl Med Assoc 1993;85:217.
6. Beckett WS. Epidemiology and etiology of lung cancer. Clin Chest Med 1993;14:1.
7. Friedenreich CM, Howe GR, Miller AB, Jain MG. A cohort study of alcohol consumption and risk of breast cancer. Am J Epidemiol 1993;137:512.
8. Szabo E, Mulshine J. Epidemiology, prognostic factors and prevention of lung cancer. Curr Opin Oncol 1993;5:302.
9. Davila DG, Williams DE. The etiology of lung cancer. Mayo Clin Proc 1993;68:170.
10. Kabat GC. Recent developments in the epidemiology of lung cancer. Semin Surg Oncol 1993;9:73.
11. Clifford C, Kramer B. Diet as risk and therapy for cancer. Med Clin North Am 1993;77:725.
12. Herbsman N, Hornsby-Lewis L. The effects of diet on colon cancer. Gastroenterology 1993;105:604.
13. Byers T. Dietary trends in the United States, relevance to cancer prevention. Cancer 1993;72(Suppl 3):1015.
14. Hursting SD, Margolin BH, Switzer BR. Diet and human leukemia: An analysis of international data. Prev Med 1993;22:409.
15. Rose DP. Diet, hormones and cancer. Annu Rev Public Health 1993;14:1.
16. Harris CC, Hollstein M. Medical progress: Clinical implications of the p53 tumor-suppressor gene. N Engl J Med 1993;329:1318.
17. Weinberg RA. Tumor suppressor genes. Science 1991;254:1138.
18. Steele GD Jr., Winchester DP, Menck HR, Murphy GP. Clinical highlights from the National Cancer Data Base: 1993. CA Cancer J Clin 1993;43:71.
19. Boring CC, Squires TS, Tong T. Cancer statistics, 1993. CA Cancer J Clin 1993;43:7.
20. Garfinkel L. Current trends in breast cancer. CA Cancer J Clin 1993;43:5.
21. Miller BA, Feuer EJ, Hankey BF. Recent incidence trends for breast cancer in women and the relevance of early detection: An update. CA Cancer J Clin 1993;43:27.

Chapter 4
Mechanisms of Cancer Pain

Benjamin W. Johnson, Jr. and Winston C. V. Parris

The basic causes of pain resulting from neoplastic processes are usually divided into three categories[1]:

1. Pain caused by the tumor
2. Pain caused by the cancer therapy
3. Pain that is totally unrelated to the cancer

This chapter examines the first two of these causes of pain in cancer patients regarding the pathophysiologic mechanisms of nociception, in addition to a brief mention of therapy based on the mechanisms of cancer pain.

Cancer Pain Due to the Tumor

The pain caused by tumor invasion can usually be attributed to a mechanical etiology, but neurohumoral mechanisms also play a role in sensitizing nerves to the mechanical effects of encroachment of the tumor on previously normal tissue.[2–4] We will examine the painful effects of tumor growth on bone, nerve, visceral, vascular, myofascial, and mucosal tissues.

Bone Pain

It is widely recognized that cancer pain caused by the invasion of bony structures is probably the most common etiology of tumor-related pain.[5–7] Although the exact mechanisms of pain production are unknown, it is believed that tumor invasion of bone provokes an inflammatory response from the body that results in alterations in bone metabolism and autocoid production.[8–10] Tumor-induced osteoclastic activity produces prostaglandins E_1 (PGE_1) and E_2 (PGE_2), which may induce osteolysis as well as sensitize peripheral nerve endings, thus sensitizing the organism to nociceptive input. Although the bone cortex and marrow are not thought to be pain-sensitive structures, myelinated and nonmyelinated nerve fibers are known to exist in bone, especially in the periosteum. The absence of pain-sensitive neurons in the bony cortex and medulla could explain the frequent observation that vertebral metastases may be asymptomatic until the tumor penetrates the cortex and invades the periosteum or causes compression of neural elements. The analgesic action of nonsteroidal anti-inflammatory drugs (NSAIDs) in these patients is probably due to the inhibitory effects these compounds have on prostaglandin synthesis. It is thought that NSAIDs inhibit cyclo-oxygenase, thus halting the formation of the arachidonic acid cascade. Prostaglandin synthesis does not seem to be a significant factor in the bony pain resulting from myeloma and lymphoma; therefore, the benefit of NSAIDs is not as significant as with "solid" tumors. Osteoclastic-inhibiting compounds probably exert their analgesic efficacy by preventing the formation of autocoids, which are known to adversely modify the response characteristics of nerve tissue to noxious or nonnoxious stimulation. Drugs such as corticosteroids, biphosphonates, cytotoxic chemotherapy, calcitonin, plicamycin, and strontium 89 and modalities such as radiotherapy are used to treat bony pain resulting from osteoclastic activity.[8, 9] Corticosteroids, in particular, are known to inhibit phospholipase A_2, which normally modulates the liberation of arachidonic acid from cellular membranes, thus initiating the arachidonic acid cascade. Autocoids are local tissue "hormones" (i.e., cytokines, potassium, bradykinin, interleukin-1, growth factors, osteoclastic-activating factor, tumor necrosis factors, and parathyroid hormone-like peptides) released as a result of osteoclastic and inflammatory activities. These substances seem to play an important role in sensitizing neural tissue to mechanical, chemical, and thermal stimuli. Autocoids lower discharge thresholds of the neuronal membrane, produce exaggerated responses to suprathreshold nociceptive stimuli, and provoke tonic impulse discharges in normally silent nociceptors. Thus, autocoids could be responsible for the translation of innocuous stimuli into nociceptive impulses.

In addition to the two mechanisms mentioned earlier for the etiology of bone pain in cancer patients, pathologic fractures can be a significant source of pain for the cancer patient. This is especially notable in the axial spine, a frequent location for metastatic lesions of numerous neoplastic processes, where either vertebral compression fractures or spinal instability can be a significant source of pain. The usual mechanism of pain from pathologic fractures is either trauma to the periosteum, compression of peripheral nerves, or compression of the spinal cord. For these patients, tumor resection and spine stabilization must be added to the pain control regimen for optimal treatment.

Pain originating from the joint often arises as a reaction to inflammatory processes provoked by the malignant process. The myelinated group III and nonmyelinated IV fibers can be sensitized by inflammatory tissue autocoids (bradykinin, prostaglandins, serotonin, histamine) to relay input from even slight joint movement that can be interpreted as pain.

In summary, the etiology of bony pain can be attributed to two additive and possibly synergistic mechanisms: (1) invasion or stretching of the pain-sensitive periosteum and (2) the sensitization of nerves in bony tissue that are normally pain-insensitive by autocoids produced during osteoclastic activity. Effective treatment results from inhibiting the osteolytic activity, minimizing the effect of heightened peripheral neuron sensitivity, or stabilizing pathologic fractures.

Neurogenic Pain

Disruption of nerve axons, either by compression or infiltration, can create chronic neurogenic pain syndromes that are severe and often resistant to therapy.[11–13] Although the initiation of acute neurogenic pain by tumor infiltration or bony collapse causing edema or ischemia is well accepted, knowledge of the true pathophysiology remains elusive.[14]

Tumor Compression of Central Nervous System Neurons

Compression of central nervous system (CNS) neurons by an expanding tumor mass produces edema, ischemia, and necrosis, resulting in local degeneration of the axon and myelin sheath with consequent phagocytosis of axonal debris by macrophages. Recent laboratory investigations using biologic tracers transported via the neuronal anterograde microtubular system suggest that traumatic events can result in a focal impairment of microtubular transport that eventually causes local axonal swelling and local lobulation, followed by rupture of the axon "cylinder."[11] This chronic axonal damage ranges from disruption of axoplasmic transport to delayed axonal rupture owing to the internal release of putative neurotransmitters (i.e., acetylcholine, glutamate, aspartate, etc.) and autocoids. With the release of these substances into the extracellular milieu, it is not surprising that the trigeminal afferents supplying cerebral vasculature may be sensitized and become a source of painful stimulus transduction. In addition, compression and distortion of intracranial vessels and dura mater can also be a stimulus for nociceptive input. After therapeutic measures such as surgery or radiotherapy, glial cells proliferate, forming a glial scar, which may prevent new axonal formation and restoration of central connections.[15] In addition, glial cells absorb any remaining fragments of myelin and axonal degenerative debris. Within 1 day of injury (including surgery), the nerve terminal and its mitochondria begin to swell; within 6–7 days, the glial cells push the ineffective terminal away from its connections to other neurons.

Tumor compression of the spinal cord occurs most often in lymphomas and carcinoma of the lung and breast. The etiology of the compression can be traced to several causes:

1. Deformity or collapse of vertebral body or pedicle
2. Direct extension of tumor into the epidural space from vertebral metastasis
3. Direct spread from paravertebral lymph nodes through the intervertebral foramina
4. Hematogenous spread
5. Intramedullary metastasis
6. Intrinsic tumors

The classic clinical presentation of spinal cord compression results from the selective sensitivity of the spinal cord tracts to mechanical pressure, as well as from the initial pressure on the anterior aspects of the spinal cord resulting from extension of the tumor from the vertebral body.[16] The presence of either edema or ischemia can accelerate the development of clinical signs and symptoms. The following list shows the usual clinical sequence observed with tumor compression of the spinal cord:

1. Pain (the initial presentation in 94% of patients)
2. Weakness
3. Sensory deficits including numbness and paresthesia
4. Loss of sphincter control

Multifocal spreading of systemic cancer to the leptomeninges via hematogenous spread to the arachnoid, rupture of brain parenchymal metastases, or direct spread from the epidural space occurs in approximately 8% of all cancer patients, especially in breast and lung cancer patients. The most common painful symptoms are headache (50%), acute low back pain (50%), and sharp radicular pain (30%).

Once present in the meninges, the cancer can produce painful sequelae by the following mechanisms:

1. Obstructive hydrocephalus
2. Invasion of nerve roots
3. Infiltration or ischemia of focal brain/spinal cord neurons
4. Reactive meningeal inflammation, with release of neuron-sensitizing tissue autocoids

Cranial Neuropathies in Cancer Patients

Head and neck cancers often invade and spread along the perineural sheath, causing myelin and ax-

onal degeneration.[14] In addition, neuronal edema and regional ischemia may result from compression of cranial nerves within bony canals, specifically at the base of the skull (jugular foramen syndrome), clivus (vertex headache with neck flexion), hypoglossal canal, and the sphenoid sinus. Entrance of the cranial nerve pain fibers (typically V, VII, IX, and X) into the CNS with the cervical plexus may produce a concurrent cervical plexopathy and cranial neuropathy.

Peripheral Neuropathies

Peripheral Neuropathic Pain Caused by Cancer

Brachial plexopathy due to tumor invasion occurs in 2–5% of patients with malignant lung lesions.[14] Breast and bronchial tumors seem to produce a majority of these lesions. Lesions of the lower elements of the brachial plexus (i.e., C-8 to T-1) are the most likely affected, but the entire plexus can be involved in many of these situations. Pain is the presenting symptom in brachial plexopathy for most patients. The characteristic moderate-to-severe aching pain of the shoulder girdle that radiates along the ulnar nerve distribution is usually aggravated by motion of the upper extremity.

Some mechanisms of tumor involvement include:

1. Focal mass in the region of the brachial plexus
2. Diffuse soft tissue infiltration of the brachial plexus
3. Paravertebral mass extension into the plexus
4. Tumor involvement of adjacent cervical vertebrae

The possibility of radiotherapy-induced brachial plexopathy, as well as radiation-induced nerve sheath tumors should also be considered in the differential diagnosis of peripheral neuropathic lesions caused by cancer.

Lumbosacral plexopathy usually results from either tumor extension from bone or from compression of the plexus against the pelvis by presacral soft tissue tumors. As with brachial plexopathy, pain is a presenting symptom for most patients, preceding numbness, weakness, and reflex asymmetry. The pain can arise from tumor encroachment of the upper lumbar plexus (L-2 to L-4) such as colorectal cancer involving the pelvic wall, wherein patients develop pain in the anterolateral or anteromedial thigh. Tumors can also arise from deep in the medial aspect of the true pelvis and invade or compress the lower lumbar plexus (L-5 to S-1) as in sarcoma, where pain is experienced in the buttock and lower leg. The entire lumbar plexus (L-2 to S-2) can be involved as in genitourinary tumors. Sacral involvement is typically caused by invasion of bladder, gynecologic, or colonic tumors and may manifest as sacral pain, painful rectal tenesmus, impotence, and urinary incontinence.

Tumor infiltration of the perineural cleft is one common cause of cancer-induced painful peripheral neuropathies, especially involving intercostal nerves and paravertebral or retroperitoneal spaces. Aside from tumor invasion and compression, painful syndromes can result from paraneoplastic syndromes such as paraproteinemias and carcinomatous neuropathies.[17] The most common neural injuries can be classified as a neuropraxis (i.e., in that the nerve trunk is intact, but not functioning). The degeneration of an axon is not an isolated event because surrounding neurons with synaptic attachments often show corresponding degenerative changes.

Within hours after sufficient damage, the distal segment begins to degenerate because of the loss of axoplasmic transport of vital elements from the cell body. The path of degeneration may be anterograde or retrograde. Anterograde changes may include sensitization of the wide dynamic range (WDR) neurons of the dorsal horn of the spinal cord. The subsequent release of excitatory amino acids (i.e., glutamate) by excitatory interneurons or nociceptors in the dorsal horn reaches the *N*-methyl-D-aspartate receptors and thereby facilitates the central summation of nociceptive input ("windup" phenomenon), which then sensitizes the spinothalamic tract cells.[11] The resulting neuronal dysfunction may be interpreted as pain by higher order neurons.

Injury to an axon by tumor infiltration may change the normally passive conducting properties of the axon to those of an ectopic chemical or mechanically induced source of aberrant action potentials. Axons in a state of demyelination, degeneration, or regeneration may manifest spontaneous electrical activity and are exquisitely sensitive to norepinephrine in the extracellular space. A single action potential in an injured axon may produce multiple electrical discharges from the damaged area. This phenomenon is known as "after-discharge" and may not only be a significant source of painful sensation, but may also modify contiguous neurons by altering ionic composition of the local extracellular milieu. Reflected axon spikes, an abnormal type of conduction resulting from varying rates of conduction within a single axon due to alteration of axonal diameter or myelination, can result in a self-propagating "circus" excitation from a single stimulus. Axonal cross talk has also been proposed as a possible mechanism for neuropathic pain. The presence of electrical junctions between axons in degenerating and regenerating axonal segments has been documented in recent investigations by Raminsky. If a low-threshold mechanical afferent is joined to a nociceptive axon, stimulation by light touch could be interpreted clinically as pain or hyperesthesia.

Drugs inhibiting mitosis, such as vincristine, are associated with sensorimotor neuropathies such as jaw pain, burning dysesthesias of the hands and feet, and allodynia when administered to cancer patients.[18, 19] Microtubules are the thickest of the neuron's cytoskeletal fibers, and are oriented along the length of the axon. Secretory residues, containing neurotransmitters manufactured in the soma of the neuron, are believed to be transported along the microtubules to the axon's terminal end, where they are released into the synaptic cleft. The microtubular system also transports neurosecretory by-products retrograde from the terminal end of the axon to the soma of the neuron for remanufacture. Microtubular disruption is a proposed mechanism by which the cellular toxins vincristine and colchicine exert their desired clinical effects. Inhibiting rapid axoplasmic transport by microtubular disruption prevents the neuron from engaging in synaptic transmission, creating a situation similar to deafferentation.

Peripheral nerve pathology, such as tumor infiltration, compression, or ischemia, can reduce the ability of afferent discharges reaching the dorsal horn to modify the activity of contiguous neurons—a characteristic known as the *dorsal root reflex*. The activation of electrically silent synapses between dorsal horn cells can apparently be unmasked abruptly by peripheral axonal injury, so that when a given axon is unable to conduct an action potential, the dorsal horn cell receives input from a different axon and adopts its receptive field.

Visceral Pain Caused by Cancer

Infiltration of Hollow Viscera

The stimuli required to activate the afferent visceral nociceptors contained within the splanchnic nerves include the following[20, 21]:

1. Torsion or traction of the mesentery
2. Distention or contraction of a hollow viscus
3. Irritation of the mucosal and serosal surfaces
4. Obstruction
5. Ischemia
6. Spasm of smooth muscle

Severe obstruction and distention result when tumor infiltration, traction, or compression compromises the outlet of hollow viscera such as the stomach, intestine, biliary tract, ureters, bladder, or uterus. The consequent isometric contractions and distention cause the characteristic diffuse, poorly localized pain, which may be referred to dermatomes supplied by the same spinal segments (Table 4-1). The distension can result in visceral ischemia, which exacerbates the pain. Mucosal ulceration of the gastrointestinal tract can cause hemorrhage, which increases peristaltic activity and can also increase the visceral pain already present.

Infiltration of Solid Viscera

Stretching of the capsule of solid viscera such as the liver, kidney, and spleen activates the afferent nociceptors present in the fascia. Tumor-induced hemorrhage into a solid viscera can also cause distention of the capsule, resulting in pain. In addition, tumor-induced necrosis provokes the release of algogenic tissue autocoids such as potassium, bradykinins, interleukins, and adenosine triphosphate, which sensitize the nerves to mechanical and chemical stimuli.

Tumor Encroachment of Vascular Structures

Infiltration and obstruction of blood and lymph vessels often produces a combination of venous engorgement, tissue edema, perivascular lymphangitis, ischemia, and reactive vasospasm, causing a diffuse, nonlocalized pain that does not follow a recogniz-

Table 4-1. Locations of Pain Referred from Visceral Structures

Organ	Referred Pain Location
Pancreas	Back, paraspinal muscles
Endometrium	Back, paraspinal muscles
Liver	Right shoulder
Prostate	Abdomen or leg

able peripheral nerve distribution. Examples include the superior vena caval syndrome resulting from obstruction of vascular structures draining the head and neck, edema of the upper extremity resulting from cancer of the breast with axillary lymphadenopathy, and edema of the lower extremity due to obstruction of vascular structures by pelvic lymphadenopathy.

Tumor Invasion of Mucosal Surfaces

Debilitating pain can result from the inflammation, ulceration, and necrosis caused by cancerous invasion of mucosal surfaces such as the lips, mouth, pharynx, and gastrointestinal and genitourinary tracts.[22–24] Algogenic tissue autocoids cause sensitization of the rich supply of cutaneous nociceptors, which are responsible for the excruciating pain.

Mechanisms of Pain Caused by Cancer Therapy

Postsurgical Pain Syndromes

The underlying mechanisms of pain production in these syndromes are both peripheral and central in nature, involving a deafferentation-like phenomenon.

Postamputation Pain

Pain in the stump of the amputated limb and phantom limb pain can develop as a result of a combination of central and peripheral mechanisms. The noxious stimulation caused by transecting the related peripheral nerves causes an acute afferent barrage of action potentials known as an "injury discharge," which sensitizes the WDR neurons of the dorsal horn. This brief phenomenon is thought to be a harbinger of the eventual development of a neuropathic pain syndrome. Although the occurrence of phantom limb phenomenon is common after amputation of a limb or other tissue (i.e., bowel, nose, breast), the development of phantom pain is quite variable (reported incidence ranging from 2–97%) and is often resistant to treatment. The proposed pathophysiology includes peripheral, spinal, central, and "psychological" mechanisms.

Peripheral mechanisms of phantom pain include the following causes: (1) spontaneous activity in neuromata and WDR neurons in the dorsal horn of the spinal cord; (2) ephaptic connections between afferent and efferent neurons; and (3) altered conduction velocities in damaged neurons.

The following includes some spinal mechanisms of phantom pain: (1) increased sensitivity of dorsal horn neurons to afferent stimuli, and (2) loss of high threshold mechanoreception with replacement by low threshold mechanoreceptors, resulting in hyperesthesia or hyperpathia.

Central mechanisms of phantom pain include the following items:

1. Simmel's argument for the presence of a "central body map" and Melzack's concept of the "body neuromatrix" suggest that an absence or distortion of modulating input from the missing body part may provoke output from the brain that is interpreted as pain.
2. Also to be considered are the cognitive aspects of the interpretation of phantom limb sensations. If these abnormal sensations are considered unpleasant by the amputee, the experience could conceivably be labeled as pain.

Postthoracotomy Pain Syndrome

Postthoracotomy pain syndrome is characterized by lancinating pains with dysesthesias and hypesthesias along the surgical scar and related intercostal nerve dermatomes. The usual mechanism seems to be surgical trauma to the intercostal nerves, either by axonotmesis or neuropraxia from retractor compression.

However, mechanisms involving the intrinsic musculoskeletal elements of the chest wall and the extrinsic chest wall musculature can be involved.

Myofascial pain due to intraoperative positioning, surgical retraction, and surgical incision of muscle with subsequent neuroma formation and scar entrapment can also occur. Although this syndrome occurs infrequently, it is a debilitating problem that interferes greatly with the quality of life of cancer patients. Occasionally, the pain can result in disuse of the ipsilateral upper extremity and cause significant disability and atrophy.

Postmastectomy Pain Syndrome

Operative trauma to the intercostobrachial and other upper thoracic nerves can provoke pain dysesthesias and hypesthesias involving the posterior arm, axilla, and anterior chest. The pain is usually described as being burning and band-like in nature. As with the postthoracotomy pain syndrome, the postmastectomy syndrome can result in significant atrophy of the ipsilateral upper extremity due to disuse from pain avoidance behavior.

Postchemotherapy Pain Syndromes

Peripheral Neuropathic Pain

As mentioned previously, treatment of cancer with *Vinca* alkaloids (vincristine and vinblastine) can result in a painful symmetric polyneuropathy, arthralgia, and myalgia at therapeutic doses. The mechanism is believed to be related to the functional interruption of the axonal microtubular transport system, which could conceivably create a deafferentation-like syndrome.

Steroid-Induced Aseptic Necrosis of Bone

Aseptic necrosis of the hip, shoulder, or both can result in severe dull, aching pain of a "constant" nature. Glucocorticoid administration seems to be the most likely cause, but the mechanism is not well understood.

Steroid Withdrawal Syndrome

Discontinuing systemic glucocorticoid therapy can result in a pseudorheumatism involving myalgias and arthralgias, which is resolved by reinstituting steroid therapy.

Mucositis

Excruciatingly painful, intractable pain of the mucosal surfaces of the nasopharynx and oropharynx can occur after chemotherapy and radiotherapy.[15, 18, 21] The supposed mechanisms for this phenomenon are biochemical changes in nociceptive elements of the mucosal surface.

Herpes Zoster and Postherpetic Neuralgia

The mechanism of this severe and debilitating neurogenic pain syndrome is believed to be the extensive damage by the herpes zoster virus to the afferent neurons in the affected dermatomes.

Postradiation Pain Syndromes

Postradiation Plexopathy

Exposure to radiation therapy can induce fibrosis of tissues surrounding the brachial, cervical, or lumbosacral nerve plexuses with distressing results.[15] The development of increasing diffuse, constant burning pain with paresthesias and dysesthesias from 6 months to 20 years after exposure is characteristic of this syndrome. The proposed mechanism is chronic progressive constrictive obstruction of neuronal axoplasmic transport, with subsequent degeneration and deafferentation.

Postradiation Myelopathy

Two forms of this condition are recognized: transient and chronic. The transient form develops over 4 months and resolves in 2–36 weeks. The chronic form develops over 5–13 months after radiation exposure to the head, neck, and mediastinum. Pain and dysesthesias are often the presenting symptoms and are usually present in the region of spinal cord damage. The mechanism of pain production is uncertain, but probably involves central mechanisms.

Table 4-2. Paraneoplastic Pain Syndromes

Pain	Paraneoplastic Disorder
Myalgia	Dermatomyositis
	Myopathy
	Polymyositis
Arthralgia/myalgia	Rheumatoid arthritis
	Polymyalgia rheumatica
Bone pain	Hypertrophic osteoarthropathy (Marie-Bamberger disease)
Ischemic pain	Blood hypercoagulability (thromboembolic phenomenon)

Radiation-Induced Nerve Tumors

Brachial and lumbosacral plexuses exposed to radiotherapy can develop neural tumors that may produce severe burning pain in the related dermatome.

Paraneoplastic Pain Syndromes

These pain syndromes can accompany malignant disease processes and are apparently provoked by them.[16] The cancers known to be associated with paraneoplastic pain syndromes include the following types:

1. Bronchogenic
2. Gastric
3. Breast
4. Pancreatic
5. Prostatic
6. Ovarian
7. Hepatic
8. Acute leukemia
9. Lymphomas

The paraneoplastic syndromes include the painful disorders listed in Table 4-2.

The mechanisms of cancer pain, in general, reflect the result of the influence of the neoplastic process on the body, or the effect of therapy directed against the cancer. For example, the neurogenic pain syndromes arise from nerve damage due to tumor infiltration, compression, ischemia, or chemotoxicity of the affected nerves; postsurgical pain syndromes result from nerve damage due to the controlled trauma of surgical procedures. In spite of the many possible mechanisms of cancer pain, it is encouraging to note that sufficient therapeutic modalities are available to treat virtually all patients suffering from cancer pain. As future research efforts produce additional knowledge concerning the mechanisms of cancer pain, it is anticipated that application of the acquired knowledge will result in improved cost-effective treatment for all patients experiencing cancer pain.

References

1. Foley KM. Pain Syndromes in Patients with Cancer. In JJ Bonica, V Ventafridda (eds), Advances in Pain Research and Therapy (Vol. 2). New York: Raven, 1979;59.
2. Levine JD, Taiwo YO, Heller PH. Cancer Pain: The Contribution of Mediators Underlying Inflammatory Pain. In RC Chapman, KM Foley (eds), Current and Emerging Issues in Cancer Pain: Research and Practice. New York: Raven, 1993;21.
3. Payne R. Anatomy, physiology and neuropharmacology of cancer pain. Med Clin North Am 1987;71:153.
4. Janig W. Neurophysiological mechanisms of cancer pain. Recent Results Cancer Res 1984;89:45.
5. Bonica JJ, Ventafridda V,Twycross RG. Cancer Pain. In JJ Bonica (ed), The Management of Pain (2nd ed). Philadelphia: Lea & Febiger, 1990;400.
6. Ventafridda V, Caraceni A. Cancer Pain. In PP Raj (ed), Current Review of Pain. Philadelphia: Current Medicine, 1994;155.
7. Caillet R. Pain Mechanisms and Management. Philadelphia: Davis, 1993.
8. Bonjour JP, Rizzoli R. Pathophysiological aspects and therapeutic approaches of tumoral osteolysis and hypercalcemia. Recent Results Cancer Res 116:29, 1987.
9. Burckhard P, Thiebaud D, Perey L, et al. Treatment of tumor-induced osteolysis by APD. Recent Results Cancer Res 116:54, 1987.
10. Portenoy RK. Cancer pain: Pathophysiology and syndromes. Lancet 1992;339:1026.
11. Johnson BW, Parris WCV. Mechanisms of Neuropathic Pain. In PP Raj (ed), Current Review of Pain. Philadelphia: Current Medicine, 1994;179.
12. Wall PD. Neurological mechanisms in cancer pain. Cancer Surv 1988;7:127.
13. Clouston PD, DeAanelis LM, Posner JB. The spectrum of neurological disease in patients with systemic cancer. Ann Neurol 1992;31:268.
14. Scott JF. Carcinoma Invading Nerve. In PD Wall, R Melzack (eds), Textbook of Pain. New York: Churchill Livingstone, 1989;598.
15. Banfi A. Radiation-Induced Complications. In G Bonadonna, G Robustelli della Cuna (eds), Handbook of Medical Oncology (3rd ed). St. Louis: Mosby-Year Book, 1988.
16. Lee SI, Phillips LH II, Jane JA. Somato-somatic referred pain caused by suprasegmental spinal cord tumor. Neurology 1991;41:928.
17. Robustelli della Cuna G. Paraneoplastic Syndromes. In G Bonadonna, G Robustelli della Cuna (eds), Handbook of Medical Oncology (3rd ed). St. Louis: Mosby-Year Book, 1988.
18. Valagussa P. Side Effects from Drug Therapy. In G Bonadonna, G Robustelli della Cuna (eds), Handbook of Medical Oncology (3rd ed). St. Louis: Mosby-Year Book, 1988.
19. Bonadonna G. Chemotherapy-Induced Complications. In G Bonadonna, G Robustelli della Cuna (eds), Handbook of Medical Oncology (3rd ed). St. Louis: Mosby-Year Book, 1988.
20. Baines M, Kirkham SR. Cancer Pain. In PD Wall, R Melzack (eds), Textbook of Pain. New York: Churchill Livingstone, 1989;590.
21. Gebhart GF. Visceral Pain Mechanisms. In RC Chapman, KM Foley (eds), Current and Emerging Issues in Cancer Pain: Research and Practice. New York: Raven, 1993;99.
22. Schubert MM. Measurement of Oral Tissue Damage and Mucositis Pain. In RC Chapman, KM Foley (eds), Current and Emerging Issues in Cancer Pain: Research and Practice. New York: Raven, 1993;247.
23. Aaronson NA, Beckmann J (eds). The Quality of Life of Cancer Patients. New York: Raven, 1987.
24. Herzberg AJ, Murphy GF. Painful tumors of the skin. J Dermatol Surg Oncol 1993;19:250.

Chapter 5

Assessment of the Cancer Pain Patient

Winston C. V. Parris

Even though cancer continues to increase in the United States and worldwide, modest strides have been made to treat this disease. Some of the new therapeutic modalities used to treat cancer are effective, others are promising, but many are not effective. The fact that so many therapeutic regimens are available attests to the reality that, for most cancers, no one therapeutic option is singularly effective most of the time. One major shortcoming of cancer management is the undertreatment of pain.[1] This factor has been universally recognized and has been addressed at several levels including the World Health Organization (WHO).[2] The U.S. government recently acknowledged the implications of chronic undertreatment in cancer pain patients, with the result that the Agency for Health Care Policy and Research (AHCPR) (an agency for the U.S. Department of Health and Human Services) convened a panel of experts on cancer pain management both from within and out of the government to develop guidelines to help practitioners better manage cancer pain. Released in March 1994, these guidelines[3] have served not only to highlight the inadequacies of cancer pain management but also to offer specific recommendations to health care providers. One fundamental deficiency of cancer pain management is inadequate assessment of cancer pain. Von Roenn et al.[4] reviewed oncology physician attitudes and practice in cancer pain management and found that inadequate pain evaluation and deficient follow-up assessment were the greatest impediments to effective management of cancer pain patients. Thus, it is clear that the problem is much greater in the nonspecialist medical community than in the or-

ganized and specialist practices. This study and others [5-7] have shown that thorough initial and follow-up assessments of cancer pain patients are important cornerstones for effective pain management. This chapter highlights the need for assessment and offers a strategy for the practical assessment of the cancer pain patient. Although there are many techniques that are appropriate and suitable for cancer pain assessment, it is important to have a particular strategy that is simple and reproducible and can be administered within the guidelines of a multidisciplinary team concept.

The major goal of pain assessment is to develop a schema whereby the most appropriate diagnostic and therapeutic considerations are defined for a particular patient, so that the pathogenesis of the cancer can be determined and an effective plan of pain treatment outlined. There are several impediments to effective assessment of cancer pain.[8] These impediments include:

1. The lack of effective communication between the patient and health care providers
2. The absence of a common language to define pain
3. Psychological, cultural and social barriers that contribute to underreporting or misreporting of pain and its characteristics
4. The multidisciplinary nature of pain and the complexity of its subjective characterizations
5. Inadequate pain measurement strategies

Although a great deal must be done in the future to solve the puzzle of cancer and management of cancer pain, there is enough information currently available and adequate therapeutic tools to at least make satisfactory progress into the effective management of cancer pain.

It is important to review the epidemiology of pain in cancer patients before discussing possible pain assessment methods. In 1990, the WHO published a document on cancer pain relief and palliative care that showed that there are approximately 14 million people worldwide living with cancer today.[2] About one-third of these patients have inadequate treatment for pain or no treatment at all. It has been demonstrated that as cancer progresses, so does the prevalence and increasing intensity of pain.[9] Further, cancer pain increases as metastatic spread increases and also as aggressive therapy is administered to patients.[10] These therapeutic measures may include surgery, radiotherapy, chemotherapy, pharmacologic therapy, and biological therapy. A simple but thorough assessment of the pain on a continuing basis would help highlight the inadequacy of treatment and would serve to enhance the effective nature of the therapeutic strategies outlined for those patients.

Another important consideration in the assessment of the cancer patient is the knowledge of the relationship between a particular cancer syndrome and its propensity to produce pain. Some tumors are commonly associated with pain, e.g., cancer of the pancreas, bone tumors, multiple myeloma, and breast cancers, whereas leukemia and lymphoma per se are not usually associated with pain (Table 5-1). An analysis of daily frequency of pain, mood scale score, intensity of worst pain, frequency of worst pain, interference with sleep, and quality of life measures are important indices for evaluating pain in the cancer patient. Thus, it is clear that a numerical characterization of pain is just one of many facets that have to be evaluated as one assesses the complete pain picture in a particular cancer patient.

Cancer pain may be assessed under the following schema: (1) pretreatment assessment, (2) intratreatment (concurrent) assessment, (3) posttreatment assessment.

In using this outline, it is important that the pain team or health care providers managing a particular pain patient retain some flexibility, because no two patients are alike. Further, it is important to have a good understanding of specific common cancer-related pain syndromes that usually affect cancer patients. Knowledge of these syndromes (see Chapter

Table 5-1. Types of Cancer Associated with Pain: Adult Group (N = 143)

Type	Number of Patients	Percentage of Patients*
Breast	46	52
Lung	30	45
Bone	6	85
Oral cavity	12	80
Gastrointestinal	20	40
Genitourinary, male	10	75
Genitourinary, female	14	70
Lymphoma	4	20
Leukemia	1	5

*Percentage of the total number of patients admitted with the tumor type.
Source: Reprinted with permission from D Doyle, G Hanks, N MacDonald. Oxford Textbook of Palliative Medicine. New York: Oxford University Press, 1993.

23), their pathogenesis, and their general course would help enhance therapeutic strategies designed to deal more effectively with the pain. Cancer pain is too complex to effectively categorize into neat compartments. However, Foley[11] has offered a classification that is a useful therapeutic guide for pain management. In this classification, patients with cancer pain are divided into five groups:

1. Patients with acute cancer-related pain
2. Patients with chronic cancer-related pain
3. Patients with preexisting chronic pain and cancer-related pain
4. Patients with a history of drug addiction in cancer-related pain
5. Dying patients with cancer-related pain

This classification prioritizes the basis for treatment and includes not only therapeutic but also prognostic implications. In addition, it provides guidelines for the urgency with which the therapeutic issues have to be addressed, the need for greater empathy and sensitivity in dealing with patients, and the rate at which realistic goals should be set.

The Edmonton Staging System for cancer pain[12] was designed to evaluate the possible chances of providing pain relief for cancer patients. Patients were classified based on seven clinical features: presence of incident pain, pain mechanism, cognitive function, previous exposure to opioids, psychological distress, tolerance to opioids, and a history of alcoholism or drug abuse. This classification has been shown to identify potential problem patients and appropriate therapy for pain relief. Preliminary studies assessing its value are encouraging, and it may be used more frequently in the future.

Pretreatment Assessment

Pain History

A detailed history should be obtained from the patient, either on initial interview or shortly thereafter. Patients may be uncomfortable, too sleepy, or exhausted from a prior investigation or a procedure to give a coherent historical account of their pain. Thus, it is important to get a detailed interview when the most information may be obtained. It is also helpful to have a family member present to assist with the information-gathering process and to generally support the patient. The history should include the following items:

1. The location of the pain, including the possibility of more than one location
2. The onset and time course of the pain
3. Characterization of pain with attempts to differentiate whether the pain is musculoskeletal, neurogenic, vascular, or visceral in nature
4. Exacerbating and relieving factors affecting the pain
5. The intensity of the pain described in the patient's own words
6. The signs and symptoms associated with the pain
7. The impact of pain on the patient's psychological state
8. The impact of pain on the activities of daily living including sleep, recreational activity, eating, sex, work, and so forth
9. The response of pain to previous analgesic interventions
10. The response of pain to current analgesic interventions

Pain Measurement

It is necessary to obtain a measurement of the patient's pain that is as precise as possible in quantifiable and reproducible terms. The particular instrument(s) used to measure the patient's

pain perception should be influenced by how familiar the user is with the instrument and by how familiar the patient is with the intended objective. The following are some of the pain assessment instruments available for measuring cancer pain:

1. Numeric verbal rating scale[13]
2. Visual analog scale [14]
3. The five-point descriptive pain intensity scale (using no pain, mild pain, moderate pain, severe pain, very severe pain)
4. Emory Pain Estimate Model[15]
5. Memorial Pain Assessment Card[16] (Figure 5-1)
6. Wisconsin Brief Pain Inventory[17]
7. McGill Pain Questionnaire[18]
8. Pain assessment diary
9. Pain drawings[19]
10. Edmonton staging system for cancer pain

It is important for the caregiver to believe the patient's complaint of pain but also to be sensitive to the patient's subjective expression of his or her pain. It is not uncommon for the patient to demonstrate semantic verbalization regarding perception of the pain while dramatizing or exaggerating the features of that pain.[20] Although these features are more characteristic of patients with chronic nonmalignant pain, some cancer pain patients, whose disease processes are not very progressive and whose behavioral factors overshadow the physical factors, may express the features of "pain behavior." In my opinion, these patients are definitely in the minority of cancer pain patients.

When assessing cancer pain patients, one should keep in mind that not all patients are literate enough to reliably understand the objective of the visual analog scale or similar pain measurement instruments. Further, not all patients speak or understand English. The Pakistan Coin Pain Scale[21] is a pain assessment scale that attempts to compensate for potentially low literacy rates. It is used in rural Pakistan where the literary rate is quite low. As part of the scale, the currency of Pakistan (rupee) is used by the patient to quantify his or her pain. This same flexibility is used in assessing pain in children. The "Oucher,"[22] which uses a continuum of faces from a very happy face (no pain) with progressive decreasing happy faces, culminating with a very distressed face (most pain), is used effectively to assess pain in pediatric patients.

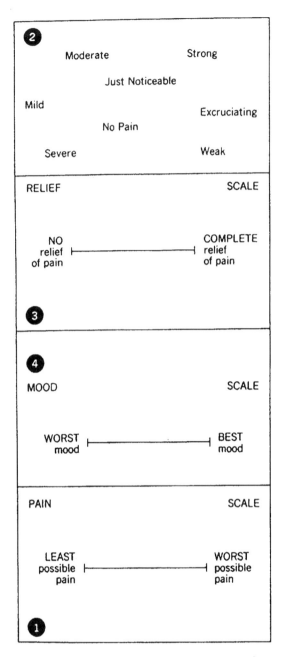

Figure 5-1. The Memorial Pain Assessment Card. (Reprinted with permission from B Fishman, S Pasternack, S Wallenstein, RW Houde, et al. The Memorial Pain Assessment Card: A valid instrument for the evaluation of cancer pain. Cancer 1987;60:1151.)

Physical and Neurologic Examination

A thorough physical examination is important to provide data to corroborate the information obtained from the history. The relationship between physical findings and pain history provides the basis for determining the presence of the disease, its progression, and to help anticipate its outcome. Knowledge of the patterns of referred pain in a particular syndrome helps direct the physical examination and, consequently, the evaluation process. For example, knowledge of the relationship between carcinoma of the lung (Pancoast's tumor) and upper extremity pain (secondary to sympathetic nervous system mediastinal invasion) may enhance the understanding of the pain origin and its distribution,[23] and may also facilitate the acquisition of meaningful laboratory and radiologic investigation to support that diagnosis. It is important to stress the fundamentals of physical examination and to use them in every examination. These time-honored fundamentals include inspection, palpation, percussion, and auscultation of the region being examined. The neurologic examination and the examination of the musculoskeletal system are important so as to attempt to determine the role of the central nervous system in the pathogenesis of pain. These examinations should include evaluation of sensory loss, motor dysfunction, the presence of allodynia and hyperesthesia, the degree of muscle spasm, patient coordination and gait, and the overall mental status. The findings from these evaluations provide a solid basis for making an accurate physical diagnosis.

Psychological Evaluation

In most evaluations of the cancer pain patient, psychological assessment is deferred until the patient is more comfortable and the presenting pain is better controlled. In some cases, it should be abbreviated considerably, or completely eliminated at least initially. Unlike the nonmalignant chronic pain patient, the degree of urgency for pain relief and the impact of the treatable emotional stresses on pain is relatively less in the cancer pain patient. This does not mean that death, dying, and family-related issues are not important in the cancer pain patient but rather that it is more appropriate to deal with them after the physical pain has been controlled or decreased. In many circumstances, the patient has not had time to grieve or express emotions relating to the cancer. An objective of the psychological assessment is to give the patient an opportunity to express these emotions. The psychological assessment should also attempt to evaluate the effect of cancer and related pain on the quality of life. Specific measures to assess quality-of-life issues should be implemented at that time.

Several psychological instruments may be used to assess the cancer pain patient. They include:

1. A Symptom Checklist 90[24]
2. Quality of Life Measurement[25]
3. Spielberger Anxiety Trait[26]
4. The Beck Depression Inventory[27]
5. Multiaxial Pain Inventory[28]
6. Varni-Thompson Pediatric Pain Questionnaire[29]
7. Sickness Impact Profile[30]
8. Behavioral Pain Profile[31]
9. Functional Assessment Screening Questionnaire[32]
10. Pain Disability Index[33]
11. Millon Behavioral Health Inventory[34]

Which instrument to use should be decided by the clinical psychologist and should be predicated on the state of disease and progression of that disease. Some well-known psychological assessment tools (e.g., the Minnesota Multiphasic Personality Inventory) may be inappropriate for use in cancer patients, whereas others (e.g., Multiaxial Pain Inventory and the McGill Pain Questionnaire) are too long for use in the patient population.

Diagnostic Evaluation

In the average consultative environment, the cancer patient is usually referred to a pain clinic or pain control center for pain management. In most circumstances, the patient has received extensive laboratory, radiologic, and neurologic investigations and the extent of the disease, its location, progression, and complication are well known and well documented. In these circumstances, further evaluations are usually unnecessary unless the previously mentioned tests were obtained more than 6 months previously, or if new signs and symptoms have developed. In these cases and in patients who have not been thoroughly investigated, it may then be appropriate to perform another series of tests to determine the location and the extent of the disease process.

The following diagnostic investigations represent some of the studies that may be used to evaluate cancer pain patients.

1. Computed tomography (CT) is useful for obtaining a detailed visualization of soft tissue on bone in a two-dimensional view. It is also useful in directing needle placement for biopsy and nerve block therapy (e.g., celiac plexus block). It is also useful for defining early bone changes in patients with cancer.[35]
2. Magnetic resonance imaging (MRI) is the most useful diagnostic test for evaluating cancer pain patients.[36]
3. Plain radiographic films are useful screening tools.
4. Bone scan is useful in determining bony abnormalities before these changes may be seen on a plain radiograph.
5. The use of tumor markers and other blood tests including carcinogenic embryonic antigen is quite useful in ovarian, lung, and breast cancer.
6. Neurophysiologic testing may be useful.
   a. Electromyography
   b. Nerve conduction studies
   c. Somatosensory auditory and visual evoked potential studies
7. Thermography may be helpful.
8. Appropriate biochemical investigations (i.e., urine, blood sugar, cholesterol) and renal and hepatic function studies may be necessary.

Psychosocial Assessment

In the treatment of the cancer pain patient, it is necessary to obtain a psychosocial assessment of the patient and to determine his or her quality of life before the onset of cancer pain.[37]

It is important to determine the significance of pain to the patient and family and their expectation of treatment in the long- and short-term. The coping strategies used by some patients to deal with the onset of cancer should be evaluated so as to determine those factors (positive or negative) that might have an effect on the patient's coping mechanisms. The useful coping skills should be enhanced and any negative pain behavior should be discouraged. The economic status and funding sources of the patient should be determined in order to optimize therapy without bureaucratic impediments. A discussion regarding the patient's perception of opioids, stimulants, and other relevant medications should be obtained. An evaluation of the patient's understanding on the role of government regulation of controlled substances should be obtained and, above all, attempts must be made to determine the patient's perception of the meaning of the pain both to the patient and his or her family.

Pharmacologic Evaluation

Most cancer pain patients are taking several medications by the time they are referred to a pain control center for pain management. These medications should be determined along with the dosage, efficacy, and incidence of side effects and adverse effects. Attempts should be made to discontinue unnecessary or harmful medications and to streamline the care toward enhancing pharmacologic efficacy.

Some medications are usually administered to cancer pain patients not only to treat the pain but also to treat the cancer itself.[38] If any doubt exists as to whether a particular medication will be useful, it is probably more appropriate and more courteous to discuss it with the physician prescribing the medication before discontinuing the medication.

Listed below are some medications that are commonly administered to typical cancer pain patients:

1. Strong narcotic analgesics[39] (e.g., morphine, hydromorphone, MS Contin)
2. Weak opioids (e.g., codeine, oxycodone, oxycontin)
3. Nonsteroidal anti-inflammatory agents (e.g., ketorolac, trilisate)[40]
4. Tricyclic antidepressants[41]
5. Centrally acting agents (e.g., carbamazepine, dilantin)[42]
6. Agents acting on neuropathic pain (e.g., mexilitine, bretylium, gabapentin, labetalol)[43, 44]
7. Agents administered via infusion (narcotics, lidocaine,[45] local anesthetics)
8. Agents administered in nerve block therapy (local anesthetics, steroids)
9. Miscellaneous agents (e.g., capsaicin, baclofen, calcitonin, substance P antagonists)[46]

A working knowledge of the pharmacology of these agents is important, so as to determine therapeutic efficacy and unacceptable side effects. It is clear that an increase in the amount of narcotics prescribed may be necessary to control pain.

Plan of Management

After history taking and physical examination, a pain diagnosis is made. In addition to the physical diagnosis, a management plan should be outlined to the patient and family so that realistic expectations of possible outcomes may be clearly understood. An estimate of the risk to benefit ratio of the different therapeutic options should be explained to the patient. The patient should also be assured that he or she will not be allowed to suffer continued pain even if the initial plan of management does not provide immediate pain relief. The therapeutic options outlined to the patient should reflect the multidisciplinary nature of the team. The following are some therapeutic options that may be discussed with the patient and family:

1. The use of nonnarcotic and narcotic analgesics on a time-contingent basis after using the WHO three-step ladder recommendation for analgesic use in cancer pain patients[47] (85–90% of patients are managed effectively using this regimen)
2. Nerve block therapy[48]
3. Cryotherapy (thermal neurolysis)[49]
4. Neurolytic blocks[50]
5. Implantation of various neuraxial stimulating devices[51]
6. Implantation of intrathecal and epidural catheters attached to pump devices submerged under the skin, so as to ensure extreme efficacy of the nerve blocks[52]
7. Palliative surgical procedures[53]
8. Aggressive radiotherapy
9. Physical measures
10. Psychological interventions
11. Analgesic adjuvants
12. Hospice consultation (when appropriate)

Intratreatment (Concurrent) Therapy

After a therapeutic plan is instituted, it is important to have a systematic intratreatment assessment of the pain. This lets the caregiver adjust individual doses and make any necessary changes to enhance therapeutic efficacy. Assessments should occur at regular intervals after initiating the therapeutic plan. Concurrent pain assessments should be determined at regular intervals after the treatment plan has been initiated, at suitable intervals after each pharmacologic intervention has been made, and after each report of new pain. Assessments using those guidelines would be used to determine which modalities are effective and which are not useful.

Posttreatment Assessment

At the end of active therapeutic interventions with various modalities, it is imperative to have a mechanism in place for follow-up pain assessments. It is important to make the patient feel comfortable in obtaining further pain consultation if it should become necessary in the future. To this end, clear lines of communication should be established and the patient should feel comfortable in activating those communication lines. If, on the other hand, the patient's pain is uncontrolled and the disease progression is rapid to the point of becoming terminal, then it is appropriate to initiate contacts with the hospice movement after clear discussion and explanation with the family. The services of a pastor, social worker, good friends, family, and other persons close to the patient may help make that goal comfortable. The need to discuss personal issues (e.g., wills, last wishes, etc.) should be encouraged and the patient's pain should be reevaluated. It is likely that new pain sites may develop and the characteristics of the old pain may change. Clear, thorough explanations and active participation in the process go a long way in helping the patient follow the rationale for therapeutic interventions.

In patients with selected cancer pain syndromes, it is necessary to understand the pathogenesis of those syndromes and to appreciate their time, course, and possible outcomes. In so doing, an understanding of the relationship of the disease process with pain may be communicated effectively to the patient and preemptive steps may be taken to minimize the pain before the full impact is experienced.

There are several specific cancer-related pain syndromes that are associated with cancer and a detailed knowledge of these conditions can facilitate the effective management of cancer pain in some patients. Some of these syndromes are presented in the following list:

1. Pain due to metastatic involvement of bony structures
2. Herpes zoster and postherpetic neuralgia
3. Peripheral neuropathies including radiation neuritis, chest pain secondary to Pancoast's tumor, breast cancer, abdominal pain, pain secondary to chemotherapy including nausea, vomiting, and oral mucositis

It is important for health care providers to evaluate cancer patients' pain, assess the characteristics of that pain, and determine the patient's perception of that pain. It is appropriate to assess pain after each therapeutic intervention and as the patient's general condition improves or worsens. Thus, comprehensive pain assessment in the cancer patient enables the health care provider to be more effective in controlling the pain while helping patients deal with their perception of the inevitability of cancer pain.

References

1. Bonica JJ. Treatment of Cancer Pain: Current Status and Future Need. In HL Fields, R Dubner, R Cervero (eds), Proceedings of the Fourth World Congress on Pain; Seattle, Washington, August 31 to September 5, 1984. Advances in Pain Research and Therapy (Vol. 9). New York: Raven, 1985;589.
2. World Health Organization. Cancer pain relief and palliative care. Report of a WHO expert committee (World Health Organization Technical Report Series, 804). Geneva, Switzerland: World Health Organization, 1990;1.
3. Management of Cancer Pain. Clinical Practice Guideline. AHCPR Publication No. 94-0592, Rockville, MD: Agency for Health Care Policy and Research, Public Health Service, US Department of Health and Human Services, March 1994.
4. Von Roenn JH, Cleeland CS, Gonin R, et al. Physician attitudes and practice in cancer pain management: A survey from the Eastern Cooperative Oncology Group. Ann Intern Med 1993;119:121.
5. Wagner G. Frequency of pain in patients with cancer. Recent Results Cancer Res 1984;89:64.
6. Ventafridda GV, Caraceni AT, Sbanotto AM, et al. Pain treatment in cancer of the pancreas. Eur J Surg Oncol 1990;16:1.
7. Walsh TD. Oral morphine in chronic cancer pain. Pain 1984;18:1.

8. Cleeland CS. Barriers to the management of cancer pain. Oncology 1987;1(Suppl 2):19.

9 Ferrell BA, Ferrel BR, Osterweil D. Pain in the nursing home. J Am Geriatric Soc 1990;38:409.

10. Elliott K, Foley KM. Neurologic pain syndromes in patients with cancer. Neurol Clin 1989;7:333.

11. Foley KM. The treatment of cancer pain. N Engl J Med 1985;313:84.

12. Bruera E, MacMillan K, Hanson J, et al. The Edmonton Staging System for cancer pain: Preliminary report. Pain 1989;37:203.

13. Gracely RH, Wolskee PJ. Semantic functional measurement of pain: Integrating perception and language. Pain 1983;15:389.

14. Houde RW. Methods for measuring clinical pain in humans. Acta Anaesthesiol Scand 1982;74(Suppl):25.

15. Brena SF, Koch DL, Moss RM. The reliability of the emory pain estimate model. Anesthesiol Rev 1976;3:28.

16. Fishman B, Pasternak S, Wallenstein SL, et al. The Memorial Pain Assessment Card: A valid instrument for the evaluation of cancer pain. Cancer 1987;60:1151.

17. Daut RL, Cleeland CS, Flanery RC. Development of the Wisconsin brief pain questionnaire to assess pain in cancer and other diseases. Pain 1983;17:197.

18. Melzack R. The McGill pain questionnaire: Major properties and scoring methods. Pain 1975;1:357.

19. McCaffery M, Beebe A. Pain: Clinical manual for nursing practice. St. Louis: Mosby, 1989.

20. Brena SF, Chapman SL. The "Learned Pain Syndrome": Decoding a patient's signals. Postgrad Med 1981;69:53.

21. Salim BM. Pakistan Coin Scale [letter]. Pain 1993; 52:373.

22. Beyer JE, Wells N. Assessment of Cancer Pain in Children. In RB Patt (ed), Cancer Pain. Philadelphia: Lippincott, 1993;57.

23. Cleeland CS, Cleeland LM, Dar R, Rinehardt LC. Factors influencing physician management of cancer pain. Cancer 1986;58:796.

24. Derogatis LR. SCL-90: Administration Scoring and Procedures Manual for the Revised Version. Baltimore: Clinical Psychometric Research, 1977.

25. Miaskowski C, Donovan M. Implementation of the American Pain Society Quality Assurance Standards for Relief of Acute Pain and Cancer Pain in oncology nursing practice. Oncol Nurs Forum 1992;19:411.

26. Spielberger CC. Manual for the State-Trait Anxiety Inventory, Form Y. Palo Alto, CA: Consulting Psychologists Press, 1983.

27. Beck AT, Steer RA. Beck Depression Inventory Manual. The Psychological Corporation. New York: Harcourt Brace Jovanovich, 1987.

28. Millon T. Millon Clinical Multiaxial Inventory-II (MCMI-II) Manual. Minneapolis, MN: National Computer Systems, 1991.

29. Varni JW, Thompson KL. The Varni-Thompson pediatric pain questionnaire. Unpublished manuscript, 1985.

30. Bergner M, Bobbitt RA, Carter W, et al. The Sickness Impact Profile: Development and final revision of a health status measure. Med Care 1981;19:787.

31. Dalton JA, Feuerstein M. Fear, alexythymia and cancer pain. Pain 1989;38:159.

32. Millard RW. The functional assessment screening questionnaire: Application for evaluating pain-related disability. Arch Phys Med Rehabil 1989;70:303.

33. Tait RC, Pollard CA, Margolis RB, et al. The pain disability index: Cyclometric and validity data. Arch Phys Med Rehabil 1988;68:438.

34. Millon T, Green CJ, Meagher RB. Millon Behavioral Health Inventory Manual (3rd ed). Minneapolis, MN: National Computer Systems, 1982.

35. Gilbert RW, Kim JH, Posner JB. Epidural spinal cord compression from metastatic tumor: Diagnosis and treatment. Ann Neurol 1978;3:40.

36. Byrne TN. Spinal cord compression from epidural metastases. N Engl J Med 1992;327:614.

37. American Pain Society, Committee on Quality Assurance Standards. Standards for monitoring quality of analgesic treatment of acute pain and cancer pain. Oncol Nurs Forum 1990;17:952.

38. Cleeland CS. Management of cancer pain. Clin Cancer Briefs 1985;7:3.

39. Foley KM. Changing Concepts of Tolerance to Opioids: What the Cancer Patient Has Taught Us. In CR Chapman, KM Foley (eds), Current and Emerging Issues in Cancer Pain: Research and Practice. New York: Raven, 1993;331.

40. Roth SH. Merits and liabilities of NSAID therapy. Rheum Dis Clin North Am 1989;15:479.

41. France RD. The future for antidepressants: Treatment of pain. Psychopathology 1987;20(Suppl 1):99.

42. Beaver WT, Wallenstein SL, Houde RW, Rogers A. A comparison of the analgesic effects of methotrimeprazine and morphine in patients with cancer. Clin Pharmacol Ther 1966;7:436.

43. Ford SR, Forrest WH, Eltherington L. The treatment of reflex sympathetic dystrophy with intravenous regional bretylium. Anesthesiology 1988;68:137.

44. Parris WCV, Harris R, Lindsey K. Use of intravenous regional labetalol in treating resistant reflex sympathetic dystrophy. Pain 1987;4(Suppl):S206.

45. Edwards WT, Habib F, Burney RG, Begin G. Intravenous lidocaine in the management of various chronic pain states: A review of 211 cases. Reg Anesth 1985;10:1.

46. Sunshine A, Olson NZ. Non-Narcotic Analgesics. In PD Wall, R Melzack (eds), Textbook of Pain (2nd ed). New York: Churchill Livingstone, 1989;670.

47. Ventafridda V, Caraceni A, Gamba A. Field-Testing of the WHO Guidelines for Cancer Pain Relief: Summary Report of Demonstration Projects. In KM Foley, JJ Bonica, V Ventafridda (eds), Proceedings of the Second International Congress on Pain. Advances in Pain Research and Therapy (Vol. 16). New York: Raven, 1990;451.

48. Cousins MJ, Bridenbaugh PO (eds). Neural Blockade in Clinical Anesthesia and Management of Pain (2nd ed). Philadelphia: Lippincott, 1987;1171.

49. Lipton S, Miles J, Williams N, Jones NB. Pituitary injection of alcohol for widespread cancer pain. Pain 1978;5:73.

50. Rodriguez-Bigas M, Petrelli NJ, Herrera L, West C. Intrathecal phenol rhizotomy for management of pain in recurrent unresectable carcinoma of the rectum. Surg Gynecol Obstet 1991;173:41.

51. Miles J, Lipton S, Hayward M, et al. Pain relief by implanted electrical stimulators. Lancet 1974;1:777.

52. Waldman SD. Implantable drug delivery systems: Practical considerations. J Pain Symptom Manage 1990;5:169.

53. White JC, Sweet WH. Pain and the Neurosurgeon. A Forty-Year Experience. Springfield, IL: Thomas, 1969.

Chapter 6

Comprehensive Medical Management: Opioid Analgesia

Paolo L. Manfredi, Sharon M. Weinstein,
Sonja W. Chandler, and Richard Payne

Role of Opioids in the Management of Cancer Pain

It has been more than a decade since the World Health Organization (WHO) established the primary role of opioid analgesia in cancer pain relief. The three-step analgesic ladder[1, 2] (Figure 6-1) outlines the titration of nonopioid, opioid, and adjuvant analgesics, alone or in combination, to meet the needs of the individual patient. This approach is effective in lessening the pain in 71–97% of patients.[3–6] Still, satisfactory relief is not provided for most of the estimated 4 million patients worldwide with cancer-related pain.[7] The inappropriate use of opioids is the main reason for this unnecessary suffering. The underuse of opioids is related to a lack of education in medical, nursing, and pharmacy schools and to the public's misconceptions about opioid drugs.

The clinical pharmacology (pharmacokinetic properties, duration of analgesia, and potency) of the drugs commonly used to treat pain is relatively simple. Pharmacologic dependence and tolerance, still poorly understood, are clinically important for only a small number of patients. A more critical point is the negative societal perception of palliative care as the "last resort." Because of this attitude, financial and human resources are usually devoted to the acute care of patients with cancer, with little impact on the disease course but with great economic and spiritual expenditure for patients, their families, and society in general.

Endogenous Opioids and Their Receptors

Over the last 20 years, much has been learned about the endogenous opioid system. The demonstration that the profound analgesia produced by electric stimulation of the brain[8] was reversed by naloxone[9] implied the presence of endogenous opioids. Exogenous opioids mimic the action of these naturally occurring opioid peptides (enkephalins, dynorphins, endorphins)[10] through recognition of common receptors. Each endogenous peptide is derived from a genetically distinct precursor polypeptide and has a characteristic anatomic distribution.

Opioids modify central processing of nociceptive inputs by interacting with specific cellular receptors, of which several subtypes are now recognized. Opioid receptors, first hypothesized to exist in 1954,[11] were demonstrated experimentally in 1973.[12] The development of specific radioligands and selective antagonists allowed the recognition of different classes of receptors implicated in the production of analgesia. Mu-receptors, subdivided into mu_1 and mu_2,[13, 14] are the binding sites responsible for morphine-induced analgesia. Mu_1-receptors predominate at the supraspinal level. The areas of the brain with a high density of opioid receptors include the periaqueductal gray matter, the locus ceruleus, and the nucleus of raphe magnus.[15, 16] In the dorsal horn of the spinal cord, morphine analgesia is mediated by mu_2-receptors. There is a synergistic analgesic effect from the concomitant activation of

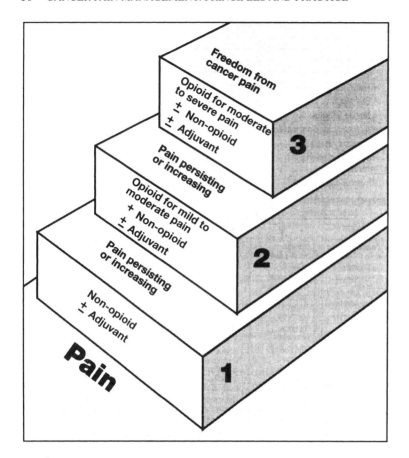

Figure 6-1. The World Health Organization Three-Step Analgesic Ladder. (Reprinted from Management of Cancer Pain: Clinical Practice Guideline No. 9. U.S. Department of Health and Human Services, Public Health Service, 1994.)

supraspinal and spinal systems.[17] Other actions of morphine are also related to the interaction with specific receptors. Respiratory depression is mediated by mu_2-receptors in the brain stem,[18, 19] whereas constipation is mediated by mu_2-receptors within the brain[20, 21] and in the intestinal plexus.[22] Theoretically, a drug specific for mu_1-receptors would not affect respiratory rate or intestinal motility. There is evidence that the reinforced behavior observed in rats self-administering morphine is mediated by action at mu_1-receptors.[23] In addition to supraspinal and spinal morphine analgesia, a peripheral mechanism is suggested by the report of profound analgesia from intra-articular injection of morphine following arthroscopic knee surgery, without evidence of significant systemic absorption.[24] Morphine also interacts with kappa- and delta-receptors, although its affinity for these receptors is much lower[23] (i.e., a higher concentration of morphine is necessary to occupy these binding sites as compared with the mu sites).

In contrast, pentazocine and nalbuphine produce analgesia by interacting with kappa-receptors.[23] The dynorphins are the endogenous ligands for these receptors.[25]

Delta-receptors were discovered to be densely localized in the vas deferens of the mouse. They are also present at the spinal and supraspinal levels. The natural ligands of the delta-receptors are the enkephalins.[26]

After opioids activate mu- and delta-receptors, a guanine nucleotide regulatory protein (G protein) couples the receptors to effector proteins. These effector proteins activate potassium channels, hyperpolarizing neuronal membranes.[27] G proteins are negatively coupled to adenyl cyclase, preventing the synthesis of cyclic adenosine monophosphate and thus decreasing neuronal excitability.[28] Kappa-receptors are coupled to G proteins that inhibit voltage-sensitive calcium channels. This might imply reduced transmitter release from nerve terminals. There are at least five families of G proteins, and each G protein has three subunits that undergo complex interactions with each other to modulate receptor and effector activities.[29] When an exogenous opioid is administered and opioid receptors are coupled to G proteins, the acute pharmacologic effects of the drug are manifested.

Pharmacologic tolerance is defined as diminishing physiologic effect of the same dose or the requirement of increasing doses to produce the same physiologic effect. It usually develops after repeated administration of a drug. With chronic morphine use, a functional uncoupling of opioid receptors from G proteins occurs and the acute effects of the drug decrease. As a result, tolerance develops and higher doses of opioid are needed to trigger the second messenger response.[30, 31] Tolerance to analgesia may occur in conjunction with tolerance to other opioid pharmacologic effects. An increase in dose will usually restore analgesia without increasing side effects. The N-methyl-D-aspartate (NMDA) receptors are a subclass of excitatory amino acid receptors that, once activated, produce calcium influx in neurons. Experimentally, NMDA receptor antagonists inhibit tolerance to the analgesic effect of morphine.[32] Ketamine, a general anesthetic with NMDA receptor antagonist activity, has been shown to induce analgesia in patients who do not respond to high doses of morphine.[33, 34] In addition to uncoupling opioid receptors from G proteins, chronic opioid administration decreases the synthesis of endogenous opioid peptides. Abrupt discontinuation of the exogenous opioid causes opioid-responsive neurons to enter a phase of rebound hyperexcitability. The increased firing of these neurons is the cellular mechanism of the opioid withdrawal syndrome. Eventually, G protein–opioid receptor coupling and endogenous opioid synthesis are restored and the withdrawal syndrome and tolerance are reversed.

Drugs that bind to opioid receptors are classified as agonists (e.g., morphine) if they produce analgesia, and as antagonists (e.g., naloxone) if they block the action of an agonist, i.e., they possess affinity for opioid receptors but not analgesic efficacy. Agonist-antagonists (e.g., pentazocine) produce analgesia by interacting with a specific receptor (e.g., kappa), but they also bind to other receptors (e.g., mu) where they can block the action of other agonists. Partial agonists (e.g., buprenorphine) bind to receptors and produce analgesia but, unlike morphine, they exhibit a ceiling effect. Increasing doses do not result in increasing analgesic effect.[35] The clinical use of mixed agonist-antagonists is limited because they tend to produce dysphoria and hallucinations. These effects are mediated by kappa-receptors[36] and nonopioid sigma-receptors.[37] Mixed agonist-antagonists and partial agonists both will cause a withdrawal syndrome when administered to the patient taking chronic opioid agonists. Antagonists are used as an antidote for opioid poisoning. They should be used judiciously in pain patients on chronic opioid therapy because they will cause acute withdrawal and immediate reemergence of pain.

Opioid Analgesics

The chemical structures of the opioid analgesics are shown in Figure 6-2.

Opioid Agonists for Mild-to-Moderate Pain

It is clinically useful to classify opioids as weak or strong, to be used for mild-to-moderate or moderate-to-severe pain (Table 6-1), depending on their relative potency. Weak opioids are used for less severe pain. Their efficacy is limited by an increased incidence of side effects at higher doses (e.g., nausea and constipation with codeine; central nervous system excitation with propoxyphene). When weak opioids are used in a fixed oral dose mixture with a nonopioid analgesic such as acetaminophen or aspirin, their efficacy is limited by the maximal safe dose of the acetaminophen or aspirin. Weak opioids are the second rung of the analgesic ladder. Strong opioids are indicated for more severe pain. They have a wide therapeutic range and no ceiling effect for analgesia: Higher doses produce an increasing level of analgesia. Strong opioids are the third rung of the analgesic ladder. Although it may appear simplistic, the approach of titration of opioids has been shown to provide effective analgesia for the vast majority of cancer patients.

Codeine, an alkaloid of opium, is the prototype of the weak opioid analgesics. Although a parenteral preparation is available, codeine is nearly always given orally, often in a fixed mixture with a nonopioid analgesic. A 200-mg dose is equipotent to 30 mg of morphine. The affinity of codeine for mu-recep-

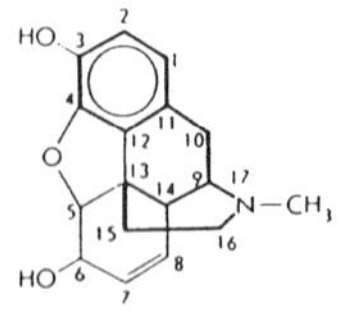

Morphine

Figure 6-2. A. Structures of opioids and opioid antagonists chemically related to morphine. B. Structures of phenylpiperidine opioids. C. Structures of methadone and propoxyphene. (Reprinted with permission from Cancer Pain Relief [2nd ed]. Geneva: World Health Organization, 1996.)

STRUCTURES OF OPIOIDS AND OPIOID ANTAGONISTS CHEMICALLY RELATED TO MORPHINE

NONPROPRIETARY NAME	CHEMICAL RADICALS AND POSITIONS			OTHER CHANGES †
	3 *	6 *	17 *	
Morphine	—OH	—OH	—CH$_3$	—
Heroin	—OCOCH$_3$	—OCOCH$_3$	—CH$_3$	—
Hydromorphone	—OH	=O	—CH$_3$	(1)
Oxymorphone	—OH	=O	—CH$_3$	(1),(2)
Levorphanol	—OH	—H	—CH$_3$	(1),(3)
Codeine	—OCH$_3$	—OH	—CH$_3$	—
Hydrocodone	—OCH$_3$	=O	—CH$_3$	(1)
Oxycodone	—OCH$_3$	=O	—CH$_3$	(1),(2)
Nalorphine	—OH	—OH	—CH$_2$CH=CH$_2$	—
Naloxone	—OH	=O	—CH$_2$CH=CH$_2$	(1),(2)
Naltrexone	—OH	=O	—CH$_2$ ◁	(1),(2)
Buprenorphine	—OH	—OCH$_3$	—CH$_2$ ◁	(1),(2),(4)
Butorphanol	—OH	—H	—CH$_2$ 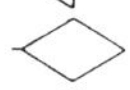 ◇	(2),(3)
Nalbuphine	—OH	—OH	—CH$_2$ ◇	(1),(2)

* The numbers 3, 6, and 17 refer to positions in the morphine molecule, as shown above.
† Other changes in the morphine molecule are as follows:
  (1) Single instead of double bond between C7 and C8.
  (2) OH added to C14.
  (3) No oxygen between C4 and C5.
  (4) *Endoetheno* bridge between C6 and C14; 1-hydroxy-1,2,2-trimethylpropyl substitution on C7

A

STRUCTURES OF PHENYLPIPERIDINE OPIOIDS

COMPOUND	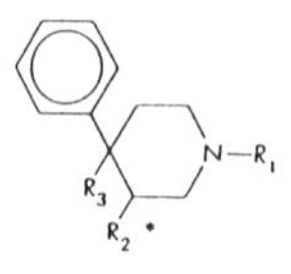 R$_1$	R$_3$
Meperidine	—CH$_3$	—COCH$_2$CH$_3$ ‖ O
Fentanyl	—CH$_2$CH$_2$— ◯	—N—C—CH$_2$CH$_3$ † ‖ O

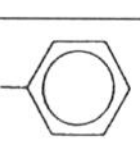

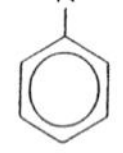

* R$_2$ = H, except in alphaprodine, where R$_2$ = CH$_3$.
† The sole *para* substitution on the piperidine ring is as shown.

B

tors is several thousand-fold less than that of morphine.[23] The half-life of codeine is 2.5–3.0 hours; approximately 10% of orally administered codeine is demethylated to morphine; free and conjugated morphine can be found in the urine. The analgesic action may be due to codeine's conversion to morphine,[38]

although analgesic structure activity studies do not support this hypothesis.[39] Constipation is the main side effect at the usual therapeutic dosages (30–60 mg every 4 hours). Codeine has an antitussive effect.

Hydrocodone is a codeine derivative available in the United States only in combination with aceta-

Methadone

Propoxyphene

C

Table 6-1. Opioid Dose Equivalents

Drug Route	Dose Equivalents (mg)	Duration (hrs)
Morphine		
Orally	30	3–4
Intravenously	10	3–4
Oxycodone		
Orally	30	3–4
Hydromorphone		
Orally	7.5	3–4
Intravenously	1.5	3–4
Levorphanol		
Orally	4	6–8
Intravenously	2	6–8
Methadone		
Orally	20	6–8
Intravenously	10	6–8

Source: Adapted from A Jacox, DB Carr, R Payne, et al. Management of Cancer Pain. Clinical Practice Guideline No. 9. AHCPR Publication No. 94-0592. Rockville, MD: Agency for Health Care Policy and Research, U.S. Department of Health and Human Services, Public Health Service, March 1994.

minophen or aspirin. It is thought to approximate the potency of oxycodone, although good data are lacking.

Propoxyphene is a synthetic analgesic that is structurally related to methadone. Propoxyphene is approximately equipotent to codeine as an analgesic but lacks codeine's antitussive properties. Propoxyphene binds to mu-receptors. Its duration of analgesia is 3–5 hours. The half-life is 6–12 hours and its major metabolite is norpropoxyphene, which has a half-life of 30–36 hours and may be responsible for some of the observed toxicity. Nor-

propoxyphene has local anesthetic effects similar to those of lidocaine, and high doses may cause cardiac arrhythmias. Seizures occur more often with propoxyphene intoxication than with morphine intoxication. Naloxone antagonizes the toxic effects of propoxyphene.[40] Propoxyphene is irritating to blood vessels and soft tissues when used parenterally; inadvertent injection into the brachial artery has resulted in tissue damage requiring amputation of digits. In conclusion, propoxyphene is difficult to use and offers no significant advantage over other opioids.

Meperidine, a synthetic phenylpiperidine-derivative mu-agonist with anticholinergic properties, is the most commonly prescribed analgesic for acute pain and is widely used for chronic pain. The medical reasons for this preference are unclear, but it probably reflects the perpetuation of common practice. The lesser increase in pressure in the common bile duct with administration of meperidine as compared with morphine[35] has not been shown to be clinically advantageous. However, the central nervous system excitatory effects that appear after chronic meperidine use are well substantiated. The accumulation of the metabolite normeperidine causes multifocal myoclonus and grand mal seizures,[41] which are not reversed by naloxone. The half-life of meperidine is 3 hours. Meperidine is in part demethylated to normeperidine, the only active metabolite, which has a half-life of 15–30 hours. Normeperidine accumulates after chronic treatment, particularly in cancer patients with renal dysfunction.[42, 43] Short-term treatment with meperidine has been associated with mild negative alterations in various elements of mood.[44] When meperidine is given to patients being treated with monoamine oxidase (MAO) inhibitors, two different patterns of toxicity have been observed: (1) severe respiratory depression or (2) excitation, delirium, hyperpyrexia, and convulsions. The equianalgesic dose of 10 mg of parenteral morphine is 75–100 mg of meperidine. The oral-to-parenteral ratio is 4 to 1. Meperidine's use by either route is rarely justified.

Oxycodone is a semisynthetic derivative of thebaine, an opium alkaloid. Because of its high bioavailability (>50%), oxycodone is suitable for oral administration and, by this route, is equipotent to morphine and ten times more potent than codeine.[38, 45] Parenterally, intensity and duration of analgesia are 25% less than with morphine.[38] Oxycodone has a half-life of 2–3 hours and a duration of action of 3–4 hours. Like codeine, oxycodone is demethylated and conjugated in the liver and excreted in the urine.[38] Part of its analgesic action is mediated by active metabolites. Oxycodone has been considered a weak analgesic because of its use in a fixed combination with acetaminophen or aspirin. These combinations limit its dosage to 10 mg every 4 hours. When oxycodone is used as a single agent, it has no ceiling effect for analgesia. The oral potency of oxycodone approximates that of morphine, but it reportedly has fewer side effects than morphine.[45–47] The availability of oxycodone in 5-mg tablets permits careful dose titration. Oxycodone is a versatile and flexible drug that can be used to treat any type of pain that requires an opioid analgesic.[39, 47, 48]

Opioid Agonists for Moderate-to-Severe Pain

Morphine, a phenanthrene derivative, is the prototype opioid agonist. All other opioids are compared with morphine when determining their relative analgesic potency. Morphine is the drug of choice for the treatment of severe pain associated with cancer.[1] As with other "strong" opioids, there is no ceiling to the analgesic effect; however, side effects (particularly sedation and confusion) may intervene before optimal analgesia is achieved. Morphine is metabolized in the liver where it undergoes glucuronidation at the 3 and 6 positions (see Chapter 9). Morphine-3-glucuronide (M3G) and morphine-6-glucuronide (M6G) accumulate with chronic morphine administration.[49] M6G binds to mu-receptors, with an affinity similar to that of morphine.[50] M6G also binds to delta-receptors, which may account for its higher analgesic

potency[51]: M6G is 3.7 times more potent than morphine when administered subcutaneously and 45 times more potent when administered in the cerebral ventricles.[50] However, only 0.077% of this metabolite crosses from the systemic circulation into the cerebrospinal fluid.[52] In single-dose morphine studies, the relative oral-to-parenteral potency ratio is 6 to 1.[53] After chronic use, the ratio changes to 3 to 1,[54] which is probably due to the accumulation of active metabolites. There is experimental[55] and clinical[56] evidence that M3G, which has negligible affinity for opioid receptors and does not produce analgesia, has excitatory effects on neurons and can cause myoclonus and rarely a hyperalgesic state. These effects may be mediated by different receptor mechanisms.[57] The half-life of morphine is about 2 hours; the half-life of M6G is somewhat longer.[35] The duration of analgesia is 4 hours. Slow-release preparations of morphine (see Chapter 8), which permit a twice a day regimen, are safe and effective.[58] They are generally best used after dose titration with immediate-release morphine sulfate. Morphine metabolites are eliminated by glomerular filtration. They do, however, accumulate in patients with renal failure, thus leading to an increased incidence of side effects.[59] Morphine should be used with caution in patients with renal failure. For these patients, a larger time interval between doses is recommended. However, one should consider using an alternative opioid to ensure that no complications arise.

Heroin is a semisynthetic lipid-soluble opioid analgesic prepared by diacetylating morphine. It is rapidly metabolized to 6-acetyl-morphine and morphine. In fact, after oral administration, neither heroin nor 6-acetyl-morphine can be detected in plasma.[60] Heroin does not have any demonstrated advantages over morphine.[61, 62] In conclusion, the administration of heroin is a less efficient way of delivering morphine.

Hydromorphone is semisynthetic phenanthrene-derivative opioid agonist commercially available as a highly water soluble salt. When administered parenterally, 1.5 mg of hydromorphone is equipotent to 10 mg of morphine. Hydromorphone is somewhat shorter acting agent, but it has a higher peak effect. Its bioavailability is 30–40%, with an oral-to-parenteral ratio of 5 to 1.[63] Because of its high potency and water solubility, hydromorphone is the drug of choice for subcutaneous administration. Continuous subcutaneous infusion and continuous intravenous infusions of hydromorphone have a similar spectrum of analgesia and side effects.[64]

Levorphanol is a synthetic opioid agonist structurally related to the phenanthrene-derivative opioids. It is a potent mu-agonist but also binds delta- and kappa-receptors.[23, 65] When administered parenterally, 2 mg of levorphanol is equipotent to 10 mg of morphine.[66] The drug also has good oral efficacy with an oral-to-intramuscular ratio of 2 to 1. It has a half-life of 12–30 hours[67] and a duration of analgesia of 4–6 hours; therefore, repeated administration is associated with accumulation. A dose reduction may be required 2–4 days after starting the drug to avoid side effects from drug accumulation. For the same reason, it may be best to avoid using levorphanol in patients with impaired renal function or encephalopathy. Levorphanol is useful as a second-line drug for patients who cannot tolerate morphine.

Methadone is a synthetic diphenylheptane-derivative mu-agonist.[35] It is an inexpensive and effective analgesic; its use is limited by the need for a careful individualized dose and interval titration. In single parenteral doses, methadone is equipotent to morphine. The oral bioavailability of methadone ranges from 41–99% and its duration of analgesia is 4–6 hours.[68] It is rapidly absorbed from the gastrointestinal tract with measurable plasma concentrations within 30 minutes after oral administration.[69] The plasma level declines in a biexponential manner, with a half-life of 2–3 hours during the initial phase and 15–60 hours during the terminal phase.[70] This biexponential decline accounts for the relatively short analgesic action and the tendency for drug accumulation with repeated dosing. When urine pH is above 6.0, renal clearance of methadone is significantly decreased[71]; patients with cancer and patients 65 years of age or older may have decreased clearance.[72] Because it is excreted almost exclusively in the feces, methadone has been proposed as a safe and effective analgesic for patients with chronic renal failure.[73] Plasma protein binding and rate of hepatic extraction also influence the highly variable half-life.[71, 72] Despite these and other factors that necessitate careful individual titration, methadone is an effective second-line drug for patients who experience unrelieved pain and intolerable side effects with morphine.[74, 75] One-tenth of the daily morphine dose is recommended as the starting methadone dose (not to exceed 100 mg), given at intervals to be determined by the patient, but not more than once every 3 hours. A

reduction in dose and increased dose interval are often needed during the first days of treatment to prevent side effects from drug accumulation.[74] Because of its low cost, methadone could be useful in developing countries or for patients requiring very high doses of opioids. The rare patient who is allergic to morphine might benefit from methadone.

Fentanyl is a synthetic phenylpiperidine-derivative opioid agonist that interacts primarily with mu-receptors.[35] It is 80 times more potent than morphine and highly lipophilic. These properties render it suitable for the transdermal route of administration. The use of transdermal fentanyl has become popular since its first clinical study with cancer pain patients.[76] Its use should be limited to patients with chronic pain who are unable to take drugs orally and do not require a rapid dose titration. The transdermal fentanyl therapeutic system delivers drug continuously to the systemic circulation for up to 72 hours. The skin permeability constant of fentanyl is about 0.0021 ml per minute per cm^2,[77] which is 60–120 times lower than the regional blood flow to the skin of the chest.[78] A special rate-controlling membrane provides additional control of drug release. Only extreme conditions, such as the cutaneous blood supply being completely cut off, would therefore influence absorption. The transdermal absorption of fentanyl is the same from chest, abdomen, and thigh.[79] A skin reaction at the application site is found in 4% of patients[78]; no skin sensitization has been observed. After application of the transdermal patch, the systemic absorption is very low in the first 4 hours, increases during the next 4–8 hours, and remains relatively constant with a coefficient of variation of 28% from 8–24 hours.[80] The probable reason for the initial delay is the time required to establish a reservoir of fentanyl in the stratum corneum. Fentanyl reaches steady-state concentrations within 12–24 hours from application. Adjustments according to efficacy and toxicity can therefore be made on a daily basis. Following removal of the transdermal patch, the serum fentanyl concentration decreases about 50% in approximately 16 hours. This apparently long half-life is probably due to the slow washout of the cutaneous reservoir. These considerations translate clinically to a delay of several hours in the onset of analgesia after an initial application, and a persistence of analgesia and side effects long after removal of the transdermal system. In patients with chronic pain, after a variable period of titration,

Table 6-2. Chronic Opioid Therapy: Comparisons of Equianalgesic Average Wholesale Price[a]

Drug	Dose	Schedule	Daily Average Wholesale Price[b]
Mild-to-moderate pain: oral administration[c]			
Codeine	60 mg	q4hr	$4.12
Oxycodone	10 mg	q4hr	$2.94
Moderate-to-severe: oral administration			
Morphine, immediate release	30 mg	q4hr	$2.49
Morphine, slow release	90 mg	q12hr	$7.44
Hydromorphone	8 mg	q3hr	$7.18
Levorphanol	4 mg	q6hr	$3.81
Methadone	5 mg	q8hr	$0.18
Moderate-to-severe pain: transdermal administration			
Fentanyl	100 µg/hr	q72hr	$8.67
Moderate-to-severe pain: intravenous continuous/ patient-controlled analgesia administration			
Morphine	2.5 mg/hr (60 mg/d)		$3.80
Hydromorphone	0.5 mg/hr (12 mg/d)		$4.49
Levorphanol	0.3 mg/hr (8 mg/d)		$9.36
Methadone	0.3 mg/hr (8 mg/d)		$1.43

[a]Average wholesale prices were averaged for all suppliers using the 1994 edition of Red Book, Medical Economics Data, Montvale, NJ. Costs to patients are variable and approximately 10–20% above average wholesale prices for outpatients and 50–200% above average wholesale prices for inpatients. Costs to pharmacies are based on product volume discounts and can be considerably less than average wholesale prices.

[b]Daily average wholesale prices represent the mean of the average wholesale prices for available products multiplied by the number of doses in a 24-hour period.

[c]Equianalgesic doses in the mild-to-moderate pain section are not intended for comparison with the moderate-to-severe pain doses.

it is possible to obtain relatively constant serum fentanyl concentrations comparable with continuous intravenous or subcutaneous infusions of the drug.[81] Fentanyl also can be used via the epidural and intrathecal routes. Recently, the use of oral transmucosal fentanyl has been proposed for the treatment of breakthrough pain. In a study of this route, initial pain relief was noted within a few minutes and maximum effect within 20–30 minutes.[82]

Principles of Opioid Analgesic Use

Formulating a Treatment Plan

Onset, peak, and duration of analgesia vary with the drug, route of administration, and individual patient. The recognition of this variability allows the appropriate choice of drug, route, and schedule. When switching from one opioid to another, one-half to two-thirds of the calculated equianalgesic dose is recommended as the initial dose owing to

incomplete cross-tolerance.[83] The standard opioid conversion charts, based on single-dose studies (see Table 6-1), should be used with caution when considering continuous administration of oral or parenteral long-acting opioids, such as methadone and levorphanol. The comparisons for long-term equianalgesic doses and costs of commonly used oral and parenteral opioids are shown in Table 6-2. Opioids recommended for cancer pain management are listed in Table 6-3. Opioids not recommended for cancer pain management are listed in Table 6-4.

In patients with acute severe pain, parenteral morphine is the opioid of choice.[1] The drug should be titrated to effect, until either analgesia or intolerable side effects develop, with boluses repeated every 15 minutes if necessary. The concomitant use of an anti-inflammatory drug is often warranted.[1] An antiemetic might be needed. When the pain intensity decreases to a bearable level, a continuous infusion of morphine should be started. The initial hourly dose can be obtained

Table 6-3. Opioids Recommended for Cancer Pain Management

Mild-to-moderate pain
  Codeine
  Oxycodone
Moderate-to-severe pain
  Morphine
  Oxycodone
  Hydromorphone
  Methadone
  Levorphanol
  Fentanyl

Table 6-4. Opioids Not Recommended for Cancer Pain Management

Buprenorphine
Butorphanol
Dezocine
Nalbuphine
Pentazocine
Meperidine

by dividing the total loading dose by four (the duration of analgesia after single morphine doses is approximately 4 hours[68]). It is important to remember that this is only an estimate and does not take into account individual variability. Considerable adjustment of the infusion rate may be needed in the first few hours. Patients receiving chronic opioid therapy often require very high doses to control acute exacerbations of pain. An infusion pump with a device for self-administration of extra doses of medication every few minutes (patient-controlled analgesia [PCA]) should be used if available.[84] The PCA dose can be as high as the hourly rate during the titration phase and if incident pain is prominent. The continuous basal rate should be adjusted frequently based on the patient's report of efficacy and the PCA usage. When venous access is problematic, the subcutaneous route may be used instead. It is good practice to avoid the intramuscular route. Once the acute pain exacerbation is controlled, the medication should be changed to the oral route. If the oral route is impracticable, the transdermal system may be used.[76] The oral transmucosal route may be effective for rescue doses, but the absorp-

tion is usually inadequate for more sustained relief. The same may be true for the rectal route, which also may be uncomfortable for the patient and the caregiver. Long-term intravenous opioid administration can be used in patients with central venous access devices who cannot take drugs orally.[85] Long-term subcutaneous administration is an effective alternative.[86]

The epidural, intrathecal, and intracerebroventricular routes are reserved for patients who fail to respond to a careful sequential trial of different opioids and adjuvants.

In patients with mild-to-moderate pain, oral analgesics such as oxycodone or codeine are appropriate choices.[1, 2] Use of fixed combinations with nonopioid analgesics is generally not advisable because they might limit the careful individualized titration, which is the basis of therapeutic success.

Opioids should be administered regularly, even if the patient must be awakened from sleep, at intervals based on the duration of analgesia for the given drug.[83, 87] This approach will keep the patient's pain at a tolerable level, which often allows a reduction in the total amount of medication taken in a 24-hour period.

Adjuvant analgesics should be used early in the pain treatment course[1] because they allow a higher ratio of analgesia to side effects by lowering the opioid dose. Like opioids, they should be administered at regular intervals. Acetaminophen or a nonsteroidal anti-inflammatory drug should always be given unless contraindicated. Steroids might be highly effective for treating pain from direct tumor invasion of neural, somatic, and visceral structures.[88] The side effects of steroids are numerous and well known but often of lesser consequence in the terminal stages of cancer. Anticonvulsants have been used for lancinating, paroxysmal pains and antidepressants for dysesthetic pains, although no controlled studies determining their efficacy in the cancer population are available. Stimulants and antihistamines might provide additional analgesia while treating side effects.[89] Neuroleptics and benzodiazepines are useful in certain patients. The use of ketamine has reportedly been effective (possibly by reversing tolerance) when the pain does not respond to massive doses of opioids.[34, 35] Its use for chronic pain is still experimental, however.

Opioid Side Effects

Tolerance to a drug implies the need to continuously increase the dose in order to obtain the desired effect. It is a complex and incompletely understood phenomenon that is clinically important in only a small number of patients. Our experience has taught us that when pain is stable, tolerance to the analgesic effects of opioids does not generally develop.[90] Our understanding of the influence of pain on the development of tolerance comes also from laboratory studies, where arthritic rats self-injected less morphine than pain-free rats. Moreover, the arthritic rats' dose remained stable, whereas pain-free rats escalated their dose.[91] The need for rapid escalation of the opioid dose in cancer patients with pain is almost always associated with new or ongoing tissue injury.[90] Although tolerance to the different opioid effects develops at different rates, it is usually possible to titrate the opioid dose to the amount that works for the individual patient, without encountering any limiting side effects. The cross-tolerance among different opiates is incomplete. Analgesia but also side effects might develop when switching to a different strong opioid at an equianalgesic dose.[83] A 30–50% dose reduction of the calculated equianalgesic dose and a gradual upward titration are therefore recommended.

Physical dependence is an altered physiologic state produced by repeated administration of a drug. This condition necessitates the continued administration of the drug to prevent the appearance of the withdrawal symptoms characteristic of the particular drug. When opioids are abruptly discontinued, the withdrawal syndrome consists of lacrimation, rhinorrhea, restlessness, and tremors.[92] These symptoms are usually mild and do not have the dramatic appearance of the withdrawal syndrome seen in the psychologically dependent patient. Patients who have received repeated dosages of morphine every day for 1 or 2 weeks will have mild and often unrecognized withdrawal symptoms when the drug is stopped. Symptoms are delayed and even less pronounced with opioids that have a long half-life, such as methadone and levorphanol. However, if an opioid antagonist is administered, symptoms of withdrawal may appear after a single dose.[92] In patients with cancer receiving long-term opioid therapy, naloxone should be administered only when the suspicion of overdose is strong and the symptoms are life-threatening. Appropriate counseling and a gradual tapering of the opioid over a few days will effectively prevent the development of a withdrawal syndrome.

Psychological dependence is described as a compulsive drug-seeking behavior and an overwhelming involvement in drug procurement and use. Only the superficial observer will misinterpret the behavior of a patient with severe unrelieved pain as indicative of psychological dependence. This distinction is important in regard to the treatment of the patient with cancer, because there is a misconception that drugs, instead of psychosocial factors, are the sole culprit in psychological dependence. With cancer patients, the problem is not stopping the drug but starting it in the setting of an often overwhelming concern about dependence. A statement such as "I don't want to become an addict" from patients in severe pain from advanced cancer is not uncommon. Lengthy counseling does not always abate the fears that come from a lifetime of experience in an opiophobic society. The rarity of psychological dependence following opioid treatment in a medical setting has been clearly documented in a study involving 11,882 patients who received at least one opioid preparation; only four patients were identified as abusing the prescribed drugs.[93] The analysis of drug-intake patterns in patients with cancer suggests that psychological dependence occurs rarely in this population.[90] An exception is patients with a history of psychological dependence that antedates the cancer.

Respiratory depression, which is mediated by mu_2-receptors in the brain stem,[18] is the most feared opioid side effect; the respiratory centers become less responsive to carbon dioxide.[35] Tolerance to this effect develops rapidly. It is now known that pain is a potent antagonist of opioid-induced respiratory depression, and that clinically relevant respiratory depression is rare in the setting of acute and chronic pain. The prerequisite for the development of respiratory depression is a relative overdosage, usually in the opioid-naive patient. Stupor or frank coma is usually associated with this condition. Respiratory depression is not a concern when the patient is alert and especially if he or she is in pain. If the pain is suddenly relieved by an analgesic procedure, the opioid dose must be adjusted to avoid a relative overdose.[94] In patients with advanced cancer, opioid overdose is an uncommon cause of encephalopathy. In a patient with terminal delirium, opioid antagonists should be used with extreme caution, if at all. When reversal of opioid effect is desirable, naloxone, an opioid antagonist, should be given intravenously with careful monitoring. If the patient has been receiving long-term opioid therapy, it is good practice to dilute 0.4 mg of naloxone in 10 ml of normal saline and inject it slowly, titrating the dose to effect. This careful titration will prevent the precipitation of severe withdrawal symptoms. Symptoms of withdrawal after administration of an antagonist are more severe than those seen on discontinuation of an opioid. Because naloxone has a half-life of 1 hour, [35] repeated injections might be needed in the event of morphine overdose. A continuous intravenous drip should be used to antagonize opioids with a longer half-life. Excessive drug intake is a rare cause of encephalopathy and respiratory depression in patients with cancer who are receiving a stable dose of opioids. It is difficult to imagine a worse experience for a dying patient than withdrawal symptoms, severe breakthrough pain, and inability to communicate because of encephalopathy. The risk of opioid-induced respiratory depression in patients with cancer is more relevant when opioids are used in conjunction with other respiratory depressants to control distressing breathlessness.

Constipation, unlike respiratory depression, is a common side effect of opioid use. Tolerance to the constipating effects does not usually develop. Opioids decrease gastric, biliary, pancreatic, and intestinal secretions and the propulsive motility of the stomach and intestine. This results in delayed passage of increasingly viscous stool. Central[20] and peripheral[21, 22] opioid receptor mechanisms are implicated. Careful assessment of bowel function and dietary habits, combined with a laxative regimen, must be part of ongoing management. Again, an individualized regimen is the key to therapeutic efficacy. Oral naloxone, which is almost completely inactivated in the liver,[35] has been used in an attempt to block the peripheral action of opioids on the gastrointestinal tract, and therefore reverse constipation.[95, 96] It should be used (1) only in selected patients, (2) in conjunction with laxatives, and (3) preferably in a controlled experimental setting.

Vomiting after opioid administration is thought to be caused by direct stimulation of the chemoreceptor trigger zone for emesis in the area postrema of the medulla.[35] If nausea precedes vomiting, or if nausea is unaccompanied by vomiting, an increased vestibular sensitivity or delayed gastric emptying could also play a role. A vestibular component is suggested by the fact that nausea is uncommon in recumbent patients but occurs in 40% of ambulatory patients after parenteral administration of 15 mg of morphine.[35] It is still unclear whether these effects involve specific opioid receptors because it has not been established whether they are reversed by naloxone.[23] Tolerance to this effect is the rule, and generally the nausea will subside in 2–3 days. M6G may be implicated in some patients with protracted nausea.[97] Only patients with a history of prior opioid-induced nausea should be given antiemetics prophylactically. Inadequately treated constipation may also be a cause of persistent nausea.

Sedation is common when opioids are first started or when the dose is increased. It is often the limiting side effect during rapid titration for acute pain exacerbation. Many physicians who use opioids only for procedure-related pain may think that sedation always accompanies pain relief. Fortunately, for most patients, sedation is only a transitory effect.[98] Opioid-induced sedation must be differentiated from the predictable deep sleep that follows pain relief in sleep-deprived patients. Excessive sedation is frequently seen when patients have mild or no pain at rest but have severe pain during activity. Stimulants like dextroamphetamine and methylphenidate[89] can counteract opiate-induced sedation; they may also provide an additive analgesic effect.[99]

Confusion can be caused or aggravated by opioids and may range from mild impairment in concentration to frank delirium with disorientation, disorganized thinking, perceptual distortions, and hallucinations. Hallucinations in the context of intact cognitive function have also been described.[100] Other common causes of altered mental status must be excluded. When the confusional state is due to opioids, it generally follows a recent increase in dose and will resolve as the dose is reduced. Discontinuation of the opioid or administration of naloxone will result in severe pain and withdrawal symptoms, and should therefore be avoided.

Dysphoria is probably more common than euphoria following opioid administration in patients with cancer. Dysphoria appears to be mediated by kappa-receptors.[36] Partial agonists and mixed agonist-antagonists can cause dysphoria and hallucinations by binding to nonopioid sigma-receptors.[37] As a rule, these drugs should not be used to treat cancer pain. Meperidine has also been associated with dysphoria.[41]

Myoclonus and seizures are side effects associated with long-term opioid use. However, these side effects do not occur when large doses of potent opioids are used to produce anesthesia for surgery.[35] Central nervous system toxicity may be due to accumulation of excitatory metabolites, which have been demonstrated with propoxyphene,[40, 42] meperidine,[41, 43] and morphine.[55] Myoclonus and seizures also may result from escalating doses of other opioids. Myoclonus is fairly common and is not troublesome to all patients. It may be treated symptomatically with benzodiazepines. Generalized tonic-clonic seizures are infrequent; when induced by morphine, methadone, or propoxyphene they can be stopped by naloxone.[35] Seizures from meperidine use may be exacerbated by naloxone,[43] suggesting a different drug-receptor interaction.[101]

Urinary retention induced by opioids is due to inhibition of the voiding reflex and increased tone of the external sphincter.[35] Catheterization is sometimes required following therapeutic doses of opioids. Tolerance to this effect develops rapidly.

Pruritus and diaphoresis are frequent but minor side effects, usually occurring after parenteral administration. They are due in part to the release of histamine. The urticaria at the injection site caused by morphine and meperidine is not blocked by naloxone.[35] A primary neuronal mechanism for pruritus is suggested by the itching that occurs after spinal administration of opioids that do not induce histamine release.[102] This effect is reversed by naloxone.

Hypotension is due to direct histamine release and to a specific action on opioid receptors. It is partially blocked by H_1 antagonists and more effectively reversed by naloxone.[35] Peripheral vasodilatation and inhibition of baroreceptor reflexes may cause orthostatic hypotension. In the recumbent patient, hypotension induced by opioids is a risk only in the presence of hypovolemia.

Pulmonary edema associated with opioid administration was described by Osler more than 100 years ago.[103] Only three cases of noncardiogenic pulmonary edema have been reported in patients with cancer who are receiving escalating opioid doses.[104]

Chest wall rigidity severe enough to compromise respiration is not uncommon during anesthesia with fentanyl,[105] but it has not been described during treatment for pain.

Increased tone at Oddi's sphincter with an increase in the common bile duct pressure is a well-known effect of morphine. It has been suggested that morphine can aggravate the pain from biliary colic.[35]

Xerostomia is a common complaint of patients receiving opioids. Frequent, small sips of water will usually alleviate this symptom. Pilocarpine can be used in selected patients, preferably in an experimental setting.

Cough suppression is mediated by opioid receptors in the medulla.[35] In the awake patient, its significance is limited to the relief of distressing dry cough.

The effects of opioids on neuroendocrine function are well described.[106] They are rare and usually transient. The clinical significance of opioid effects on the immune system is unclear.[107] The miotic effect of toxic doses of opioids is well known. Miosis is due to an excitatory effect on the autonomic segment of the oculomotor nuclear complex in the midbrain.[35] Meperidine is an exception, causing mydriasis at toxic doses. Long-term effects of chronic opioid use on intellectual function have not been demonstrated.

Opioids do not mask pain from new or ongoing tissue injury.[90] Substantial clinical experience with cancer patients suggests that medical emergencies such as acute abdomen and myocardial infarction will not go unrecognized in a patient on a stable opioid regimen.

Early treatment with opioids does not preclude effective pain management as cancer progresses. It is therefore recommended that pharmacologic analgesic agents be used aggressively regardless of the stage of the disease so as to improve quality of life. Of course, the medical treatment of pain must be individualized to become an integral part of the overall medical care of the cancer patient.

References

1. World Health Organization (WHO). Cancer Pain Relief. Geneva: WHO, 1986.
2. World Health Organization (WHO). Cancer Pain Relief and Palliative Care: Report of a WHO Expert Committee. Geneva: WHO, 1990.
3. Ventafridda V, Tamburini M, Caraceni A, et al. A validation study of the WHO method for cancer pain relief. Cancer 1987;59:851.

4. Schug SA, Zech D, Dorr U. Cancer pain management according to WHO guidelines. J Pain Symptom Manage 1990;1:27.

5. Takeda F. Results of field testing in Japan of the WHO Draft Interim Guidelines on Relief of Cancer Pain. Pain Clin 1986;1:83.

6. Grond S, Zech D, Schug SA, et al. Validation of the World Health Organization guidelines for cancer pain relief during the last days and hours of life. J Pain Symptom Manage 1991;6:411.

7. Stjernsward J, Teoh N. Current status of the Global Cancer Control Program of the World Health Organization. J. Pain Symptom Manage 1993;8:340.

8. Reynolds DV. Surgery in the rat during electrical anaesthesia induced by focal brain stimulation. Science 1969;164:4445.

9. Akil H, Mayer DJ, Liebeskind JC. Antagonism of stimulation-produced analgesia by naloxone, a narcotic antagonist. Science 1974;191:961.

10. Evans CJ, Hammond DL, Frederickson RCA. The Opioid Peptides. In Pasternak GW (ed), The Opiate Receptors. Clifton Park, NJ: Humana, 1988;23.

11. Beckett AH, Casy AF. Synthetic analgesics: Stereochemical considerations. J Pharm Pharmacol 1954;6:986.

12. Pert CB, Snyder SH. Opiate receptor demonstrated in nervous tissue. Science 1973;179:1011.

13. Wolozin BL, Pasternak GW. Classification of multiple morphine and enkephalin binding sites in the central nervous system. Proc Natl Acad Sci U S A 1981;78:6181.

14. Pasternak GW, Wood PL. Multiple mu receptors. Life Sci 1986;38:1889.

15. Lewis VA, Gerbhardt GF. Evaluation of the periaqueductal gray (PAG) as a morphine specific locus of action and examination of morphine induced and stimulation produced analgesia at coincident PAG loci. Brain Res 1977;124:283.

16. Bodnar RJ, Williams CL, Lee SJ, Pasternak JW. Role of mu_1 opiate receptor in supraspinal opiate analgesia: A microinjection study. Brain Res 1988;447:25.

17. Advokat C. The role of descending inhibition in morphine induced analgesia. Trends Pharmacol Sci 1988;9:330.

18. Ling GSF, Spiegel K, Nishimura S, Pasternak GW. Dissociation of morphine's analgesic and respiratory depressant actions. Eur J Pharmacol 1983;86:487.

19. Ling GSF, Spiegel K, Nishimura S, Pasternak GW. Separation of opioid analgesia from respiratory depression: Evidence for different receptor mechanisms. J Pharmacol Exp Ther 1985;232:149.

20. Heman JS, Williams CL, Burks TF, et al. Dissociation of opioid antinociception and central gastrointestinal propulsion in the mouse: Studies with naloxazine. J Pharmacol Exp Ther 1988;245:238.

21. Paul D, Pasternak GW. Differential blockade by naloxazine of two mu opiate actions: Analgesia and inhibition of gastrointestinal transit. Eur J Pharmacol 1988;149:403.

22. Ginzler AR, Pasternak GW. Multiple mu receptors: Evidence of mu_2 sites in the guinea pig ileum. Neurosci Lett 1983;39:51.

23. Pasternak GW. Pharmacological mechanisms of opioid analgesia. Clin Neuropharmacol 1993;16:1.

24. Stein C, Comisel K, Haimeri E, et al. Analgesic effect of intraarticular morphine after arthroscopic knee surgery. N Engl J Med 1991;325:1123.

25. Chavkin C, James IF, Goldstein A. Dynorphin is a specific endogenous ligand of the kappa opiate receptors. Science 1982;215:413.

26. Lord JAH, Waterfield AA, Hughes J, Kosterlitz HW. Endogenous opioid peptides: Multiple agonists and receptors. Nature 1977;267:495.

27. North RA. Opioid receptor types and membrane ion channels. Trends Neurosci 1986;9:114.

28. Schoffelmeer ANM, Van Vliet BJ, DeVries TJ, et al. Regulation of brain neurotransmitter release and of adenylate cyclase activity by opioid receptors. Biochem Soc Trans 1992;20:449.

29. Rosenthal W, Heschler J, Trautwein W, Schultz G. Control of voltage dependent Ca^+ channels by G protein coupled receptors. FASEB J 1988;2:2784.

30. Su YF, Wong CS, Russel RD, et al. Mechanisms of Opioid Tolerance. In CE Short, A Van Poznak (eds), Animal Pain. New York: Churchill Livingstone, 1990;259.

31. Trujillo KA, Akil H. Opiate tolerance and dependence: Recent findings and synthesis. New Biol 1991;3:915.

32. Trujillo KA, Akil H. Inhibition of morphine tolerance and dependence by the NMDA receptor antagonist MK-801. Science 1991;251:85.

33. Laird D, Llovel T. Paradoxical pain [letter]. Lancet 1993;341:241.

34. Kanamaru T, Saeki S, Katsumata N, et al. Ketamine infusion for control of pain in patients with advanced cancer. Masai 1990;39:1368.

35. Jaffe JH, Martin WR. Opioid Analgesics and Antagonists. In AG Gillman, TW Rall, AS Nies, P Taylor (eds), Goodman and Gillman's: The Pharmacologic Basis of Therapeutics. New York: Pergamon, 1990;485.

36. Millan MJ. μ-Opioid receptors and analgesia. Trends Pharmacol Sci 1990;11:70.

37. Quirion R, Chicheportiche R, Contreras PC, et al. Classification and nomenclature of phenilciclidine and sigma receptor sites. Trends Neurosci 1987;10:444.

38. Beaver WT, Wallenstein SL, Rogers A, Houde RW. Analgesic studies of codeine and oxycodone in patients with cancer. Comparison of oral with intramuscular codeine and oral with intramuscular oxycodone. J Pharmacol Exp Ther 1978;207:92.

39. Beaver WT, Wallenstein SL, Rogers A, Houde RW. Analgesic studies of codeine and oxycodone in patients with cancer. Comparison of intramuscular oxycodone with intramuscular morphine and codeine. J Pharmacol Exp Ther 1978;207:101.

40. Inturrisi CE, Colburn WN, Verebey K, et al. Propoxy-phene and norpropoxyphene kinetics after single and repeated doses of propoxyphene. Clin Pharmacol Ther 1982;31:157.

41. Kaiko RF, Foley KM, Grabinski PY, et al. Central nervous system excitatory effects of meperidine in cancer patients. Ann Neurol 1983;13:180.

42. Chan GLC, Matzke GR. Effects of renal insufficiency on the pharmacokinetics and pharmacodynamics of opioid analgesics. Drug Intell Clin Pharm 1987;21:773.

43. Szeto HH, Inturrisi CE, Houde R, et al. Accumulation of normeperidine, an active metabolite of meperidine, in patients with renal failure and cancer. Ann Intern Med 1977;86:738.

44. Kantor TG, Hopper M, Laska E. Adverse effects of commonly ordered oral narcotics. J Clin Pharmacol 1981;21:1.

45. Kalso E, Vanio A. Morphine and oxycodone for cancer pain. Clin Pharmacol Ther 1990;47:639.

46. Kalso E, Vanio A. Hallucinations during morphine but not during oxycodone treatment [letter]. Lancet 1987;2:912.

47. Glare PA, Walsh TD. Dose-ranging study of oxycodone for chronic pain in advanced cancer. J Clin Oncol 1993;11:973.

48. Poyhia R, Vainio A, Kalso E. A review of oxycodone's clinical pharmacokinetics and pharmacodynamics. J Pain Symptom Manage 1993;8:63.

49. Sawe J, Svensson JO, Rane A. Morphine metabolism in cancer patients on increasing oral doses—No evidence of autoinduction or dose-dependence. Br J Clin Pharmacol 1983;16:85.

50. Pasternak GW, Bodnar RJ, Clarcke JA, Inturrisi CE. Morphine-6-glucuronide, a potent mu agonist. Life Sci 1987;41:2845.

51. Oguri K, Yamada-Mori Y, Shigezane J, et al. Enhanced binding of morphine and nalorphine to opioid delta receptor by glucuronite and sulphite conjugations at the 6-positions. Life Sci 1987;41:1457.

52. Portenoy RK, Khan E, Layman M, et al. Chronic morphine therapy for cancer pain: Plasma and cerebrospinal fluid morphine and morphine-6-glucuronide concentrations. Neurology 1991;41:1457.

53. Houde RW, Wallenstein SL, Beaver WT. Evaluation of Analgesics in Patients with Cancer Pain. In L Lasagna (ed), International Encyclopedia of Pharmacology and Therapeutics (Vol. 1). New York: Pergamon, 1966;59.

54. Twycross R. The use of narcotic analgesics in terminal illness. J Med Ethics 1975;1:10.

55. Labella FS, Pinsky C, Havlicek V. Morphine derivatives with diminished opiate receptor potency show enhanced central excitatory activity. Brain Res 1979;174:263.

56. Morley JL, Miles JB, Wells JC, Bowsher D. Paradoxical pain [letter]. Lancet 1992;340:1045.

57. Smith MT, Watt JA, Cramond T. Morphine-3-glucuronide—A potent antagonist of morphine analgesia. Life Sci 1990;47:579.

58. Kaiko RF. Controlled-release oral morphine for cancer-related pain: The European and North American experiences. Adv Pain Res Ther 1990;14:171.

59. Osborne RJ, Joel SP, Slevin ML. Morphine intoxication in renal failure: The role of morphine-6-glucuronide. Br Med J 1986;292:1548.

60. Saltzburg D, Inturrisi CE, Greenslade R, et al. Blood profiles of heroin and metabolites during repeated oral administration in cancer pain patients. Proc Am Soc Clin Oncol 1988;S73(Suppl):278.

61. Twycross RG. Choice of strong analgesics in terminal cancer: Diamorphine or morphine? Pain 1977;3:93.

62. Kaiko RF, Wallenstein SL, Rogers AG, et al. Analgesic and mood effects of heroin and morphine in cancer patients with postoperative pain. N Engl J Med 1981; 304:1501.

63. Houde RW. Clinical analgesic studies of hydromorphone. Adv Pain Res Ther 1986;8:129.

64. Moulin DE, Kreeft JH, Murray-Parsons N, Bouquillon AI. Comparison of continuous subcutaneous and intravenous hydromorphone infusions for management of cancer pain. Lancet 1991;337:465.

65. Tive L, Ginsberg K, Pick CG, Pasternak GW. Kappa$_3$ receptors and levorphanol analgesia. Neuropharmacology 1992;9:851.

66. Houde RW, Wallenstein SL, Beaver WT. Clinical measurement of pain. In G DeStevens (ed), Analgesics. New York: Academic, 1976;75.

67. Dixon R. Pharmacokinetics of levorphanol. Adv Pain Res Ther 1986;8:217.

68. Beaver WT, Wallenstein SL, Houde RW, Rogers A. A clinical comparison of the analgesic effects of methadone and morphine administered intramuscularly and of oral and parenterally administered methadone. Clin Pharmacol Ther 1967;8:415.

69. Meresaar U, Nillson MI, Holmstrand J, Anggard E. Single dose pharmacokinetics and bioavailability of methadone in man studied with a stable isotope method. Eur J Clin Pharmacol 1981;20:473.

70. Sawe J. High dose morphine and methadone in cancer patients. Clinical pharmacokinetic consideration of oral treatment. Clin Pharmacol 1986;11:87.

71. Inturrisi CE, Colburn WA, Kaiko RF, et al. Pharmacokinetics and pharmacodynamics of methadone in patients with chronic pain. Clin Pharmacol Ther 1987;41:392.

72. Plummer JL, Gourlay GK, Cherry DA, Cousins MJ. Estimation of methadone clearance: Application in the management of cancer pain. Pain 1988;33:313.

73. Kreek MJ, Schecter AJ, Gutjahr CL, Hecht M. Methadone use in patients with chronic renal disease. Drug Alcohol Depend 1980;5:195.

74. Morley JS, Watt JWG, Wells JC, Miles JB, et al. Methadone in pain uncontrolled by morphine [letter]. Lancet 1993;342:1243.

75. Galer BS, Coyle N, Pasternak GW, Portenoy RK. Individual variability in the response to different opioids: Report of five cases. Pain 1992;49:87.

76. Miser AW, Narang PK, Dothage JA, et al. Transdermal fentanyl for pain control in patients with cancer. Pain 1989;37:15.

77. Michaels AS, Chandrasekaran SK, Shaw JE. Drug permeation through human skin: Theory and in vitro experimental measurements. Am Inst Chem Eng 1975;21:986.

78. Hwang SS, Nichols KC, Southam MA. Transdermal Permeation: Physiological and Physiochemical Aspects. In KA Lehmann, D Zech (eds), Transdermal Fentanyl. Berlin: Springer, 1991;1.

79. Roy SD, Flynn GL. Transdermal delivery of narcotic analgesics: pH, anatomical and subject influences of cutaneous permeability of fentanyl and sufentanil. Pharm Res 1990;7:842.

80. Varvel JL, Shafer SL, Hwang SS, et al. Absorption characteristics of transdermally administered fentanyl. Anesthesiology 1989;70:928.

81. Southam M, Gupta B, Knowles N, Hwang SS. Transdermal Fentanyl: An Overview of Pharmacokinetics, Efficacy and Safety. In KA Lehmann, D Zech (eds), Transdermal Fentanyl. Berlin: Springer, 1991;107.

82. Fine PG, Marcus M, Just De Boer A, Van der Oord B. An open label study of oral transmucosal fentanyl citrate (OTFC) for the treatment of breakthrough cancer pain. Pain 1991;45:149.

83. Foley KM. The treatment of cancer pain. N Engl J Med 1984;313:84.

84. Citron ML, Johnston-Early A, Boyer M, et al. Patient-controlled analgesia for severe cancer pain. Arch Intern Med 1986;46:734.

85. Portenoy R. Continuous infusion of opioid drugs in the treatment of cancer pain: Guidelines for use. J Pain Symptom Manage 1986;1:223.

86. Bruera E, Chadwick S, Bacovsky R. Continuous subcutaneous infusion of narcotics using a portable disposable pump. J Palliat Care 1985;1:45.

87. Payne R, Foley KM. Advances in the management of cancer pain. Cancer Treatment Reports 1984;68:173.

88. Bruera E, Roca E, Cedaro L, et al. Action of oral methylprednisolone in terminal cancer patients: A prospective randomized double blind study. Cancer Treatment Reports 1985;69:751.

89. Bruera E, Brenneis C, Chadwick S, et al. Methylphenidate associated with narcotics for the treatment of cancer pain. Cancer Treatment Reports 1987;71:67.

90. Kanner RM, Foley KM. Patterns of Narcotic Use in a Cancer Pain Clinic. In RB Millman, P Cushman, JH Lowinson (eds), Research Developments in Drug and Alcohol Use. New York: New York Academy of Sciences, 1981;161.

91. Lyness WH, Smith FL, Heavner JE, et al. Morphine self administration in the rat during adjuvant induced arthritis. Life Sci 1989;45:2217.

92. Jaffe JH. Drug Addiction and Drug Abuse. In AG Gillman, TW Rall, AS Nies, P Taylor (eds), Goodman and Gillman's: The Pharmacologic Basis of Therapeutics. New York: Pergamon, 1990;485.

93. Porter J, Hershel J. Addiction rare in patients treated with narcotics [letter]. N Engl J Med 1980;302:123.

94. Hanks GW, Twicross RG, Lloyd JW. Unexpected complication of successful nerve block. Anaesthesia 1981;36:37.

95. Robinson BA, Johansson L, Shaw J. Oral naloxone in opioid associated constipation [letter]. Lancet 1991;338:581.

96. Culpepper-Morgan JA, Inturrisi CE, Portenoy R, Kreek M. Oral naloxone treatment of narcotic induced constipation. NIDA Res Monogr 1989;95:399.

97. Hagen NA, Foley KM, Cerbone DJ, et al. Chronic nausea and morphine-6-glucuronide. J Pain Symptom Manage 1991;6:125.

98. Bruera E, Macmillan K, Hanson J, MacDonald N. The cognitive effects of the administration of narcotic analgesics in patients with cancer pain. Pain 1989;39:13.

99. Foley KM, Inturrisi CE. Analgesic drug therapy in cancer pain: Principles and practice. Med Clin North Am 1987;71:207.

100. Bruera E, Schoeller T, Montejo G. Organic hallucinosis in patients receiving high dose of opiates for cancer pain. Pain 1992;48:397.

101. Umans JG, Inturrisi CE. Antinociceptive activity and toxicity of meperidine and normeperidine in mice. J Pharmacol Exp Ther 1982;223:203.

102. Duthie DJR, Nimmo WS. Adverse effects of opioid analgesic drugs. Br J Anaesth 1987;59:61.

103. Cooper A, White D, Matthay R. Drug-induced pulmonary disease. Am Rev Respir Dis 1986;133:488.

104. Bruera E, Miller MJ. Noncardiogenic pulmonary edema after narcotic treatment for cancer pain. Pain 1989;39:297.

105. Monk J. Sufentanil: A review. Drugs 1988;36:249.

106. Howlett TA, Rees LH. Endogenous opioid peptides and hypothalamo-pituitary function. Annu Rev Physiol 1986;48:527.

107. Sibinga NES, Goldstein A. Opioid peptides and opioid receptors in cells of the immune system. Annu Rev Immunol 1986;6:219.

Chapter 7

Appropriate Management of Cancer Pain: Not the Second Order of Business Anymore

John M. Flexner

One merely has to examine the headlines of our voluminous office magazines and papers to know that something is happening. The April 1994 issue of *Oncology News (International)* has as its headline: "Government Releases Its Clinical Practice Guidelines on Management of Cancer Pain." Likewise, the front page of its sister publication, *Oncology Times,* reads "MDs Still Get Low Marks for Pain Relief." The cover also has a summary of the Agency for Health Care Policy and Research, U. S. Public Health Service's Cancer Pain Guidelines, the same agency referred to by *Oncology News.* The March 1994 issue of *Oncology* has an article on "Current Management of Pain in Patients with Cancer" as well as one on "Phantom Pain." The March 1994 issue of the *New England Journal of Medicine* has an article entitled "Pain and Its Treatment in Outpatients with Metastatic Cancer" and a special report on "New Clinical Practice Guidelines for the Management of Pain in Patients with Cancer."

Just last year, the Eastern Cooperative Oncology Group (ECOG) reported the results of a survey of all ECOG physicians with patient care responsibilities (medical oncologists, hematologists, oncological surgeons, and radiation therapists). These physicians care for more than 70,000 cancer patients. The results were reported in the *Annals of Internal Medicine* (July 1993). They showed that cancer patients still are not receiving adequate relief from their pain. The American Cancer Society has undertaken a pain initiative in more than 30 states under the auspices of an ad hoc pain committee. Their objective is to educate, assess, and correct the deficiencies in cancer pain management, including most of the major hospitals where cancer is treated. This lack of appropriate care continues today throughout the country. Indeed, although appropriate and effective care of cancer pain may be a short way off, the progress being made today is dramatic. For the past 20–30 years, we have been aware that cancer patients are undertreated. The reasons for this are numerous; however, dating back to the studies by Marks and Sachar in 1973,[1] it was apparent that fear of addiction and the untoward effects of "big time" narcotics were factors profoundly influencing the hesitancy of house staffs to prescribe appropriate analgesics. Consequently, meperidine (Demerol) was used almost exclusively in inappropriate cases or in subpharmacologic amounts. In the study by Marks and Sachar, it was noted that no patient received more that 90 mg of Demerol at any one time, and most received appreciably less. Interns learned about pain management from their residents, those residents from the residents before them, and so on. This practice has been labeled "prescribing by custom." Several studies followed, all with the same appalling results—the undertreatment of cancer pain in these unfortunate patients.[2–4] In addition to the house staff and attending physicians, nurses also were part of this phobic approach of "using the least of the mildest."[5] Aggressive use of opiates was indeed a rare occurrence, except by the nationally renowned university-based cancer centers. These institutions enjoyed the luxury of a pain management program with a director who oftentimes was a subspecialist, neurologist, oncologist, or anesthesiologist. These individuals perceived the scope of the problem earlier than most, as evidenced by the reviews by Foley[6] and Portenoy[7] from Sloan Kettering Cancer Center that appeared in peer review journals in the late 1970s and early 1980s. Little attention was given to these reviews, as shown by recent surveys. However, it was a start of what was termed "The Pain Revolution." Bonica reviewed approximately 9,000 pages from 12 or 13 cancer texts that were available in the late 1970s and early 1980s and could find only 17 pages devoted to management of cancer pain, 13 of which were found in one text.[8] Why has this problem persisted despite the formation of pain clinics in nearly every major hospital and the advent of several pain journals as well as journals on symptomatic care plus the emergence of board-certified pain experts in every city who belong to pain societies that meet all over the world and discuss cancer-related pain? The World Health Organization (WHO) states that it has three goals in its approach to cancer: (1) cure if possible, (2) prevention, and (3) adequate relief of cancer pain. What have been the so-called barriers to the last of the WHO goals?

The recent ECOG survey has condensed its findings into four major areas, including physicians, nurses, patients, and the role of their respective families. Its findings concern the training, experience, phobias, and taboos inherent in these groups. However, the federal government and its policy of "Just Say No" has spilled over from the street corners into our hospital wards and clinics. The major barriers to adequate pain management according to the ECOG survey[9] are presented here:

1. Physicians' attitudes, poor pain assessment, limited experience and education regarding pain management, and reluctance to prescribe drugs such as opiates, even though they know that these drugs are appropriate in cancer patients are some reasons for inadequate pain management. More than half of the 1,200 cancer specialists surveyed thought that pain control was inadequate in their institution and many mentioned that up to 25% of their cancer patients died in pain. The majority (85%) thought that their cancer patients were grossly undermedicated for pain.

2. The patients on the other hand were reluctant to take opioids for fear that this was the "last or final rites." They likened opiates to euthanasia or mercy killing. They believed that if their disease required large doses of narcotics that they must be in the "terminal phase" of their illness. In addition, they feared addiction and dependency. The families of most patients seconded this decision in most cases. They were also unsure of what was legal and what was illegal as far as narcotic medication was concerned. In regard to the latter, Hill of the M.D. Anderson Cancer Center has stated[10]:

> The actions that should be taken to relieve cancer pains involve changing the concepts and behaviors of persons treating pain and the attitude of patients, family, and friends toward this pain. We know there is presently an ongoing new body of knowledge about pain in cancer and it should be presented in a convincing manner. We should develop strategies to change drug laws and regulations where needed to help regulators differentiate between the legitimate medical use of narcotics and the abuse of them.

Dr. Stewart Grossman of John Hopkins Medical Center concurs and adds,[11] "Let no extensive monotony of opiate prescribing pattern by governmental agency deter physicians from providing adequate management of pain relief." This point cannot be overemphasized.

In addition to the barriers outlined previously, pain experts have noted repeatedly that most physicians lack a broad understanding of cancer pain pathophysiology, as well as in-depth understanding of the pharmacology of narcotic analgesics. The few experts on cancer pain have had little effect on changing the views held by many physicians regarding pain management. What then is the impact of constant, unrelieved cancer pain on the patient? It is a strong, negative force that tends to give cancer patients decreased confidence in the health care system. It may ultimately lead to treatment rejection, depression, and even suicidal ideation. The lack of adequate pain control has a far-reaching effect not only on the suffering patient, but also on the inpatient experience and the family itself. Oftentimes, the family is demoralized that nothing is being done to lessen the patient's pain.

It is therefore vitally important that the pain management approach be one that includes good medical, psychological, and spiritual care, as in the hospice experience. This intervention requires the multidisciplinary approach of hospital and community resources, social workers, and all professionals who are involved in the total holistic policy of dealing with cancer patients and their many problems.

It is important to stress the importance of pain assessment because this area of pain management has been lacking in the past. Much information has been written and spoken about the indications, pharmacology, and side effects of analgesics. The common attitude has been, "The right dose, by the right route, at the right time." However, little attention has been directed toward appropriate pain assessment. Nurses and staff are meticulous about recording vital signs, temperature and weight changes, and other changes that are thought to be of little relevance to the cancer pain patient. Chemotherapeutic, antibiotic, endocrine, or therapeutic protocols are rigidly adhered to and meticulously recorded in the chart. Yet, when a cancer pain patient requires narcotics for pain, little can be found in the chart other than the original order or any subsequent order that would alter the dosage or time interval.

Assessment should be the foundation of any therapeutic plan to treat cancer pain. It is important to establish a baseline of pain control that can be rigorously adhered to and to determine the putative mechanisms of the cancer pain. The appropriate interventions are selected first (most commonly, pharmacologic) and then the therapeutic response is evaluated. This is recorded on a designated (permanent part of the medical record) pain (flow) sheet day by day. The medical history, physical examination, laboratory evaluation, and cancer therapy are all integral parts of pain assessment because they often play a role in determining the etiologic factors for the pain. A psychological and social evaluation of the patient and the patient's family and environmental situation should also be made. There should be an appropriate pain scale (e.g., a numeric scale, or pictorial representation of happy and sad faces or colors) for judging the intensity of the pain and its subsequent relief. The pain history should include the approximate site of pain, what makes it worse or better, its temporal pattern, any present therapy, and past experience with pain management, either satisfactory or unsatisfactory. By definition, the proper pain assessment requires a multidisciplinary approach and a written process that outlines treatment and evaluation. The various team members need role definitions and a way to receive feedback from the patient. Solutions to problems should be described on this form. The pain team, including the attending physician, should meet regularly to discuss the treatment of the patient. A designated physician will be responsible for prescribing and managing the narcotics. The team nurse also helps plan pain management, pharmacologic and nonpharmacologic. He or she oversees the actual drug administration in addition to documenting and evaluating the efficiency of the treatment plan. The psychosocial assessment is performed by the social worker who also oversees any psychosocial intervention. The social worker is also responsible for activation of local resources needed to support overall patient care. The chaplain provides spiritual support. The patient's family is included in *all* phases of the overall decision-making process. Collectively, all members of the team are advocates for the patient. Open communication is the byword and the team should help dispel the customary myths so prevalent regarding drugs such as morphine.

Proper knowledge of the sound principles of pain control requires a working knowledge of analgesics: the right drug at the right dose at the right time interval via the right route. The oral route is, of course, preferable. However, as Foley has stated so succinctly, "The dose that works is the dose that works." It is extremely important to know the differences between parenteral and oral doses of narcotics, as well as their side effects. Constipation is the most often overlooked side effect and is responsible in many incidences for exaggeration of abdominal cancer pain. Nausea also needs attention and may temporarily prohibit the use of opiates. Respiratory depression is the least oftern encountered side effect (but most feared) and only presents a problem with parenteral, intrathecal, or subdural routes. If pharmacologic interventions fail, a reassessment is appropriate. Is the patient receiving the appropriate dose at the appropriate level with the appropriate analgesic by the best route possible? Is the patient compliant? Are the side effects (nausea, constipation, sedation) unacceptable? Does the patient feel guilty about using opiates? Would an adjunctive drug help? Is an antidepressant, steroid, or anxiolytic drug needed? Would social or psychological intervention help the patient feel better? Is a nerve block, transcutaneous electrical nerve stimulator unit, or neurosurgical approach needed? The treatment plan must be tailored to fit the individual needs of each patient. The Bill of

Rights for cancer patients needs to be reinforced. It states the following:

1. I have the right to have my pain relieved by health professionals, friends, family and others around me.
2. I have the right to have my pain controlled, no matter what its cause or how severe it may be.
3. I have the right to be treated with respect at all times. When I need medication for pain, I should not be treated like a drug abuser.
4. I have the right to have pain resulting from treatment and procedures prevented or at least minimized.

We have made real progress in the treatment of cancer pain in the past few years. The tenets of good cancer pain management will soon be implemented in many of our institutions that provide care for cancer patients. We still have a long way to go, however. As pointed out in the guidelines stated by the Agency for Health Care Policy and Research, U.S. Public Health Service (March 1994):*

> Pain is commonly undertreated.
> An aggressive approach to pain control is necessary.
> Barriers may prevent proper control of cancer pain.
> Pain can be controlled.
> Pain must be assessed properly.
> Begin with the least invasive option.
> The guidelines were developed by a private-sector expert panel and are based on science and expert opinion.

In conclusion, it is appropriate to again quote Foley: "At the present time there are only a few highly trained physicians in cancer pain management, psycho-oncology or palliative care whose main interest is to place the high priority on pain management, symptoms control, and psychological support for patients with advanced disease."[12] It is hoped that cancer pain management will become as effective and matter of fact as are antibiotics for infectious diseases.

References

1. Marks RM, Sachar EJ. Undertreatment of medical inpatients with narcotic analgesics. Ann Intern Med 1973;78:178.
2. Charap AD. The knowledge, attitudes and experience of medical personnel treating pain in the terminally ill. Mt Sinai J Med 1978;45:561.
3. Weiss OF, Sriwatanakuls S, Alloza JC, et al. Attitudes of patients, house-staff and nurses toward postoperative analgesic care. Anesth Analg 1983;62:70.
4. Cleeland CS, Cleeland LB, Dar R, et al. Factors influencing physician management of cancer pain. Cancer 1986;58:796.
5. Sriwatanakuls S, Weiss OF, Alloza JC, et al. Analysis of narcotic analgesic usage in the treatment of postoperative pain. JAMA 1983;250:926.
6. Foley KM. The treatment of cancer pain. N Engl J Med 1985;313:34.
7. Portenoy RK. Practical aspects of pain control in the patient with cancer. CA Cancer J Clin 1988;38:7.
8. Bonica JJ. Advances in Pain Research and Therapy. New York: Raven, 1983.
9. Von Roenn JH, Cleeland CS, Gonin R, et al. Physician attitudes and practice in cancer pain management. A survey from the Eastern Cooperative Oncology Group. Ann Intern Med 1993;119:121.
10. Hill CS Jr. Pain management in a drug oriented society. Am J Med 1989;63(Suppl.):2383.
11. Grossman SA, Sheidler VR, Sweeden K, et al. Correlation of patient and caregiver ratings of cancer pain. J Pain Symptom Manage 1991;6:53.
12. Foley KM. The relationship of pain and symptom management to patient requests for physician assisted suicide. J Pain Symptom Manage 1991;6:289.

---

* These guidelines are available by calling (1-800-4-CANCER) and asking for *Management of Cancer Pain: A Quick Reference Guide for Clinicians.*

Chapter 8
The Use of Controlled-Release Opioids

Robert F. Kaiko

Introduction

Cancer pain requires aggressive management and subtly optimized therapy, fine-tuned to individual needs. The goals include acceptable pain control with minimal side effects, prevention of "breakthrough" pain, relief from pain-associated suffering (including anxiety and depression), and patient rehabilitation.[1-3] The approach chosen must be flexible enough to accommodate an often rapid change in pain status while also striving for stabilized palliation.

Despite present-day clinical and social strides in the management of cancer-related pain, many patients still suffer needlessly[4, 5] not because their discomfort is untreatable, but because it is inadequately treated.[4, 6-11] Opioids, which are capable of both modifying the perception of pain and the reaction to it,[12] are the most effective analgesics for the relief of chronic moderate-to-severe pain. Yet, physicians often underprescribe morphine or other opioids because of improper application of available knowledge concerning these drugs.[4, 5, 9, 13-17] Fear of addiction or poor understanding of the implications of tolerance or physical dependence, phenomena that need not be feared or confused with addiction, are part of the problem. Although poor pain assessments and reluctance to give medication pose major barriers to success, the reluctance by patients to report pain and to take effective medication may worsen their plight.[17] Nevertheless, most patients with cancer[4, 18, 19] (as many as 90%)[4, 13, 18] could achieve pain control through proper pharmacologic treatment.

This chapter discusses the optimal use in cancer patients of controlled-release opioid preparations available in the United States (see manufacturer's prescribing information for each before use). These products include morphine sulfate for oral administration every 12 or 8 hours (MS Contin Tablets, The Purdue Frederick Company, Norwalk, CT, and Oramorph SR, previously known as Roxanol SR, Roxane Laboratories, Inc., Columbus, OH; in this chapter, only the designation Oramorph SR is used for this product, even though cited documents refer to Roxanol SR). An additional controlled-release opioid formulation for oral use, which contains oxycodone hydrochloride (OxyContin Tablets, Purdue Pharma L.P., Norwalk, CT), became available in early 1996, when this chapter had already been submitted for publication. For obvious reasons, it encompassed only the state-of-the-art controlled-release opioids available at the time of writing. The brief following discussion of controlled-release oxycodone tablets, which promise to have a major impact on the therapy of persistent moderate-to-severe pain, was subsequently added. This preparation, the importance of which is becoming increasingly evident in an accumulating body of published literature (bibliography available on request), merits more extensive discussion than possible in this chapter.

In addition to preparations for oral use, controlled-release opioid products include a transdermal system that delivers fentanyl over a 48- to 72-hour period (Duragesic Transdermal system, Janssen Pharmaceutica, Inc., Titusville, NJ).

Controlled-release opioid medication facilitates analgesia on a regular around-the-clock rather than on an "as needed" basis, with each dose administered before the effect of the last has faded.[1, 6, 13, 20, 21] A fixed dosage schedule has many advantages over as needed dosing for patients with chronic pain. It eliminates much of the pain, anxiety, and frustration associated with as needed dosing,[1, 22, 23] and may permit smaller doses of opioids because less drug is required to prevent the recurrence of pain than to relieve it.[1, 24] The right amount for each patient is the amount that controls pain but does not cause unacceptable side effects. After a clinical assessment of the pain syndrome, the physician must determine the most effective strategy to manage it,[18] while keeping in mind that individualization is the key to optimal pain control.

When opioid analgesics are indicated, the cause and type of pain,[25] both of which have major implications for therapy, dictate the treatment modalities. Although it is best to use only a single opioid, additional nonopioid analgesics and adjuvants may significantly enhance palliation. The multidimensional nature of the cancer pain experience (which is influenced by cognitive, emotional, socioenvironmental, and nociceptive factors) warrants management that is also multimodal.[26] Antineoplastic measures, where indicated, are important therapy for pain caused by the tumor.[25] Somatic therapies directed at nociception may lessen the debilitating psychological aspects of cancer pain. Likewise, psychosocial therapies may have an effect on nociception.[26]

Regardless of the type of analgesic chosen, its benefits can be maximized by carefully choosing the initial dose and all subsequent titrations against the patient's level of pain and other effects and by appropriate control of adverse effects. If the response to therapy is less than predicted or if exacerbation of pain occurs, the physician should reassess the treatment approach or search for a possible new cause of the pain.[27]

The oral route of analgesic administration, i.e., that recommended by the World Health Organization and other authorities,[1, 6, 12, 13] satisfies the needs of most cancer patients.[25] Besides the avoidance of painful injections, the advantages of oral administration to patients include simplicity, convenience, economy, and stable opioid blood levels. Additional benefits include relative safety, patient independence and control with mobility, and duration of effect.[1, 6, 12, 13, 28, 29, 32, 33]

Oral opioids are as effective as parenteral opioids (provided there is appropriate dosage adjustment) and can control the pain of most patients with advanced cancer until their final days or hours of life.[15, 30] The controlled-release delivery of oral opioids has the added advantages of less frequent dosing (every 12 or 8 hours), improved medication compliance, and reduced sleep disturbance. This approach allows the patient full freedom of movement and requires minimal intrusion into his or her life.

One must keep in mind, however, that, as with any oral opioid, suspected or confirmed paralytic ileus is an absolute contraindication to any oral opiod, including morphine and oxycodone. In addition, the controlled-release tablets discussed in the next section must be ingested whole rather than chewed or crushed so as to avoid rapid release and the potential absorption of a toxic dose of opioid. Some patients, such as those truly unable to swallow or those experiencing untreatable emesis, cannot use oral therapy.

Controlled-Release Oral Morphine Sulfate

The chronology of oral controlled-release morphine therapy encompasses treatment initiation and dose titration based on the patient's level of pain. After an appropriate dose is established, it is necessary to monitor and reassess the individual's pain and response to treatment. The patient may require titration again due to a change in his or her status. Titration should be performed until adequate pain control or unacceptable side effects occur. Controlled-release oral morphine may be supplemented by a dose of a short-acting morphine for breakthrough pain (intermittent exacerbations of pain that can occur spontaneously) and by coadministration of a nonopioid analgesic and analgesic adjuvants or both once the initial titration establishes an appropriate morphine dosage. When adjusting dosing, the dosing interval should never exceed 12 hours, because the administration of large single doses may lead to acute overdose. Patients who require or prefer 8-hour doses should take one-third of the total daily dosage every 8 hours.

Initiation of Therapy

It is critical to choose the initial dosing regimen of controlled-release morphine sulfate for each patient individually, taking into account his or her prior analgesic treatment experience. Although it is impossible to enumerate every consideration when selecting the initial regimen of oral controlled-release morphine, attention should be given to (1) the daily dose, potency, and precise characteristics of the prior opioid, if any (e.g., whether it is a pure agonist or mixed agonist-antagonist), (2) the reliability of the relative potency estimate used to calculate the needed dose of morphine, (3) the degree of opioid tolerance, if any, and (4) the general condition and medical status of the patient. The following dosing recommendations, therefore, should only be considered suggested approaches based on the series of clinical decisions designed to manage each patient's pain.

Opioid-Naive Patients (Those Using Controlled-Release Morphine as the First Opioid Analgesic) and Patients with Unstable Pain and Medical Status

It is usually advisable to begin a treatment regimen with immediate-release morphine tablets or solution. After establishment of the safe and effective 24-hour immediate-release dose, patients can substitute half that quantity of controlled-release oral morphine every 12 hours. As experience is gained, adjustments can be made to obtain an appropriate balance among pain relief, opioid side effects, and the convenience of the dosing schedule (see section on Dose Titration).

Patients Receiving Fixed-Combination Products

Patients receiving low-dose fixed-combination opioid analgesics, such as medications containing oxycodone hydrochloride plus aspirin or acetaminophen, should start controlled-release morphine therapy with 12-hourly doses of 15 or 30 mg (as two 15-mg tablets if available, to provide more titration options), depending on prior opioid dosage, pain control, and side effects. If pain persists, each 12-hourly dose should be increased by 15 or 30 mg until the pain is controlled; if the patient needs less than 30 mg every 12 hours, but has been started on that amount, the dose can be adjusted downward. A starting dose of 30 or 60 mg , as two 30-mg tablets every 12 hours of the controlled-release medication, titrated upward as indicated, is recommended for those previously treated with high doses of fixed combination analgesics. If

Table 8-1. Multiplication Factors for Converting from Oral Potent Opioids to Controlled-Release Morphine Sulfate

Prior Oral Opioid	Multiplication Factor*
Morphine	1
Hydromorphone	4
Methadone	1.5
Levorphanol	7.5
Meperidine	0.1
Oxycodone (alone)	1

*These multiplication factors are derived from well-controlled relative analgesic potency studies. Prior use of more than one opioid requires that each opioid be considered when estimating the oral morphine dosage. These multiplication factors apply only to the substitution of oral controlled-release morphine sulfate for other oral opioid regimens and not to the reverse conversion. In both situations, the objective is to estimate the new dose conservatively to avoid greater intensity of pharmacologic effects.

the patient needs less than 60 mg of morphine every 12 hours, the dose can be adjusted downward.

Conversion from Oral or Parenteral Strong Opioids

Patients already receiving strong opioid analgesics will require controlled-release morphine dosages greater than those needed by patients receiving nonopioids or fixed-combination analgesics. A complete and thorough knowledge of their recent opioid dosage is critical for selecting the initial dose of oral controlled-release morphine.

It is important to determine drug conversion dosages carefully. Because of uncertainty about and intersubject variation in the relative estimates of opioid potency and incomplete cross-tolerance, initial dosing regimens of MS Contin Tablets should be conservative. It is better to underestimate the 24-hour requirement of oral morphine than to overestimate it. Tables 8-1 and 8-2 can serve as a guide in calculating oral morphine dosages. The conversions provided in the tables use the more conservative parenteral-to-oral morphine equianalgesic milligram dose ratio of 1 to 3.

The daily doses of all concurrently used prior opioids are multiplied by the appropriate multiplication factor from Tables 8-1 (oral) and 8-2 (parenteral), and the results are added to obtain the daily

Table 8-2. Multiplication Factors for Converting from Parenteral Opioids to Controlled-Release Morphine Sulfate

Prior Parenteral Opioid	Multiplication Factor*
Morphine	3
Hydromorphone	20
Methadone	3
Levorphanol	15
Meperidine	0.4

*These multiplication factors are derived from well-controlled relative analgesic potency studies and conservatively assume that 30 mg of orally administered morphine is equianalgesic to 10 mg intramuscular morphine.[20, 82] Prior use of more than one opioid requires that each opioid be considered when estimating the oral morphine dosage. These multiplication factors apply only to the substitution of oral controlled-release morphine sulfate for parenteral opioid regimens and not to the reverse conversion. In both situations, the objective is to estimate the new dose conservatively and to avoid greater intensity of pharmacologic effects.

Table 8-3. Appropriate Tablet Strengths of Controlled-Release Morphine Sulfate for Initial Dosing or Dose Titration

Every 12 Hours* Dose Requirement (mg)	MS Contin Tablet Strength (mg)
Less than 60	15 or 30
60 to less than 120	30 or 60
120 to less than 300	60 or 100
300 to less than 400	100 or 200
400 or more	200

*Some patients may require or prefer every 8-hour dosing, in which case the total daily requirement of controlled-release morphine sulfate tablets should be divided by three and administered every 8 hours.

Table 8-4. Suggested Titration Ladder

12-Hourly Dosage of Controlled-Release Morphine Sulfate (mg)*	Individual Doses of Immediate-Release Morphine Sulfate Added for Breakthrough Pain (mg)
30	10
60	20
90	30
120	40
180	60
240	80
300	100
400	130
500	150
500+	150+

* Increase the dose, not the dosing frequency, using increments approximating 50% of low doses and 25% of higher doses of controlled-release morphine sulfate. These increases are permitted as often as every 24 hours, if needed.

dosage of oral controlled-release morphine sulfate (which is halved for every 12-hour administration). (See Table 8-3 for recommended MS Contin Tablet strengths for the first prescription.) Upward or downward titration should proceed as indicated.

Dose Titration

Dose titration is important to analgesic treatment throughout its entire course, beginning with the initial dosages. It is the critical element in cancer pain therapy because of the large interindividual variability in analgesic requirements that characterizes such patients.[31] The following general principles apply to dose titration of oral controlled-release morphine sulfate.

Stepwise Progression of Analgesic Therapy

The dosage should be titrated as necessary to control pain, while maintaining the 12-hourly interval, until either adequate pain control or unacceptable side effects occur. The step-by-step plan depicted in Table 8-4 is a guide to this process. This strategy broadly involves initial titration of the daily dosage, indicated increase in dosage (as often as once a day if needed), management of breakthrough pain with immediate-release morphine, and further increases of controlled-release morphine dosage as required. Throughout this process, side effects are managed prophylactically or therapeutically. If signs of excessive opioid effects appear early in a dosing interval, the next dose should be reduced; if side effects persist, they should be treated. If titration leads to inadequate analgesia (i.e., breakthrough pain late in the dosing interval), the interval may be shortened to 8 hours. Alternatively, oral controlled-release morphine therapy may be supplemented by a dose of short-acting morphine (see Table 8-4 and the section entitled "Immediate-

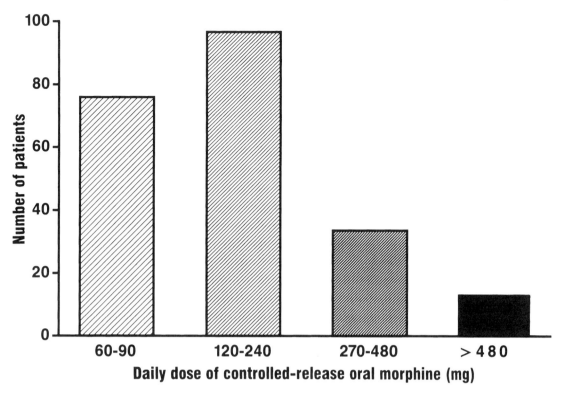

Figure 8-1. Mean daily dose of controlled-release oral morphine administered to 218 cancer patients; data from nine dose titration studies conducted in the United States. (Reprinted with permission from RK Kaiko, R Grandy, B Oshlack, et al. The United States experience with oral controlled-release morphine [MS Contin Tablets]: Parts I and II. Review of nine dose titration studies and clinical pharmacology of 15-mg, 30-mg, 60-mg, and 100-mg tablet strengths in normal subjects. Cancer 1989;63:2348.)

Release Rescue Medication") or a nonopioid analgesic. It is important to note that the as needed dose of immediate-release morphine is approximately one-fourth to one-third of the 12-hour dose of controlled-release morphine.

The dosage of oral controlled-release morphine should not exceed that which controls pain with few or no supplemental rescue doses of immediate-release morphine needed and without unacceptable side effects. The appropriate dosage varies widely with the individual, as illustrated in composite data from a total of 218 cancer patients[32] in nine dose titration studies (Figure 8-1). Some tolerant patients are able to take up to several thousand milligrams per day without any significant problems[22]; nevertheless, such dosage escalation should not be undertaken lightly and not without appropriate assessment of effects and dosage adjustments.

Titration leads to initial stabilization of pain on a particular dosage, after which time tablet strengths

can be changed, as appropriate to reduce the number of tablets ingested.

Appropriate Tablet Strengths for Different Doses

Table 8-3 relates ascending 12-hour dose requirements in the titration process to tablet strength. Combinations of tablet strengths may be used where appropriate.

Immediate-Release Rescue Medication

Immediate-release morphine sulfate (e.g., MSIR tablets or oral solution, The Purdue Frederick, Co.) must be available for breakthrough and incident pain. Breakthrough pain (defined as flair-ups of underlying pain during regularly administered analgesic therapy) may occur[33] if plasma drug levels are insufficient, such as late in a dosing interval. Incident pain is related to specific activities, such as eating, defecation, walking, or socializing. The rationale for selecting morphine sulfate rather than another opioid as the immediate-release rescue drug is predicated on the accurate calculation of its dosage as a more or less constant fraction of a given daily dose of morphine, as well as the consistency, in terms of pharmacologic effects and metabolism, of both the controlled-release form and immediate-release rescue medication.

To prevent or modify anticipated incident pain, the immediate-release opioid should be given 1 hour prior to the pain-causing activity. Immediate-release morphine should be administered as needed, but not more frequently than every 4 hours at about one-fourth to one-third the 12-hour dose of the controlled-release formulation. If the patient needs more than two doses per day of rescue medication, the physician should consider increasing the dose of the controlled-release medication. It is almost always appropriate to increase the daily dose rather than to reduce the dosing interval. When immediate-release morphine is used often for incident pain, upward titration of the 12-hour controlled-release morphine dosage is not usually indicated.

Stabilization

Although usually a temporary state for cancer pain patients, stabilization is the maintenance of consistent, undiminished efficacy with no exacerbation of pain over a reasonable segment of time, permitting constant analgesic therapy both in terms of dosage and frequency of administration. Each patient's understanding of stabilization depends on the degree of pain and severity of side effects accepted. Some patients find that even moderate pain represents an improvement over their previous pain experience and are willing to tolerate it, perhaps, thereby, averting distressing side effects, whereas others will accept side effects in return for a pain-free state. Still others achieve the ideal result, i.e., complete analgesia without side effects. Although the patient may be stabilized, it is still essential to have a continued availability of rescue medication available.

The two primary reasons for destabilization are exacerbation of the disease process and development of tolerance. Pain monitoring may lead to investigation of disease status as the possible cause of a change in pain status. By careful monitoring and skillful communication, the individuals charged with

the patient's pain management are sometimes the first to suspect that the course of the disease has worsened. Regardless of the cause of destabilization, appropriate dose titration can resolve the problem.

Conversion from Controlled-Release Oral Morphine to Parenteral Opioids

If patients are no longer able to swallow and parenteral opioids are chosen to replace oral morphine, a ratio of 6 mg oral to 1 mg parenteral drug is appropriate, unlike the ratio (3 to 1) suitable for conversion in the opposite direction. In both cases, the objective is to estimate the new dose conservatively.

Special Populations

Children

Dosing guidelines for the available controlled-release morphine products have not been established in children. According to product prescribing information,[34] Oramorph SR has not been evaluated in this population and is not recommended for pediatric use. MS Contin Tablets, although used in limited pediatric studies, have not been systematically evaluated in children.

Some investigators believe that children eliminate morphine less effectively and are more sensitive to its respiratory depressant effect than adults.[35] However, the pharmacokinetics and effect on respiration of morphine in children, at least those older than 5–6 months, appear comparable with those in adults.[35–37] Available data show that the plasma clearance of morphine is significantly higher in children and older infants than in neonates,[36, 38] and that the neonates can form glucuronide conjugates with morphine less readily.[36]

Certain investigators have used oral controlled-release morphine sulfate (the formulation in MS Contin Tablets) successfully for cancer-related pain in children.[39, 40]

The Elderly

The pharmacodynamic effects of morphine may vary more in older adults than in younger populations. Patients differ widely in the effective initial dose, rate of development of tolerance, and the frequency and intensity of associated adverse effects with increasing doses. It is important to individualize dosages carefully for elderly patients.

Generally, the elderly show increased sensitivity to morphine, apparently because of altered disposition of the drug.[41] Increases in age are associated with increases in duration of analgesia. Morphine-induced respiratory depression occurs most frequently in elderly and debilitated individuals and those suffering from conditions accompanied by hypoxia or hypercapnia, where even moderate therapeutic doses may dangerously decrease pulmonary ventilation. [34]

Patients with Impaired Hepatic Function

Hepatic metabolism appears to be responsible for most of the clearance of morphine from the body. Patients with hepatic dysfunction may have reduced drug clearance and increased oral bioavailability. Morphine has been reported to cause excessive sedation and even precipitate hepatic encephalopathy in patients with liver cirrhosis. This finding prompted Hasselstrom et al. [42] to study its disposition after a single oral 10-mg dose and a 4-mg intravenous dose in six patients who had this disease (of unspecified severity) but did not exhibit actual signs of encephalopathy. The cirrhotic patients demonstrated a mean oral availability of 100% as compared with 40% in patients with normal liver function and an elimination half-life of 4.4 hours versus 2.3 hours for the normal controls, respectively. Although the electroencephalographic pattern did not deteriorate, some patients did report experiencing sedation. The investigators concluded that the high oral bioavailability and prolonged elimination half-life of morphine in patients with hepatic cirrhosis warrant cautious dosing despite the absence of electroencephalographic effects.

Unlike Hasselstrom, Patwardhan et al. [43] found the disposition and elimination of morphine to be unaffected by moderate-to-severe cirrhosis, as compared with normal subjects. These investigators administered a single intravenous dose of 0.15 mg per kg, with a maximum of 15 mg. Whereas sedation was present in normal subjects, it was only mild, with no evidence of hepatic coma in the cirrhotic group. The mean plasma concentration–time profiles of unchanged morphine and morphine glu-

curonide were qualitatively and quantitatively similar in both groups, with levels of conjugated drug declining more slowly than those of unchanged drug. The cirrhotic patients showed decreased clearance and a prolonged elimination half-life of indocyanine green (a drug transported to bile without metabolic transformation), from which the presence of intrahepatic or extrahepatic shunting was inferred. The authors suggested significant extrahepatic glucuronidation as a possible reason for the seemingly normal metabolism and pharmacokinetics of morphine in the cirrhotic patients. However, they cautioned that prolonged use of this drug might lead to different results. They also stressed the need for further study before the routine use of morphine in patients with hepatic disease could be justified.

In a subsequent review, Säwe[44] pointed to recommendations in the literature for cautious morphine dosing in patients with hepatic dysfunction, regardless of the reported effects of such impairment on the drug's metabolism and pharmacokinetics. These views were based on clinical evidence of increased sensitivity to the pharmacodynamic effects of morphine, and of its increased oral bioavailability, among such patients.

Patients with Impaired Renal Function

Although hepatic metabolism appears to be responsible for clearance of most of the morphine from the body, it has been claimed that patients with chronic renal failure are more sensitive to the pharmacologic effects of morphine than normal subjects, and that these patients experience a prolonged duration of action of the drug.[45]

Some controversy remains regarding the disposition of morphine in the presence of impaired renal function, particularly as a result of different analytical techniques used and their varied specificity for unchanged morphine.[45] The demonstration of a variable volume of distribution but normal clearance of unchanged morphine in patients with renal failure[45, 46] led to speculation regarding the possible role of morphine metabolites.[47] Although patients with renal failure metabolize morphine normally, its metabolites are not readily eliminated in oliguric or anuric states,[46] and thus can accumulate.[47, 48] A preliminary study has found marked accumulation of morphine-3-glucuronide.[44] Even though morphine is primarily metabolized to inactive metabolites,

Table 8-5. Single-Dose Pharmacokinetic Comparison of Two Controlled-Release Morphine Sulfate Preparations*

	MS Contin Tablets	Oramorph SR	Significance of Difference
C_{max} (ng/ml)	29.4	16.8	*P* < 0.0001
T_{max} (hr)	2.7	2.2	NS
AUC_{0-12} (ng/ml × hr)	147	116	*P* < 0.01
AUC_{0-24} (ng/ml × hr)	176	159	NS

*Mean values: n = 18.
C_{max} = maximum plasma morphine concentration; T_{max} = time to C_{max}; AUC_{0-12} and AUC_{0-24} = area under 12- and 24-hour plasma morphine curve, respectively; NS = not significant; hr = time after administration.
Source: Adapted from RF Kaiko, R Grandy, JJ Savarese, et al. Comparative Bioavailability of Two Controlled-Release Oral Morphine Tablets [abstract]. In The American Pain Society. Sixth General Meeting. Program, Abstracts, and Meeting Information. Chicago: The American Pain Society, 1986;79.

renal disease can result in markedly reduced elimination of the active metabolite, morphine-6-glucuronide. Accumulation of this conjugate can lead to clinical signs of opioid intoxication.[47]

Although titration should be sufficient to deal with slowly changing or reduced renal function, discontinuation of morphine is indicated in patients who have unstable renal function or who are anephric.

Differences Between MS Contin Tablets and Oramorph SR

MS Contin Tablets are marketed in numerous countries, having been first introduced in the United Kingdom in 1981. Numerous published clinical studies have evaluated MS Contin, including many well-controlled, multiple-dose studies and a large number of less well-controlled studies.

The two formulations have different physical, pharmacokinetic, and clinical characteristics. As detailed in the following section, results of biopharmaceutical studies indicate that the two products are not bioequivalent. In addition, clinical differences were observed in single-dose efficacy studies, but it remains to be determined whether these differences are evident in repeated dose studies. These findings illustrate the profound effects that a delivery system of even inert components can have on a formulation's performance as compared with other products with the same active drug substance at the same milligram dose.

Pharmacokinetics

Two single-dose bioavailability studies in healthy volunteers [49, 50] initially demonstrated pharmacokinetic differences between MS Contin Tablets and Oramorph SR tablets. They showed that MS Contin Tablets yield a substantially higher maximal plasma morphine concentration (C_{max}), and a significantly higher 0- to 12-hour bioavailability (area under 12-hour plasma morphine curve, AUC_{0-12}) relative to Oramorph SR, and, therefore, a lack of bioequivalence. Table 8-5 and Figure 8-2 present the results of one of these investigations,[50] a definitive sequential crossover study in which a single two-tablet dose was used in normal subjects, which demonstrates that the two preparations are not bioequivalent.

On the other hand, the authors of a steady-state study claim that their investigation shows bioequivalence between the two formulations.[51] The difference in C_{max} at steady state was not as prominent as in the foregoing single-dose trial; however, the plasma time curves presented are clearly not superimposable or bioequivalent. Morphine concentration rose more rapidly, whereas the extent of absorption was comparable. The time to maximal concentration (T_{max}) differed by more than 26%.

There are also differences regarding the effects of food intake on the pharmacokinetics of Oramorph SR and MS Contin Tablets.[52, 53] Data from a study in which MS Contin Tablets were administered to normal subjects after a morning fast or after a high-fat morning meal in a single 30-mg

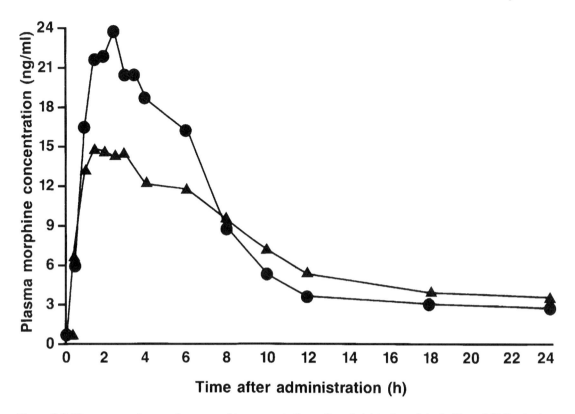

Figure 8-2. Time course of mean plasma morphine concentrations after administration of single 60-mg MS Contin doses (two 30-mg tablets) (●) and Oramorph SR (▲) to 18 normal young male adults. (Reprinted with permission from RF Kaiko, R Grandy, JJ Savarese, et al. Comparative Bioavailability of Two Controlled-Release Oral Morphine Tablets [abstract]. In The American Pain Society. Sixth General Meeting. Program, Abstracts, and Meeting Information. Chicago: The American Pain Society, 1986;79.)

dose yielded superimposable curves with no significant effects of the food on any of the pharmacokinetic values obtained (AUC, C_{max}, and T_{max}).[53] A separate study involving Oramorph SR showed a significantly greater AUC on dosing with a high-fat morning meal ($P < 0.05$).[52] Additional dosing with Oramorph SR during an evening fast yielded a similar AUC but a significantly longer T_{max} relative to dosing during a morning fast. Maximal concentrations and apparent elimination half-lives did not differ significantly among the three treatment groups.

Clinical Experience

In one open-label study a clinical comparison was made of orally administered MS Contin Tablets and Oramorph SR tablets in 37 patients with advanced cancer. The patients received 60–420 mg of morphine daily in 30-mg tablets, for 2–80 days.[54] Oramorph SR was given at 6- to 10-hour intervals and MS Contin Tablets every 8–14 hours. The patients were followed primarily at home under the supervision of a local hospice care team. Thirty-five of the 37 patients obtained good-to-excellent analgesia (only two required rescue medication), and 17 of 19 patients who took the tablets for 20 or more days achieved stable dosage schedules. The authors concluded that MS Contin Tablets were preferable because of their smaller tablet size and longer duration of analgesic effect. None of the 37 patients experienced any serious complications from the therapy.

The difference between MS Contin Tablets and Oramorph SR in the extent of clinical experience was also evident on separate comparison of each drug with immediate-release morphine. Clinical data accumulated in well-controlled double-blind and open studies or gathered empirically, consistently demonstrated at least equal efficacy and safety of morphine in the Contin system relative to immediate-release oral morphine. One published report describes a controlled clinical investigation of Oramorph SR.[55] This study was a two-center, double-blind, randomized, crossover, repeated-dose comparison of 12-hourly Oramorph SR and immediate-release oral morphine sulfate solution, every 4 hours, in 27 hospitalized completed patients with chronic pain from advanced cancer. The investigators observed no substantial difference between the two regimens with respect to efficacy and side effects.

Tablet Size and Strength

MS Contin Tablets are significantly smaller than Oramorph SR tablets. Both preparations come in 30-, 60-, and 100-mg strengths. MS Contin Tablets are additionally available as 15-mg and 200-mg tablets.

Conversion from Controlled-Release Oral Morphine to Other Opioids

Although oral opioids are as effective as parenteral opioids when given in appropriately adjusted dosages, poor pain control with oral morphine due to inadequate dosage is widely, though erroneously, ascribed to the inferiority of the oral drug over the parenteral drug. This assumption, based on myth rather than valid criteria, may stem from the well-known lesser bioavailability of the oral forms, for which dosage adjustments can compensate. Orally administered morphine is now recognized as an effective analgesic when taken in appropriate doses.[1, 6, 12, 13, 18, 20, 56] Unless delivery of opioid analgesics by this route is inappropriate (as in patients truly unable to swallow or patients experiencing untreatable emesis), the routine use of invasive therapy should be avoided. A recent survey[57] demonstrated the need for more specific criteria and guidelines for this form of analgesia. It found that many patients who are able to swallow are nevertheless transferred from oral analgesics to invasive routes in the erroneous belief that these routes are more effective. This common misconception stems from widespread unawareness that considerably higher oral doses than parenteral doses are required for equianalgesic potency to compensate for differences in bioavailability.[24] Nevertheless, if the oral route becomes unfeasible, other options including rectal, subcutaneous, intravenous, and transdermal administration of opioids are available (the latter in the form of the controlled-release fentanyl system [Duragesic]). This strong opioid preparation may be a useful alternative to continuous subcutaneous opioid infusion in relatively stable patients.[31] According to the manufacturer, the relative analgesic potency of transdermally delivered fentanyl to morphine approximates 1 to 20 to 1 to 30 in patients with acute pain who are not tolerant to opioids.[34]

Controlled-Release Oxycodone (OxyContin Tablets)

Overview

The present section (which was added after this chapter's submission for publication, and just shortly before its appearance in print), is primarily based on the current prescribing information for OxyContin Tablets. (Relevant citations from the published literature are available on request.) As previously stated, controlled-release oral oxycodone hydrochloride (OxyContin Tablets) became available in the United States in early 1996 for the management of moderate-to-severe pain, where use of an opioid analgesic is appropriate for more than a few days. This formulation, which is suitable for pain associated with cancer or with certain nonmalignant conditions such as osteoarthritis or low-back disorders, is available in small tablets of different strengths that are dose proportional for both maximum plasma oxycodone concentration and extent of absorption.

Controlled-release oral oxycodone combines advantageous characteristics of both the active drug substance and the delivery system to provide the efficacy and safety of immediate-release oral oxycodone with the convenience of 12-hour dosing. Like morphine and other pure agonist opioids, the oxycodone drug substance has no ceiling effect for analgesia and allows upward dose titration as individually needed and tolerated. The oral bioavailability as compared with the parenteral bioavailability of oxycodone is among the highest reported in the literature for commonly used opioids, and more than twice that of morphine, due to less presystemic metabolism. In controlled-release oxycodone, the delivery system ensures the measured release of OxyContin from the tablet matrix via a dual-release mechanism, which allows biphasic absorption. This pattern is characterized by initial prompt release and absorption of oxycodone within 1 hour of dosing, followed by a more protracted phase that ensures effective blood concentrations over a 12-hour interval. Normal volunteers exhibited one absorption half-life of oxycodone at 0.6 hours and a second at 6.9 hours with OxyContin Tablets, as compared with a single half-life of absorption of 0.4 hours associated with use of immediate-release oxycodone. The purpose of the dual-release mechanism is to prolong analgesia without compromising either its early onset or its degree when compared with immediate-release oxycodone. Results of controlled clinical studies are consistent with this pattern, showing onset of analgesia within 1 hour of dosing in most patients, with pain control continued over the following 12 hours. In spite of its prolonged analgesic action, controlled-release oxycodone yields peak and trough plasma oxycodone concentrations similar to those obtained with immediate-release oxycodone at equivalent total daily doses, though with a 50% reduction in the rate of fluctuation (one instead of two peaks per day). Stable pain control is achieved early in the course of treatment every 12 hours with OxyContin Tablets, evidently due to the attainment of steady-state plasma oxycodone concentrations within 24–36 hours after the start of dosing. Pharmacokinetic and pharmacodynamic evaluations demonstrated dose-plasma concentration-effect relationships of this preparation.

Food has no significant effect on the absorption of oxycodone from OxyContin Tablets, in contrast to immediate-release oxycodone preparations. Oxycodone release from the tablets is pH-independent.

OxyContin Tablets are an appropriate opioid formulation with which to start and stay in a stepwise, progressive pain management scheme. Oxycodone in fixed-combination products is well established for use in Step 2 of the World Health Organization (WHO)[6] pain management program. However, dose titration with fixed combinations is limited by the toxicity associated with the nonopioid component. As a single-entity agent, controlled-release oxycodone escapes this limitation and can be titrated to the appropriate level for pain control. It can be coadministered with a variety of nonopioid analgesics and adjuvants, each at the appropriate dose and schedule.

Well-controlled clinical studies have clearly and consistently demonstrated the analgesic efficacy and safety of controlled-release oxycodone every 12 hours for moderate-to-severe pain due to cancer or nonmalignant disorders, such as osteoarthritis and low-back disorders. In two double-blind parallel-group studies involving cancer patients, controlled-release oxycodone administered every 12 hours demonstrated analgesic efficacy equivalent to that of immediate-release oxycodone given four times daily at equivalent total daily doses. Peak and trough plasma concentrations were similar to those with the immediate-release drug. With titration to analgesic effect and proper use of rescue medication, nearly every patient achieved adequate pain control with OxyContin Tablets. The controlled-release drug also showed equivalent efficacy to immediate-release oxycodone, dosed four times daily, at the same total daily doses, in a double-blind crossover trial. In most patients, doses of both preparations could be titrated to stable, acceptable pain control within 2 days.

Initiation of Therapy

The previously listed important considerations in the initiation of controlled-release oral morphine therapy also pertain to controlled-release oxycodone, including the patient's general condition and medical status, dosage, potency and kinds or prior analgesics, and the prior opioid exposure and opioid tolerance. Care should be taken to use low initial doses of OxyContin Tablets in patients who are not already opioid tolerant, especially those under concurrent treatment with muscle relaxants, sedatives, or other medications that act on the central nervous system. As with morphine, individualized initiation of the dosage regimen is critical.

Patients Not Already Taking Opioids (Opioid Naive)

Clinical trials have shown that patients may initiate analgesic therapy with OxyContin Tablets. A reasonable starting dose for most patients who are opioid naive is 10 mg every 12 hours. If a nonopioid analgesic, such as aspirin, acetaminophen, or a NSAID is being provided, it may be continued. If the current nonopioid is discontinued, early upward

Table 8-6. Multiplication Factors for Converting the Daily Dose of a Prior Opioid to the Daily Dose of Oral Oxycodone*

Prior Opioid	Oral	Parenteral
Oxycodone	1	—
Codeine	0.15	—
Fentanyl	Transdermal[†]	Transdermal[†]
Hydrocodone	0.9	—
Hydromorphone	4	20
Levorphanol	7.5	15
Meperidine	0.1	0.4
Methadone	1.5	3
Morphine	0.5	3

*In mg/day prior opioid × factor = mg/day oral oxycodone. To be used only for conversion to oral oxycodone. For patients receiving high-dose parenteral opioids, a more conservative conversion is warranted. For example, for high-dose parenteral morphine, use 1.5 instead of 3 as a multiplication factor.
[†]Conversion from Fentanyl Transdermal System (TS) to OxyContin Tablets. Eighteen hours following the removal of the transdermal fentanyl patch, patients can be initiated on OxyContin. Although there has been no systematic assessment of such conversion, a conservative oxycodone dose, approximately 10 mg every 12 hours of OxyContin, should be initially substituted for each 25 µg/hr fentanyl transdermal patch. The patient should be followed closely for early titration as there is limited clinical experience with this conversion.

dose titration of OxyContin Tablets may be required using standard conversion ratios (Table 8-6), and the 24-hour dose divided in half for 12-hourly administration. The dose should be rounded down for the tablet strengths available (10-, 20-, and 40-mg tablets). All other around-the-clock opioid drugs should be discontinued when controlled-release opioids are initiated.

Conversion from Fixed-Ratio Opioid/Nonopioid Combination Drugs

Patients who are taking one to five tablets/capsules/caplets per day of a regular strength fixed-combination opioid/nonopioid should be started on 10–20 mg of OxyContin every 12 hours. For patients taking six to nine tablets/capsules/caplets, a starting dose of 20–30 mg every 12 hours is suggested and for those taking 10–12 tablets/caplets/capsules daily, 30–40 mg of oxycodone every 12 hours should be considered. The nonopioid may be continued as a

separate drug. Alternatively, a different nonopioid analgesic may be selected. If the decision is made to discontinue the nonopioid, consideration should be given to early upward titration of OxyContin Tablets.

Patients Currently on Opioid Therapy

If a patient has been receiving opioid-containing medications prior to OxyContin therapy, the composite total daily dose of the other opioids should be determined.

1. Using standard conversion ratio estimates (see Table 8-6) multiply the milligram per day of the previous opioids by the appropriate multiplication factors to obtain the equivalent total daily dose of oral oxycodone.
2. Divide this 24-hour oxycodone dose in half to obtain the twice a day (every 12 hours) dose of OxyContin.
3. Round down to a dose that is appropriate for the tablet strengths available.
4. Discontinue all other around-the-clock opioid drugs when OxyContin therapy is initiated.

No fixed conversion ratio is likely to be satisfactory in all patients, especially patients receiving large opioid doses. The recommended doses shown in Table 8-6 are only starting points, and close observation and frequent titration are indicated until patients are stable on the new therapy.

Conversion from Transdermal Fentanyl to Controlled-Release Oral Oxycodone

OxyContin treatment can be initiated 18 hours following the removal of the transdermal fentanyl patch.
Although there has been no systematic assessment of such conversion, a conservative oxycodone dose, approximately 10 mg every 12 hours of OxyContin, should be initially substituted for each 25 µg of fentanyl transdermal patch. The patient should be followed closely for early titration as there is only limited clinical experience with this conversion.

Dose Titration

The short elimination half-life and time to steady state of oxycodone, as well as the controlled-release characteristics of OxyContin Tablets, are reasons why the preparation can be readily used for dose titration; immediate-release oxycodone is not required for titration but only as rescue medication.

Table 8-7 outlines the suggested titration process for OxyContin Tablets, which requires availability of a supplementary short-acting opioid (e.g., immediate-release oxycodone tablets or solution) as rescue medication for breakthrough and incident pain. Rescue oxycodone supplements should be given as needed but not more often than every 6 hours, in approximate individual doses of 25–33% of the 12-hourly dose of controlled-release oxycodone. If more than two rescue doses are required per 24 hours, the treating health care provider should consider increasing the dose. To prevent or modify incident pain, immediate-release oxycodone should be administered 1 hour before its anticipated occurrence.

After establishing a safe and effective 24-hour dose, the health care provider must periodically reassess the patient's pain response to treatment. A change in pain status may require further dose titration. Different tablet strengths of OxyContin may be combined in individual doses. Even when the patient is stabilized, the continued availability of rescue medication is essential.

The analgesic oral dose of controlled-release oxycodone varies widely with the individual. Even though administration every 12 hours of equal (symmetric) morning and evening doses is appropriate for the majority of patients, some may benefit from unequal (asymmetric) morning and evening dosing tailored to their pain pattern.

Maintenance Therapy

The intent of the titration period is to establish a patient-specific 12-hour dose that will maintain adequate analgesia without unacceptable side effects for as long as pain relief is required. Should pain recur, the dose can be incrementally increased to reestablish control, using therapy adjustments as outlined previously. During chronic therapy, the continued need for around-the-clock opioid therapy should be reassessed periodically (e.g., every 6–12 months, as appropriate).

Clinical studies have shown a lack of significant accumulation of oxycodone or its metabolites during long-term administration of OxyContin Tablets.

Table 8-7. OxyContin Titration Guide

Tablet Strength (mg)	OxyContin Tablets (mg Every 12-Hour Dose)	IR Oxycodone Dose for Rescue (mg)
10	10*	5
	20	5
	30	10
20	40	10
	60	15
40	80	20
	120	30

Note: Continue titrating, if necessary, using these guidelines: Titrate the dose if more than two rescue doses per day are needed. Titrate dosage every 1–2 days, if necessary. Increase the every 12-hours dose by 25–50%, if necessary; do not increase the dosing frequency. Manage breakthrough pain with IR oxycodone at one-fourth to one-third the 12-hourly OxyContin dose. Elevate the OxyContin dose when more than two rescue doses are required per day.
*For patients taking OxyContin, 10 mg every 12 hours, the next titration step should be 20 mg every 12 hours and breakthrough pain should be managed with immediate-release oxycodone, 5 mg.

The preparation can be used safely and effectively as maintenance therapy during chronic analgesic management.

Special Populations

Children

Safety and effectiveness in pediatric patients younger than 18 years have not been established with this dosage form of oxycodone. However, oxycodone has been used extensively in the pediatric population in other dosage forms, as have the excipients used in this formulation. No specific increased risk is expected from the use of this form of oxycodone in pediatric patients old enough to safely take tablets if dosing is adjusted for body weight.

The Elderly

In controlled pharmacokinetic studies in elderly subjects (older than 65 years) the clearance of oxycodone appeared to be slightly reduced. Compared with young adults, the plasma concentrations of oxycodone were increased by approximately 15%.

In clinical trials with appropriate initiation of therapy and dose titration, no untoward or unexpected side effects were seen based on age, and the usual doses and dosing intervals are appropriate for the geriatric patient. As with all opioids, the starting dose should be reduced to one-third to one-half the usual doses and careful dose titration is warranted.

Gender Differences

In pharmacokinetic studies, opioid-naive female subjects demonstrate up to 25% higher average plasma concentrations and a greater frequency of typical opioid adverse events than male subjects, even after adjustment for body weight. The clinical relevance of a difference of this magnitude is low for a drug intended for chronic usage at individualized dosages, and there was no male to female difference detected for efficacy or adverse events in clinical trials.

Patients with Hepatic Impairment

Study of OxyContin Tablets in patients with hepatic impairment indicates higher plasma oxycodone concentrations in this population than in those with normal hepatic function. The initiation of therapy at one-third to one-half the usual doses, and careful dose titration, are warranted.

Patients with Renal Impairment

In patients with renal impairment, as evidenced by decreased creatinine clearance (<60 ml per minute), the concentrations of oxycodone in the plasma are approximately 50% higher than in subjects with normal renal function. Dose initiation should follow a conservative approach and dosages should be adjusted according to the clinical situation.

Controlled-Release Transdermal Fentanyl

It should be appreciated that based on reports of unacceptable "misuse," the dosage and administration guidelines for transdermal fentanyl were revised toward more restricted usage in 1994. It is, therefore, imperative to consult all current labeling for the product.

The fentanyl patch (Duragesic Transdermal System) was initially investigated in a well-controlled acute pain model in perioperative studies involving surgical procedures expected to produce various intensities of pain. An open prospective survey was also conducted in patients with cancer-related pain. Based on results of these trials, transdermal fentanyl was found to be effective in both populations, but was considered unsuitable for postoperative pain because of a 4% incidence of hypoventilation in these patients.[34] On January 17, 1994, the manufacturer of Duragesic notified health care professionals of the previously mentioned revised product labeling, prompted by several patient deaths since the introduction of this product in 1991.[58] The fatalities included a 9-year-old child after a tonsillectomy and a 17-year-old adolescent after a "wisdom tooth" extraction. Based on the possibility of life-threatening hypoventilation, the warning notice issued listed the following contraindications for Duragesic[58]: (1) acute or postoperative pain, including that after outpatient surgery, (2) mild or intermittent pain that can otherwise be managed by "lesser means" such as acetaminophen-opioid combinations, nonsteroidal analgesics, or short-acting opioids administered as needed, and (3) use of doses exceeding 25 μg per hour at the initiation of opioid therapy. (See also warnings later in this chapter concerning restricted use of Duragesic in children younger than 12 years old or in patients younger than 18 years old who weigh less than 50 kg.)

Transdermal fentanyl is administered in the form of a rectangular transparent unit that adheres to the skin. As with oral controlled-release opioid analgesics, doses must be individualized and should be reassessed at regular intervals. Although offering some advantages over certain other routes of drug delivery, such as the possibility of very infrequent administration, the transdermal system also has potentially serious, possibly even life-threatening, disadvantages, largely related to the pharmacokinetic properties.

Pharmacokinetic Characteristics as Related to Efficacy and Safety

Pharmacokinetic considerations are paramount when using the patch. Because of individual differences in skin permeability and body clearance of fentanyl, serum concentrations show wide individual variations, as graphically illustrated in the product's labeling.[34] Peak serum levels, and hence maximum pain control, occur no sooner than 1–3 days after contact with the skin.[34, 59, 60]Alternative analgesia must be provided during this period or longer, because 6 days or more may pass before the steady state is reached,[59, 60] i.e., after two or more sequential 72-hour applications.[34] Dosing guidelines provide for adjustment not more often than every 6 days (after initial titration on the third day).[59] After removal of the fentanyl patch, systemic absorption from the skin continues slowly, with the elimination half-life averaging about 17 hours[60] or more (as long as 34 hours) in individual cases.[59] The prolonged half-life after removal may pose difficulties in reversing adverse reactions rapidly.[61]

Serum concentrations derived from the fentanyl patch could theoretically increase by as much as one-third when body temperature is 102°F, because increases in temperature cause more fentanyl to be released and also produce increased skin permeability.[60] Therefore, patients wearing the fentanyl patch who develop a fever should be monitored for opioid side effects, and the dose should be adjusted if necessary.[58] The current information on the Duragesic Transdermal System requires that patients be advised to avoid exposing the application site to direct heat sources, including electric blankets, heating pads, heat lamps, saunas, and hot tubs.

Choice of Initial Doses

As with oral morphine, attention should be given to (1) the daily dose, potency, and characteristics (pure agonist or agonist-antagonist) of any prior opioid, (2) the reliability of the relative potency estimate used to calculate the needed fentanyl dose, (3) the degree of preexisting tolerance, if any (the most important factor in determining the appropriate initial dose), and (4) the patient's general condition and medical status. During the initial application of Duragesic, patients should have short-acting analgesics available until therapeutic serum fentanyl concentrations are attained. Thereafter, some patients still may require periodic supplemental doses of other short-acting analgesics for breakthrough pain.

Opioid-Naive Patients

Because most patients in the clinical trials conducted have been converted to this system from other opioids, there has been no systemic evaluation of Duragesic as an initial opioid analgesic in the management of chronic pain. In the absence of opioid tolerance, the initial dose must not exceed 25 μg per hour (see also previously mentioned notice of January 17, 1994[58]).

Patients Receiving Oral or Parenteral Opioids

The manufacturer recommends calculation of the analgesic requirement for the previous 24 hours, and conversion of this amount to the equianalgesic 24-hour dose of morphine and then to the corresponding dose of fentanyl (see conversion tables B and C from the product prescribing information[34]). The conversion ratio from oral morphine to Duragesic is conservative, and 50% of patients are likely to require a dose increase after initial application of the system.

Dose Titration

The initial fentanyl dosage may be increased after 3 days. Thereafter, upward titration may continue at 6-day intervals until analgesic efficacy is attained. Supplementary doses of a short-acting analgesic are usually needed during upward titration.[34] Appropriate dosage increments should be based on the daily dose of supplementary opioids, using the ratio of 90 mg every 24 hours of oral morphine to a 25 μg per hour increase in the fentanyl dose; doses greater than 25 μg per hour are indicated for use only in opioid-tolerant patients.[34] Multiple Duragesic systems may be used for delivery rates in excess of 100 μg per hour.

The majority of patients are adequately maintained with transdermal fentanyl, administered every 72 hours. A small number of patients require application of the system every 48 hours. It may take up to 6 days after a dose is increased for the patient to reach equilibrium on the new dose of Duragesic. Therefore, patients should maintain this new dose through two applications before any further increase occurs.[34]

Discontinuation

Some patients will require a change to other opioid therapy when the dose of fentanyl exceeds 300 μg per hour. To initiate conversion, remove the patch and begin treatment with half the equianalgesic dose of the new opioid 12–18 hours later (it takes 17 hours or more for the fentanyl serum concentration to decrease by 50% after the system is removed). Titrate the dose of the new analgesic based on the reported pain intensity until adequate analgesia occurs. For patients requiring discontinuation of opioids, gradual decrements are recommended because it is not known at what dose level the opioid may be discontinued without producing the signs and symptoms of abrupt withdrawal.[34]

Special Populations

Children

The safety and efficacy of the fentanyl transdermal system in children has not been established.[34] The most recent labeling contraindicates the use of Duragesic in children younger than 12 years of age or in individuals younger than 18 years of age who weigh less than 50 kg, except in an authorized investigational research setting.[58]

Elderly, Cachectic, or Debilitated Patients

Results of a pilot study of the pharmacokinetics of intravenous fentanyl in geriatric patients indicate that the clearance of fentanyl may be greatly reduced in patients older than 60 years. The relevance of these findings to transdermal use of fentanyl is presently unknown. Because elderly, cachectic, or debilitated patients may have altered pharmacokinetics owing to altered clearance, poor fat stores, or muscle wasting, they should not receive initial doses of transdermal fentanyl higher than 25 µg per hour unless they are already taking more than 135 mg of oral morphine per day or an equivalent dose of another opioid.[34]

Patients with Renal or Hepatic Disease

Insufficient information exists at present to permit recommendations regarding the use of this transdermal system in patients with impaired renal or hepatic function. If administered to these patients, it should be used with caution because of the hepatic metabolism and renal excretion of fentanyl.[34]

Issues Relevant to Oral and Transdermal Controlled-Release Opioid Therapy

Tolerance, Dependence, and Abuse Potential

The use of opioid analgesics may result in tolerance, physical dependence, and psychological dependence (addiction). These designations, although used interchangeably, differ in meaning and hence, to a large extent, in related clinical issues of importance.

Tolerance and physical dependence, often erroneously confused with addiction, are both easily manageable pharmacologic phenomena. When they occur, they usually do not develop to a clinically significant degree until several weeks of continued opioid usage, and are not criteria of abuse or addiction to opioids. Addiction, on the other hand, is not a pharmacologic phenomenon and is difficult to manage.

Tolerance

Tolerance refers to the need for increasingly larger doses of opioids to produce the same degree of analgesia,[62–64] or to diminished analgesia with the same dose in the absence of other causes for increased pain, such as disease progression. The first sign of tolerance is usually a decreased duration of effective analgesia, with reduced intensity of analgesia occurring subsequently.

Tolerance can be demonstrated in animals and humans[65] and may develop rapidly, slowly, or not at all. However, this phenomenon may occur more rapidly with parenteral doses than with oral doses,[63] and in addicts rather than nonaddicts.[4] Often the patient is labeled a "clock watcher," a sign frequently mistaken for early addiction. Fear of tolerance often interferes with aggressive opioid treatment. However, tolerance to the analgesic effects of morphine is not a significant problem in the treatment of chronic cancer pain.[66–68] Some increase in the required oral opioid dosage occurs with time, but it is relatively small on the average,[68] with substantial patient-to-patient variation. Doses required for chronic pain often stabilize after increasing gradually,[4] but other patterns have been identified.

When strong opioids are used appropriately, tolerance is rarely a practical problem,[30, 69] as long as appropriate titration procedures are followed. When it does occur, it is normally dealt with by merely increasing the opioid dosage. Pharmacologically, tolerance represents a shift to the right in a dose-response relationship without any change in slope, whereby the original desirable opioid effect can be regained. The existing degree of tolerance is a critical factor in guiding the administration of oral controlled-release morphine in chronic pain patients and in opioid-tolerant cancer patients; however, factors such as perception of pain, extent of disease, and differences in drug metabolism also contribute to the marked individual variation (as much as 50-fold or more) in the analgesic oral dosage of morphine required for cancer-related pain.

When tolerance does develop to opioid analgesia, it concurrently develops to the side effects of concern at a comparable rate. For example, no evidence exists to suggest that tolerance develops more rapidly to the analgesic effect than to the respiratory depressant action. Only pupillary constriction and constipation are subject to slower development of tolerance than the analgesia.

After withdrawal has been completed in previously physically dependent patients, tolerance to opioids largely disappears, and many addicts have taken fatal overdoses by resuming their previous intake immediately after undergoing withdrawal.[38]

Physical Dependence

Physical dependence refers to the phenomenon of withdrawal that occurs when opioid use is abruptly discontinued or when an opioid antagonist (such as naloxone), a mixed agonist-antagonist (pentazocine, etc.), or a partial agonist (buprenorphine) is administered. It develops not only with opioids, but also after chronic administration of several other drug classes, and is often mistakenly confused with psychological dependence or addiction.

The characteristic manifestations of the abstinence syndrome due to abrupt opioid withdrawal are well known. During the first 24 hours, these symptoms include lacrimation, rhinorrhea, yawning, perspiration, mydriasis, and other symptoms. These events often increase in severity over the next 72 hours, during which a host of other signs and symptoms may also occur, including severe cardiovascular events. Because of excessive loss of fluids through sweating, vomiting, and diarrhea, there is usually marked weight loss, dehydration, ketosis, and disturbance in acid-base balance. Cardiovascular collapse can occur. Without treatment, most observable signs

and symptoms disappear in 5–14 days; however, a phase of secondary or chronic abstinence symptoms appears to take place, characterized by insomnia, irritability, and muscular aches, which lasts from 2–6 months. If treatment for physical dependence on controlled-release oral morphine is necessary, the patient may be detoxified by gradual reduction of the dosage. Gastrointestinal disturbances or dehydration should be treated appropriately.

The abrupt withdrawal of opioids is often much less disabling than the abrupt withdrawal of other drugs that produce physical dependence.[70] For example, a severe withdrawal syndrome consisting of seizures and delirium, which can be life-threatening, can occur after abrupt cessation of barbiturate or benzodiazepine use.[71, 72]

When an opioid is used to manage cancer pain, physical dependence should not present a problem if patients are warned not to stop taking the drug abruptly and a tapering schedule is used when dose reduction is indicated.[73] At least 25% of the previous daily dose, with further gradual titration, usually will prevent withdrawal symptoms.[17, 42]

When withdrawal symptoms are precipitated by the administration of a drug with opioid-antagonist activity, the onset of signs and symptoms of abstinence is almost immediate and the intensity is more severe than in the absence of such drugs.

Psychological Dependence (Addiction)

Psychological dependence or addiction signifies a pattern of compulsive drug-seeking behavior that leads to an overwhelming preoccupation with the procurement and use of a substance, beyond that associated with accepted medical practice. Fear of opioid addiction is a major consideration limiting the use of appropriate doses of opioid analgesics in cancer pain management,[13, 17, 74] due to lack of understanding of the distinction between physical dependence, tolerance, and psychological dependence, including unawareness that a patient can be physically dependent on an opioid analgesic without being addicted.

Although repeated use of opioids can indeed be habit forming, individuals who take these drugs for analgesia only rarely become addicted in the absence of prior substance abuse,[4, 16, 42, 75–79] as evident from epidemiologic surveys involving thousands of patients. In addition, opioids do not lead to psychological dependence in terminally ill patients.[4, 12, 16, 42, 75–77, 79] The clinical data demonstrate that, in the absence of any history of substance abuse, addiction is rare in the cancer pain patient.[8]

According to Wesson et al.,[80] addicts in need of opioid analgesia require a different treatment strategy than nonaddicted patients. A written plan should be negotiated with the patient that specifies allowable medications and doses, amounts to be dispensed, policies regarding refills, and replacement of medications reported "lost," as well as frequency of office visits, prohibitions (e.g., against receiving prescriptions from other physicians), and addiction treatment (e.g., psychotherapy and attendance at 12-step recovery meetings). The plan, which basically amounts to a contract with the patient, should specify the potential consequences of nonadherence to its requirements. The patient should sign this acknowledgment agreement, and receive a copy, as should other physicians or consultants involved with his or her care. The original should be placed in the patient's chart.

A pattern of drug-seeking behavior similar to that seen in patients with true psychological dependence, known as pseudoaddiction, is an iatrogenic syndrome caused by undermedication of pain. Typically, the syndrome begins with inadequate pain management, e.g., when an analgesic of insufficient potency is administered on an as needed basis. The patient develops feelings of anger in response and makes increasing demands for analgesics.

Opioid-Associated Side Effects and Their Management

Common Side Effects

Dose-limiting opioid-associated side effects may interfere with optimal pain management and hence with attainment of adequate analgesic levels.[7] The side effects of opioids, such as constipation, nausea and vomiting, and sedation, should therefore be anticipated, and aggressive and early measures should be taken to control them.[22, 27, 81–83]

Constipation is a particularly common and troublesome opioid-associated side effect and should be managed aggressively with the prophylactic regularly scheduled use of laxatives.[22, 82, 83] Indeed, each patient requires individualized laxative titration. All patients regularly dosed with opioids should be maintained on a laxative regimen from the start of therapy. Most patients will need a bowel stimulant (e.g., standardized senna concentrate) combined with a stool softener,[84, 85] with dose titration as needed to a maximum of four tablets twice a day in the case of this preparation.[86] Some patients may need additional laxatives or enemas. Dietary modification may be beneficial. Those not responding to escalating therapy over 3–4 days should be checked for impaction.

The nausea sometimes observed on initiation of morphine therapy is usually transient and often subsides within a few days and may be controlled by positional and dietary measures and antiemetics. Nausea from the use of one type of opioid does not mean it will occur with all such drugs.[7] In addition, nausea can sometimes be due to constipation, which should be prevented as advised previously. Patients should be provided with prescriptions for low-dose antiemetics for as needed use; prophylactic use of antinauseants is not recommended because of associated sedation.[87]

Sedation, which may occur during initiation of morphine therapy, usually subsides within a few days. It occurs most commonly during the dose titration period and is rarely caused by the opioid alone in patients previously stabilized on an opioid regimen.[7] In many cases, sedation may be due to sleep deprivation from previously uncontrolled pain. Some affected patients may benefit from short periods of morning amphetamine administration.

Respiratory Depression

Chronic cancer pain patients previously treated with opioids for prolonged periods or tolerant to them can use these drugs without significant risk of respiratory depression.[7, 17] One reason is that tolerance to this most feared effect of opioids will also develop.[17] Respiratory depression occurs most commonly in the nontolerant patient after acute administration of an opioid and is associated with other signs, such as sedation and mental cloudiness.[7] If it indeed occurs with chronic opioid therapy, another cause is frequently present. The most common cause is an unrecognized pulmonary process, such as pneumonia, embolism, or pulmonary edema.[88]

As for the available oral controlled-release opioids (e.g., morphine and oxycodone), clinically significant respiratory depression is uncommon with these drugs, provided that the doses are properly titrated to provide adequate pain relief,[89] even to the large doses used to manage severe cancer pain.[90, 91] This relates to the fact that morphine is a relatively selective drug that produces respiratory depression at doses above the analgesic threshold.[89] In addition, pain, which is also a powerful respiratory stimulant, counteracts opioid-induced respiratory depression.[92]

It is too early to form conclusions concerning the prevalence of respiratory depression in cancer patients being treated with transdermal fentanyl. Hypoventilation has been observed in 2% of 153 cancer patients treated with this system,[60] and the patch's manufacturer recently reported patient deaths apparently associated with hypoventilation related to use of Duragesic.

Opioids should be used with caution in patients with impaired respiratory function. These patients are at greater risk of experiencing respiratory depression in response to usual therapeutic doses of morphine.[17] Symptomatic respiratory depression should be treated with opioid antagonists, such as naloxone, of which repeated doses may be required (see product prescribing information). Caution should be exercised in patients who may be physically dependent, to prevent precipitation of withdrawal symptoms.

Drug Interactions

Opioids should be used with caution and in reduced dosage in patients who are currently receiving other central nervous system depressants including sedatives or hypnotics, general anesthetics, phenothiazines or other tranquilizers, sedating antihistamines, and alcohol, because respiratory depression hypotension and profound sedation or coma may result. When such combined therapy is contemplated, the dose of one or both agents should be reduced in accordance with product labeling.

Opioid analgesics may enhance the neuromuscular blocking action of skeletal muscle relaxants and may produce an increased degree of respiratory depression.

Overdosage and Its Management

With all opioids (including oral controlled-release drugs of this class and transdermal fentanyl), over-dosage can occur in unusual circumstances. In such situations, unacceptable side effects, such as respiratory depression and excessive sedation, can be reversed with specific narcotic antagonists, typically naloxone, by carefully following guidelines in the prescribing information for each opioid product.

Conclusions

Of the few controlled-release opioid products available in the United States, two are controlled-release morphine sulfate formulations for oral use in patients with moderate-to-severe pain, which differ from each other in their delivery systems, tablet sizes and strengths, and pharmacokinetic and therapeutic performance. The third and newest controlled release opioid for oral use in patients with moderate-to-severe pain is controlled-release oxycodone. This product, which is expected to have a major impact on pain management, uses a dual drug-release mechanism that allows early onset and extended duration of analgesia. A controlled-release opioid preparation for transdermal delivery of fentanyl, which is of potential value for patients unable to take oral medication, has the advantage of infrequent and noninvasive application, but also has certain significant risks and other disadvantages, mainly related to its pharmacokinetic and associated pharmacodynamic characteristics. The lack of an extensive history of chronic use and information concerning its effects in special patient populations renders attempts to assess the system's value in cancer pain management premature at this time.

Acknowledgment

The author thanks Liane K. Schein for helping to prepare this manuscript.

References

1. Health and Public Policy Committee, American College of Physicians. Drug therapy for severe, chronic pain in terminal illness. Ann Intern Med 1983;99:870.
2. Inturrisi CE. Management of cancer pain: Pharmacology and principles of management. Cancer 1989; 63:2308.

3. Houde RW. Management of Pain [abstract]. In American Cancer Society National Conference: The Primary Care Physician and Cancer. Washington, DC, 1982.

4. Melzack R. The tragedy of needless pain. Sci Am 1990;262:27.

5. Melzack R. The Tragedy of Needless Pain: A Call For Social Action. In R Dubner, GF Gebhart, MR Bond (eds), Proceedings of the Vth World Congress on Pain. Elsevier, Amsterdam, 1988;1.

6. World Health Organization. Cancer Pain Relief and Palliative Care. Geneva: WHO, 1990.

7. Coyle N, Foley KM. Alterations in Comfort: Pain. In SB Baird, R McCorkle, M Grant, (eds), Cancer Pain Nursing. Philadelphia: Saunders, 1991;782.

8. Expert Advisory Committee on the Management of Severe Chronic Pain in Cancer Pain. A Monograph on the Management of Cancer Pain. No. H42-2/5-1984E. Ottawa, Canada: Department of National Health and Welfare, 1984;5.

9. Bonica JJ. Treatment of Cancer Pain. Current Status and Future Needs. In HL Fields, R Dubner, F Cervero (eds), Advances in Pain Research and Therapy (Vol. 9). New York: Raven, 1985;589.

10. Twycross RG, Lack SA (eds). Myths About Morphine. In Symptom Control in Far Advanced Cancer: Pain Relief. London: Pitman, 1983;223.

11. Portenoy RK. Cancer pain. Epidemiology and syndromes. Cancer 1989;63:2298.

12. McGivney WT, Crooks GM. The care of patients with severe chronic pain in terminal illness. JAMA 1984;251:1182.

13. World Health Organization. Cancer Pain Relief. Geneva: WHO, 1986.

14. Friedman DP. Perspectives on the medical use of drugs of abuse. J Pain Symptom Manage 1990;5(Suppl.):S2.

15. Rane A, Säwe J, Dahlstrom B, et al. Pharmacological treatment of cancer patients with special reference to oral use of morphine. Acta Anaesthesiol Scand (Suppl.) 1982;74:97.

16. Kanner RM, Foley KM. Patterns of narcotic drug use in a cancer pain clinic. Ann NY Acad Sci 1981;362:161.

17. Von Roenn JH, Cleeland CS, Gonin R, et al. Results of a physician's attitude toward cancer pain management survey by ECOG. Proc Am Soc Clin Oncol 1991;10:326.

18. Foley KM. The treatment of cancer pain. N Engl J Med 1985;313:84.

19. Ventafridda V, Tamburini M, Caraceni A. A validation study of the WHO method for cancer pain relief. Cancer 1987;59:850.

20. Abramowitcz M, Aaron H (eds). Drug treatment of cancer pain. Med Letter Drug Ther 1982;24:95.

21. Portenoy RK. 3-Step analgesic ladder for management of cancer pain. Surg Prac News 1988.

22. Levy MH. Oral Controlled-Release Morphine: Guidelines for Clinical Use. In C Benedetti, et al. (eds), Advances in Pain Research and Therapy (Vol. 14). New York: Raven, 1990;285.

23. Moertel CG. Treatment of cancer pain with orally administered medications. JAMA 1980;244:2448.

24. Jaffe JH, Martin WR. Opioid Analgesics and Antagonists (Chap. 21) and Jaffe JH, Drug Addiction and Drug Abuse (Chap. 22). In Goodman and Gilman's: The Pharmacological Basics of Therapeutics (8th ed). New York: Pergamon, 1990;485.

25. Jacox A, Carr DB, Payne R, et al. Management of Cancer Pain. In TW Rall, AS Nies, et al (eds), Clinical Practice Guideline No. 9. AHCPR Publication No. 94-0592. Rockville, MD: Agency for Health Care Policy and Research, Department of Health and Human Services, March 1994.

26. Breitbart W, Holland J. Psychiatric Aspects of Cancer Pain. In KM Foley, JJ Bonica, V Ventafridda, et al. (eds), Advances in Pain Research and Therapy (Vol. 16). New York: Raven, 1990;73.

27. Levy MH. Pain management in advanced cancer. Semin Oncol 1985;12:394.

28. Portenoy RK, Foley KM. Chronic use of opioid analgesics in nonmalignant pain: Report of 38 cases. Pain 1986;25:171.

29. Portenoy RK. Management of cancer pain. Presented at the Ninth Scientific Meeting of the American Pain Society, St. Louis, MO, October 1990.

30. Twycross RG. Clinical experience with diamorphine in advanced malignant disease. Int J Clin Pharmacol Ther Pharmacol 1974;9:184.

31. Portenoy RK. Drug therapy for cancer pain. Am J Hospice Palliat Care 1990;7:10.

32. Kaiko RF, Grandy R, Oshlack B, et al. The United States experience with oral controlled-release morphine (MS Contin Tablets): Parts I and II. Review of nine dose titration studies and clinical pharmacology of 15-mg, 30-mg, 60-mg and 100-mg tablet strengths in normal subjects. Cancer 1989;63:2348.

33. Portenoy RK, Hagen NA. Breakthrough pain: Definition, prevalence and characteristics. Pain 1990;41:273.

34. Physicians' Desk Reference, Montvale, NJ: Medical Economics Data Production Co., 1994;48:1083, 1160, 1821, 2023.

35. Olkkola KT, Maunuksela E-L, Korpela R, et al. Kinetics and dynamics of postoperative intravenous morphine in children. Clin Pharmacol Ther 1988;44:128.

36. Choonara IA, McKay P, Hain R, et al. Morphine metabolism in children. Br J Clin Pharmacol 1989;28:599.

37. Dahlstrom B, Bolme P, Feychting H, et al. Morphine kinetics in children. Clin Pharmacol Ther 1979;26:354.

38. American Medical Association. AMA Drug Evaluations (6th ed), Chicago: American Medical Association, 1986;57.

39. Goldman A, Bowman A. The role of oral controlled-release morphine for pain relief in children with cancer. Palliat Med 1990;4:279.

40. Richter R, Sittl R, Fengler R, et al. First results of a German multicenter study concerning pain therapy in

incurable pediatric cancer patients [abstract]. J Pain Symptom Manage 1989;4(Suppl.):S5.

41. Kaiko R, Wallenstein SL, Rogers AG, et al. Narcotics in the elderly. Med Clin North Am 1982;66:1079.

42. Hasselstrom J, Eriksson LS, Persson A, et al. Morphine metabolism in patients with liver cirrhosis [Abstracts II]. Third World Conference on Clinical Pharmacology and Therapeutics, Stockholm. July 27 to August 1, 1986;101.

43. Patwardhan RV, Johnson RF, Hoyumpa A Jr., et al. Normal metabolism of morphine in cirrhosis. Gastroenterology 1981;81:1006.

44. Säwe J. High-dose morphine and methadone in cancer patients. Clinical pharmacokinetic considerations of oral treatment. Clin Pharmacokinet 1986;11:87.

45. Aitkenhead AR, Vater M, Achola K, et al. Pharmacokinetics of single-dose i.v. morphine in normal volunteers and patients with end-stage renal failure. Br J Anaesth 1984;56:813.

46. Säwe J. Morphine and Its 3- and 6-Glucuronides in Plasma and Urine During Chronic Oral Administration in Cancer Patients. In KM Foley, CE Inturrisi (eds), Opioid Analgesics in the Management of Clinical Pain. Advances in Pain Research and Therapy (Vol. 8). New York: Raven, 1986;45.

47. Bodenham A, Shelly MP, Park GR. The altered pharmacokinetics and pharmacodynamics of drugs commonly used in critically ill patients. Clin Pharmacokinet 1988;14:347.

48. Chan GLC, Matzke GR. Effects of renal insufficiency on the pharmacokinetics and pharmacodynamics of opioid analgesics. Drug Intell Clin Pharm 1987;21:773.

49. Kaiko RF, Grandy R, Savarese JJ, et al. Comparative bioavailability of controlled-release oral morphine tablet for eight vs twelve-hour analgesia [abstract]. Acta Pharmacol Toxicol 1986;59(Suppl.):97.

50. Kaiko RF, Grandy R, Savarese JJ, et al. Comparative Bioavailability of Two Controlled-Release Oral Morphine Tablets [abstract]. In The American Pain Society. Sixth General Meeting. Program, Abstracts, and Meeting Information. Chicago: The American Pain Society, 1986;79.

51. Shepard KV. Review of a Controlled-Release Morphine Preparation Roxanol SR. In KM Foley, JJ Bonica, V Ventafridda (eds), Advances in Pain Research and Therapy (Vol. 16). New York: Raven, 1990;191.

52. Kaiko R, Grandy R, Thomas G, Goldenheim P. A single-dose study of the effect of food ingestion and timing of dose administration on the pharmacokinetic profile of 30-mg sustained-release morphine sulfate tablets. Curr Ther Res 1990;47:869-878.

53. Kaiko RF, Lazarus, H, Cronin C, et al. Controlled-release morphine bioavailability (MS Contin Tablets) in the presence and absence of food. Hospice J 1990;6:17.

54. Sherman LM. The use of sustained-release morphine in a hospice setting. Pharmatherapeutica 1987;5:99.

55. Walsh TD, MacDonald N, Bruera E, et al. A controlled study of sustained-release morphine sulfate tablets in chronic pain from advanced cancer. Am J Clin Oncol 1992;15:268.

56. RG Twycross, SA Lack (eds). Oral Morphine Sulfate. In Symptom Control in Far Advanced Cancer: Pain Relief. London: Pitman, 1983;167.

57. Kaiko RF. Survey of parenteral PCA use indicating inappropriate utilization. Poster presentation at August 1991 Meeting of American Academy of Pain Management, Baltimore, MD.

58. Klausner MA (Janssen Pharmaceutical Research Foundation). Notice to health care professionals regarding revised prescribing information for Duragesic, January 17, 1994.

59. Miser AW, Narang PK, Dothage JA, et al. Transdermal fentanyl for pain control in patients with cancer. Pain 1989;37:15.

60. Manufacturer's full prescribing information for DURAGESIC (fentanyl transdermal system) CII. Piscataway, NJ: Janssen Pharmaceutica.

61. Payne R, Moran K, Southam M. The Role of Transdermal Fentanyl in the Management of Cancer Pain. In FG Estafanous (ed), Opioids in Anesthesia (Vol. II). Boston: Butterworth-Heinemann, 1991;215.

62. Foley KM, Inturrisi CE. Analgesic drug therapy in cancer pain: Principles and practice. Med Clin North Am 1987;71:207.

63. Weissman DE, Burchman SL, Dinndorf PA, et al. Handbook of Cancer Pain Management (3rd ed). Milwaukee, WI: Wisconsin Cancer Pain Initiative, 1992.

64. Foley KM. Controversies in cancer pain: Medical perspectives. Cancer 1989;63:2257.

65. Hanks GW, Twycross RG. Pain: The physiological antagonist of opioid analgesics. Lancet 1984;1:1477.

66. Walsh TD. Oral morphine in chronic cancer pain. Pain 1984;18:1.

67. Reynolds JEF (ed), Martindale: The Extra Pharmacopoeia (29th ed). London: The Pharmaceutical Press, 1989;1310.

68. Cancer pain management: A dialogue. Selections from Opioid Analgesics in the Management of Clinical Pain. An International Workshop held at Memorial Sloan-Kettering Cancer Center, July 29–30, 1983;1.

69. Cancer Pain Relief and Palliative Care. Geneva: World Health Organization. Technical Report Series 804, 1990.

70. Hoskin PJ, Poulain P, Hanks GW. Controlled-release morphine in cancer pain. Anaesthesia 1989;44:897.

71. Alexander L, Luterman A, Dyess D, et al. MS Contin, an Oral Morphine Preparation for Post Burn Analgesia. In Proceedings of the American Burn Association (22nd Annual Meeting). Las Vegas, NV, 1990;22:206.

72. Lang E, McCloud K, Childs L, et al. Preliminary Evaluation of Controlled-Release Morphine (MS Contin) for Background Analgesia in Burn Patients. In Proceedings of the American Burn Association (22nd Annual Meeting). Las Vegas, NV, 1990;22:50.

73. Brookoff D, Palomano R, Callans D. Management of sickle cell pain with controlled release morphine [abstract]. American Pain Society Eighth Annual Scientific Meeting, Phoenix, AZ, 1989;54.

74. Regnard CB, Randell F. Controlled-Release Morphine in Advanced Cancer Pain. In E Wilkes (ed), Advances in Morphine Therapy. The 1983 International Symposium on Pain Control. International Congress and Symposium Series 64. London: R Soc Med, 1984;141.

75. Porter J, Jick H. Addiction rare in patients treated with narcotics. N Engl J Med 1980;302:123.

76. Perry S, Heidrich G. Management of pain during debridement: A survey of U.S. burn units. Pain 1982;13:267.

77. Medina JL, Diamond S. Drug dependency in patients with chronic headache. Headache 1977;17:12.

78. Taddeini L, Rotschafer JC. Pain syndromes associated with cancer: Achieving effective relief. Postgrad Med 1984;75:101.

79. Portenoy RK. Chronic opioid therapy in nonmalignant pain. J Pain Symptom Manage 1990;5(Suppl.):S46.

80. Wesson DR, Ling W, Smith DE. Prescription of opioids for treatment of pain in patients with addictive disease. J Pain Symptom Manage 1993;8:289.

81. Ferrell B, Wisdom C, Wenzl C, et al. Effects of controlled-release morphine on quality of life for cancer pain. Oncol Nurs Forum 1989;16:521.

82. Warfield CA. Evaluation of dosing guidelines for the use of oral controlled-release morphine (MS Contin Tablets). Cancer 1989;63:2360.

83. Warfield CA. Guidelines for the use of MS Contin Tablets in the management of cancer pain. Postgrad Med J 1991;67(Suppl. 2):S9.

84. Hill CS. Doctor-patient crisis: Pain—How much is too much? Prim Care Cancer 1988;8:27.

85. Goughnour BR, Arkinstall WW, Stewart JH. Analgesic response to single and multiple doses of controlled-release morphine tablets and morphine oral solution in cancer patients. Cancer 1989;63:2294.

86. Portenoy RK, Maldonado M, Fitzmartin R, et al. Oral controlled-release morphine sulfate: Analgesic efficacy and side effects of a 100 mg tablet in cancer pain patients. Cancer 1989;63:2284.

87. Levy MH. Comprehensive cancer pain management. Curr Probl Cancer 1992;16:337.

88. Derbyshire DR, Vater M, Maile CID, et al. Non-parenteral postoperative analgesia. A comparison of sublingual buprenorphine and morphine and morphine sulfate (slow release) tablets. Anaesthesia 1984;39:324.

89. Mignault GG, Latreille J, Viguie F, et al. Cross over double blind efficacy assessment of morphine sulfate Contin (MSC) given q 12 vs q 8 hours [abstract]. Pain 1990;(Suppl. 5):S180.

90. Kossman B, Dick W, Bowdler I, et al. Modern Aspects of Morphine Therapy. In E Wilkes (ed), Advances in Morphine Therapy. The 1983 International Symposium on Pain Control. International Congress and Symposium Series 64. London: Royal Soc Med, 1984;73.

91. Goth A. Narcotic and Analgesic Drugs (Chap. 29), Contemporary Drug Abuse (Chap. 30), and Appendix A. Drug Blood Concentrations. In Medical Pharmacology (11th ed), St. Louis: Mosby, 1984;319,758.

92. Bates T, Kearney M. Sustained Release Morphine Sulfate Tablets for Longer-Term Pain Control of Terminal Illness. In P Band, J Stewart, T Towson (eds), Advances in the Management of Chronic Pain. The International Symposium on Pain Control. Toronto: Purdue Frederick, 1986;57.

Chapter 9

Morphine Metabolites

Piotr K. Janicki

Role of Morphine in Cancer Pain Treatment

Currently, there are many compounds that produce analgesia and other effects similar to those produced by morphine. Some of these compounds may have some special properties, but none has proved to be clinically superior in relieving pain. Morphine still remains the standard narcotic drug of choice for chronic, cancer-related pain and also the standard agent against which new analgesics are assessed.[1] Morphine and related mu-opioid receptor agonists produce their major effects on the central nervous system (CNS) and the bowel by acting as agonists, particularly at mu-receptors. However, they also have appreciable affinity for delta- and kappa-receptors. Morphine-induced analgesia is due to actions at several sites within the CNS, including spinal and supraspinal sites. Furthermore, when administered via the intra-articular route, morphine has been shown clinically to be effective for postoperative pain relief following arthroscopy.[2, 3]

In principle, there is enough information to support the effective use of morphine for cancer pain. However, improvements need to be made to educate the physician about morphine indications and its pharmacologic and pharmacokinetic properties. This is especially important considering the recent findings that the analgesic activity of morphine and the incidence of morphine-induced side effects can be produced in the body as a result of complex interactions of the parent drug (i.e., morphine) with its pharmacologically active metabolites.

Pharmacokinetics of Morphine and Formation of Metabolites

Morphine is readily absorbed from almost all accessible administration sites (i.e., gastrointestinal tract and after intravenous, intramuscular, subcutaneous, or even peripheral intra-articular injection). Oral doses of morphine have less effect than parenteral doses, owing to the significant first-pass metabolism in the liver (i.e., the bioavailability of the oral preparations of morphine is only about 25%). The time–effect curve varies with the route of administration; therefore, the duration of action of orally administered drugs is often somewhat longer than other routes. If adjustments are made for variability of first-pass metabolism and clearance, it is possible to achieve adequate pain relief by orally administered morphine.[4] Satisfactory analgesia in cancer patients has been associated with a broad range of steady-state concentrations of morphine in plasma (16–364 ng per ml). Because of its short duration of action (4 hours), conventional morphine has to be given every 4 hours, which is not always acceptable for the long-term treatment of chronic cancer pain in outpatients. However, slow-release morphine tablets have been developed that maintain plasma levels within a therapeutically effective range for 12 hours. Twice daily administration of morphine shows in steady-state a peak-to-trough variation that reduces the possible side effects of high plasma levels and the breakthrough pain of low plasma levels.

Morphine is considered to be an intermediate drug, i.e., subject to pronounced presystemic elimination. Morphine is metabolized to several metabolites, most of them having some pharmacologic activity (Table 9-1). The metabolic pathways of morphine, including its O-transmethylation to codeine, demethylation to normorphine, diglucuronidation to morphine-3,6-diglucuronide, conjugation to morphine-3-sulfate, and formation of morphine-ethereal-sulfate, appear to have minor pharmacokinetic and pharmacologic significance. During oral or systemic administration of morphine in humans, glucuronidation (i.e., conjugation with glucuronic acid) at the phenolic and alcoholic hydroxyl groups at position 3 and 6, respectively, occurs mainly in the liver. UDP-Glucuronosyl transferase (UDPGT) was identified as the enzyme responsible for production of glucuronides from morphine.[5] There is now overwhelming evidence that UDPGTs exist as a multigene family (at least 11 different forms have been identified), resulting in a range of isoenzymes. Morphine is metabolized to morphine-3-glucuronide (M3G) by more than one UDPGT isoenzyme (Figure 9-1). Recently, however, a functional heterogeneity has been observed between the isoenzymes responsible for the glucuronidation of morphine in the 3- and 6-positions.[6] Therefore, the possibility exists that differences in M3G or morphine-6-glucuronide (M6G) production could represent a differential development of these UDPGTs. Although the liver is the major site of metabolism, evidence of extrahepatic glucuronidation of morphine has been reported. Enterohepatic cycling of morphine has been described in rats and dogs. Glucuronides can be deconjugated by the colonic flora after having been excreted via the bile to the gut lumen, where the parent compound can be subsequently reabsorbed. Morphine, M3G, and M6G have all been found in bile.[7, 8] This metabolic processing results in the formation of M3G and M6G, which may be found in large concentrations in plasma. In fact, during chronic morphine administration, circulating concentrations of M3G and M6G markedly exceed those of morphine itself because hepatic metabolism converts approximately 70% of morphine into M3G (55%) and M6G (15%). In adults, chronic oral administration of morphine produces variable plasma ratios of M3G to M6G, with reported mean ratios of 10 to 1,[9] 6 to 1,[10] and 5 to 1.[11] A study that used a single

Table 9-1. Metabolites of Morphine

Morphine-3-glucuronide*
Morphine-3,6-glucuronide
Normorphine*
Normorphine-6-glucuronide (?)
Methylmorphine (codeine)*
Ether sulfate of morphine (?)
Morphine-3-sulfate (?)

*Pharmacologically active metabolites.

intravenous dose of morphine in adults found a plasma M3G to M6G ratio of 8 to 5.[12] The ratio of M3G to M6G found in neonates is 3 to 1, which is markedly lower than previously demonstrated in adults or children.[13]

Recent evidence suggests that M3G and M6G production is significantly influenced by the route of morphine administration. After a single intravenous dose of morphine, the molar ratio of M6G to M3G to morphine in plasma was significantly lower than oral morphine administration.[14] Morphine metabolite-to-parent drug molar ratios after sublingual and buccal morphine administration were not significantly different than ratios after oral administration.[14] After oral administration of single-dose morphine, M6G and M3G were found to be present at concentrations higher than those achieved with rectal dosing.[15] These data suggest that rectal administration of morphine is associated with significant avoidance of hepatic biotransformation. Patients receiving orally adminstered morphine had significantly greater amounts of M3G and M6G than patients subjected to chronic systemic morphine administration. In our own study involving terminal cancer patients, some patients receiving orally administered morphine for a prolonged time had a significantly higher ratio of M3G to M6G to morphine in urine than patients receiving morphine systemically.[16]

Although the primary site of action of morphine is in the CNS, only small quantities of morphine actually cross the blood–brain barrier in adults. Compared with other more lipid-soluble opioids such as codeine, heroin, and methadone, morphine crosses the blood–brain barrier at a considerably lower rate. Among opioids, morphine is relatively water-soluble. This would also be expected in its glucuronide metabolites. Recently, however, an unexpected high

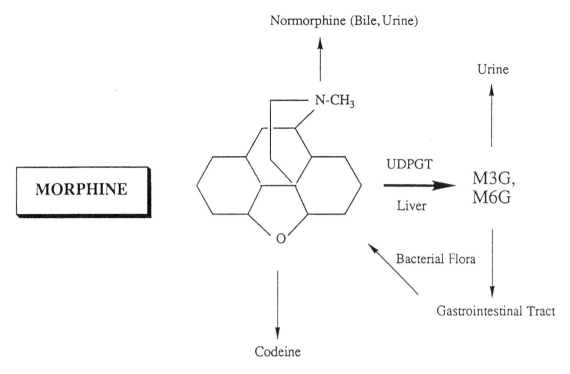

Figure 9-1. Major metabolic pathways of morphine metabolism in humans.

lipophilicity has been reported for M3G and M6G, which implies that a significant blood–brain barrier passage may also occur.[17]

Pharmacologic Properties of Morphine Metabolites

M3G and M6G are both pharmacologically active. M6G has a relatively high affinity for the mu-opioid receptors and has been shown to be considerably more potent than morphine in behavioral analgesic tests.[17, 18] M6G has also been shown to dose dependently inhibit the C-fiber evoked responses of convergent dorsal horn neurons with a potency ratio of 13 to 1 compared with morphine. The analgesic activity of morphine may be due to its 6-glucuronide formed in vivo. M6G could be found in the cerebrospinal fluid (CSF) after morphine administration. It is unclear yet whether this M6G is derived from glucuronidation of morphine in the brain or from M6G that has entered the brain from the blood.[19–22]

In contrast, M3G shows no affinity for the mu-opioid receptor and is presumed to be devoid of analgesic activity as suggested in behavioral antinociceptive tests and in electrophysiologic studies on dorsal horn nociceptive neurons.[23] However, despite this apparent lack of activity, intracerebroventricular or intraperitoneal M3G has been reported to antagonize the analgesic activity of morphine in various animal pain models.[24, 25] Similarly, M3G has been found to antagonize M6G-induced antinociception and ventilatory depression in the rat. Intrathecal administration of M3G (or morphine) in experimental animals induces allodynia and hyperalgesia, and progressively higher doses of M3G produce a range of adverse effects in experimental animals including excessive grooming behavior, tremors, and wet dog shakes.[17, 26] Allodynia is a condition in which an ordinarily innocuous stimulus is perceived as being painful. Thus, after intrathecal administration of morphine or M3G to rats, a light tactile stimulus applied to the flank caused aggressive behavior suggestive of a pain state. M3G and the 3-sulfate conjugate of morphine were 10–50 times more potent than morphine. This effect is not mediated by an opioid receptor. The central excitatory effects of M3G may complicate the interpretation of behavioral measures of antinociception and may interfere with the analgesic activity of morphine itself. The concentration of M3G in the blood of patients taking morphine exceeds that of morphine itself by approximately 20-fold, whereas the concentration of M6G is twofold higher than morphine. Recently, the pharmacologic effects of M3G were shown not to be directly produced at the spinal cord level. It is therefore possible that M3G could act at nonspinal sites to attenuate morphine analgesia.[23] Thus, the analgesic effect of morphine is probably the result of complex interactions between the drug and its two main metabolites.

Involvement of Metabolites in Morphine-Induced Side Effects

M6G is eliminated from the body via urinary excretion. The slow elimination of glucuronides is important for patients with impaired renal function. High plasma levels of M6G were observed in patients with renal failure several days after termination of morphine treatment.[27, 28] These patients may experience more metabolite-related side effects. These high plasma levels (without measurable plasma morphine concentrations) were accompanied by respiratory depression, sedation, and vomiting, which could be reversed by naloxone, an opioid receptor antagonist. The most serious complications reported in patients with impaired renal function are encephalopathy and myoclonus.[27] Recently, the M6G to morphine ratio in these patients was shown to correlate with increased blood urea nitrogen or creatinine levels. Furthermore, a significant difference was observed between the prevalence of myoclonus in patients receiving orally adminstered morphine and those patients receiving parenterally administered morphine, with a threefold greater frequency in patients receiving oral morphine.[27] These observations indicate that cumulative properties of glucuronides exist in the patients taking high morphine doses and with impaired renal clearance.[29]

The most distressing side effects of repeated morphine administration include drowsiness, constipation, and nausea and vomiting. Recent studies in animals[30] and humans[31] have shown that M6G produces more nausea than morphine itself. Constipation is the most annoying side effect of prolonged morphine use.[4] Tolerance to the analgesic and sedative effects develops faster than the tolerance to the constipation and other peripheral side effects. Several published studies have shown that the intestine does become at least partially tolerant to the constipating effect of morphine. Moreover, clinical observations have suggested that morphine does not induce tolerance to its constipating action. Our clinical impression is that the tolerance to morphine in the gut does not occur when morphine is administered orally to cancer patients. On the other hand, the relatively fast development of tolerance (as evidenced by the lack of constipation) was observed after systemic administration of morphine.[32, 33] Several investigators[14, 16, 28] have shown that different metabolic patterns of morphine will occur when it is administered orally as compared with systemically. M6G has been shown to be the prevalent metabolite after prolonged oral administration of morphine.[32, 33] This M6G is described as more potent in producing analgesia than morphine itself and, more importantly, in producing inhibition of the gastrointestinal transit.[34] The differences in the metabolite formation between systemic and oral morphine administration could be explained by the fact that, in the latter route, morphine is subjected to much higher conversion into glucuronides within the liver after reaching it through the portal circulation. Moreover, several studies in the rat [32, 33] have shown that the metabolism of morphine in the gut wall contributes to the overall presystemic extraction of morphine. It is safe to speculate therefore that, in the oral route of administration, M6G in plasma could more severely inhibit the gastrointestinal tract than in the systemic method of prolonged morphine administration.

Morphine Metabolites and Paradoxical Pain

The literature has reported an increasing number of cases in which chronic pain patients do not respond as expected to powerful opioids.[35–37] Most of these cases are patients with malignant diseases, but some involve patients with such nonmalignant conditions as neurogenic pain of various origins. These cases of nociceptive pain that are unresponsive to opiates have become known as "paradoxical pain" or "overwhelming pain syndrome." In the case of neurogenic pain (exemplified by postherpetic neuralgia, trigeminal neuralgia, painful diabetic neuropathy, reflex sympathetic dystrophy, and central [thalamic] pain), there is no direct nociceptor stimulation. The nociceptive impulses are generated as a result of neuronal dysfunction and do not follow classic pain pathways. Not surprisingly, such pains are not very susceptible to the action of conventional analgesics, including opiates. Hyperalgesia, hyperesthesia, or other neuropathic pain syndromes in cancer patients, unresponsive to even large doses of morphine, may sometimes be accompanied by myoclonus.[38] Although there are only a few clinical descriptions of the relationship among hyperalgesia, myoclonus, and high doses of morphine, experimental findings from animal studies indicate that morphine, or its metabolites, plays a causative role in the observed behavioral syndrome. High doses of morphine microinjected intrathecally in rats have been shown to produce hyperalgesia and hypesthesia as opposed to the analgesia that is found at lower doses.

Morphine is metabolized in the liver to M3G and M6G, both of which can modulate pain response. M6G is a much more potent analgesic than morphine itself. However, M3G antagonizes the opioid activity (including analgesia) of M6G in various experimental conditions. Thus, the analgesic response of patients to morphine appears to depend on their M3G to M6G ratio, with M6G being responsible for the analgesic effect. This ratio in plasma has been reported in several case reports of patients with malignant disease who were taking oral doses of slow-release morphine for long periods. The ratio usually ranges from 4.5 to 5.0 to 1.

It is not known if interindividual differences in the metabolite ratios in patients are inherent or are induced by disease, drugs, or age. Further, it is also not known (1) what the normal range of ratio is when morphine is given to opioid naive subjects and (2) what plasma levels of morphine and M6G are associated with effective analgesia. Pharmacokinetic studies indicate that, with chronic dosing, plasma levels of both M3G and M6G are higher than those of morphine itself.[39] The route of morphine administration can also influence the observed ratio of morphine and its metabolites. The concentration ratios of morphine to its active metabolite M6G and to its inactive metabolite M3G are higher after prolonged oral administration than after systemic administration. Patients receiving oral doses of morphine produced significantly higher amounts of M6G than patients subjected to chronic systemic morphine treatment.

There is no report that links the M3G to M6G ratio in plasma during intrathecal morphine administration to the analgesic effectiveness of morphine. Little is known about the glucuronide metabolites and their concentration in CSF and plasma after intrathecal morphine administration. Morphine metabolite concentrations were higher in plasma than in CSF, and the plasma to CSF ratios for M6G and M3G were 1 to 0.08 and 4 to 1, respectively, suggesting that M6G penetrates the blood–brain barrier more easily than M3G.[19] In a study[40] in which morphine and M6G were measured in the CSF of cancer patients receiving chronic morphine treatment, plasma contained approximately twice as much M6G as morphine, whereas CSF contained only one-fifth to one-third as much. These data suggest that M6G in plasma is redistributed in CSF, but to a far lesser extent than morphine. The metabolite concentrations observed in plasma of patients after intrathecal morphine administration probably reflect hepatic biotransformation of free morphine in the plasma. Even if morphine glucuronidation has been demonstrated in postmortem human brain tissue, the rate of glucuronidation in these tissue samples was very low compared with those in liver. Some recent reports indicate, however, that morphine metabolites can be formed directly in vivo in CSF after cerebroventricular administration of morphine.[20] Nevertheless, the role of morphine metabolites as excitatory agents producing hyperalgesia and myoclonus remains an unresolved question.

High levels of M3G have been demonstrated during chronic systemic and intraspinal morphine administration in humans.[37, 38] This finding is consistent with its effects in rodents, in which M3G is a potent antagonist of the antinociceptive effects of M6G and morphine. Thus, the accumulation of M3G in the CNS may result in hyperalgesia and myoclonus. The mechanism of this action is not known but may involve nonopioid receptor mechanisms. If hyperalgesia and myoclonus responses are due to a nonopioid receptor effect exerted by morphine or its metabolites, then the use of nonmorphine-related opioids for cancer patients requiring increasing high doses of opioids or for those patients not responding to long-term morphine treatment may be relevant and worthy of therapeutic monitoring.

References

1. World Health Organization. Cancer Pain Relief. Geneva: WHO, 1986.
2. Lawrence AJ, Joshi GP, Michalkiewicz A, et al. Evidence for analgesia mediated by peripheral opioid receptors in inflamed synovial tissue. Eur J Clin Pharmacol 1992;43:351.
3. Stein C, Comisei K, Haimerl E, et al. Analgesic effect of intraarticular morphine after arthroscopic knee surgery. N Engl J Med 1991;325:1123.
4. Dethlefsen U. Systemic Opiate Treatment. In J Chrubasik, M Cousins, E Martin (eds), Advances in Pain Therapy (Vol. 1). Berlin: Springer, 1992;18.
5. Miners JO, Lillywhite KJ, Birkett DJ. In vitro evidence for the involvement of at least two forms of human liver UDP-glucuronosyltransferase in morphine-3-glucuronidation. Biochem Pharmacol 1988;37:2839.
6. Mullder GJ, Coughtrie MHH, Burchell B. Glucuronidation. In GJ Mullder (ed), Conjugation Reactions in Drug Metabolism. London: Taylor-Francis, 1990;1.
7. Hanks GW, Wand PJ. Enterohepatic circulation of opioid drugs. Is it clinically relevant in the treatment of cancer patients? Clin Pharmacokinet 1989;17:65.
8. Hasselstrauom J, Sauawe J. Morphine pharmacokinetics and metabolism in humans. Enterohepatic cycling and relative contribution of metabolites to active opioid concentrations. Clin Pharmacokinet 1993;24:344.
9. Hand CW, Blunnie WP, Claffey LP, et al. Potential analgesic contribution from morphine-6-glucuronide in CSF. Lancet 1987;2:1207.
10. Venn RF, Michalkiewicz A, Hardy P, Wells C. Concentrations of morphine, morphine metabolites and peptides in human CSF and plasma. Pain 1990;(Suppl. 5):S188.
11. McQuay HJ, Carroll D, Faura CC, et al. Oral morphine in cancer pain: Influences on morphine and metabolite concentration. Clin Pharmacol Ther 1990;48:236.
12. Hasselstrauom J, Eriksson S, Persson A, et al. The metabolism and bioavailability of morphine in patients with severe liver cirrhosis. Br J Clin Pharmacol 1990;29:289.
13. Choonara I, Lawrence A, Michalkiewicz A, et al. Morphine metabolism in neonates and infants. Br J Clin Pharmacol 1992;34:434.
14. Osborne R, Joel S, Trew D, Slevin M. Morphine and metabolite behavior after different routes of morphine administration: Demonstration of the importance of the active metabolite morphine-6-glucuronide. Clin Pharmacol Ther 1990;47:12.
15. Babul N, Darke AC. Disposition of morphine and its glucuronide metabolites after oral and rectal administration: Evidence of route specificity. Clin Pharmacol Ther 1993;54:286.
16. Janicki PK, Erskine WAR, James MFM. The route of prolonged morphine administration affects the pattern of its metabolites in the urine of chronically treated patients. Eur J Chem Clin Biochem 1991;29:391.
17. Mullder GJ. Pharmacological effects of drug conjugates: Is morphine-6-glucuronide an exception? Trends Pharmacol Sci 1992;13:302.
18. Hanna MH, Peat SJ, Woodham M, et al. Analgesic efficacy and CSF pharmacokinetics of intrathecal morphine-6-glucuronide: Comparison with morphine. Br J Anaesth 1990;64:547.
19. Bigler D, Broen Christensen C, Eriksen J, Jensen NH. Morphine, morphine-6-glucuronide and morphine-3-glucuronide concentrations in plasma and cerebrospinal fluid long-term high-dose intrathecal morphine administration. Pain 1990;41:15.
20. Sandouk P, Serrie A, Scherrmann JM, et al. Presence of morphine metabolites in human cerebrospinal fluid after intracerebroventricular administration of morphine. Eur J Drug Metab Pharmacokinet 1991;3:166.
21. Samuelsson H, Hedner T, Venn R, Michalkiewicz A. CSF and plasma concentrations of morphine and morphine glucuronides in cancer patients receiving epidural morphine. Pain 1993;52:179.
22. Schneider JJ, Ravenscroft PJ, Cavenagh JD, et al. Plasma morphine-3-glucuronide, morphine-6-glucuronide and morphine concentrations in patients receiving long-term epidural morphine. Br J Clin Pharmacol 1992;34:431.
23. Hewett K, Dickenson AH, McQuay HJ. Lack of effect of morphine-3-glucuronide on the spinal antinociceptive actions of morphine in the rat: An electrophysiological study. Pain 1993;53:59.
24. Ekblom M, Gardmark M, Hammarlund-Udenaes M. Pharmacokinetics and pharmacodynamics of morphine-3-glucuronide in rats and its influence on the antinociceptive effect of morphine. Biopharm Drug Dispos 1993;14:1.
25. Smith MT, Watt JA, Cramond T. Morphine-3-glucuronide—A potent antagonist of morphine analgesia. Life Sci 1990;47:579.
26. Gong QL, Hedner J, Bjorkman R, Hedner T. Morphine-3-glucuronide may functionally antagonize morphine-6-glucuronide induced antinociception and ventilatory depression in the rat. Pain 1992;48:249.
27. Tiseo PJ, Thaler HT, Lapin J, et al. Morphine and cancer pain: Relationship between renal function, side effects and the metabolite morphine-6-glucuronide [abstract]. 12th Annual Scientific Meeting of the American Pain Society 1993;93512.
28. Peterson GM, Randall CT, Paterson J. Plasma levels of morphine glucuronides in the treatment of cancer pain: Relationship to renal function and route of administration. Eur J Clin Pharmacol 1990;38:121.
29. Portenoy RK, Foley KM, Stulman J, et al. Plasma morphine and morphine-6-glucuronide during chronic morphine therapy for cancer pain: Plasma profiles, steady-state concentrations and the consequences of renal failure. Pain 1991;47:13.

30. Thompson PI, Bingham S, Andrews PL, Patel N, et al. Morphine-6-glucuronide: A metabolite of morphine with greater emetic potency than morphine in the ferret. Br J Pharmacol 1992;106:3.

31. Hagen NC, Foley KM, Cerbone DJ, et al. Chronic nausea and morphine-6-glucuronide. J Pain Symptom Manage 1991;6:125.

32. Janicki PK, Erskine WAR, James MFM. The route of morphine administration affects the development of tolerance in relation to gastric emptying in rats: Is morphine-6-glucuronide involved? Clin Exp Pharmacol Physiol 1991;18:193.

33. Janicki PK, Erskine R, James MFM. Different effects of systemic vs oral methods of prolonged morphine administration on gastrointestinal motility and morphine metabolic pattern in rat. Res Commun Subst Abuse 1992;13:167.

34. Janicki PK, Erskine WAR, Budd K. Differences in opioid fractional receptor occupancy (FRO) for morphine and morphine-6-glucuronide (M6G) in isolated guinea-pig ileum (GPI) in normal and morphine tolerant animals. Pharm Pharmacol Lett 1993;2:199.

35. Arner S, Mayerson BA. Lack of analgesic effect of opioids on neuropathic and idiopathic forms of pain. Pain 1988;33:11.

36. Bowsher D. Paradoxical pain. When the metabolites of morphine are in the wrong ratio. Br Med J 1993;306:473.

37. Morley JS, Miles JB, Wells JC, Bowsher D. Paradoxical pain. Lancet 1992;340:1045.

38. Sjogren P, Jonsson T, Jensen NH, et al. Hyperalgesia and myoclonus in terminal cancer patients treated with continuous intravenous morphine. Pain 1993;55:93.

39. Saauwe J. Morphine and Its 3- and 6-Glucuronides in Plasma and Urine During Chronic Administration in Cancer Patients. In KM Foley, CE Inturrisi (eds), Advances in Pain Research and Therapy. New York: Raven, 1986;45.

40. Portenoy RK, Khan E, Layman M, et al. Chronic morphine therapy for cancer pain: Plasma and cerebrospinal fluid morphine and morphine-6-glucuronide concentrations. Neurology 1991;41:1457.

Chapter 10
The Sympathetic Nervous System

Allen H. Hord

Invasion or compression of somatic structures (including nerves) or side effects of cancer treatment (surgery and chemotherapy), which may also damage somatic tissue, account for most cases of cancer pain. Involvement of the sympathetic nervous system as a primary cause of cancer pain is infrequent. However, a review of the sympathetic nervous system and its involvement in cancer pain is important for three reasons. First, visceral afferent nerves travel with sympathetic efferent nerves. Although the visceral afferents are not part of the autonomic nervous system, a knowledge of the anatomy of the sympathetic nerves is important to understanding visceral pain and the use of nerve blocks for its treatment. Second, the reflex sympathetic dystrophy (RSD) syndrome may develop from cancer or surgery for cancer. Because RSD must be recognized early and treated differently from other types of cancer-related pain, a review of its presentation and therapy is necessary. Finally, cancer-related pain syndromes, such as phantom limb pain and postherpetic neuralgia, may be improved by sympathetic blockade.

Anatomy

The sympathetic nervous system consists of a portion of the visceral efferent (autonomic) nervous system whose activities include generalized vasoconstriction, cardiac acceleration, and a decrease in peristalsis of the gut and contraction of its sphincters (Figure 10-1). These functions activate body re-

sources for the "fight or flight" response. A brief review of the anatomy of the sympathetic nervous system follows. (See references 1–3 for a more in-depth review of the entire autonomic system.)

Unlike somatic peripheral nerves, there are two neurons in the pathway between the spinal cord and visceral organs. Cell bodies of the preganglionic neurons are located in the intermediolateral cell column of the thoracic and upper lumbar spinal cord. The preganglionic axons have diameters from 1.5–4.0 μm. They are usually thinly myelinated and exit the spinal column via the ventral roots of the spinal nerves with the first thoracic through third lumbar spinal nerves. After exiting the foramen, they branch off as the white rami communicans to reach the sympathetic trunk in the paravertebral region. After reaching the sympathetic trunk, fibers may synapse with second-order neurons at the same spinal level or make synapses at more cephalad or caudad levels within the sympathetic trunk. In addition, first-order neurons may pass through the sympathetic trunk without interruption to make synapses in peripheral autonomic ganglia.

The preganglionic fibers synapse with second-order neurons in paravertebral or peripheral ganglia. The preganglionic neuron may synapse with 20 or more postganglionic neurons, thus accounting for diffuse autonomic response from central stimulation. Postganglionic axons are generally unmyelinated C-fibers. The postganglionic sympathetic nerves innervate all sweat glands, erector muscles of hairs, and muscular walls of blood vessels, in addition to the viscera. There is evidence that

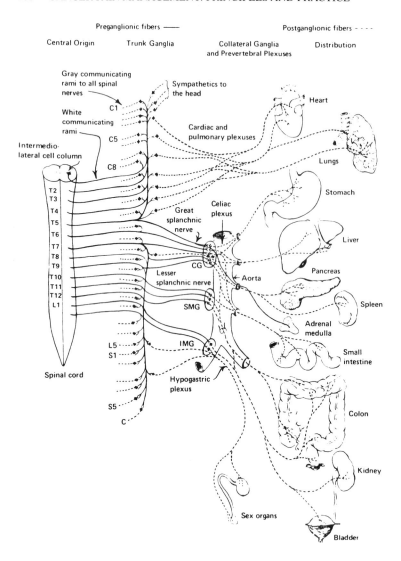

Figure 10-1. Anatomy of the sympathetic nervous system. (CG = celiac ganglion; SMG = superior mesenteric ganglion; IMG = inferior mesenteric ganglion.) (Reprinted with permission from JG Chusid [ed], Correlative Neuroanatomy & Functional Neurology [19th ed]. Los Altos, CA: Lange, 1985;163.)

synapses also occur within spinal nerves and completely bypass the sympathetic trunks.[4, 5] This may account for the incomplete sympathectomy following surgical removal of the sympathetic chain itself.

Sympathetic nerve fibers exit the sympathetic trunk to rejoin the spinal nerve proximal to the white rami communicans. Because most of the nerve fibers are postganglionic, the nerve has a gray appearance and is called the gray rami communicans. Almost all of the fibers of the gray rami that return to the spinal nerve are postganglionic axons. Axons of second-order neurons do not necessarily exit at the same spinal level as their neuron. They may ascend or descend before leaving the sympathetic trunk. Due to ascent and descent of both pre-

ganglionic and postganglionic fibers, considerable overlap exists between adjacent spinal levels and there is little segmentalization of the sympathetic nervous system. In addition to peripheral innervation through spinal nerves, postganglionic sympathetic fibers may distribute directly to viscera or may be carried peripherally by communication with the blood vessels adjacent to the sympathetic trunk.

Paravertebral Plexuses

The paravertebral sympathetic trunk extends from the base of the skull to the coccyx. From the cervical to the lumbar regions, the trunks are located bilaterally on the anterolateral surface of the vertebral body. At the level of the coccyx, the trunks meet anteriorly as the ganglion impar. The cervical sympathetic trunk is generally divided into the superior, middle, and cervicothoracic (stellate) ganglia. The superior cervical ganglion is the largest of the three. It is located at the level of the second and third cervical vertebrae. The middle cervical ganglion is the smallest and is usually found at the level of the sixth cervical vertebra. The cervicothoracic (stellate) ganglion is a fusion of the lower cervical and first thoracic ganglia and is located anterolateral to the longest colli muscle at the level of the seventh cervical vertebra and first rib. The ganglion is located in close proximity to the lung apex inferiorly, the carotid artery anteriorly, the longest colli muscle posteromedially, and the anterior scalene muscle laterally. Preganglionic sympathetic fibers destined for the superior and middle cervical ganglia traverse the cervicothoracic ganglion without interruption.

Sympathetic innervation of the head and neck is derived mostly from T-1 to T-3, whereas preganglionic fibers supplying the upper limbs are derived from T-2 to T-6. Postganglionic fibers travel with the brachial plexus to the upper extremity. The blood vessels of the upper extremity receive their sympathetic innervation from the adjacent brachial plexus.

Surgical sympathectomy to the upper limb can be accomplished by interrupting the rami communicans of the second and third thoracic ganglia. Most of the vasoconstrictor fibers to the limb are located at this level. The white ramus to the first thoracic (or cervicothoracic) ganglion is preserved, because little innervation of the upper limb comes from this spinal level; however, innervation of the head is mostly derived from this level. After synapsing in the middle and upper cervical ganglia, the postganglionic sympathetic fibers supply vasomotor and sudomotor control of the face and neck, in addition to innervating the dilator pupillae and nonstriated muscle of the upper and lower eyelids. Therefore, interruption of these fibers by stellate ganglion block or surgical denervation of T-1 lead to Horner's syndrome, which consists of miosis, ptosis, and enophthalmus.

The thoracic portion of the sympathetic chain consists of several ganglia. Commonly, the ganglia are located anterior to the heads of the rib and posterior to the parietal pleura. Branches from the first five ganglia supply the thoracic aorta, pulmonary plexus, and cardiac plexus. Branches of the lower seven ganglia make up the greater and lesser splanchnic nerves. These nerves travel inferiorly and anteriorly to form the periaortic plexus. The greater splanchnic nerve ends in the cephalad portion of the celiac ganglion, whereas the lesser splanchnic nerve supplies a lower part of the celiac ganglion that is sometimes separately identifiable as the aorticorenal ganglion. These preganglionic fibers pierce the crus of the diaphragm to reach the aorta. They may be blocked before reaching the celiac ganglion as in the retrocrural approach to neurolysis of the celiac plexus.

The lumbar portion of the sympathetic chain is found in the retroperitoneal connective tissue on the anterolateral surface of the vertebral column at the anteromedial surface of the psoas major. It passes posterior to the iliac arteries to reach the pelvic area where it is located anteriorly to the sacrum and medially to the anterior sacral foramina. Four branches—the lumbar splanchnic nerves—leave the lumbar sympathetic trunk to join the celiac, mesenteric, and superior hypogastric plexuses. Branches from the most caudad lumbar splanchnic nerves also form a plexus along the iliac arteries. Branches from the sacral portion of the sympathetic trunk give off branches to the inferior hypogastric plexus and to the roots of the somatic nerves, which form the sacral plexus. Preganglionic sympathetic fibers to the lower limb originate in the lower three thoracic and upper two to three lumbar segments of the spinal cord. Because the preganglionic fibers travel caudad through the sympathetic trunk, a surgical sympathectomy can be accomplished by removing the lumbar sympathetic trunk and ganglia between L-1 and L-3.

Celiac and Other Intra-abdominal Plexuses

The celiac plexus is located at the level of the twelfth thoracic and the upper portion of the first lumbar vertebra. It consists of a network of sympathetic nerves and two discreet ganglia. The plexus is located on the anterior surface of the abdominal aorta and crura of the diaphragm, and surrounds the base of the celiac and superior mesenteric arteries. From the celiac plexus, branches extend to the intra-abdominal viscera and form multiple secondary plexuses, including the phrenic, splenic, hepatic, left

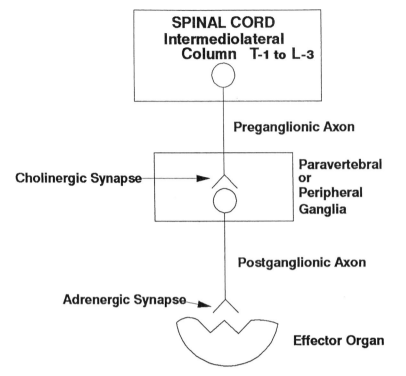

Figure 10-2. Schematic representation of the sympathetic nervous system.

gastric, intramesenteric, adrenal, testicular or ovarian, and superior and inferior mesenteric plexuses.

The superior mesenteric plexus is an extension of the celiac plexus inferiorly, which surrounds the superior mesenteric artery. It distributes along the artery to the small intestine and the ascending and transverse colon. In addition, its branches innervate the pancreas. The periaortic plexus is called the aortic plexus as it extends inferiorly. At the level of the inferior mesenteric artery, its name then changes to the inferior mesenteric plexus, which innervates the descending colon. The superior hypogastric plexus is located more caudad at the bifurcation of the abdominal aorta. It receives branches from the more cephalad aortic plexuses and from the third and fourth lumbar splanchnic nerves. The hypogastric nerves extend along the common iliac artery and its branches to form the inferior hypogastric plexus. Branches from the superior hypogastric plexus innervate the left part of the transverse colon and the descending and sigmoid colon. The inferior hypogastric plexus innervates a majority of pelvic viscera and gives rise to multiple minor plexuses and ganglia.

Pharmacology of the Sympathetic Nerves

There are two synapses within the extraspinal portion of the sympathetic nervous system. The first synapse is between the preganglionic and postganglionic neurons and occurs at the level of the sympathetic trunk or peripheral ganglia. This synapse is cholinergic in nature. Acetylcholine is released from the preganglionic neurons and binds to receptors on the postsynaptic neuron, causing depolarization. Acetylcholine is quickly metabolized by acetylcholinesterase to choline and acetate. Essentially, no acetylcholine reaches the systemic circulation. The postganglionic neuron may be either cholinergic or adrenergic. All postganglionic sympathetic nerves are adrenergic except those innervating the sweat glands and vasodilator neurons to skeletal muscle blood vessels. All other postganglionic sympathetic neurons release norepinephrine at their synapse with the effector organ (Figure 10-2). In the nerve ending, tyrosine is converted to dopamine, which is subsequently converted to norepinephrine by dopamine beta-hydroxylase. The norepinephrine is stored in

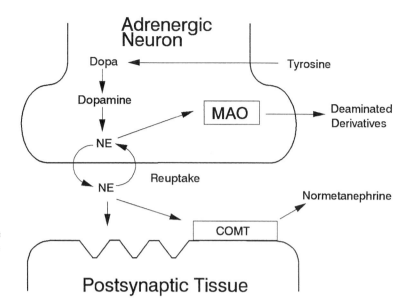

Figure 10-3. Pharmacology of the adrenergic synapse. (NE = norepinephrine; MAO = monoamine oxidase; COMT = catechol-o-methyl transferase.)

presynaptic vesicles until depolarization. After being released into the junctional cleft, norepinephrine binds to its receptor on the postjunctional membrane of the effector organ (Figure 10-3). Norepinephrine is removed from the junctional cleft by metabolism by catechol-o-methyl transferase or monoamine oxidase. In addition, norepinephrine is actively reabsorbed into the adrenergic neuron for reuse. Blockade of the reuptake of norepinephrine into the prejunctional cell increases levels of norepinephrine in the junctional cleft. This reuptake can be prevented by use of cocaine or tricyclic antidepressants. The release of norepinephrine into the junctional cleft from the presynaptic vesicles can be blocked by guanethidine and bretylium. Both guanethidine and bretylium depend on active uptake into the adrenergic neuron, which can be blocked by cocaine or antidepressants by the same mechanism that prevents norepinephrine reuptake.

The adrenal medulla is densely innervated by both myelinated and unmyelinated preganglionic neurons. The axons originate at the level of T-8 to L-1 and traverse the sympathetic trunk, celiac ganglion, and suprarenal plexus before reaching the adrenal gland. The axons terminate at synapses with chromaffin cells that, on stimulation, release epinephrine and norepinephrine into the systemic circulation.

Visceral Pain

Afferent visceral sensation is transmitted by both myelinated and unmyelinated nerve fibers. They have been called the sensory counterpart of the autonomic nervous system efferents.[3] Visceral structures are generally insensitive to cutting or crushing, but are extremely sensitive to stretching and distraction and are probably involved in visceral sensations of hunger, nausea, and bladder and rectal fullness. Visceral pain is usually described as diffuse aching or cramping and may be accompanied by referred pain. Referred pain is thought to occur by activation of the somatic afferent at the same level of the spinal cord where the visceral afferent axons enter the spinal cord.

The cell bodies of the visceral afferent fibers are located in the dorsal root ganglia, as spinal nerves, along with somatic nerve cell bodies. Their axons are short and synapse with interneurons and neurons of ascending pathways in the dorsal horn of the spinal cord. The afferent nerve dendrites are extremely long from visceral structures to the ganglion. They are intimately interspersed within the sympathetic nerves, but do not make synapses within the peripheral or paravertebral ganglia. Visceral afferent sensation may be interrupted by local anesthetic or neurolytic blockade. Techniques of plexus blockade for visceral pain management are discussed in Chapter 11.

Sympathetically Mediated Pain and Cancer

Cancer may result in a clinical syndrome that is causalgic in nature and responds to sympathetic interruption.[6] Hupert has reported a series of patients who fulfilled Bonica's criteria for causalgia, except that they had no history of missile trauma.[7] Symptoms include burning pain, hyperalgesia, allodynia, vasomotor changes, sudomotor changes, and pilomotor changes. Radiographs may demonstrate patchy periarticular demineralization and generalized osteoporosis in the limb typical of the dystrophic stages of RSD. Successful treatment of pain by sympathetic interruption with local anesthetics, and long-term relief with either a series of blocks or with neurolysis, have been reported.[6–8]

Diagnosis

If sympathetically mediated pain (SMP) is suspected, the patient should be examined for the presence of autonomic instability. Measurement of temperature with infrared telethermometry (thermography) records skin temperature instantaneously, with greater than 0.1°C accuracy over areas as small as a few square millimeters. Unfortunately, peripheral skin blood flow is very sensitive to any physical or emotional stimuli, and a thermogram represents only one point in time. Despite its shortcomings, thermography has improved in the past 10 years. In a retrospective study of 803 chronic pain patients, Uematsu attempted to use thermography to differentiate organic pain. The results were ambiguous.[9] Karstetter found that 32% of RSD patients had affected limbs that were warmer than the unaffected limb by 1°C or more, whereas 62% had colder limbs.[10] Sherman found that thermography was a good way to monitor changes in pain level and in the symmetry of heat patterns. He also used it to document the effectiveness of sympathetic blocks.[11] Uematsu found clear evidence of thermographic change, after lidocaine blockade of peripheral nerves in monkeys; however, in patients with RSD, thermography did not give definitive diagnoses.[12] Recently, Sherman et al. found that thermography alone was not appropriate for diagnosis of RSD.[13] Thermal asymmetry and direction of temperature change were not consistent between patients or for patients tested on more than one occasion.

Cold challenge has also been a valuable source for evaluation of patients with RSD, because cold intolerance is a common symptom. Either thermographic evaluation or direct temperature measurement may be used, but methods of cold challenge vary widely. A standardized protocol, the isolated cold stress test, has been developed that avoids such inconsistencies. The patient's hands or feet are placed through portals into a refrigerator while skin temperature is continuously measured. After 20 minutes of exposure to a temperature of 6–10°C, the extremity is allowed to rewarm at room temperature. Normal volunteers have a transient 2–5°C decrease in temperature from a baseline of above 30°C (type I response). After evaluating 96 patients with complaints of pain, numbness, or cold intolerance of the hand(s), Koman et al. defined two abnormal temperature-response curves (types II and III).[14] All patients with the diagnosis of RSD were found to have type III patterns with baseline temperatures less than 28.5°C, rapid cooling to 8–13°C below baseline, and slow rewarming to baseline or below. Recently, Koman and colleagues have been monitoring tissue blood-flow by laser Doppler during the isolated cold stress test and believe that this measure of microvascular response to cold challenge is superior to skin temperature measurement alone. However, direct measures of peripheral blood flow, including laser Doppler, may be too complex or expensive for routine clinical use.

As an indicator of sympathetic cholinergic response, sweating can be measured using sympathogalvanic skin impedance changes. Moisture can be demonstrated by ninhydrin, cobalt blue, or starch iodide. Recently, quantitative sudomotor axon reflex test has been used. A perspex capsule is placed on the skin and the increase in humidity of air blown through the capsule is measured. Acetylcholine is then iontophoresed into the skin and, following a brief latency period, the resulting sweat output is measured. The sweat droplets are evaporated and the humidity change is measured. The time interval is then continuously integrated and converted to absolute units using a derived equation. The affected side may have either higher or lower sweat output. Low et al. found that men had three times more sweat output than women.[15] A major improvement has been the simultaneous recording of axon reflex stimulation using acetylcholine electrophoresis because it provides a dynamic recording of the sweat response with the indices of latency, volume, and amplitude.

Sympathetic blockade has long been recommended for diagnosis (and treatment) of SMP. However, sympathetic blockade as a test for RSD may lead to false-negative results because of inadequate sympathetic nerve block or false-positive results because of inadvertent somatic block. To overcome these obstacles, Arner and Raja et al. propose phentolamine as a diagnostic aid. Raja et al. compared local anesthetic sympathetic blocks (LASB) to intravenous phentolamine (25–35 mg total) in 20 patients with chronic pain and hyperalgesia who were suspected of having SMP.[16] Patients were given phentolamine or LASB in randomized order on different days. The patient and an observer recording pain scores were unaware of the times and doses of intravenous phentolamine boli. Decreases in spontaneous and stimulus-evoked pain appeared to parallel the administration of increasing doses of phentolamine. In addition, the degree of pain relief following phentolamine correlated extremely well with the relief obtained from LASB (Figure 10-4). In a similar study, Arner gave intravenous phentolamine (5–15 mg) as a continuous infusion over 5–10 minutes to both adults and children with pain and evidence of sympathetic dysfunction.[17] Intravenous regional guanethidine blocks were performed on each patient several days later. A highly significant correlation between response to phentolamine and response to guanethidine was found in adults and children. The advantages of intravenous phentolamine over LASB for the diagnosis of SMP include the ability to assess placebo response, the lack of potential for somatic block, the low rate of complications, and the minimal pain of the procedure.

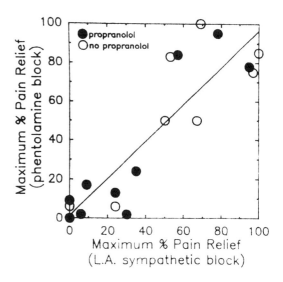

Figure 10-4. Correlation of maximum pain relief after local anesthetic sympathetic ganglion block and phentolamine block ($n = 18$, $r = 0.84$). (Reprinted with permission from SN Raja, R-D Treede, KD Davis, JN Campbell. Systemic alpha-adrenergic blockade with phentolamine: A diagnostic test for sympathetically maintained pain. Anesthesiology 1991;74:691.)

Treatment Modalities

Physical Therapy

The importance of physical therapy in patients with SMP cannot be overstated. Most cases of early RSD can be either averted or successfully treated by physical therapy before they are even diagnosed. In more advanced cases, mobility and function of the affected limb are maintained with hopes of avoiding the severe osteoporosis, contractures, and mus-

cular atrophy seen in the second and third stages. Unfortunately, some patients are intolerant of joint manipulation because of the pain associated with even the mildest levels of physical therapy.[18–20] Hand and wrist splints commonly have been used in the therapy of RSD. In the latter two stages of the disease, splints appear to limit contracture formation in some patients but exacerbate disease progression and pain in others. Unreliable results also have been noted with the use of heat or ice packs.[19–21] Deep friction massage has shown encouraging results in the relatively few patients who can tolerate such manipulation.[19] Daily ultrasonic stimulation has also been reported to be effective in a small series of patients.[22]

Transcutaneous electrical nerve stimulation (TENS) is another form of therapy that has been used to control pain in RSD patients. The TENS unit selectively activates the large A-type fibers. According to the "gate-control theory" of pain transmission, stimulation of A fibers causes decreased activity of wide dynamic range neurons in the spinal cord and, therefore, a decrease in pain. Although several investigations involving the use of TENS in children with RSD have reported excellent results,[23, 24] most studies on adult patients have reported long-lasting relief in only 25% of patients.[25–27] However, Robaina has reported good-to-excellent results with TENS in 20 of 29 patients with long-standing RSD.[28] Eighty percent of patients had "notable" relief, with an average reduction in pain intensity of 70%. Reports of exacerbation of RSD pain during TENS therapy are not unusual.[19, 29]

Psychological Therapy

Although a full discussion of the psychological aspects of RSD can be found elsewhere,[30] it is still important to mention the need for routine psychological evaluation of patients with RSD so that individualized therapy can be started early in the course of the disease. In addition to the common psychosocial problems that accompany cancer pain, patients with SMP also experience periods of anxiety and stress. It is believed that release of endogenous catecholamines in response to anxiety and stress results in direct stimulation of sensitized alpha-adrenergic receptors in the affected extremity. Therefore, reducing anxiety by minimizing family conflicts and stressful work and social situations is therapeutic.

Pharmacologic Therapy

Although more specific methods of treatment of SMP are described in the following sections, there should be no hesitation in using opioids and nonsteroidal anti-inflammatory drugs in patients with cancer and SMP. Pharmacologic therapy for SMP can be used as a first-line treatment, although sympathetic blocks should be considered early in the course of the disease, if more conservative medical treatment fails. Numerous medications have been used to treat SMP, but few have proved to be widely efficacious. I have included in this discussion only those that I think are appropriate for cancer patients.

Corticosteroids

Steinbrocker et al.[31] reported the use of loading doses of corticotropin and cortisone (100 and 200 mg per day, respectively) for 3–10 days before reducing the dose by small increments to 45–50% of the original dose for the treatment of "shoulder-hand syndrome." Therapy was continued for approximately 6 months, and pain relief was reported in 9 of 13 patients, whereas 2 of 13 had therapy-related complications. One group from Denmark reported excellent results with oral prednisone at 30 mg per day for no more than 12 weeks in a double-blind, randomized, placebo-controlled study.[32] The current recommendation for steroid therapy is oral prednisone given at high initial doses (40–60 mg) for 4–6 weeks followed by tapering of the dose over 2–4 weeks.

Alpha-Adrenergic Antagonists

In view of current etiologic theories, treatment of SMP with $alpha_1$-adrenergic blockade should be successful. $Alpha_1$-receptor blockade, with agents such as prazosin and phenoxybenzamine, has been shown to be beneficial for some patients. However, in many patients, alpha-adrenergic blockade results in hypotension, reflex tachycardia, fatigue, and dizziness.[33, 34] The intravenous administration of phentolamine, a mixed $alpha_1$-$alpha_2$-antagonist, has been recommended as a diagnostic test for SMP.[35, 36] If the phentolamine test result is positive, a trial of prazosin is initiated. The dose should be titrated upward until pain is relieved or symptoms such as orthostasis are limited. Patients with SMP seem to tolerate prazosin very well. I usually start with 3 mg per day (1 mg three times a day) and increase weekly by 3 mg per day to a maximum dosage of 15 mg per day. Terazosin has also been used for treating SMP and, in my experience, is better tolerated than prazosin.[37]

Local Anesthetic Blockade

Local anesthetic blockade of the sympathetic ganglia can be used to treat RSD or to predict the response to surgical sympathectomy. More than 80% of patients with RSD have been reported to respond to a series of sympathetic blocks combined with physical therapy.[38–40] Lower recovery rates are seen in patients with long-standing pain[41] or with partial major peripheral nerve injury (causalgia).[39] These lower recovery rates can be expected in the patient with cancer because of the presence and progression of tumor infiltration that sustains the SMP. Bonica reports a 50% long-term success rate with sympathetic blocks for the treatment of causalgia.

Pain relief usually lasts longer than the duration of local anesthetic blockade, although patients rarely experience permanent pain relief from a single block. Usually, a series of blocks is performed as long as pain continues to decrease, or the period of pain relief after each block continues to increase. When intermittent sympathetic ganglion blocks fail to give long-term relief, an intravenous regional (IVR) block or a continuous sympathetic block should be tried. If the pain is not temporarily relieved by sympathetic blockade, the diagnosis of SMP should be questioned. It is possible for the patient to have symptoms consistent with RSD but the pain is independent of the sympathetic nervous system (sympathetically independent pain).

Stellate ganglion blocks are generally used for diagnostic and prognostic blocks because sensory blockade is avoided. For a series of therapeutic blocks, stellate ganglion, brachial plexus, or cervical epidural blocks can be used. Some authors recommend the use of brachial plexus blocks for a more complete sympathetic block to the arm. Theoretically, sympathetic innervation from as low as T-4 may be missed with stellate ganglion blocks, especially with low-volume injections. However, skin temperature or other measures of sympathetic function can be used to ensure adequate sympathetic blockade.

For the reasons stated previously, lumbar sympathetic blocks are preferred over epidural or peripheral nerve blocks for diagnostic and prognostic investigations of the leg. Unlike stellate ganglion block (where a Horner's syndrome usually accompanies a successful block), there are no obvious physical signs accompanying sympathetic blockade. Therefore, it is important to document successful needle placement with fluoroscopy or objective measurements of sympathetic blockade. If fluoroscopic guidance is used, injection of a contrast medium should confirm placement of the needle tip in the retroperitoneal space, anterior and lateral to the vertebral body. Although some authors have recommended that three separate needles be used at L-2, L-3, and L-4, we found that a single injection at L-2 or L-3 is sufficient.

Intravenous Regional Sympathetic Blocks

The use of guanethidine by an IRV (Bier block) technique for causalgia was reported by Hanning-ton-Kiff in 1974.[42] Guanethidine selectively inhibits peripheral sympathetic nerve transmission. It is transported by the norepinephrine pump into the presynaptic vesicles of the postganglionic adrenergic neurons. After causing an initial release of norepinephrine, guanethidine prevents the reuptake of norepinephrine from the synaptic cleft and inhibits further release of norepinephrine. This biphasic effect is seen clinically as an initial increase in sympathetic tone followed by a prolonged decrease in sympathetic activity. Although the oral use of guanethidine for RSD has been described, systemic side effects such as postural hypotension, dizziness, nausea, and diarrhea are common.[43] Administration of intravenous guanethidine (10–20 mg) into a limb isolated by a tourniquet produces a high concentration in the adrenergic neurons of the affected extremity while minimizing systemic side effects. Concurrent administration of tricyclic antidepressants may interfere with the uptake of guanethidine into presynaptic vesicles. The effect of guanethidine is specific to patients with SMP, because only adrenergic neurons are blocked. Wahren et al. found that patients with sympathetically independent pain had no change in vibration-produced allodynia following IVR guanethidine, whereas patients with SMP had normalization of their heat, cold, and vibration pain thresholds following IVR guanethidine.[44]

The mean duration of chemical sympathectomy after IVR guanethidine is 3 days following the first treatment and 6 days following the second.[45–48] An increasing duration of sympathetic blockade may be seen with a series of treatments. Hannington-Kiff has postulated that repeated administration of guanethidine leads to an accumulation of guanethidine in sympathetic nerve endings, causing retraction of axons from their effector sites.[49]

Like guanethidine, bretylium accumulates in postganglionic adrenergic neurons and inhibits conduction by preventing norepinephrine release. Ford et al.[50] described the use of IVR bretylium for treatment of RSD. They used 1 mg bretylium per kg and obtained pain relief and subjective warmth in the extremity for 7–21 days following the first treatment in four patients. Subsequent treatments resulted in pain relief lasting from 25 days to 7 months. This low dose of bretylium appears to be virtually without side effects. In our experience, sympathetic blockade following IVR bretylium (1.5 mg per kg) lasted 2 weeks to 7 months in patients who received only 6–24 hours of relief after multiple sympathetic ganglion blocks with local anesthetic. The average duration of pain relief greater than 30% was 20 days[51] (Figure 10-5), although permanent relief of symptoms of RSD has been seen. The major side effects of IVR bretylium are hypertension and tachycardia from the initial release of norepinephrine, followed by orthostatic hypotension from chemical sympathetic blockade. Orthostatic hypotension can be prevented by the intravenous administration of 750–1,000 ml of saline or lactated Ringer's solution, following an IVR block. Because of its minimal toxicity, ready availability, and apparent efficacy, bretylium is currently being used for IVR chemical sympathectomy.

IVR sympathetic blockade is appropriate in patients who have SMP that is distal to the axilla or groin. Patients who have procedures performed for peripheral tumors (e.g., osteogenic sarcoma, melanoma, schwannoma, etc.) may have SMP that does not extend above the tourniquet. However, most patients with SMP related to cancer will have proximal pain that is not amenable to IVR sympathetic blocks.

Epidural and Somatic Blocks

Patients with stage III RSD do not obtain adequate analgesia for physical therapy with sympathetic blockade alone, because pain from manipulation of fibrotic joints and muscles is carried by A-alpha nerve fibers. In addition, patients with cancer may be expected to have coexisting somatic sources of pain due to tumor infiltration. Somatic sources of pain may be important in perpetuating a cycle leading to sympathetic overactivity. Therefore, coexisting problems directly related to tumor, or unrelated problems, such as tendinitis, carpal tunnel syndrome, and ulnar nerve entrapment should be treated concurrently by appropriate methods, such as steroids or surgical decompression. Although this pain is difficult to control, continuous somatic nerve blockade combined with physical therapy may offer the only hope of pain relief and rehabilitation.[52]

Intermittent somatic blocks with local anesthetic have sometimes been used to treat refractory cases of RSD. Gibbons et al. reported a series of 25 patients who were treated with interscalene blocks for upper extremity pain.[53] Stellate gan-

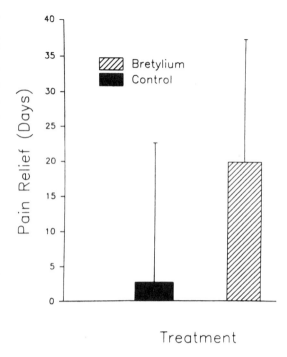

Figure 10-5. Days of pain relief (duration) with drugs used for intravenous blockade. Control group received lidocaine alone; Bretylium group received lidocaine plus bretylium. (Reprinted with permission from AH Hord, MD Rooks, BO Stephens, et al. Intravenous regional bretylium and lidocaine for treatment of reflex sympathetic dystrophy: A randomized, double-blind study. Anesth Analg 1992;74:818.)

glion blocks had previously been performed in eight of the patients. Although six patients had some response to stellate blocks, none had obtained long-term relief of pain. Of the 25 patients treated with interscalene blocks, 17 had RSD. Eleven of the patients with RSD had significant pain relief on follow-up. Nine of the 11 had increased range of motion. Therefore, somatic blockade of the brachial plexus should be considered in those patients who are refractory to sympathetic block or who have a restricted range of motion. Any patient with a range-of-motion deficit when tested during general or regional anesthesia should be considered for continuous somatic blockade. In addition, there may be patients with both sympathetically dependent and independent pain who will need sensory analgesia in order to tolerate physical therapy. These patients will need intermittent or continuous somatic blockade.

Specific Cancer Pain Syndromes and Sympathetically Mediated Pain

Pancoast's Tumor

Tumors of the superior pulmonary sulcus (Pancoast's tumor) often lead to an SMP syndrome at some time during the course of the disease. Pancoast originally postulated that tumors of the superior sulcus were of nonpulmonary origin. However, later investigators have reported that the most superior sulcus tumors are pulmonary in origin and occur in men.[54] Pancoast's tumors represent only 3% of all lung tumors.[55] Almost all patients with Pancoast's tumor have severe intractable pain,[56] which is initially described as a deep ache in the shoulder and scapula. Later, as damage to the lower trunks of the brachial plexus occurs by tumor infiltration or compression, neuralgic pain extends into the forearm and hand. Paresthesias, dysesthesias, and hypesthesias are commonly present. Compression or destruction of the cervicothoracic sympathetic chain by tumor may result in a Horner's syndrome. As tumor invasion progresses, sensory and motor neurologic deficits become more extensive and deafferentation pain is more prominent.

Signs of hyperalgesia, allodynia, or vasomotor changes may indicate causalgic pain resulting from partial injury to the brachial plexus. Dystrophic changes may be present, although they are often difficult to differentiate from the effects of the brachial plexus injury and subsequent disuse. Edema results from causalgia or venous or lymphatic obstruction, and symptoms may be palliated by radiation therapy or high-dose steroids. Pain should be eliminated or decreased by sympathetic blockade until the pain from the neural invasion itself becomes most prominent or deafferentation occurs. Neurolysis may be performed when technically feasible. However, tumor invasion of the paravertebral space can prevent normal spread of local anesthetics or neurolytic substances.

Lumbar Plexus Invasion

Symptoms of lumbar plexus invasion parallel those resulting from brachial plexus invasion. Tumors that commonly result in lumbar plexus invasion include those of the prostate, bladder, uterus, cervix, or colon. Infiltration and compression of the plexus occur from direct extension of tumor from the primary site or from adjacent lymph nodes or bone. The distribution of the pain varies because the tumor may invade the plexus at any level. When causalgic pain occurs, it may be technically easier to perform sympathetic neurolysis than with Pancoast's tumors, because preganglionic fibers of the sympathetic chain can usually be interrupted above the level of tumor invasion.

Cancer-Related Pain Syndromes and Sympathetic Blockade

Phantom Limb Pain

Large studies have shown the incidence of phantom limb pain (PLP) to be from 60–85%.[57–60] The incidence of PLP increases with more proximal amputations. Wall reported PLP in 88% of patients following hemipelvectomy or hip disarticulation for cancer.[61] Severe pain was present in 36% of these patients. Roth and Sugarbaker reported a 68% incidence of PLP after hemipelvectomy and 40% after hip disarticulation, whereas above-knee and below-knee amputations were associated with a 19% and 0% incidence, respectively.[62]

Nerve blocks are commonly used to treat PLP and reportedly they have a high success rate.[63] Trigger-point or direct stump injections and sympathetic, peripheral nerve, and major conduction blocks have all been used to treat the pain. However, most amputees report either no effect or minor temporary changes with nerve blocks.[60] Only 14% of amputees report even a significant temporary change; less than 5% report a large permanent change or complete cure.[60] The use of neural blockade in the treatment of PLP is based on anecdotal reports in the literature. Blankenbaker reported his experiences in treating PLP with sympathetic blockade[64] and concluded that sympathetic blocks are successful if amputees are treated soon after the onset of PLP. Although this assertion is unsupported by controlled studies, many researchers think that a diagnostic sympathetic block should be performed in amputees who describe throbbing pain in the phantom limb or stump, or who have symptoms of sympathetic overactivity or vascular compromise. Although local anesthetics provide only temporary relief in most patients, some obtain prolonged relief of pain.

The usual course of PLP is to remain unchanged or to improve.[60, 65] Up to 56% of patients report improvement or complete resolution.[60] Therefore, when symptoms of PLP increase in severity or begin later than 1 month postamputation, the reasons should be investigated. There have been two reports of angina that presented as pain referred to the phantom left arm.[66, 67] Radicular pain in the phantom limb may be associated with disc herniation,[68] or it may be triggered by reactivation of herpes zoster or by recurrence of cancer.[69, 70] Any patient who has undergone amputation due to cancer should have an evaluation for metastatic disease if PLP significantly increases.

Postmastectomy Syndrome

Postmastectomy pain syndrome (PMPS) occurs in 4–6% of patients following breast surgery.[71] It is most commonly associated with radical mastectomy, although it can occur any time that there is extensive dissection of axillary nodes. It is thought to result from damage to the intercostobrachial nerve during surgery. The intercostobrachial nerve is a division of the T-2 intercostal nerve that innervates the proximal medial arm from the axilla to the elbow. It is located subcutaneously in the axilla and can be easily damaged or severed during axillary dissections. The result is a neuralgia characterized by burning pain in the axilla, medial arm, and anterior chest. Lancinating pains in the medial arm are common, and hyperesthesia, dysesthesia, hyperalgesia, allodynia, or hypoesthesia in the intercostobrachial nerve distribution may occur. Even contact of the arm with the chest wall or clothing may be uncomfortable. Movement of the arm may be painful, such that the arm is voluntarily immobilized.

In treating patients with PMPS, it is important to restore range of motion to the arm and shoulder by providing adequate pain relief. SMP may develop in the limb if treatment is delayed. Initial treatment is with oral analgesics, tricyclic antidepressants, T-2 intercostal nerve blocks, epidural blocks, and neuroma infiltration. TENS may be useful for patients who can tolerate it. Continuous epidural analgesia or neuroablative procedures (dorsal root entry zone or rhizotomy) are indicated in severe cases that do

not respond to conservative therapy. For those patients who develop a frozen shoulder from prolonged immobilization, interscalene blocks followed by closed manipulation and aggressive physical therapy are needed to restore function.

When SMP develops, it usually takes the appearance of a variant of RSD called the shoulder-hand syndrome. Pain is primarily located in the proximal arm and shoulder, with dystrophic changes in the hand and forearm. Edema may be present due to either RSD or venous or lymphatic obstruction in the axilla. In cases of PMPS where hyperalgesia and allodynia are prominent and not relieved by oral medications and intercostal nerve blocks, diagnostic sympathetic blockade by intravenous phentolamine test or stellate ganglion block should be performed. If the results indicate the presence of SMP, a trial of oral alpha-adrenergic blockade or a series of sympathetic blocks should be initiated. IRV blocks are usually not appropriate because allodynia does not allow tourniquet placement and most of the pain may be located proximal to the level of the tourniquet. A limited trial of continuous epidural analgesia with local anesthetics or opioids should be considered if intermittent sympathetic blocks fail to adequately facilitate range of motion and physical therapy.

Postthoracotomy Pain Syndrome

This syndrome is characterized by pain that may be associated with sensory loss in an intercostal nerve distribution following thoracotomy. Such pain is common following thoracotomy, but usually resolves within 2 weeks. It has been proposed that crush injury, or section of the nerve, occurs intraoperatively, leading to a fibrotic neuropathy and subsequent intercostal neuralgia. However, Kanner et al. have shown that most cases of persistent pain following thoracotomy for cancer are recurrent disease.[72] In a study that followed 117 cancer patients after thoracotomy, the authors found that postthoracotomy pain resolved in 26% of patients within 1 month, 28% within 2 months, and another 28% within the follow-up period after surgery. The remaining patients had pain that increased in the postoperative period and was usually associated with recurrent tumor. In addition, 13 of the patients with initial resolution of pain (11%) had recurrence of pain associated with recurrent tumor. The study emphasizes the fact that persistent or recurrent postthoracotomy pain almost always signifies recurrence of tumor. However, occasionally, there are patients who have persistent pain following thoracotomy with no evidence of recurrence. The incidence in our practice has declined noticeably in the last 7 years and we are unsure whether this is due to changes in surgical technique or to preemptive effects of the use of epidural analgesia in nearly all patients undergoing thoracotomy for the last 5 years.

Pain can be located in the scar and chest wall or in a radicular pattern corresponding to an injured intercostal nerve. The quality and intensity of the pain varies, depending on the etiology. Patients may describe paresthesias, dysesthesias, hyperesthesias, or allodynia. RSD may develop in the ipsilateral upper extremity, and an adhesive capsulitis may occur. If pain persists or recurs, a diagnostic workup including computed tomography or magnetic resonance imaging should be performed to rule out recurrent tumor.

Because the pain usually resolves within 2 months (in the absence of recurrent tumor), treatment is directed toward symptomatic relief and preservation of range of motion of the upper extremity. TENS may reduce pain from intercostal neuralgia by stimulation of adjacent (intact) intercostal nerves. Physical therapy should be initiated to maintain upper extremity range of motion and to begin desensitization procedures if hyperesthesia and allodynia are present. Tricyclic antidepressants may be useful for promoting analgesia and sleep. A trial of anticonvulsants, such as carbamazepine, phenytoin, or clonazepam, should be considered for patients who have intermittent lancinating pains. Posterior intercostal nerve block with local anesthetic provides analgesia during the recovery phase and may hasten resolution of the pain. However, when pain recurs, treatment with oral opioids, epidural analgesia, or neuroablative procedures should be considered if intercostal blocks do not give long-term relief.

Acute Herpes Zoster and Postherpetic Neuralgia

Acute Herpes Zoster

Herpes zoster occurs commonly in patients with cancer. The herpes varicella-zoster virus is a DNA virus that is thought to remain latent in the dorsal root ganglion after the initial infection (chickenpox). In otherwise immunocompetent patients, the incidence of zoster increases with age and is thought to be a result of decreasing immune surveillance.[73] In patients who are immunocompromised by cancer or by its treatment modalities, zoster is more common and severe than in the general population. Patients with lymphoma or leukemia and those who undergo radiation and chemotherapy are most likely to develop zoster. Systemic distribution is thought to occur most frequently in patients with deficient T-cell function.[74]

Pain is usually the first symptom of zoster and increases in severity during the first week. The pain is commonly described as itching and burning, and occasionally sharp or lancinating. Within 5 days of the onset of pain, vesicals erupt in a dermatomal pattern. Hyperesthesia is prominent while vesicles are present. The vesicles crust over and heal within 3 weeks and pain gradually subsides, except in those patients who develop postherpetic neuralgia. Hemorrhagic inflammation of the peripheral nerve and dorsal root ganglion occurs, with resulting wallerian degeneration of axons. Preferential destruction of large fibers may predispose to postherpetic pain.[75]

Several antiviral agents have been used to treat acute herpes zoster. In particular, vidarabine and acyclovir have proved to be effective in shortening the duration of symptoms and preventing complications, such as dissemination.[76] When vidarabine is used within 72 hours of rash onset, it appears to decrease the extent of cutaneous distribution and to prevent systemic spread. A decrease in both acute pain and postherpetic neuralgia was suggested. Treatment requires hospitalization for intravenous infusion and is recommended only for immunosuppressed patients. By inhibiting viral DNA polymerase, acyclovir prevents dissemination and hastens healing in normal and immunosuppressed patients. More recently, two more antiviral drugs have been released for treatment of herpes zoster. Valacyclovir is a prodrug that is rapidly converted to acyclovir in the liver.[77] Acyclovir levels are improved because of rapid absorption. Valacyclovir is indicated for the treatment of herpes zoster in immunocompetent adults. Valacyclovir should be given at a dose of 1 g three times daily for 7 days, starting at the earliest signs of herpes zoster. Famcyclovir is also a prodrug that is rapidly metabolized to pencyclovir.[78] In treatment of herpes zoster, famcyclovir has been shown to accelerate lesion healing and reduce the duration of viral shedding. It has been clearly shown to result in faster resolution of postherpetic neuralgia at doses of 500 or 750 mg three times daily for 7 days. Both valacyclovir and famcyclovir are also active against herpes simplex viruses 1 and 2. Because systemic spread is rare in immunocompetent patients, antiviral agents are only officially recommended in those with disease- or drug-induced immunosuppression.

Corticosteroids may be used to lessen the tissue (including nerve) injury that may lead to chronic pain following herpes zoster. Steroids have also been shown to decrease the acute pain of herpes zoster and to speed the resolution of pain.[74, 79–81] However, the effect of steroids on vesicle resolution and prevention of systemic spread is controversial. There is concern about the possibility of further immunosuppression with corticosteroids in the already immunocompromised patient, but this has not been observed clinically. There have been positive anecdotal reports of using subcutaneous injection of steroids under the vesicles but no clear evidence that healing is more rapid.[82]

Most studies on the use of sympathetic blocks for treatment of acute herpes zoster have been uncontrolled. In two such studies, patients were treated within 2 weeks of the onset of zoster lesions with local anesthetic sympathetic ganglion blocks.[83, 84] The authors report pain relief in from 85–90% of patients. Patients required one to four sympathetic blocks to achieve pain relief. Unfortunately, it appears that the timing of the blocks was critical. Only 40% of patients had pain relief if treated more than 2 weeks after zoster erupted. Raj has reported a series of patients who underwent stellate ganglion block for the treatment of acute zoster pain in the trigeminal nerve distribution.[82] Dramatic and lasting pain relief was obtained in 77% of patients and vesicular lesions dried more quickly than in untreated patients. Epidural blocks with local anesthetics have also been used successfully within the first 7 weeks of herpes zoster.[85] Ninety percent to 100% of patients obtained relief within the first 24 hours after the block and there were no patients with postherpetic neuralgia (PHN) on long-term follow-up. Other somatic blocks, particularly intercostal blocks, have been frequently used to control acute pain.

Postherpetic Neuralgia

Persistent pain following the healing phase of acute herpes zoster is called PHN. It occurs in less than 10% of patients following zoster, but is far more common in the elderly. Up to 37% of patients over 60 years of age have pain for more than 1 year.[86] PHN is more common following zoster in the ophthalmic division of the trigeminal nerve than in a spinal nerve distribution. Pain is described as a constant aching or burning. Although hyperalgesia and allodynia may be present, more commonly the patient's skin is hypesthetic. Paresthesias may also be present.

PHN has been treated with multiple drugs and nerve blocks, and controlled studies have supported the use of tricyclic antidepressants to promote analgesia and sleep.[87] Phenothiazines such as fluphenazine have been used in combination with antidepressants, but evidence for their efficacy is still needed. A trial of anticonvulsants, such as carbamazepine, phenytoin, gabapentin, or clonazepam, should be considered when intermittent lancinating pains are present. Opioid analgesics may be partially effective in relieving pain. In patients with persistent PHN, long-acting opioids, such as continuous-release morphine or methadone, should be used to promote a more stable level of analgesia. Especially in the patient with a limited life expectancy, there should be no fear of addiction.

The pain of PHN can be managed with somatic and sympathetic blocks, but there is little evidence of their long-term efficacy. Because zoster usually occurs in the thoracic and trigeminal nerve distributions, intercostal, epidural, and stellate ganglion blocks are most commonly used. Nerve blocks may be used to temporarily relieve patients with severe pain while oral analgesics are adjusted. Although I do not usually recommend neurolytic blocks for the treatment of PHN, they may have a limited role in palliative treatment of patients with limited life expectancy due to cancer. Cryoanalgesia is preferable to chemical neurolysis, due to the low incidence of neuralgia from the procedure.

The literature on the use of sympathetic blocks for prevention of PHN is mostly anecdotal. There are no controlled studies. However, some of the studies mentioned previously report an incidence of PHN that is lower than in the general population who are not treated with sympathetic blocks.[82, 83] It is postulated that sympathetic blockade relieves pain and prevents nerve damage and subsequent neuralgic pain by relieving vasospasm in perineural vasculature. As with PLP, it appears that sympathetic blocks may have a role in prevention, but rarely in the treatment of well-established pain.

References

1. Bonica JJ. Definitions and Taxonomy of Pain. In JJ Bonica (ed), The Management of Pain (Vol. 1). Malvern, PA: Lea & Febiger, 1990;18.

2. Chusid JG (ed), Correlative Neuroanatomy & Functional Neurology (19th ed). Los Altos, CA: Lange, 1985.

3. R Warwick, PL Williams (eds), Gray's Anatomy (35th British ed). Philadelphia: Saunders, 1973.

4. Kuntz A. Autonomic Nervous System (4th ed). Philadelphia: Lea & Febiger, 1953.

5. Mitchell GAG. Anatomy of the Autonomic Nervous System. London: Livingstone, 1953.

6. Wilson PR, Wedel DJ. Role of Pain Clinic in Bone Cancer Pain. In FH Sim (ed), Diagnosis and Management of Metastatic Bone Disease: A Multidisciplinary Approach. New York: Raven, 1988;109.

7. Hupert C. Recognition and treatment of causalgic pain occurring in cancer patients. Pain Abstracts (Vol. 1). Second World Congress on Pain, Montreal Canada, August 27 to September 1, 1978.

8. Bonica JJ. Causalgia and Other Reflex Sympathetic Dystrophies. In JJ Bonica (ed), The Management of Pain (Vol. 2). Malvern, PA: Lea & Febiger, 1990;220.

9. Uematsu S, Hendler N, Hungerford D, et al. Thermography and electromyography in the differential diagnosis of chronic pain syndromes and reflex sympathetic dystrophy. Electromyogr Clin Neurophysiol 1981; 21:165.

10. Karstetter KW, Sherman RA. Use of thermography for initial detection of early reflex sympathetic dystrophy. J Am Podiatr Med Assoc 1991;81:198.

11. Sherman RA, Barja RH. Thermographic correlates of chronic pain: Analysis of 125 patients incorporating evaluations by a blind panel. Arch Phys Med Rehabil 1987;68:273.

12. Uematsu S. Thermographic imaging of cutaneous sensory segment in patients with peripheral nerve injury. J Neurosurg 1985;62:716.

13. Sherman RA, Karstetter KW, Damiano M, Evans CB. Stability of temperature asymmetries in reflex sympathetic dystrophy over time and changes in pain. Clin J Pain 1994;10:71.

14. Koman L, Nunley J, Goldner J, et al. Isolated cold stress testing in the assessment of symptoms in upper extremity: Preliminary communication. J Hand Surg 1984;3:305.

15. Low PA, Caskey PE, Tuck RR, et al Quantitative sudomotor axon reflex test in normal and neuropathic subjects. Ann Neurol 1983;14:573.

16. Raja SN, Treede R-D, Davis KD, Campbell JN. Systemic alpha-adrenergic blockade with phentolamine: A diagnostic test for sympathetically maintained pain. Anesthesiology 1991;74:691.

17. Arner S. Intravenous phentolamine test: Diagnostic and prognostic use in reflex sympathetic dystrophy. Pain 1991;46:17.

18. Duncan K, Lewis RC, Racz G, Nordyke MD. Treatment of upper extremity reflex sympathetic dystrophy with joint stiffness using sympatholytic bier blocks and manipulation. Orthopedics 1988;11:883.

19. Schutzer S, Gossling H. Current concepts review: The treatment of reflex sympathetic dystrophy syndrome. J Bone Joint Surg Am 1984;66:625.

20. Schwartzman R, McLellan T. Reflex sympathetic dystrophy: A review. Arch Neurol 1987;44:555.

21. Hodges DL, McGuire TJ. Burning and pain after injury: Is it causalgia or reflex sympathetic dystrophy? Postgrad Med 1988;83:187.

22. Portwood MM, Lieberman JS, Taylor RG. Ultrasound treatment of reflex sympathetic dystrophy. Arch Phys Med Rehabil 1987;68:116.

23. Richlin DM, Carron H, Rowlingson JC, et al. Reflex sympathetic dystrophy: Successful treatment by transcutaneous nerve stimulation. J Pediatr 1978;93:84.

24. Stilz R, Carron H, Sanders DB. Case history number 96: Reflex sympathetic dystrophy in a 6-year-old: Successful treatment by transcutaneous nerve stimulation. Anesth Analg 1977;56:438.

25. Meyer GA, Fields HL. Causalgia treated by selective large fibre stimulation of peripheral nerve. Brain 1972;95:163.

26. Owens S, Atkinson ER, Lees DE. Thermographic evidence of reduced sympathetic tone with transcutaneous nerve stimulation. Anesthesiology 1979;50:62.

27. Wall PD, Sweet WH. Temporary abolition of pain in man. Science 1967;155:108.

28. Robaina FJ, Rodriguez JL, de Vera JA, Martin MA. Transcutaneous electrical nerve stimulation and spinal cord stimulation for pain relief in reflex sympathetic dystrophy. Stereotact Funct Neurosurg 1989;52:53.

29. Withrington RH, Parry CBW. The management of painful peripheral nerve disorders. J Hand Surg 1984;9-B:24.

30. Haddox JD. Psychological Aspects of Reflex Sympathetic Dystrophy. In M Stanton-Hicks (ed), Pain and the Sympathetic Nervous System (Vol. 7). Norwell: Kluwer, 1990;207.

31. Steinbrocker O, Neustadt D, Lapin L. Shoulder-hand syndrome: Sympathetic block compared with corticotropin and cortisone therapy. JAMA 1953;153:788.

32. Christensen K, Jensen EM, Noer I. The reflex sympathetic dystrophy syndrome response to treatment with systemic corticosteroids. Acta Chir Scand 1982;148:653.

33. Carter SA. Finger systolic pressures and skin temperatures in severe Raynaud's syndrome: The relationship to healing of skin lesions and the use of oral phenoxybenzamine. Angiology 1981;32:298.

34. Porter JM, Snider RL, Bardana EJ, et al. The diagnosis and treatment of Raynaud's phenomenon. Surgery 1975;77:11.

35. Raja SN, Treede R-D, Davis KD, Campbell JN. Systemic alpha-adrenergic blockade with phentolamine: A diagnostic test for sympathetically-maintained pain. Anesthesiology 1991;74:691.

36. Arner S. Intravenous phentolamine test: Diagnostic and prognostic use in reflex sympathetic dystrophy. Pain 1991;46:17.

37. Stevens DS, Robins VF, Price HM. Treatment of sympathetically maintained pain with terazosin. Reg Anesth 1993;18:318.

38. Abram SE. Pain of Sympathetic Origin. In PP Raj (ed), Practical Management of Pain. Chicago: Year Book, 1986;451.

39. Bonica JJ. Causalgia and Other Reflex Sympathetic Dystrophies. In JJ Bonica, JC Liebeskind, D Albe-Fessard (eds), Advances in Pain Research and Therapy (Vol. 3). New York: Raven, 1979;141.

40. Carron H, Weller RM. Treatment of post-traumatic sympathetic dystrophy. Adv Neurol 1974;4:485.

41. Abram SE, Anderson RA, Maitra-D'Cruze AM. Factor predicting short-term outcome of nerve blocks in the management of chronic pain. Pain 1981;10:323.

42. Hannington-Kiff JG. Intravenous regional sympathetic block with guanethidine. Lancet 1974;1:1019.

43. Tabira T, Shibasaki H, Kuroiwa Y. Reflex sympathetic dystrophy (causalgia) treatment with guanethidine. Arch Neurol 1983;40:430.

44. Wahren LK, Torebjoaurk E, Nystroaum B. Quantitative sensory testing before and after regional guanethidine block in patients with neuralgia in the hand. Pain 1991;46:23.

45. Davidoff G, Morey K, Amann M, Stamps J. Pain measurement in reflex sympathetic dystrophy syndrome. Pain 1988;32:27.

46. Driessen JJ, Van Der Werken C, Nicolai PA, Crul JF. Clinical effects of regional intravenous guanethidine (Ismelin) in reflex sympathetic dystrophy. Acta Anaesthesiol Scand 1983;27:505.

47. Hannington-Kiff J. Pharmacological target blocks in hand surgery and rehabilitation. J Hand Surg 1984;9:29.

48. McKain C, Urban BJ, Goldner JL. The effects of intravenous regional guanethidine and reserpine. J Bone Joint Surg Am 1983;65:808.

49. Hannington Kiff J. Antisympathetic Drugs in Limbs. In PD Wall, R Melzack (eds), Textbook of Pain. New York: Churchill Livingstone, 1984;566.

50. Ford SR, Forrest WH, Eltherington L. The treatment of reflex sympathetic dystrophy with intravenous regional bretylium. Anesthesiology 1988;68:137.

51. Hord AH, Rooks MD, Stephens BO, et al. Intravenous regional bretylium and lidocaine for treatment of reflex sympathetic dystrophy: A randomized, double-blind study. Anesth Analg 1992;74:818.

52. Hord AH, Raj PP. Treatment of stage III reflex sympathetic dystrophy. Reg Anesth 1987;12:102.

53. Gibbons JJ, Wilson PR, Lamer TJ, Elliott BA. Interscalene blocks for chronic upper extremity pain. Clin J Pain 1992;8:264.

54. Berrino F. Epidemiology of Superior Pulmonary Sulcus Syndrome (Pancoast Syndrome). In JJ Bonica, V Ventafridda, CA Pagni (eds), Advances in Pain Research and Therapy (Vol. 4). New York: Raven, 1982;15.

55. Kanner RM, Martini N, Foley KM. Incidence of Pain and Other Clinical Manifestations of Superior Pulmonary Sulcus Tumor (Pancoast's tumor). In JJ Bonica, V Ventafridda, CA Pagni (eds), Advances in Pain Research and Therapy (Vol. 4). New York: Raven, 1982;27.

56. Watson PN, Evans RJ. Intractable pain with lung cancer. Pain 1987;29:163.

57. Jensen TS, Krebs B, Nielsen J, et al. Phantom limb, phantom pain and stump pain in amputees during the first 6 months following limb amputation. Pain 1983;17:243.

58. Parkes CM. Factors determining the persistence of phantom pain in the amputee. J Psychosom Res 1973;17:97.

59. Sherman RA, Sherman CJ. Prevalence and characteristics of chronic phantom limb pain among American veterans. Results of a trial survey. Am J Phys Med 1983;62:227.

60. Sherman RA, Sherman CJ, Parker L. Chronic phantom and stump pain among American veterans: Results of a survey. Pain 1984;18:83.

61. Wall R, Novotny-Joseph P, MacNamara TE. Does preamputation pain influence phantom limb pain in cancer patients? South Med J 1985;78:34.

62. Roth YF, Sugarbaker PH. Pains and sensations after amputation: Character and clinical significance. Arch Phys Med Rehabil 1980;61:490.

63. Sherman RA, Sherman CJ, Call NG. A survey of current phantom limb pain treatment in the United States. Pain 1980;8:85.

64. Blankenbaker WL. The care of patients with phantom limb pain in a clinic. Anesth Analg 1977;56:842.

65. Jensen TS, Borge K, Nielsen J, et al. Immediate and long-term phantom limb pain in amputees: Incidence, clinical characteristics and relationship to pre-amputation limb pain. Pain 1985;21:267.

66. Cohen H. Anginal pain in a phantom limb [letter]. Br Med J 1976;2:475.

67. Meter SW, Clintron GB, Long C. Phantom angina. Am Heart J 1988;116:1627.

68. Finneson BE, Haft H, Krueger EG. Phantom limb syndrome associated with herniated nucleus pulposus. J Neurosurg 1957;14:344.

69. Wilson PR, Person JR, Su DW, et al. Herpes zoster reactivation of phantom limb pain. Mayo Clin Proc 1978;53:336.
70. Sugarbaker PH, Weiss CM, Davidson DD, et al. Increasing phantom limb pain as a symptom of cancer recurrence. Cancer 1984;54:373.
71. Granek I, Ashikari R, Foley KM. Postmastectomy pain syndrome: Clinical and anatomic correlates. Proc Am Soc Clin Oncol 1983;3:122.
72. Kanner R, Martini N, Foley KM. Nature and incidence of postthoracotomy pain. Proc Am Soc Clin Oncol 1982;1:152.
73. Berger R, Florent G, Just M. Decrease of the lymphoproliferative response to varicella-zoster virus antigen in the aged. Infect Immunol 1981;32:24.
74. Price RW. Herpes zoster: An approach to systemic therapy. Med Clin North Am 1982;66:1105.
75. Noordenbos W. Problems pertaining to the transmission of nerve impulses which give rise to pain. Pain 1959;1:4, 68.
76. Whitley RJ, Soong SJ, Dolin R, et al. Early vidarabine therapy to control the complications of herpes zoster in immunosuppressed patients. N Engl J Med 1982;307:971.
77. Valacyclovir. Med Lett Drugs Ther 1996;38:3.
78. Barbarash RA, Nahlikje, Cunningham A, et al. Famcyclovir for the treatment of acute herpes zoster. Effects on acute disease and post herpetic neuralgia. A randomized, double blind, placebo-controlled trial. Ann Intern Med 1995;123:89.
79. Gelfand ML. Treatment of herpes zoster with cortisone. JAMA 1954;154:911.
80. Appleman DH. Treatment of herpes zoster with ACTH. N Engl J Med 1955;253:693.
81. Elliot FA. Treatment of herpes zoster with high doses of prednisone. Lancet 1964;2:610.
82. Raj PP. Pain Due to Herpes Zoster. In PP Raj (ed), Practical Management of Pain (2nd ed). St. Louis: Mosby, 1992;517.
83. Colding A. The effect of regional sympathetic blocks in the treatment of herpes zoster. Acta Anaesth Scand 1969;13:133.
84. Colding A. Treatment of pain: Organization of a pain clinic, treatment of herpes zoster. Proc R Soc Med 1973;66:541.
85. Perkins HM, Hanlon PR. Epidural injection of local anesthetic and steroids for relief of pain secondary to herpes zoster. Arch Surg 1978;113:253.
86. Maragas JM, Kierland RR. The outcome of patients with herpes zoster. Arch Dermatol 1957;75:193.
87. Watson CP, Evans RJ, Reed K. Amitriptyline versus placebo in postherpetic neuralgia. Neurology 1982;32:671.

Chapter 11

Nerve Block Therapy for Cancer Pain

Winston C. V. Parris

Several studies, including the recently released Cancer Pain Guidelines, have demonstrated that most cancer patients (50% of patients with early cancer and 75% of patients with advanced cancer) experience moderate-to-severe pain during the course of their disease. These findings have heightened sensitivity toward effective pain control in cancer patients. Several modalities have been proposed for the management of pain in cancer patients. Although not necessarily the modality of first choice, nerve block therapy is a useful and important option for pain management. This chapter discusses the rationale, prerequisites, classification, indications, contraindications, complications, and other aspects of nerve block therapy for cancer pain patients.

Why Nerve Block Therapy?

The late John J. Bonica, widely acknowledged as the father of pain medicine, proposed (and this proposal is almost universally accepted) that chronic pain management including cancer pain management is best administered under the auspices of an interdisciplinary, multispecialty, multimodal approach.[1] This approach facilitates and optimizes comprehensive pain management while ensuring flexibility, team-oriented care, and consideration of multiple modalities, all tailored to meet the therapeutic needs of the individual cancer pain patient. Although this therapeutic model is generally considered to be ideal, its absence does not necessarily mean that unidisciplinary or unimodal pain management is unacceptable. If thorough patient assessment, maintenance of proper patient selection, and triage are ensured, these unidisciplinary facilities may have a useful (but limited) role in the management of selected cancer pain syndromes, e.g., postherpetic neuralgia and radiation neuritis. Nevertheless, it is important to strive to avoid the tempting therapeutic principle that, "When you have a hammer, everything looks like a nail."

Given the general principles outlined previously, nerve block therapy is used most effectively for the following conditions:

1. To offer pain relief for patients whose pain is restricted to anatomic regions that are amenable to nerve blocks;
2. For patients who are unwilling or unable to accept other pain control modalities;
3. As diagnostic or prognostic blocks prior to neurolytic blocks in patients with limited life expectancy;
4. As a form of preemptive analgesia in cancer patients scheduled for radical surgery or amputation of body appendages;
5. For pain management in cancer-related pain syndromes, especially when a putative sympathetic basis for pain is suspected;
6. To facilitate the use of a delivery system that supplements pain control, e.g., intrathecal or epidural opioid administration;
7. As an alternative therapeutic modality when

orally or parenterally administered medications become ineffective; and

8. As a supplement to other modalities.

However, meticulous evaluation of the patient's general physical status, progress of the disease, and contemporary pain assessment along with a review of medications administered (especially pain medications) still remain the most appropriate methods to determine the patient's requirement for specific pain control. These evaluations and assessments must be repeated intermittently because of variances in the systemic condition and pain requirements of cancer pain patients.[2]

If properly selected and effectively administered, nerve block therapy may provide satisfactory-to-excellent pain relief alone or in combination with other modalities, e.g., oral opioids, parenteral medications, radiation therapy, and chemotherapy.

Prerequisites

Nerve blocks may produce significant systemic side effects in addition to exacerbating localized side effects. It is important to stress to the patient the severity of the possible systemic and local side effects and to dispel the notion that was originally perceived from anesthetic practice, i.e., that the level of vigilance may be lowered when regional anesthesia (nerve blocks) instead of general anesthesia is considered. The effects of some nerve blocks, especially spinal or epidural blocks, on the circulatory, cardiorespiratory, and central nervous system may be life-threatening if adequate prophylactic measures and thorough postblock monitoring techniques are not implemented.[3] Adequate monitoring may improve safety and limit complications of nerve blocks.

Before nerve blocks are administered, the following preconditions are recommended:

1. Adequate knowledge of the pathology or syndrome to be treated.
2. Understanding the risks and benefits concerning the nerve block, its administration, and the implications of not performing the nerve block.
3. Full knowledge of the anatomy of the region to be blocked.
4. Familiarity with the equipment to be used.

5. Understanding the pharmacology of the agents to be used.
6. A mobile cart stocked with supplies necessary for the procedure.
7. The assistance of a nurse or similar health care professional to facilitate monitoring, patient assessment, and resuscitation (in the unlikely event of a complication).
8. Appropriate drugs and equipment necessary to perform the procedure and also for possible resuscitation, if necessary.
9. Informed consent from the patient and his or her accompanying relative prior to performing the block.
10. Easy access to resuscitation equipment and pharmacologic agents to help manage complications of nerve blocks, including cardiorespiratory resuscitation.
11. Personnel adequately trained and appropriately certified in Advanced Cardiac Life Support.
12. Adequate preblock and postblock monitoring of essential vital signs (i.e., pulse, respiration, blood pressure, and so forth).

Other prerequisites may be important in selected cases. As a result, each case should be individualized and appropriate measures implemented to safeguard the particular needs of each patient.[4] Some controversy exists regarding nerve block therapy, which may have some relevance for the cancer pain patient. The typical nonmalignant chronic pain patient may have multiple psychosocial, emotional, and behavioral factors that may affect the chronic pain syndrome, thus making pain management in that patient population much more complex than pain management in the cancer pain patient. In the nonmalignant chronic pain patient, the major therapeutic goals are to promote self-reliance, to teach self-coping mechanisms, and to strive for both physical and psychological rehabilitation.[5] For these reasons, it is important to avoid reinforcement of the medical model and instead to promote an independence from drugs and the general medical infrastructure. On the other hand, in the cancer pain patient, systemic involvement either as a result of the disease or as a result of treatment of the disease (i.e., surgery, chemotherapy, and radiotherapy) may compromise the patient's general condition. To guarantee maximum aseptic precautions, this compromise may manifest as intravascular depletion, hypotension, and electrolyte and other biochemical dysfunctions. These problems could increase the risks of serious complications from nerve block therapy. Thus, it is appropriate to institute adequate intravenous access before performing nerve blocks on cancer pain patients.

The nerve block tray is important in facilitating safe and reliable procedures. The quality and specifications of the equipment used may help minimize side effects and optimize good results. A typical nerve block tray should be assembled and maintained in a sterile manner. It should consist of a "prep" compartment and a compartment containing needles, syringes, and a receptacle for drugs.[6] The prep compartment should contain a receptacle for cleansing antiseptic solutions (e.g., povidone-iodine [Betadine]) and sponge tip cleaning applicators. To maximize aseptic precautions, this compartment should be considered nonsterile and the other compartment (containing the needles, etc.,) should be considered sterile. In other words, material from the prep compartment should not be transferred into the compartment containing the drugs and vice versa so as to decrease the risks of contamination. A variety of needles should be present in the tray and these needles are usually 22-gauge needles of different lengths. A typical tray may contain needles of 2.5, 4.5, and 5.5 inches in length. The tray should also contain sponges, a pulsator syringe, and a Luer-Lok syringe. The pulsator syringe helps determine the tissue planes especially when using the "loss of resistance" technique to identify the epidural space. The Luer-Lok syringe adds a safety feature to nerve block administration by allowing local anesthetic to be administered in small volumes of 1–2 ml at a time while allowing for immediate postinjection aspiration. This technique minimizes the possibility of inadvertent intravascular injection. An antiseptic agent should be kept in a separate compartment from the local anesthetic so as to eliminate possible neurologic complications. These complications may occur if neurotoxic preservatives of the antiseptic cleansing agent were inadvertently injected intrathecally or epidurally.[7] Similar complications occurred in the United Kingdom (1954) and, consequently, adversely affected the development of regional anesthesia in that country for several decades.[8] In the United States, inadvertent intrathecal injections have been the cause of severe and irreversible neurologic sequelae.

Nerve blocks should be performed in facilities where patients can be treated comfortably and safely and where there is equipment to monitor patients after nerve blocks. There should be easy access to resuscitation equipment including endotracheal tubes, laryngoscopes, oropharyngeal airways, suction devices, electrocardiographic monitoring equipment, and defibrillation equipment. It is also important that drugs essential to resuscitation (e.g., sodium bicarbonate, epinephrine, calcium chloride, lidocaine, bretylium, atropine, and isoproterenol) be present in the facility. Appropriate intravenous fluids and their administration sets with needles should also be readily available.[9] Because central nervous system seizure activity is frequently associated with intravascular local anesthetic toxicity, it is also appropriate to have sodium thiopental and diazepam readily available to treat those complications. Diazepam is frequently used as a prophylaxis in nerve blocks that are known to be associated with a high risk of seizure activity because the drug raises the seizure threshold and, thus, may prevent the onset of seizures. When used to treat ongoing seizures, the effect of diazepam is not as rapid as sodium thiopental, which is the preferred drug (in doses of 50–75 mg) for ongoing convulsions. It is also important to have a physician skilled and credentialed in Advanced Cardiopulmonary Life Support (ACLS) present. Although it is clinically desirable and legally prudent to have that physician be an anesthesiologist, nerve block therapy is not the exclusive domain of the specialty of anesthesiology.

Mechanism of Action

The basic principles underlying the action of nerve block therapy in cancer pain patients as in other patients is the interruption of sensory and nociceptive pathways in various tissues and organs. Although the efficacy of nerve blocks in interrupting these fibers is unpredictable, nerve blocks are frequently effective in alleviating pain. Some reasons for the failure of nerve block therapy include poor technique, inappropriate selection of nerve block, inadequate drug or inappropriate dosage used for nerve block administration, anatomic variation of neural tissue (including inconsistent synapse of nerve fibers within ganglionic tissue), and physiologic dysfunction produced by either the overproduction or underproduction of various vasoactive neuropeptides. Sensory nerve blocks relieve pain and interrupt the afferent limb of normal reflex mechanisms. Thus, relatively low concentrations of local anesthetics (e.g., 0.125% or 0.25% of bupivacaine) make it possible to block those nerve fibers carrying nociceptive stimuli (i.e., unmyelinated C fibers and small A-delta fibers) without significantly impairing motor function, which is subserved by larger (A-alpha and A-beta) fibers.

It was recognized more than a century ago that nerve blocks with short-acting local anesthetics may produce pain relief that outlasts the anticipated pharmacologic duration of action of the local anesthetic by several hours, days, weeks, and even longer.[10] Although the precise mechanism of this prolonged analgesic effect is not precisely known, it is clearly not due to the simple analgesic action of the local anesthetic. This principle is exploited by neurolytic agents including alcohol and phenol, which produce prolonged pain relief by destroying neurons in the nociceptive pathways.[11]

Under normal conditions, various stimuli may exceed a given minimal potential (known as the resting potential) and initiate the development of an action potential that travels orthodromically along the external fiber of a sensory (afferent) nerve. At the end of this nerve, a synapse with another nerve fiber or with muscle (neuromuscular junction) occurs. To facilitate continued activation and, in other cases, to enhance activation and perpetuation of the original stimulus, a neurotransmitter is usually released. This released neurotransmitter could be acetylcholine, which acts via a chemical interaction on the motor endplate or the dendrites of other nerve fibers.[12] Other neurotransmitters, including norepinephrine, epinephrine, substance P, and several other neuropeptides and vasoactive substances, may help perpetuate the stimulus.[13] Some of these compounds may act as secondary neurotransmitters, which may either inhibit the basic stimulus or may potentiate the action. However, the primary purpose of local anesthetics is to inhibit the generation of an action potential, thus producing conduction blockade. This conduction blockade not only affects sensory fibers but also sympathetic and motor fibers.[14] The sensory and sympathetic fibers are the primary targets for blockade but oftentimes motor fibers are also blocked. This motor fiber blockade is not a complication but may be perceived as an undesirable side effect of nerve block therapy.

Covino proposed a schema (Table 11-1) that represents a logical approach to the sequence of events involved in local anesthetic–induced conduction blockade.[15] Local anesthetics block nerve impulses by interfering with the function of sodium channels. This action initiates depolarization of nerves, resulting in conduction blockade. In so doing, local anesthetics convert the sodium channels from a preblocked active state to an inactivated state during which the conduction of normal action potentials cease. From a molecular level, the precise mechanism of action is more complex, considering that calcium ions play a major role in translocating the adenosine triphosphate pump mechanism,[16] which is responsible for maintaining the ionic gradient of sodium and potassium across the cell membrane.

Using voltage clamp techniques, it was shown that the initial upswing of an action potential associated with a nerve impulse was initiated by an increase in permeability of the nerve membrane to sodium ions. This resulted in the inward migration of sodium ions through specific channels into the cell membrane. The initial stimulus responsible for producing the action potential causes a voltage-dependent sodium channel to open in the membrane, thus allowing sodium ions to move intracellularly. This activity produces depolarization of the nerve in the area of the open channel as the negative intracellular charge is reversed due to the entry of positive sodium ions. It has also been postulated that the action potential causes a specific change in the lipoprotein nerve membrane, which results in the opening of the sodium channel gate. The sodium channel gate is believed to consist of two proteins designated as the M and H proteins.[17–20] The action potential of an impulse culminates in the closure of the sodium channel, and the depolarization process spreads to adjunct membrane areas that, in turn, reach threshold voltage and propagate the action potential. Thus, the entire depolarization process is self-perpetuating. At the end of depolarization, potassium ion outflow commences, but that process is slower and is not actively facilitated by the adenosine triphosphate pump mechanism. The outflow of potassium ions peaks relatively long after the inward movement of sodium ion subsides. Subsequently, both

Table 11-1. Sequence of Events in Local Anestheti–Induced Conduction Blockade

---

Binding of local anesthetic molecules to receptor sites
  in the nerve membrane
Reduction in sodium permeability
Decrease in the rate of depolarization
Failure to achieve threshold potential level
Lack of development of a propagated action potential
Conduction blockade

Source: Reprinted with permission from BG Covino, DF Bush. Clinical evaluation of local anesthetic agents. Br J Anaesth 1975;47:289.

ions are restored to their initial intracellular and extracellular concentrations. It is important to note that this entire process is much more complicated than described here. New understandings of the process are being continuously discovered as more sophisticated experimental techniques are designed and implemented. However, it is depolarization and repolarization that are key factors in the propagation of an action potential.

It is thought that local anesthetics prevent the development of the action potential in a nerve by preventing sodium ions from moving intracellularly through sodium channels. The resulting anesthesia produces stabilization of the membrane because the resting membrane potential is unaffected by subsequent nerve stimulation. Binding of most local anesthetics occurs within the sodium channel after the drug enters the channel from the axoplasmic or intracellular side of the nerve membrane. Thus, penetration of the nerve membrane occurs before (internal) binding of the local anesthetics takes place. To facilitate that process, the local anesthetic penetrates the lipid structure of the cell membrane in its lipid soluble uncharged base form and then re-equilibrates in the axoplasm of the nerve into the charged cationic and uncharged free base form in accordance with the drug dissociation constant (pKa) and the pH of the axoplasm. The cationic form of the local anesthetic then enters the sodium channel from the intracellular side of the nerve membrane and binds to an anionic site within the sodium channel. This action results in physical and ionic blockade of sodium ion movements.[21] This process has been described as the hydrophilic pathway for local anesthetic action.

Local anesthetics block transmission of nociceptive stimuli differently, depending on the individual pharmacologic characteristics of the local anesthetics. The following list shows the pharmacologic characteristics[22] that may influence the activity of local anesthetics:

1. Molecular weight
2. Structural-activity relationships
3. pKa or dissociation constant
4. Lipid solubility
5. Protein binding
6. Partition coefficient
7. Equipotent concentration percent
8. Intrinsic vasodilator activity
9. Tissue diffusibility
10. Rate of local anesthetic biodegradation.

Other factors include the site of the nerve block, concentration and total mass of the drug injected, and the presence or absence of vasoconstrictor agent or other adjuvants.

Supplemental Techniques

The following techniques may be used to supplement and optimize successful nerve block therapy:

1. Radiologic localization of the needle prior to injection of drug may be accomplished either by fluoroscopic technique or by the injection of selected contrast materials (e.g., metrizamide) into the selected area prior to injection. Use of the C-arm has facilitated that process and decreased its cumbersome nature.

2. Peripheral nerve stimulation is a mechanical technique whereby a voltage 1–10 V or a current of 0.5–10.0 mA with a 1–2 pulse per second capability is used in stimulating the nerve and observing subsequent muscular response. This process not only confirms the correct placement of the needle but also is important for minimizing needle movement after that confirmation and prior to and during the injection of the drug.

3. Elicitation of paresthesia helps confirm correct needle placement. Needle placement may be associated with neuronal damage, which may produce significant sensory and motor complications. Thus, careful technique should be employed when inserting the probing needle into nerve tissue prior to nerve block therapy.

Classification

For the cancer pain patient, nerve blocks may be classified into the following categories: (1) diagnostic nerve blocks, (2) prognostic nerve blocks, (3) therapeutic nerve blocks, and (4) neurolytic nerve blocks.[23]

Nerve blocks may be given to patients prior to considering a specific therapeutic plan of management. The therapy may include additional nerve blocks, neurolytic nerve blocks, therapeutic nerve blocks, chemotherapy, radiation therapy, or surgery. Prior to initiating the particular therapy, a diagnostic nerve block of a specific nerve or nerve groups may be performed to determine the projected efficacy of the nerve block. The agents used to perform the diagnostic nerve blocks are usually short- to medium-acting local anesthetics. The concentration of the agents used depends on the intended pharmacologic objective.

Therapeutic nerve blocks are administered to patients after successful diagnostic nerve blocks or after assessment reveals that a particular nerve block might be effective in controlling pain. As a result, these blocks may be performed in patients whose life expectancy is limited or, in the case of peripheral nerves, in patients who have early to moderately advanced cancer. Any nerve block may have diagnostic implications if knowledge of the anatomy of the blocked nerve is appreciated and the pharmacology of the agent used to administer that nerve block is understood. An assessment of both the anatomic and pharmacologic implications of the nerve block therapy may yield significant information regarding the prognostic implications of the particular nerve block and its further application for enhanced therapy.

Neurolytic Nerve Blocks

Following successful diagnostic, prognostic, and therapeutic nerve blocks in patients with advanced cancer associated with severe pain and in patients with limited life expectancy, neurolytic nerve blocks may be administered to achieve pain control and, at times, palliation. The ideal patient for neurolytic nerve block therapy has a limited life expectancy, well-localized (nondiffuse) distribution of pain, and pain that is confined to one side of the body.[24] In

other words, neurolytic blocks are not usually considered appropriate for bilateral or central diffuse pain syndromes. Neurolytic blocks and their implications are discussed more extensively in Chapter 20.

Indications

As indicated previously, oral opioids represent the initial approach and, in most cases, the mainstay of pain management in cancer patients. This approach is usually effective in approximately 90–95% of patients with early to moderately advanced cancer. Nerve block therapy should be considered for patients in whom oral opioids have failed or in whom other therapeutic options are being explored, and this represents approximately 5–10% of cancer pain patients.

The indications for nerve block therapy include pain syndromes associated with cancer (i.e., herpes zoster, Pancoast's tumor, etc.), selected cancers specifically affecting the sympathetic nervous system (i.e., pancreas, bowel, uterine, or prostate cancer), and any musculoskeletal pain that is confined to a specific dermatomal distribution associated with cancer patients.

Pharmacology of Agents Used

Just about any local anesthetic or adjunctive agent may be used to implement nerve block therapy. The following list reflects agents most commonly used for nerve block therapy: (1) local anesthetics, (2) neurolytic agents, (3) steroids, and (4) miscellaneous agents.

Local anesthetics are commonly used for prognostic, diagnostic, and therapeutic nerve blocks. Their pharmacologic characteristics make them suitable for achieving several therapeutic goals in the management of cancer pain patients. Early in the twentieth century, Gasser and Erlanger demonstrated that peripheral nerves have sensory, motor, and sympathetic components.[25] A lower concentration of local anesthetics is usually employed in an attempt to facilitate sympathetic or sensory nerve block while minimizing motor blockade. A higher concentration of the same local anesthetics may induce motor blockade, which is usually reserved for anesthesia for surgical indications. The particular local anesthetic used is mainly based on the decision of the physician performing the nerve block and on the intended therapeutic objectives. The physician may make an informed selection regarding the appropriate drug if he or she has an adequate knowledge of the structure-activity relationships of various local anesthetics. The characteristics of local anesthetic that significantly influence the choice of local anesthetic include molecular structure, pKa or dissociation constant, protein-binding properties, and lipid solubility.[26]

All local anesthetics have potential side effects. Consequently, the choice of a particular local anesthetic for a particular nerve block in a given patient is influenced by the individual characteristics of the given local anesthetic. The author's preferred drug for most nerve blocks is 0.25% bupivacaine (Marcaine, Sensocaine). This drug satisfies most of the previously mentioned characteristics of local anesthetics necessary to accomplish adequate nerve blockade in the pain clinic setting, particularly for cancer pain patients. Other local anesthetics may accomplish the same effects, provided their individual pharmacologic characteristics are kept in mind. It is prudent to know the potential side effects and toxic dosages of all local anesthetics.[27] However, it is important to emphasize a few well-known complications of local anesthetics. Bupivacaine (0.75%) has reportedly caused sudden and progressive cardiovascular collapse with arrest, which is usually difficult to treat.[28] 2-Chloroprocaine, if inadvertently introduced intrathecally, may produce severe and irreversible neurologic complications.[29] On the other hand, prilocaine, in doses of 500 mg or higher, may cause methemoglobinemia.[30]

Neurolytic agents are commonly used to manage chronic intractable pain in cancer pain patients with limited life expectancy.[31] Recently, this therapy has also been used in patients with terminal human immunodeficiency virus disease. Neurolytic blocks have a few associated complications, including bowel and bladder dysfunction and motor paralysis. Patients scheduled for neurolytic blocks should have been shown to respond favorably to diagnostic nerve blocks (e.g., suprascapular or ulnar nerve block). In addition, the associated sensory or motor deficits must be acceptable to the patient. As a result, it is important to obtain informed consent from the patient and family prior to initiating any neurolytic procedure. Agents used to implement neurolytic blocks in cancer pain patients include the following:

1. Absolute alcohol[32]
2. 6% phenol in glycerine[33]
3. Glycerol[34]
4. Ammonium sulfate[35]
5. Chlorocresol
6. Hypertonic (cold) saline

Although all of these agents have potential side effects, absolute alcohol and 6% phenol in glycerine remain the two most popular agents for neurolytic blockade in most clinical practice.

Steroids[36] are used extensively to manage lumbar, cervical, thoracic, and sacrococcygeal back pain. These agents are particularly indicated for cancer patients who may develop discogenic disease. When slow-releasing steroids (depo-steroids) are used carefully, the customary biochemical complications of steroids (i.e., adrenal axis suppression, Cushing's syndrome, osteoporosis, etc.) are usually not observed. The most commonly used steroids include methylprednisolone (Depo-Medrol) and triamcinolone diacetate (Aristocort). They are usually mixed with varying volumes of local anesthetics. This combination enhances the efficacy of the epidural steroid injection. The advantage of using local anesthetics with the depo-steroid is the immediate relief following the administration of the local anesthetic since the depo-steroids do not usually provide instantaneous pain relief. Another advantage is that if an inadvertent dural puncture is made, the imminent resultant motor blockade would warn the physician of that complication sooner rather than later and appropriate therapeutic measures may be taken.

The mechanism of action of depo-steroids in pain patients is unclear. However, several theories have been advanced and are presented here:

1. An anti-inflammatory effect[37]
2. A hypothesis suggesting the presence of perispinal and intraspinal steroid receptors[38]
3. Increased phospholipase A2 activity

Although their mechanism of action remains unclear, intrathecal depo-steroids are not recommended because the presence of preservatives (benzyl alcohol, polyethylene glycol) may induce unacceptable neurologic sequelae[39] (e.g., arachnoiditis, cauda equina syndrome, transverse myelitis) as a result of the intrathecal injection.

Miscellaneous Agents

Many other agents have been used either alone or as adjuncts to facilitate nerve block therapy. These include narcotic analgesics,[40] substance P antagonist,[41] synthetic endorphins and enkephalins,[42] lioresal (Baclofen),[43] parenteral nonsteroidal anti-inflammatory agents (e.g., ketoralac), alpha$_2$-antagonist,[44] and other neuropeptides (e.g., somatostatin, calcitonin).

Complications

When properly administered, under ideal conditions, nerve block therapy is relatively safe and relatively free of complications. It is important at the outset for physicians to recognize and for patients to understand the differences between the side effects and the complications of a properly conducted nerve block. Because this difference may have significant medical and legal implications, it is important to obtain informed consent from the patient prior to performing the nerve block.

In addition, any relevant information from the patient history and physical examination should be determined, so as to avoid any situation that may adversely affect the successful outcome of the nerve block. Appropriate coagulation studies should be performed if coagulopathies are present or if the patient has been taking any anticoagulants currently or in the recent past. Several diseases including porphyria, Christmas disease, hemophilia, pyoderma gangrenosum, and so forth may enhance coagulation dysfunction and, thus, adversely affect nerve block therapy. In situations where the blocks are very necessary, meticulous informed consent regarding potential bleeding complications (i.e., hematoma and mechanical compression syndromes resulting in neurologic sequelae) should be obtained from the patient.

The more common complications of nerve blocks are presented here:

1. Cardiovascular system effects[45]
   A. Hypotension
   B. Bradycardia
   C. Arrhythmia
   D. Cardiac muscle toxicity
   E. Peripheral vascular collapse
   F. Cardiac arrest

2. Central nervous system effects[46]
   A. Coma
   B. Convulsions
   C. Loss of consciousness
   D. Tinnitus
   E. Dizziness
   F. Visual disturbances
   G. Metallic taste
   H. Circumoral and tongue numbness
3. Respiratory system effects
   A. Pneumothorax
   B. Hemopneumothorax
   C. Respiratory insufficiency
   D. Respiratory failure
4. Local tissue effects
   A. Muscle atrophy[47] (following bupivacaine)
   B. Prolonged paresthesia, sensory and motor deficits (especially following 2-chloroprocaine)[29]
   C. Methemoglobinemia (following prilocaine)[30]
   D. Infection (following poor sterile technique)
5. Miscellaneous phenomena
   A. Allergic reactions[48]
   B. Anaphylactic reactions
   C. Idiosyncratic reactions
   D. Hypersensitivity reactions
   E. Vasovagal reactions

All of these complications are possible following a nerve block. Certain complications are associated with specific nerve blocks and these are discussed in conjunction with the particular nerve block. Most complications may be avoided by meticulous attention to technical details. Further, most of these complications are reversible if diagnosed early, treated promptly, and managed with professional competence.

Specific Nerve Blocks for Cancer Pain

Nerve blocks may be administered to cancer pain patients for several reasons. The major indication is to relieve pain caused by the tumor itself or by its spread to contiguous or distant areas (metastases). Nerve blocks may also be administered to deal with the complications of cancer therapy including chemotherapy, radiation therapy, surgical therapy, or biological therapy. In addition, there are several pain syndromes associated with cancer patients for whom

Figure 11-1. Anatomy of the gasserian ganglion block. (Reprinted with permission from J Katz. Head and Neck. In P Prithvi Raj [ed], Practical Mangement of Pain [2nd ed]. St. Louis: Mosby–Year Book, 1992.)

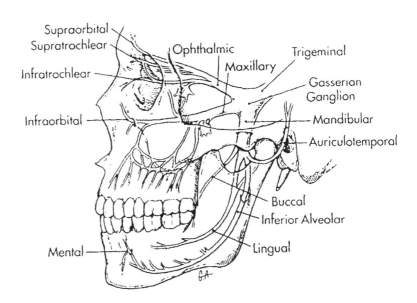

Figure 11-1. Anatomy of the gasserian ganglion block. (Reprinted with permission from J Katz. Head and Neck. In P Prithvi Raj [ed], Practical Mangement of Pain [2nd ed]. St. Louis: Mosby–Year Book, 1992.)

nerve blocks may be administered. These syndromes include herpes zoster and postherpetic neuralgia, cancer of the pancreas, and chest pain secondary to Pancoast's tumor. Nerve blocks are usually administered using a single-shot technique with the expectation that the analgesia obtained will be sustained and long-lasting. On the other hand, a continuous technique may be implemented using a catheter or similar device and the continuous or intermittent infusion of the appropriate agent to obtain pain relief.

Somatic Blocks

Somatic blocks in cancer pain patients are used primarily to diagnose and treat pain syndromes secondary to cancer or cancer therapy–related pain syndromes. Specific syndromes (e.g., postherpetic neuralgia, radiation neuritis, radiation osteitis) may be managed either solely by somatic nerve blocks or in combination with other modalities to treat the pain resulting from these syndromes.

Gasserian Ganglion Block

The gasserian ganglion or trigeminal nerve ganglion is formed by the fusion of a series of rootlets

that originate along the ventral surface of the brain stem at the mid-pons level. These rootlets pass forward within the posterior cranial fossa and leave the skull as three major divisions: the ophthalmic, maxillary, and the mandibular nerves (Figure 11-1). They innervate the head and are usually susceptible to tumor invasion, surgical manipulation, radiation neuritis, pressure, and other occurrences. Blocks of the gasserian nerve ganglion were performed more commonly in the past but their use in recent times has diminished because of the introduction of better techniques and more efficacious drugs. However, in the appropriate setting and after careful patient selection, gasserian ganglion block or block of one of its major branches may still be indicated and effective. Gasserian ganglion block should always be done with radiographic guidance to confirm needle placement. For this technique, the patient lies in a supine position with the head slightly extended. The needle is inserted approximately 1 inch lateral to the corner of the mouth and advanced through the substance of the cheek just medial to the ramus of the mandible in a slightly cephalad and medial direction. Thus, the general direction of the needle following insertion should be toward the pupil of the eye. In order to ensure proper direction and adequate placement, a finger is placed intraorally to guide the needle correctly.

The accurate placement of the needle is confirmed with fluoroscopy. At this point, the needle should be advanced until it contacts the base of the skull. Using radiographic verification, the needle is then redirected until the foramen ovale is penetrated without eliciting significant paresthesia. A diagnostic block of the gasserian ganglion may be performed by injecting 2–3 ml of a local anesthetic slowly after careful aspiration for both blood and cerebrospinal fluid. If adequate pain relief is obtained but is not sustained, then a neurolytic block with 1 ml of absolute alcohol injected in divided doses may be administered.

The gasserian ganglion may also be treated with radiofrequency lesioning, glycerol,[49] thermocoagulation, or phenol injection. The author prefers 6% phenol instead of alcohol because the latter may produce severe complications including anesthesia dolorosa, keratitis, and painful alcoholic neuritis.[50] In the past, hot water, hypertonic saline, and yttrium have been injected into the gasserian ganglion. These techniques are no longer used. Because the actual administration of a gasserian ganglion block is associated with some discomfort and occasionally severe pain, it is important to administer heavy sedation or, in some cases, a general anesthetic prior to performing this block.

Complications of gasserian ganglion block include rapid loss of consciousness, which may proceed to cardiac arrest as a result of inadvertent dural puncture. In addition to alcoholic neuritis when alcohol is used for gasserian ganglion block, the patient may also experience a numbing and irritating sensation over the entire face. This complication is minimized by performing a local anesthetic block prior to the alcohol injection. Corneal anesthesia associated with inflammatory diseases of the eye may develop and proceed undetected for a long period. Thus, frequent eye examinations are recommended following gasserian ganglion block.

Block of the Ophthalmic Division of the Trigeminal Nerve

The ophthalmic division of the trigeminal nerve divides into three major branches: the frontal, nasociliary, and lacrimal nerves. A block of the ophthalmic division is not performed commonly because it may be associated with serious complications, including keratitis. However, a block of the branches of the ophthalmic nerve may be performed in patients with postherpetic neuralgia. Supraorbital nerve block is fairly commonly performed for unilateral frontal headache.

Block of the Maxillary Nerve

Maxillary nerve block is performed with the patient lying in the supine position with the head turned away from the side to be blocked. A 3-inch needle is advanced parallel to the base of the skull until it contacts with the lateral pterygoid plate. This usually occurs approximately 1.0–1.5 inches below the skin. At that point, the needle is redirected anteriorly and superiorly in the direction of the orbit of the eye. As the needle is slowly advanced past the anterior border of the lateral pterygoid plate, a paresthesia to the upper jaw is usually experienced; 6–8 ml of a local anesthetic (0.25% bupivacaine) is injected for a diagnostic block and 1.5–3.0 ml of absolute alcohol is injected for a neurolytic block. The area innervated by the maxillary nerve includes the maxilla, maxillary antrum, teeth of the upper jaw, roof of the mouth, lower part of the nose, nasopharynx, tonsilar fossa, and the skin over the middle one-third of the face. Maxillary nerve block is usually facilitated by local anesthetic infiltration of the area inferior to the middle aspect of the zygomatic arch and by moderate intravenous sedation.

Block of the Mandibular Nerve

The mandibular nerve is the third and largest of the three branches of the trigeminal nerve. The mandibular nerve innervates the mandible, anterior two-thirds of the tongue, teeth of the lower jaw, external auditory meatus, temporal region, anterior part of the ear, temporomandibular joint, and skin over the lower one-third of the face.

The mandibular nerve is blocked by inserting a needle inferior to the midpoint of the zygomatic arch and then advancing it until the lateral pterygoid plate is reached. After contact with the lateral pterygoid plate, the needle is withdrawn slightly and redirected posteriorly toward the ear. Paresthesia to the lower jaw or to the tongue is elicited approximately 1.0–1.5 cm beyond the posterior border of the lateral pterygoid plate. This paresthesia signifies accurate placement of the needle. A local block may be achieved using 6–8 ml of local anesthetic and a neurolytic block may be obtained using 1.5–3.0 ml of absolute alcohol or 6% phenol.

Facial Nerve Block

The facial nerve (cranial nerve VII) has both sensory and motor roots. After it traverses the pons and the medulla oblongata, the facial nerve exits the skull at the stylomastoid foramen. At this point, it passes inferiorly, anteriorly, and laterally to the styloid process and, eventually, enters the body of the parotid gland. After emerging from the parotid gland, it divides into the terminal branches. The motor division of the facial nerve innervates the muscles of facial expression.

The facial nerve has small sensory branches that innervate the tissues surrounding the parotid gland and anterior to the ear. Indications for facial nerve blocks in cancer pain patients are infrequent. The facial nerve is accessible to blocking because it transverses between the mastoid process and the midpoint of the posterior border of the ramus of the mandible.

Complications of facial nerve block include facial paralyses, parotid gland trauma, block of the glossopharyngeal and vagal nerves, and puncture of the internal carotid artery and jugular vein. Careful aspiration for blood is necessary before performing this nerve block.

Block of the Vagus and Glossopharyngeal Nerves

The vagus nerve innervates the base of the tongue, epiglottis larynx above the vocal cords, and pharynx. The glossopharyngeal nerve innervates the palatine tonsils, pharyngeal wall, and posterior one-third of the tongue. Glossopharyngeal and vagus nerve blocks are usually indicated in cancer pain patients for head and neck tumors that may invade structures continuous to the vagus and in patients who develop mucositis secondary to radiation of the contiguous anatomic structures including the pharyngeal mucosa, tonsilar area, and posterior one-third of the tongue. The glossopharyngeal, vagus, spinal accessory, and hypoglossal nerves are closely related to each other in that a block of one nerve usually results in the block of one or two or all of the other nerves. The block of both nerves is performed by injecting a needle immediately below the external auditory meatus and just anterior to the border of the mastoid process. The styloid process is contacted as the needle is advanced for about 1.5–2.5 cm. At this point of contact, the needle is withdrawn and redirected slightly posteriorly to the styloid process and advanced for an additional 1 cm. Careful aspiration, prior to injecting the local anesthetics, is mandatory because the needle is usually in close proximity to the internal carotid artery and the internal jugular vein. Inadvertent puncture and subsequent injection of those structures can have dramatic cardiorespiratory implications and cause major convulsions.

Supraorbital Nerve Block

The major indication for this block is for pain confined to the unilateral forehead area. The supraorbital nerve is blocked by entering the supraorbital fossa along the supraorbital ridge and eliciting paresthesia toward the forehead and the frontal area of the skull (Figure 11-2). This nerve may be blocked using 3–4 ml of a local anesthetic and a neurolytic block can be accomplished using 1–2 ml of 6% phenol. The supratrochlear nerve is usually blocked just medial to the supraorbital nerve.

In order to protect the patient's eyes during the block, instruct the patient to close his or her eyes during the performance of the block and avoid handling syringes and needles over the patient's face. One minor, but irritating side effect is the drooping eyelid that may occur following successful block of the supraorbital nerve.

Infraorbital Nerve Block

The infraorbital nerve is a branch of the maxillary nerve that supplies sensory branches to an area inferior to the eye and lateral to the nose. An imaginary line, connecting the supraorbital, intraorbital, and submental fossae, passes through the pupil of the eye with the supraorbital fossa just lateral to the

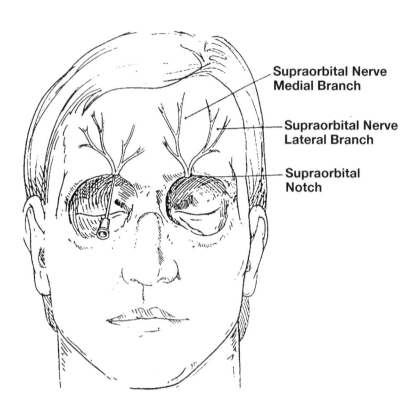

Figure 11-2. Anatomy of the supraorbital nerve and the technique of nerve blocking. (Reprinted with permission from J Katz. Head and Neck. In P Prithvi Raj [ed], Practical Mangement of Pain [2nd ed]. St. Louis: Mosby–Year Book, 1992.)

pupil, the infraorbital fossa just medial to the pupil, and the submental fossa just medial to the infraorbital fossa. This imaginary line serves as an excellent landmark when performing each nerve block.

Cervical Plexus Block

The cervical plexus is formed by the anterior or ventral primary ramus of the upper four cervical nerves. Those nerves interconnect with each other via ascending and descending branches (Figure 11-3). In cancer pain patients, this nerve block may be effective for several neck pain syndromes and for pain associated with radiation neuritis and metastatic disease of the cervical area.

Important branches of the cervical plexus include the phrenic nerve, occipital nerve, and suprascapular nerve. The occipital nerve block may be used to treat cancer pain patients with occipital headaches, and this may have diagnostic and therapeutic implications. The procedure for blocking the occipital nerve is usually performed with the patient in a sitting position and with his or her head slightly flexed. Because it innervates the posterior portion of the skull, the occipital nerve may be blocked by inserting a needle perpendicular to the superior nuchal line and close to the midline. The nerve lies close to the insertion of the semispinalis muscle and the origin of the trapezius muscle. Paresthesia is usually experienced and careful aspiration should be performed prior to injection because the occipital nerve lies in close proximity to the occipital artery.

The phrenic nerve arises from the anterior primary ramus of C-4 with minor contributions from C-3 and C-5. It passes inferiorly in the neck along the anterior surface of the anterior scalene muscle and between this muscle and the sternocleidomastoid muscle. The major indication for a phrenic nerve block in cancer patients is to diagnose and treat intractable hiccups. This symptom may be found in some patients with carcinoma of the mediastinum and lung, lymphoma patients, patients with Hodgkin's disease, and in some uremic patients. The specific technique for phrenic nerve block is insertion of a needle at the C-6 level between the sternocleidomastoid and the anterior scalene muscle. The needle is advanced medially and 8–10 ml of local

Figure 11-3. Anatomy of the cervical plexus and its relationship to the brachial plexus. (Reprinted with permission from PP Raj, U Pai, N Rawal. Techniques of Regional Anesthesia in Adults. In PP Raj [ed], Clinical Practice of Regional Anesthesia. New York: Churchill Livingstone, 1991.)

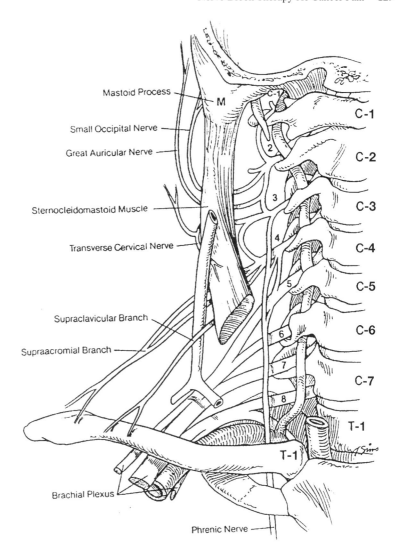

anesthetic is injected in several planes of the sternocleidomastoid muscle. This block is facilitated by using a peripheral nerve stimulator, by observing a diaphragmatic twitch, or by using fluoroscopy.

A neurolytic block of this nerve should never be contemplated because the phrenic nerve is the major nerve supplying the central portion of the diaphragm, which is the key muscle of inspiration. Bilateral phrenic nerve blocks are absolutely contraindicated.

Suprascapular Nerve Block

This nerve is blocked by introducing the needle one finger breadth (approximately 1.5–2.0 cm) above the midpoint of the spine of the scapula (Figure 11-4) and directing it laterally and inferiorly until a paresthesia is elicited at the tip of the shoulder. Eight to 10 ml of a local anesthetic may be used for a diagnostic or therapeutic block and 3–5 ml of 6% phenol may be used for a neurolytic block.[51]

Pneumothorax, a relatively infrequent complication of suprascapular block, may be avoided by asking the patient to place the hand of the side being treated on the opposite shoulder after introducing the needle approximately 2–3 mm below the skin. This action of touching the opposite shoulder serves to rotate the scapula posteriorly and laterally away from the chest wall, thus decreasing the incidence of inadvertent pneumothorax.[55]

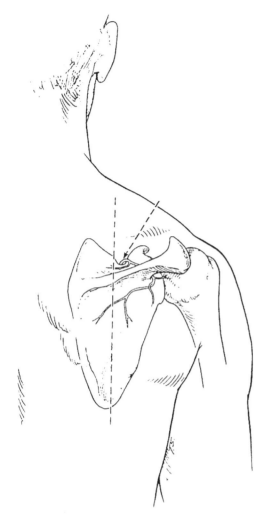

Figure 11-4. Suprascapular nerve block. (Reprinted with permission from PP Raj, U Pai, N Rawal. Techniques of Regional Anesthesia in Adults. In PP Raj [ed], Clinical Practice of Regional Anesthesia. New York: Churchill Livingstone, 1991.)

Brachial Plexus Block

The neural components of the brachial plexus include the roots, trunks, divisions, and cords, emanating from the ventral rami of C-5, C-6, C-7, C-8, and T-1, with minor contributions from C-4 and T-2. These neural structures innervate the pectoral girdle and the entire upper extremity. In cancer patients with metastatic involvement, tumor invasion (e.g., carcinoma of the lung), Hodgkin's disease, lymphoma, and in patients with radiation neuritis of the upper extremity, severe upper extremity and shoulder pain may become a major problem. A block of

the brachial plexus may help control pain either by itself or in conjunction with other modalities. The brachial plexus may be performed using four distinct techniques: (1) supraclavicular,[52] (2) infraclavicular,[53] (3) interscalene,[54] and (4) axillary.[55]

Although the supraclavicular approach is reliable, it may be associated with a small incidence of pneumothorax if meticulous attention to detail is not maintained. The infraclavicular approach is not associated with pneumothorax and is usually reserved for patients who require an infusion or continuous technique (Figure 11-5). The interscalene approach is also quite reliable but it may be associated with side effects such as hoarseness, numbness of the neck and upper extremity, and uncomfortable drooping of the eye. Serious complications include inadvertent puncture of the vertebral artery resulting in grand mal seizures, hypotension, and cardiovascular collapse with cardiac arrest. During an interscalene brachial plexus block, the stellate ganglion may be inadvertently blocked and a Horner's syndrome in addition to anhidrosis and conjunctival injection may be experienced. The axillary approach is least invasive but is also the most unreliable. However, using peripheral nerve stimulation, needle placement may be confirmed and an adequate block obtained.

Brachial plexus blocks in cancer pain patients may be used for postoperative pain management and for patients with peripheral neuropathies (including brachial plexopathy) and complex regional pain syndromes (including reflex sympathetic dystrophy) of the upper extremity. Neurolytic blocks involving the brachial plexus may also be performed for cancer pain. Brachial plexus blocks are best achieved with 10–40 ml of a local anesthetic (the amount may vary depending on the extent of the area to be blocked). Additional complications of an interscalene approach to the brachial plexus blocks include total spinal and high epidural blockade. These complications may be prevented by careful aspiration prior to injection and may be managed competently by airway control, oxygen administration, and maintenance of the blood pressure. Pneumothorax may occur following a supraclavicular brachial plexus block and treatment depends on the size of the pneumothorax. A chest radiograph and a thoracic surgical consultation should be obtained. Pneumothorax of less than

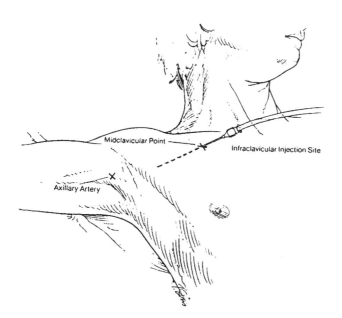

Figure 11-5. Technique of brachial plexus block by the infraclavicular approach. (Reprinted with permission from PP Raj, U Pai, N Rawal. Techniques of Regional Anesthesia in Adults. In PP Raj [ed], Clinical Practice of Regional Anesthesia. New York: Churchill Livingstone, 1991.)

10% should be treated conservatively, whereas a pneumothorax of more than 20% requires the insertion of a chest tube with appropriate drainage.

Nerve Blocks at the Elbow

The radial, median, and ulnar nerves may be blocked in the elbow individually or in combination. These blocks may be performed as adjuncts to other modalities for pain management in the forearm. The ulnar nerve is usually blocked by inserting a needle tangentially and distally at the midpoint of a line connecting the medial epicondyle with the olecranon fossa. Paresthesia radiating distally toward the hand and the fourth and fifth fingers signifies successful needle placement. The median nerve is blocked at the elbow by palpating the biceps tendon and its immediate medial structure, the brachial artery. With a finger on the brachial artery, a needle is advanced medial to the brachial artery until a paresthesia is elicited radiating distally into the hand. The median nerve is blocked at that point with approximately 5–8 ml of a local anesthetic. The radial nerve is blocked by inserting a needle 1 cm lateral to the biceps tendon and medial to the brachioradialis muscle. If paresthesia is experienced, the needle has been placed correctly. The block of these nerves at the elbow supplements regional anesthesia for the high-risk cancer patient undergoing upper extremity surgery.

Blocks of the Lumbosacral Plexus

Many patients with gynecologic and prostatic cancer, renal tumor, tumor of the gastrointestinal tract, and other tumors invading the neuraxial area develop symptoms secondary to direct tumor invasion of the spinal cord and corresponding spinal plexuses and nerves. There may also be metastatic spread from the tumor affecting those tissues and, in the cancer pain patient, it may be necessary to be more aggressive in the performance of nerve block therapy because the patient's life expectancy may be much more limited than in the patient with a chronic nonmalignant pain syndrome. It is important to make sure that the patient and his family understand the potential risks associated with the anticipated nerve block therapy. Although cancer pain patients are not usually litigious, it is still important to make sure that adequate informed consent is obtained, that proper communication is established between the patient and the physician and the physician and the family, and that a high level of vigilance and expertise is maintained before, during, and after the nerve block. Even with the most meticulously administered techniques, complications may occur. Side effects are normal and expected; however, complications are abnormal and undesirable. The potential risk of complications should be explained to the patient as part of the process for obtaining informed consent has been received. The manner in which this explanation occurs and the compassion with which it is delivered becomes an important cornerstone of a positive relationship between physician and patient.

Sciatic Nerve Block

The sciatic nerve, the largest nerve in the body (1.5–2.0 cm in width), originates from the anterior primary rami of L-4, L-5, S-1, S-2, and S-3. As it exits the pelvis, the sciatic nerve enters a tunnel located between the greater trochanter and the ischial tuberosity. The sciatic nerve is susceptible to trauma from surgical instrumentation, tumor invasion, piriformis muscle spasm, trauma from a needle, radiation injury, or from other physical forces. The roots and trunks of the sciatic nerve may be invaded by primary and secondary neoplasms. The classic presentation of the pain would be low back pain radiating down the posterior aspect of the lower extremity. In these circumstances, it is appropriate to perform a diagnostic sciatic nerve block. The results of that procedure are usually short-lasting but, in a few patients, the pain relief may have the efficacy of a therapeutic block. If analgesia obtained from diagnostic and therapeutic blocks is not long-lasting, then it is appropriate to consider a neurolytic block with absolute alcohol or with 6% phenol in glycerine in patients with advanced cancer.

Several techniques exist for blocking the sciatic nerve. The simplest approach (in the author's opinion) is to identify the midpoint of a line between the ischial tuberosity and the greater trochanter. On advancing the needle along that pathway, a paresthesia radiating down the posterior surface of the lower extremity may be elicited.[56] This technique is facilitated by placing the patient in the lateral position with the blocked side uppermost and the upper hip and knee flexed to 90 degrees. If the patient is unable to turn on his or her side because of pain, collapsed vertebra, or other reasons, the block may be performed with the patient in the supine position with the hip flexed at 90 degrees (or more, if possible) and the knee flexed at about 70–80 degrees. The needle is advanced perpendicular to the skin from the midpoint of a line between the greater trochanter and the ischial tuberosity. The end point is reached either by the eliciting paresthesia, by using a nerve stimulator, or by observing dorsiflexion of the foot. Fifteen to 20 ml of a local anesthetic is needed for adequate pain relief. A contraindication to a sciatic nerve block is local infection at the site of injection.

Modified Sciatic Nerve Block

A modified sciatic nerve block is performed in patients who have pain of the sciatic nerve distribution that is located below the knee. This approach involves the recognition that the sciatic nerve continues from the tunnel between the ischial tuberosity and the greater trochanter and passes in a distal direction surrounded by some of the large thigh muscles. In the mid-thigh compartment, it is surrounded by the semimembranosus, semitendinosus, and biceps femoris. The sciatic nerve traverses the popliteal fossa. The popliteal fossa is formed superiorly and laterally by the biceps femoris and superiorly and medially by the semimembranosus and semitendinosus. Inferiorly, both medially and laterally, the popliteal fossa is formed by the two heads of the gastrocnemius.

It is possible to block the sciatic nerve in the apex of a diamond-shaped popliteal fossa (Figure 11-6). This block is useful for young children, geriatric patients, and patients who require vascular access for chemotherapy.[57] Thus, if a needle is introduced in the apex of the popliteal fossa and is advanced in a slight lateral and cephalad direction, paresthesia may be experienced. A nerve stimulator may also be used to confirm precise needle placement.

Femoral Nerve Block

The femoral nerve originates from the anterior primary rami of L-2, L-3, and L-4. These roots form part of the lumbar plexus and run inferiorly between the psoas major and iliacus muscles. They are covered by the iliopsoas fascia, which separates the femoral nerve from the femoral artery. The femoral

mately at the midpoint of a line connecting the anterior superior iliac spine and the pubic symphysis. The femoral nerve is located approximately one finger breadth (1.5–2.0 cm) lateral to the artery. The insertion of the needle at that point and directed cephalad at an angle of 30 degrees produces paresthesia radiating distally in the anterior aspect of the thigh. A nerve stimulator may also be used to locate this nerve. Fifteen to 20 ml of local anesthetic is used to perform this block. The complications of femoral nerve block include femoral neuritis, prolonged block, hematoma, infection to the groin area, and rarely, arteriovenous fistula of the femoral vessels.

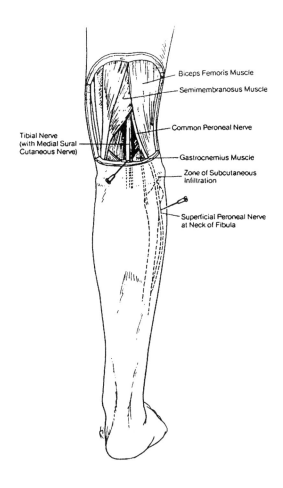

Obturator Nerve Block

The obturator nerve, like the femoral nerve, also arises from the anterior primary rami of L-2, L-3, and L-4. The obturator nerve supplies sensory innervation to the medial aspect of the thigh. It has articular branches that supply the hip and knee joints. The obturator nerve exits to the pelvis after crossing over the lateral aspect of the pelvic wall through the obturator foramen to reach the medial and superior region of the thigh. The obturator nerve has unpredictable sensory distribution and its blockade is used to manage pain in the medial aspect of the thigh. The obturator may be invaded by pelvic tumors, especially in patients with carcinomas of the cervix and prostate. Medial thigh pain may also result from radiation therapy that injures the obturator nerve.

The procedure to block the obturator nerve is performed with the patient in the supine position with the thigh abducted to make the adductor longus tendon prominent at its attachment to the pubic bone. While standing on the opposite side of the nerve to be blocked, the physician advances the needle perpendicular to the skin at a point 1 cm lateral and inferior to the pubic tubercle until the inferior pubic ramus is contacted. At this point, the needle is withdrawn and is directed laterally in a slightly superior and posterior direction. Confirmation of a successful block may be made by eliciting paresthesia or by using a nerve stimulator. Ten milliliters of local anesthetic is usually used to perform this block. Successful block produces numbness of the medial side of the thigh associ-

Figure 11-6. Course of the tibial and common peroneal nerves at the knee and the technique of blocking them. (Reprinted with permission from PP Raj, U Pai, N Rawal. Techniques of Regional Anesthesia in Adults. In PP Raj [ed], Clinical Practice of Regional Anesthesia. New York: Churchill Livingstone, 1991.)

nerve lies lateral to the artery and deep to the inguinal ligament, whereas the femoral vein is medial to the artery. Some cancer patients may experience pain in the anterior aspect of the thigh that is caused by tumor invasion or by radiation neuritis. A diagnostic or therapeutic block of the femoral nerve may be used to treat these pain syndromes. The femoral nerve ends distally as the saphenous nerve, which supplies the medial side of the leg down to the medial aspect of the foot.

The procedure to block the femoral nerve is performed with the patient in the supine position while palpating the femoral artery, which is approxi-

ated with loss of adduction and loss of external rotation of the thigh. Complications of obturator nerve block include hematoma, intravascular injection, and failure to achieve satisfactory nerve blockade.

Lateral Femoral Cutaneous Nerve Block

The lateral femoral cutaneous nerve arises from the anterior primary rami of L-2 and L-3. This nerve lies on the lateral border of the psoas major muscle and pierces the tensor fascia lata medially and inferiorly to the anterior superior iliac spine where it is usually blocked at this location. Thus, at a point approximately 2.5–3.0 cm inferiorly and medially to the anterior superior iliac spine, a needle is advanced cephalad and laterally toward the iliac crest. Paresthesia may be experienced; however, if paresthesia is not obtained, the needle is advanced until a popping sensation (signifying that the needle has gone through the tensor fascia lata) is experienced. It is important to keep in mind that the lateral femoral cutaneous nerve of the thigh lies just inferior to the tensor fascia lata. Approximately 10 ml of local anesthetic is injected after paresthesia is experienced.

The lateral femoral cutaneous nerve usually provides sensory innervation to the lateral aspect of the thigh from the hip to the knee. This innervation does not extend below the knee. Many factors may result in neuropathy of this nerve, including trauma, pressure from prolonged anesthesia in the prone position, surgical manipulation and other instrumentation, and, commonly, radiation neuritis. All patients with lateral femoral cutaneous neuropathy present with pain in the lateral aspect of the thigh.

A chronic pain syndrome associated with neuropraxia of the lateral femoral cutaneous nerve is called meralgia paresthetica.[58] This condition may be treated with a diagnostic or therapeutic block or, in select patients, neurolytic block. The lateral femoral cutaneous nerve is mainly a sensory nerve and does not have any major motor branches. Thus, unacceptable motor weakness is not likely to occur following this block. There are few complications associated with lateral femoral cutaneous nerve block because there are no important structures in close proximity to this nerve.

Common Peroneal Nerve Block

The sciatic nerve divides in the popliteal fossa into a lateral branch (the common peroneal nerve) and a medial branch (the tibial nerve). The common peroneal nerve has a deep and superficial peroneal branch. The deep peroneal nerve continues on the anterior surface of the distal end of the tibia and innervates the dorsum of the foot, including the great toe and the second toe. The superficial peroneal nerve supplies the rest of the dorsum of the foot and the other toes not innervated by the deep peroneal nerve and sural nerves. The common peroneal nerve can be blocked as it traverses the posterior surface of the head of the fibula. The correct needle placement is facilitated by eliciting paresthesia or by using a nerve stimulator.[59] Five milliliters of local anesthetic is needed to block this nerve. Complications of common peroneal block may include infection, hematoma, prolonged foot drop, and neuropathy. This block may be used in patients who have metastatic involvement of the tibia and fibula.

Ankle Block

The blockade of any of the following nerves may relieve pain in the foot (Figure 11-7), depending on the location of the pain: (1) posterior tibial nerve, (2) saphenous nerve, (3) superficial peroneal nerve, (4) deep peroneal nerve, and (5) sural nerve. Few complications are associated with these blocks.

Intercostal Nerve Block

Cancer pain syndromes associated with chest pain include postherpetic neuralgia, postmastectomy syndrome, postthoracotomy syndrome, Pancoast's tumor, and metastases to the thoracic vertebrae, lung, and thoracic cage (including the ribs).

More than 55% of patients with herpes zoster have the herpetic lesions in the chest between T-4 and T-10. Chest pain in these patients is not amenable to stellate ganglion blocks or lumbar sympathetic blocks. Instead, intercostal nerve blocks are one of the main forms of therapy for managing the chest pain. The precise dermatomal distribution is demarcated and intercostal nerve blocks are performed; one above and one below the demarcated region, including the nerves in the af-

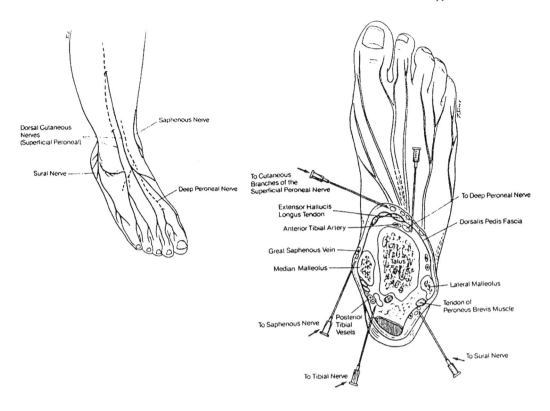

Figure 11-7. Anatomy of the tibial and peroneal nerves and their branches at the ankle and sites of block. (Reprinted with permission from PP Raj, U Pai, N Rawal. Techniques of Regional Anesthesia in Adults. In PP Raj [ed], Clinical Practice of Regional Anesthesia. New York: Churchill Livingstone, 1991.)

fected area. For example, if the lesions are between T-6 and T-9, intercostal nerve blocks are performed at the fifth, sixth, seventh, eighth, ninth, and tenth ribs. Intercostal nerve blocks are associated with the highest local anesthetic blood levels and, thus, seizures are most likely to occur after these blocks. Intercostal nerve blocks may be performed for diagnostic, prognostic, and therapeutic reasons. Intercostal nerve blocks are useful for patients with multiple myeloma associated with lytic lesions and for patients with multiple fractured ribs.

Several techniques may be used to perform intercostal nerve blocks. Ideally, the block is performed at the posterior axillary line but it may also be performed at the angle of the rib posteriorly or at the anterior axillary line anteriorly. The block is performed by palpating the inferior border of the rib and stretching the skin inferiorly while advancing a needle until it contacts the inferior aspect of the rib. With the

stretching action still maintained on the lower portion of the rib, the distal end of the needle is just "walked off" the inferior edge of the rib with minimal advancement inwardly (approximately 1–2 mm). The intercostal nerve and intercostal vessels lie in this area. After careful aspiration, approximately 3–4 ml of local anesthetic is injected in this area. Careful attention must be taken to avoid pneumothorax or, more importantly, tension pneumothorax. Complications of intercostal nerve blocks include pneumothorax, grand mal seizures, and intravascular injection leading to cardiovascular collapse.

Interpleural Analgesia

The ideal candidates for interpleural analgesia with catheter placement are patients with protracted chest pain either postoperatively or following postherpetic neuralgia and who may not have responded to intercostal nerve blocks.[60]

Central Nerve Blocks

Cancer pain patients who experience pain in a well-demarcated anatomic area may be managed initally by a diagnostic block using local anesthetics. Infrequently, a diagnostic block may have longer than expected analgesic effects. In these situations, the block may be repeated intermittently and adequate pain control experienced. In other cases, a neurolytic block may be performed and long-term pain relief obtained. This generalization is true for somatic blocks. Because of their close proximity and actual interaction with the neuraxis and its component parts, central nerve blocks are inappropriate for this therapeutic approach. Two or three decades ago, neurolytic central nerve blocks were commonly used to manage cancer pain. Unfortunately, there were unsatisfactory and unacceptable complications associated with these procedures. However, great advances have been made in cancer pain management including the advent of the potent and long-lasting narcotic analgesic agents, patient-controlled analgesia, dorsal column stimulators, and infusion pump devices. These advances have decreased the importance of central neurolytic blocks. Furthermore, central neurolytic blocks were indicated primarily for cancer pain patients whose life expectancy was limited and were almost never used in patients with nonmalignant chronic pain. It is still relevant, however, to discuss central nerve blocks because they could have some limited applicability in a few selected patients in a modern practice. The central nerve blocks to be discussed include (1) epidural blocks, (2) subarachnoid blocks, (3) cauda equina block, and (4) sacral nerve blocks.

Recently, some applications of these central nerve blocks have changed to the extent that they are still performed but their applications have changed significantly. Subarachnoid neurolytic blocks are infrequently administered; instead, specially manufactured spinal catheters are introduced and infusions of narcotic analgesics, local anesthetics, or mixtures of both are administered by bolus injections or by intermittent or continuous infusions. These infusions are facilitated by a variety of pump devices and by appropriate catheter tunneling to facilitate easy ambulation of the patient. These techniques are discussed in detail in Chapters 13 and 15.

Epidural injections may be administered at any level of the vertebral column.[61] The more frequent applications are in the lumbar area, but they are increasingly being used in the caudal area, particularly in patients with tumors originating in the pelvis or with pelvic metastases. Thoracic epidural injections are used primarily for patients with resistant postherpetic neuralgia who have not responded to other therapeutic modalities. Cervical epidural injections are infrequently used, but certain patients may receive some therapeutic benefit. Epidural injections may be performed by single-shot injections or by catheter implantation where intermittent or continuous infusions of local anesthetics or narcotic analgesics or mixtures of both may be administered. A more frequent application of epidural blocks is the implantation of stimulation devices designed to manage cancer pain. These devices are relatively expensive and, in the author's opinion, have been used indiscriminately by a few pain specialists in the past. The criteria for implantation should be meticulously observed and a trial of temporary devices should be initiated before permanent dorsal epidural stimulators are implanted.

Subarachnoid Block

The spinal cord continues from the base of the brain through the vertebral column and usually terminates at the level of L-1. The spinal cord is ensheathed by the dura mater, which contains the cerebrospinal fluid. The dural sac terminates at the level of S-2. In the neonate, the spinal cord extends lower in the lumbar region, usually to L-3 or L-4. The implication of these anatomic landmarks is that, in the adult, if the needle is inserted below L-2, it is unlikely that the spinal cord would be contacted. It is important to maintain meticulous sterility when performing a subarachnoid block. Bacterial contamination of the subarachnoid space may lead to disastrous effects including meningitis and encephalitis with major neurologic sequelae. The positioning of the patient for performance of the block helps facilitate an atraumatic entry into the subarachnoid space. Entry to the subarachnoid space may be obtained with the patient in the sitting, lateral, or jackknife position. The position used for performing a subarachnoid block in a cancer pain patient depends on the region being blocked, the technique being used, and the agent being administered. The sitting position is usually reserved for patients having a hyperbaric solution injected (e.g., 6% phenol in glycerine). In this position, a hyperbaric agent may be injected and it gravitates to the most dependent area because phenol is heavier than the cerebrospinal fluid.[62] The jackknife position is used in patients where a hypobaric solution (e.g., absolute alcohol) is used, capitalizing on the fact that the agent would have a specific gravity less than the cerebrospinal fluid. In the lateral position, the patient is manipulated so as to achieve the desired effect, depending on the baricity of the agent being used. It is important to monitor the patient after the subarachnoid block to prevent major cardiovascular complications. Vital signs should be monitored frequently for at least an hour after the performance of a block. It is important to have intravenous access in order to initiate any resuscitative measure that may become necessary after performing of the block.

Subarachnoid blocks are contraindicated in patients with blood dyscrasia, coagulopathy, infection at the injection site, or in patients with active neuropathy. It is critical to obtain informed consent from the patient and his or her family and to stress to them the possibility of motor dysfunction to the lower extremities and bladder and bowel malfunctions that may occur following subarachnoid block. Patient refusal is an absolute contraindication to performing any block, especially a subarachnoid block.

Cauda Equina Block

Cauda equina block is performed for patients with lumbosacral pain or pain in that region. This block is indicated for patients who already have bladder and bowel dysfunction (e.g., colostomy or an indwelling urethral catheter). A typical patient would be a patient with metastatic cervical cancer, uterine body cancer, ovarian cancer, prostate cancer, colon cancer, or bladder cancer. Such a patient might present with lumbosacral back pain radiating to one or both lower extremities.

During the procedure, the patient is placed in the jackknife position, with special care being taken to avoid undue pressure on the pelvis, thighs, or lower legs. The subarachnoid space is entered at the L-4 to L-5 interspace or at the L-5 to S-1 interspace. Typically, 5 ml of cerebrospinal fluid is withdrawn and 5 ml of absolute alcohol is injected slowly. The patient is then kept in that position for approximately 35–45 minutes so as to prevent the spread of alcohol in a cephalad direction and, thereafter, the patient is maintained in the supine and modest head-down position for approximately 12 hours.

Subarachnoid blocks may be associated with major complications. When neurolytic agents are used, the severity of those complications may be pronounced. Further, as subarachnoid catheters or various stimulation devices are inserted in the subarachnoid space, the incidence of infections and other complications increases. The complications of subarachnoid block include subdural hematoma,[63] epidural hematoma, neurologic trauma, anterior spinal artery syndrome, arachnoiditis, epidural abscess, profound hypotension with cardiovascular collapse, severe headache secondary to dural puncture, loss of consciousness and apnea secondary to drug effect, convulsions secondary to intravenous injection, broken catheter or broken needle, and, rarely, subdural injection. Most of these complications may be avoided if proper technique is implemented. However, after they have occurred and if recognized early, most of these complications can be managed satisfactorily without major morbidity and mortality.

Epidural Blocks

The epidural space begins from the foramen magnum where the meningeal dura fuses with the endosteal dura. Inferiorly, the epidural space is formed by the sacral coccygeal membrane, posteriorly by the arches of the lamina and the intervening ligamentum flava, anteriorly by the posterior longitudinal spinal ligament overlying the vertebral bodies and the intervertebral discs and laterally by the pedicles and the intervertebral foramina. The epidural space is largest in the midlumbar region and narrowest in the cervical region. In the lumbar area, it measures 5–6 mm whereas in the cervical space, it is from 1.5–2.0 mm. The epidural space contains fat, fibrous tissues, epidural vessels, and several traversing spinal nerves.

Epidural blocks at either the cervical, thoracic, lumbar, or caudal level may produce significant physiologic effects that depend on the level at which sympathetic blockade occurs. The epidural block affects the cardiovascular, central nervous system, respiratory, and endocrine systems.[64] In general, the higher the block the more profound the effects. In situations where it is possible to restrict the block to specific segments, the physiologic effects are limited and easily controlled; in situations when it is not possible to restrict the level of the block, the more cephalad the spread, the more profound the cardiovascular effects. These effects may be due to the following factors:

1. The loss of cardiac sympathetics due to the block of the sympathetic cardioaccelerator nerves[65]
2. The effect of the pharmacologic sympathectomy
3. The effect of local anesthetics that cause vasodilatation with peripheral vascular collapse and subsequent myocardial depression[66]
4. The vasopressor effect

All of these effects may be managed both prophylactically and, to a lesser extent, postblock. In the cancer pain patient, careful attention must be given to preblock hydration status. In patients who are intravascularly depleted, corrective replacement measures should be instituted so as to minimize profound cardiovascular effects after nerve blockade.

In the cancer patient, epidural blocks are used to administer local anesthetics and narcotic analgesics. Analgesia is provided via continuous or intermittent epidural catheter infusions. Many different pumps are available to facilitate the administration of the medication and these pump devices may be implanted subcutaneously and connected to epidural catheters via catheters that are tunneled from the site of the pump to the epidural catheter. Another method of administration of epidural block is the insertion of dorsal column stimulators[67] into the epidural space at particular levels corresponding with the pain site. These techniques are described in Chapters 13, 14, and 15. In special situations, epidural neurolytic blocks may be performed and may be associated with significant complications including dural puncture, subdural injection, massive subarachnoid injection, severe and protracted headaches, inadvertent intravenous injection, neurologic trauma, epidural hematoma, broken epidural catheter, epidural abscess, arachnoiditis, transverse myelitis, and the anterior spinal artery syndrome.[68]

Careful technique and meticulous aseptic precautions will prevent most of these complications. However, when these complications occur and are recognized early and managed promptly, the sequelae of the complications can be limited without major morbidity.

Caudal Epidural Blocks

Caudal epidural blocks may play a significant role in treating cancer patients who have sacrococcygeal pain. The etiology of the pain may be from direct tumor invasion, radiation neuritis, metastatic involvement, or postsurgical sequelae following radical surgery. Diagnostic blocks may be performed with local anesthetics, and in situations where there is satisfactory but time-limited pain relief, neurolytic caudal epidural blocks may be performed. It is possible to be more aggressive in using this block than in lumbar or thoracic epidural neurolytic blocks because most of those patients already have significant bowel and bladder dysfunction and they either have colostomies or urinary diversion procedures. Thus, potential bladder and bowel complications are not relevant in assessing those patients for caudal epidural neurolytic blocks. The author prefers to use 6% phenol in glycerine because the hyperbaricity of phenol allows the patient to be positioned so as to facilitate neurolysis of the desired nerve groups.

It is important to keep in mind that more than 40% of patients have anomalies of the sacral bones and that the sacrococcygeal hiatus may be anatomically altered in normal subjects.[69] In some patients, the sacral cornu may not be palpable and the coccygeal bones may be all merged with the sacral bones, thus distorting the anatomy.

A major consideration when performing a caudal epidural block is that the dural sac ends at S-2 in the adult and, as a result, if the catheter or needle is advanced beyond that point, subarachnoid block may inadvertently occur with disastrous consequences, especially if that complication is not recognized early. The caudal epidural space also can be used to insert catheters for infusion purposes or stimulation purposes if the lumbar region is contraindicated or inappropriate.

Sacral Block

The paired sacral nerves may be blocked individually or in groups, depending on the location of the pain. The sacral foramina are easily identified, and radiographic confirmation may always be obtained to verify their location. If diagnostic blocks are effective in sacral nerve blocks, then neurolytic sacral nerve blocks may be performed in selected groups of patients with sacral pain. These blocks are performed infrequently because a caudal epidural steroid may be simpler and easier to administer from a patient's standpoint than the multiple skin punctures that are necessary to achieve adequate analgesia with sacral nerve blocks. However, there may be situations when epidural blocks may be contraindicated and sacral nerve blocks may be indicated for the management of sacral pain.

Sympathetic Blocks

Some cancer pain patients may develop certain syndromes that may produce pain that may have a sympathetic basis. For those patients, sympathetic blocks may be performed with satisfactory results. Sympathetic nerve blocks usually used in cancer pain patients include (1) stellate ganglion blocks,[70] (2) celiac plexus blocks,[71] and (3) paravertebral lumbar sympathetic blocks.[72–74]

Stellate Ganglion Block

The stellate ganglion is formed by the fusion of the inferior cervical ganglion and the first thoracic ganglion. This fusion may exist in various stages of completion and the cell bodies of the preganglionic fibers originate in the anterior lateral horn of the spinal cord. The stellate ganglion is variable in size and is usually located in front of the neck of the first rib. It extends cephalad to the C-7 level. Thus, the stellate ganglion lies in close proximity not only to the lungs and the pleural membranes, but also to the suprapleural membrane. For this reason, the stellate ganglion is blocked at the C-6 level, which corresponds to the anatomic location of the cricoid cartilage. Because the deposited local anesthetics travel caudally toward the stellate ganglion block, this procedure is more appropriately referred to as a cervicothoracic sympathetic block rather than a stellate ganglion block. Stellate ganglion block is performed by locating the sixth transverse process (at the level of the cricoid) and palpating the carotid artery at that level.[75] The carotid artery and the anterior border of the sternocleidomastoid muscle are retracted laterally, stretching all the tissues lateral to the cricoid cartilage. Thus, subcutaneous tissue and fat should be all that separates the skin from the transverse process at that level. A needle advanced perpendicular to the skin at that level should contact the anterior tubercle of the sixth transverse process at a relatively superficial level. The needle is then withdrawn 1–2 mm and meticulous aspiration performed. If blood is observed, it is likely that the needle is in the vertebral artery. The injection of local anesthetics into the vertebral artery could produce disastrous consequences including grand mal seizures and cardiac arrest. If blood is observed, the needle should be withdrawn completely, pressure should be applied to the site for approximately 3 minutes, and a fresh attempt at the block should be made. If no blood is seen in the needle after aspiration, then the local anesthetic may be administered 1 ml at a time followed by careful aspiration. Following meticulous aspiration, 10 ml of 0.25% bupivacaine is commonly used to accomplish stellate ganglion block.

The complications associated with stellate ganglion blocks include hoarseness, dyspnea, partial brachial plexus block, intraspinal injection with cardiorespiratory arrest, and seizures from an intravascular injection. Pneumothorax is also possible if the block is performed at the C-7 level. It is important to distinguish between side effects and complications. The side effects of a successful stellate ganglion block include Horner's syndrome (meiosis, enophthalmos, ptosis), anhidrosis, nasal congestion, and conjunctival injection.

Celiac Plexus Block

The celiac plexus is a network of ganglia located in the region of T-12 and L-1. These fibers innervate the stomach, liver, pancreas, duodenum, and jejunum. Celiac plexus block is effective for relieving abdominal and back pain associated with pancreatic cancer.[76] The block may be performed unilaterally or bilaterally. If pain relief obtained is short-lived, then a neurolytic celiac plexus block using 6% phenol in

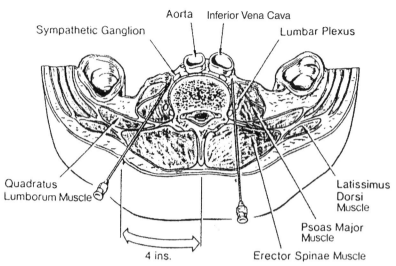

Figure 11-8. Cross-section of posterior back region showing sympathetic ganglia in relation to the major vessels, psoas major muscle, and vertebral body. (Reprinted with permission from R Rauck. Head & Neck and Trunk. In P Prithvi Raj [ed], Practical Management of Pain [2nd ed]. St. Louis: Mosby–Year Book, 1992.)

glycerine may be performed. Absolute alcohol may also be used for neurolytic celiac plexus block. Needle placement for this procedure may be confirmed by fluoroscopy of the C-arm.

Because of the relationship of the celiac plexus to the aorta and crus of the diaphragm, inadvertent puncture of both structures may produce hemorrhage and pneumothorax, respectively (Figure 11-8).[77] Other complications of celiac plexus block include trauma to the renal parenchyma with associated hematuria, profound hypotension, paraplegia,[78] grand mal seizure following inadvertent intravascular injection, hemorrhage following laceration of the inferior vena cava (on the right side), profound hypotension, anterior spinal artery syndrome, nausea and vomiting, and profound motor paralysis. These complications are even more dramatic and ominous when they follow neurolytic blocks that have used phenol or alcohol.[79] Thus, careful needle placement with confirmation by radiographic techniques is mandatory prior to the injection of a neurolytic agent into the celiac plexus.

Paravertebral Lumbar Sympathetic Blocks

Paravertebral lumbar sympathetic blocks[80] may be performed in cancer patients for the management of chronic pain syndromes of the lower extremity. Cancer pain patients may develop radiculopathy and sympathetically mediated pain following radiother-

apy, chemotherapy, and tumor invasion by primary tumor or metastatic involvement. As with other blocks, a diagnostic or therapeutic nerve block of local anesthetic is performed. If that technique provides short-lived but satisfactory pain relief, a neurolytic nerve block[81] may be performed. The sympathetic ganglia are concentrated at the L-2 level, which is identified by palpating both 12th ribs (in patients without thoracotomy). The distal ends of both ribs are connected by a line that should cross the midline at L-2. A needle inserted approximately 4–5 cm from the midline and inserted slightly medially should come into contact with the body of the vertebra. As the needle is withdrawn and redirected laterally, the needle should be in a location anterolateral to the body of L-2. A distinct sensation is felt as the needle exits the psoas major muscles. The fascial plane outside of that muscle group is the prevertebral fascial plane, which contains the paravertebral ganglia. Satisfactory needle placement is confirmed using the loss of resistance technique. This is pronounced because the negative intrathoracic pressure is extended through the prevertebral fascial plane. Twenty milliliters of 0.25% bupivacaine is customarily used to block this ganglion.

The usual indications for lumbar sympathetic block in cancer pain patients include causalgia, reflex sympathetic dystrophy, herpes zoster of the lower extremity, postherpetic neuralgia, vascular insufficiency following tumor involvement, diabetic neuropathy in some cancer pain patients, phantom limb pain, and acrocyanosis. Neurolytic lumbar sympathetic block may be performed in selected patients.

Complications of lumbar sympathetic blocks include grand mal seizures following inadvertent intravascular injections, profound hypotension with circulatory collapse, renal trauma, inadvertent subarachnoid or epidural injection with cardiorespiratory arrest, neuralgia of the lumbar somatic nerves, and, rarely, infection. Infection can be almost completely eliminated by strict observance of aseptic precautions.

Nerve block therapy is not the most important modality to treating cancer pain. However, when used effectively in appropriate patients, it may dramatically relieve and manage cancer pain. Although there are specific cancer-related pain syndromes that respond satisfactorily to specific nerve blocks, it is generally advocated that nerve blocks be used as only one of many modalities in the armamentarium of a multidisciplinary approach to cancer pain management.

References

1. Bonica JJ. The Management of Pain. Philadelphia: Lea & Febiger, 1953.
2. Cleeland CS. The impact of pain on the patient with cancer. Cancer 1984;54:2635.
3. Moore DC. Regional Block (4th ed). Springfield, IL: Thomas, 1975.
4. Dam WH. Therapeutic blockades. Acta Chir Scand 1965;343(Suppl.):89.
5. Brena SF, Chapman SL. Chronic pain: An algorithm for management. Postgrad Med 1982;72:111.
6. Parris WCV. Nerve block therapy. In Contemporary Issues in Chronic Pain Management. Boston: Kluwer, 1991;171.
7. Bonica JJ. Clinical Applications of Diagnostic and Therapeutic Nerve Blocks. Springfield, IL: Thomas, 1959.
8. Cope RW. The Wooley and Roe case. Wooley and Roe vs. the ministry of health and others. Anaesthesia 1954;9:249.
9. Standards for cardiopulmonary resuscitation (CPR) and emergency cardiac care (ECC). JAMA 1992;227 (Suppl.):883.
10. Parris WCV. Nerve block therapy. Clin Anesthesiol 1985;3:93.
11. Arner S. The role of nerve blocks in the treatment of cancer pain. Acta Anaesthesiol Scand 1982;74(Suppl.):104.
12. Ritchie JM, Ritchie B, Greengard P. The active structure of local anesthetics. J Pharmacol Exp Ther 1965;150:152.
13. Hanley MR. Substance P Antagonists. In D Bousfield (ed), Neurotransmitters in Action. Amsterdam: Elsevier, 1985;170.
14. Bonica JJ. Autonomic innervation of the viscera in relation to nerve block. Anesthesiology 1968;29:793.
15. Covino BG, Bush DF. Clinical evaluation of local anesthetic agents. Br J Anaesth 1975;47:289.
16. Langley JN, Dickinson WL. On the local paralysis of the peripheral ganglia and on the connection of different classes of nerve fibers with them. Proc R Soc 1889;46:423.
17. Rosenberg PH, Kytta J, Alila A. Absorption of bupivacaine, etidocaine, lignocaine and ropivacaine into N-heptane, rat sciatic nerve, and human extradural and subcutaneous fat. Br J Anaesth 1986;58:310.
18. Covino BG. Pharmacology of local anesthetic agents. Br J Anaesth 1986;5:701.
19. Tucker GT, Boyes RN, Bridenbaugh PO, et al. Binding of anilide-type local anesthetics in human plasma. I. Relationships between binding, physicochemical properties and anesthetic activity. Anesthesiology 1970;33:287.
20. Moore DC. The pH of local anesthetic solutions. Anesth Analg 1981;60:833.
21. Hille B. Local anesthetics: Hydrophilic and hydrophobic pathways for the drug-receptor reaction. J Gen Physiol 1977;69:497.
22. Bridenbaugh PO, Cousins MJ. Neural Blockade in Clinical Anesthesia and Management of Pain. Philadelphia: Lippincott, 1988.
23. Nathan PW, Sears TA. Effects of phenol on nervous conduction. J Physiol 1961;150:565.
24. Ferrer-Brechner T. Anesthetic techniques for the management of cancer pain. Cancer 1989;63:2343.
25. Gasser HS, Erlanger J. Role of fiber size in establishment of nerve block by pressure or cocaine. Am J Physiol 1929;88:581.
26. Akerman B, Hellberg IB, Trossvik C. Primary evaluation of the local anesthetic properties of the amino agent ropivacaine (LEA 103). Acta Anaesthesiol Scand 1977;69:497.
27. Reiz S, Nath S. Cardiotoxicity of local anaesthetic agents. Br J Anaesth 1986;58:736.
28. Albright GA. Cardiac arrest following regional anesthesia with etidocaine or bupivacaine. Anesthesiology 1979;51:285.
29. Ravindran RS, Bond VK, Tasch MD, et al. Prolonged neural blockade following regional analgesia with 2-chloroprocaine. Anesth Analg 1980;58:447.
30. Lund PC, Cwik JC. Propitocaine (Citanest) and methemoglobinemia. Anesthesiology 1965;26:569.
31. Cornblath DR. Treatment of the neuromuscular complications of human immunodeficiency virus infection. Ann Neurol 1988;23:88.
32. Gallagher HS, Yonezawa T, Hay RC, et al. Subarachnoid alcohol block. Its histologic changes in the central nervous system. Am J Pathol 1961;35:679.
33. Wood KM. The use of phenol as a neurolytic agent: A review. Pain 1978;5:205.
34. Haukanson S. Trigeminal neuralgia treated by the injection of glycerol into the trigeminal cistern. Neurosurgery 1981;9:638.

35. Lund PC. The role of analgesic blocking in the management of cancer pain: Current trends, a review article. J Med 1982;13:161.

36. Brown FW. Management of discogenic pain using epidural and intrathecal steroids. Clin Orthop 1977; 129:72.

37. Delaney TJ, Rowlingson JC, Carron H, et al. The effects of steroids on nerves and meninges. Anesth Analg 1980;59:610.

38. Dirksen R, Rutgers MJ, Coolen JM. Cervical epidural steroids can reflect sympathetic dystrophy. Anesthesiology 1987;66:71.

39. Swerdlow M, Sayle-Creer W. The use of extradural injections in the relief of lumbosciatic pain. Anaesthesia 1970;25:128.

40. Morgan M. The rational use of intrathecal and extradural opioids. Br J Anaesth 1989;63:165.

41. Regoli D, D'Orleans-Juste P, Drapeau G, et al. Pharmacological Characterization of Substance P Antagonists. In R Hakanson, F Sundler (eds), Tachykinin Antagonists. Amsterdam: Elsevier Science, 1985.

42. Bunney W, Pert C, Klee W, et al. Basic and clinical studies of endorphins. Ann Intern Med 1979;91:239.

43. Wilson PR, Yaksh TL. Baclofen is anti-nociceptive in the spinal intrathecal space of animals. Eur J Pharmacol 1978;51:323.

44. Fleetwood-Walker S, Mitchell R, Hope PJ, et al. An alpha2 receptor mediates the selective inhibition by noradrenaline of nociceptive responses of identified dorsal horn neurones. Brain Res 1985;334:243.

45. Liu P, Feldman HS, Covino BM, et al. Acute cardiovascular toxicity of intravenous amide local anesthetics in anesthetized ventilated dogs. Anesth Analg 1982;61:317.

46. Wagman IH, deJong RH, Prince DA. Effect of lidocaine on the central nervous system. Anesthesiology 1967;28:155.

47. Parris WCV, Dettbarn WD. Muscle atrophy following bupivacaine trigger point injection. Anesthesiol Rev 1988;16:50.

48. Brown DT, Beamish D, Wildsmith JAW. Allergic reaction to an amide local anesthetic. Br J Anaesth 1981;53:435.

49. Pitkin GP. Blocking the Trigeminal Nerve. In JL Southworth, RA Hingson, WM Pitkin (eds), Conduction Anesthesia (2nd ed). Philadelphia: Lippincott, 1953;360.

50. Mandl F. Aqueous solution of phenol as a substitute for alcohol in sympathetic block. J Int Coll Surg 1950;13:566.

51. Parris WCV. Suprascapular nerve block: A safer technique. Anesthesiology 1990;72:580.

52. Kulenkampff D. Anesthesia of the brachial plexus (German). Zentralbl Chir 1911;38:1337.

53. Raj PP, Montgomery SJ, Nettles D, et al. Infraclavicular brachial plexus block: A new approach. Anesth Analg 1973;52:987.

54. Winnie AP. Interscalene brachial plexus block. Anesth Analg 1970;49:455.

55. deJong RH. Axillary block of the brachial plexus. Anesthesiology 1961;22:215.

56. Labat G. Regional Anesthesia. Philadelphia: Saunders, 1930.

57. Raj PP, Pai U, Rawal N. Techniques of Regional Anesthesia in Adults. In PP Raj (ed), Clinical Practice of Regional Anesthesia. New York: Churchill Livingstone, 1991.

58. Raj PP, Pai U. Upper and Lower Extremity Blocks. In PP Raj (ed), Practical Management of Pain (2nd ed). St. Louis, MO: Mosby, 1992;743.

59. Raj PP, Rosenblatt R, Montgomery SJ. Use of the nerve stimulator for peripheral blocks. Reg Anaesth 1980;5:19.

60. Reiestad F, Stroaumskag KE. Interpleural catheter in the management of postoperative pain. Reg Anaesth 1986;11:89.

61. Murphy TM. Spinal, Epidural and Caudal Anesthesia. In RD Miller (ed), Anesthesia (2nd ed). New York: Churchill Livingstone, 1986.

62. Gregg RV, Constantin ED, Ford DJ, et al. Electrophysiologic investigation of alcohol as a neurolytic agent. Anesthesiology 1985;63:A250.

63. Dawkins CJM. An analysis of the complications of extra-dural and caudal block. Anaesthesia 1969;24:554.

64. Waldman SD. A simplified approach to the subcutaneous placement of epidural catheters for long-term administration of morphine sulfate. J Pain Symptom Manage 1987;3:163.

65. Ward RJ, Bonica JJ, Freund FG, et al. Epidural and subarachnoid anesthesia: Cardiovascular and respiratory effects. JAMA 1965;191:275.

66. Hoffman HH. An analysis of the sympathetic trunk and rami in the cervical and upper thoracic regions in man. Ann Surg 1957;145:94.

67. Cousins MJ. Acute and Postoperative Pain. In PD Wall, R Melzack (eds), Textbook of Pain (2nd ed). New York: Churchill Livingstone, 1989;284.

68. Woodham MJ, Hanna MH. Paraplegia after coeliac plexus block. Anaesthesia 1989;44:487.

69. Pederson HE, Blunck CFJ, Gardiner E. The anatomy of lumbosacral posterior rami and meningeal branches of spinal nerves (sinu-vertebral nerves). J Bone Joint Surg Am 1956;38:377.

70. Carron H, Litwiller R. Stellate ganglion block. Anesth Analg 1975;54:567.

71. Owitz S, Koppolu S. Celiac plexus block: An overview. Mt Sinai J Med 1983;50:486.

72. Mitchell GAG. Anatomy of the Autonomic Nervous System. Edinburgh: Livingstone, 1953.

73. Becket RF, Grunt JA. The cervical sympathetic ganglia. Anat Rec 1956;127:1.

74. Bonica JJ. Sympathetic Nerve Blocks for Pain Diagnosis and Therapy. New York: Breon Laboratories, 1984.

75. Carron H, Litwiller R. Stellate ganglion block. Anesth Analg 1975;54:567.

76. Leung JW, Bowen-Wright M, Aveling W, et al. Coeliac plexus block for pain in pancreatic cancer and chronic pancreatitis. Br J Surg 1983;70:730.

77. Owitz S, Koppolu S. Celiac plexus block: An overview. Mt Sinai J Med 1983;50:486.

78. Galizia EJ, Lahiri SK. Paraplegia following coeliac plexus block with phenol. Br J Anaesth 1974;46:539.

79. Brown DL, Bulley TK, Uiel EL. Neurolytic celiac plexus block for pancreatic cancer pain. Anesth Analg 1987;66:869.

80. Boas RA, Hatangdi VS, Richards EG. Lumbar sympathectomy: A percutaneous chemical technique. Adv Pain Res Ther 1976;1:685.

81. Cousins MJ, Reeve TS, Glynn CJ, et al. Neurolytic lumbar sympathetic blockade: Duration of denervation and relief of rest pain. Anaesth Intensive Care 1979;7:121.

Chapter 12

Illustrations of Common Nerve Blocks

Gülen Tangören and Winston C. V. Parris

Nerve block therapy is one of several modalities used to manage pain in cancer patients. Nerve block therapy may be used by itself or in combination with other modalities. If used appropriately and for properly selected patients, nerve block therapy may be effective in alleviating pain in cancer patients. This chapter lists in schematic fashion the indications, contraindications, complications, and the recommended agents that may be used for each nerve block.

Paravertebral Lumbar Sympathetic Block (Figure 12-1)

Indications

1. Herpes zoster below the T-10 level
2. Postherpetic neuralgia below the T-10 level
3. Radiculopathy of the lower extremity
4. Vascular insufficiency of the lower extremities
5. Sympathetically mediated pain of the lower extremities
6. Some forms of radiation neuritis

Contraindications

1. Patient refusal
2. Bleeding diatheses and other blood dyscrasias
3. Patient on anticoagulant medications
4. Patients with aortic aneurysm
5. Patients with known anomalies of spinal arterial blood supply (i.e., spinal artery syndrome of

Adamkiewicz or arteriovenous malformation of the spinal artery)
6. Patient with horseshoe kidney or polycystic kidney

Complications

1. Renal parenchymal puncture with hematuria
2. Hypotension secondary to sympathetic block
3. Profound cardiovascular collapse following inadvertent intravascular injection
4. Grand mal seizures secondary to intravascular injection
5. Puncture of the aorta (left side) and inferior vena cava (right side)
6. Injection of thoracic duct or right lymphatic duct
7. Injection of bladder in patients with horseshoe kidney or polycystic kidney
8. Failed sympathetic block
9. Paraplegia or severe motor deficits (rare)

Recommended Dose

Paravertebral sympathetic blocks may be performed using 20 ml of 0.25% bupivacaine (Marcaine). This dose can be decreased to 10–15 ml for patients who are cachectic or elderly. In certain patients, the block can be performed using fluoroscopy. An experienced physician may not need to perform a diagnostic or therapeutic paravertebral lumbar sympathetic block with fluoroscopy. However, it is mandatory to use fluoroscopy when neu-

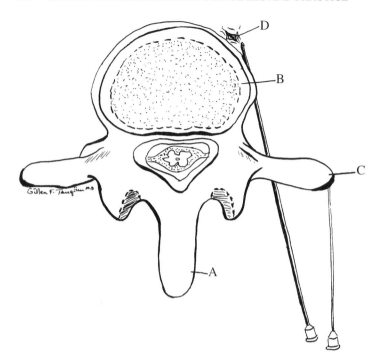

Figure 12-1. Paravertebral lumbar sympathetic block. A. Spinous process. B. Vertebral body. C. Transverse process of vertebra. D. Sympathetic ganglia.

rolytic lumbar sympathetic blocks (rarely performed) are considered.

Brachial Plexus Block (Figure 12-2)

Indications

1. Brachial plexus avulsion
2. Radiculopathy of the upper extremity
3. Brachial plexopathy
4. Radiation-induced brachial plexitis

Contraindications

1. Patient refusal
2. Anticoagulation therapy
3. Coagulopathy
4. Infection at the site of the injection (relative contraindication)

Complications

1. Pneumothorax when supraclavicular approach is used
2. Arteriovenous fistula
3. High spinal block or epidural block when interscalene approach is used
4. Seizure activity
5. Cardiovascular collapse secondary to intravascular injection

Recommended Dose

Twenty to 40 ml of 0.25% bupivacaine or 15–30 ml of 1.5% mepivacaine (Carbocaine) may be used for a single-shot administration depending on the patient's body weight and preblock physical status. For cancer pain patients who are experiencing severe shoulder and upper extremity pain (as in carcinoma of the bronchus), a brachial plexus infusion may provide satisfactory pain relief. In these circumstances, the infraclavicular approach to the brachial plexus is the preferred route.

Deep Cervical Plexus Block (Figure 12-3)

Indications

1. Anterior neck pain associated with cancer of the thyroid, pharynx, or larynx

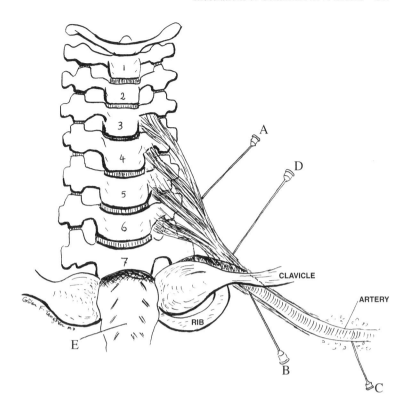

Figure 12-2. Approaches to brachial plexus block. A. Interscalene approach. B. Infraclavicular approach. C. Axillary approach. D. Supraclavicular approach. E. Sternum.

Figure 12-3. Deep cervical plexus block. A. Needles on the transverse processes of cervical vertebrae. B. Sternocleidomastoid muscle. C. Superficial cervical plexus. D. Clavicle.

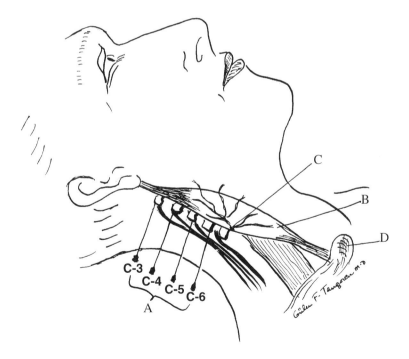

2. Postherpetic neuralgia with lesions affecting the neck area

Contraindications

1. Patient refusal
2. Local neck infection
3. Systemic infection
4. Anticoagulant therapy
5. Blood dyscrasias

Complications

1. Hypotension secondary to intravascular injections
2. Hematoma formation
3. Grand mal seizures secondary to intravascular injections

Recommended Dose

Ten to 15 ml of 0.25% bupivacaine or 10–15 ml of 1.5% mepivacaine is recommended.

Stellate Ganglion Block (Figure 12-4)

Indications

1. Sympathetically mediated pain syndromes
2. Herpes zoster with lesions above T-4 level
3. Postherpetic neuralgia lesions above T-4 level
4. Upper chest pain secondary to Pancoast's tumor
5. Phantom limb phenomenon of upper extremity
6. Postradiation neuritis
7. Pain from central nervous system lesions
8. Vascular occlusive states
9. Vascular headaches
10. Postradical neck dissection pain syndrome
11. Postmastectomy arm and chest pain

Contraindications

1. Patient refusal
2. Coagulopathy
3. Anticoagulant medication

Complications

1. Vertebral artery injection with grand mal seizures and possibly cardiac arrest
2. Carotid artery injection with major cardiorespiratory sequelae
3. Injection of the thyroid gland
4. Injection of the esophagus with possible mediastinitis
5. Transverse process osteitis
6. Persistent hoarseness secondary to recurrent laryngeal nerve blockade
7. Partial brachial plexus blockade producing prolonged motor blockade
8. Intraspinal injection (intrathecal) producing respiratory paralysis and unconsciousness
9. Pneumothorax, if the C-7 tubercle is used (especially on the right side)

Recommended Dose

Ten milliliters of 0.25% bupivacaine is recommended.

Suprascapular Nerve Block (Figure 12-5)

Indications

1. Persistent shoulder pain secondary to radiation neuritis
2. Adhesive capsulitis in cancer pain patients
3. Persistent shoulder pain secondary to mammoplasty for breast reconstruction in patients with breast carcinoma
4. Shoulder pain in postmastectomy pain syndromes

Contraindications

1. Patient refusal
2. Infections of the shoulder (relative contraindication)
3. Patients with pneumonectomy or lobectomy

Complications

1. Pneumothorax secondary to inadvertent puncture of the lungs
2. Failure of nerve block
3. Intravascular injection with cardiovascular collapse

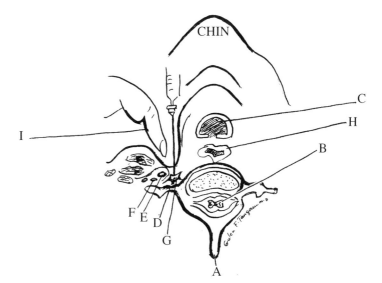

Figure 12-4. Stellate ganglion block (transverse view). A. Spinous process of sixth cervical vertebra. B. Spinal cord. C. Trachea. D. Transverse process of sixth cervical vertebra. E. Carotid artery. F. Jugular vein. G. Stellate ganglion. H. Esophagus. I. Physician's finger retracting sternocleidomastoid muscle.

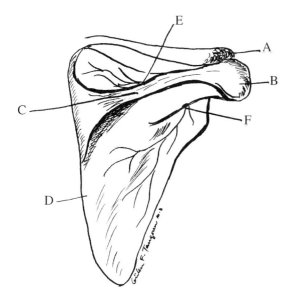

Figure 12-5. Suprascapular nerve block. A. Distal end of clavicle. B. Acromial end of scapula. C. Spine of scapula. D. Scapula. E. Suprascapular nerve. F. Infrascapular nerve.

Recommended Dose

Ten milliliters of 0.25% bupivacaine with a supplemental dose of 1 ml of 4% methylprednisolone (Depo-Medrol) in patients with inflammatory components to the pain is recommended.

Obturator Nerve Block (Figure 12-6)

Indications

1. Persistent pain of the medial aspect of the thigh secondary to carcinoma of the cervix, prostate, uterine body, and colon
2. Groin pain secondary to carcinoma of cervix and prostate
3. Groin and medial thigh pain in some patients with lymphoma and Hodgkin's disease
4. Radiation neuritis of obturator nerve in patients receiving radiotherapy

Contraindications

1. Patient refusal
2. Coagulopathy
3. Anticoagulant medication
4. Infection at the site of injection

Complications

1. Failure of nerve block
2. No other major complications

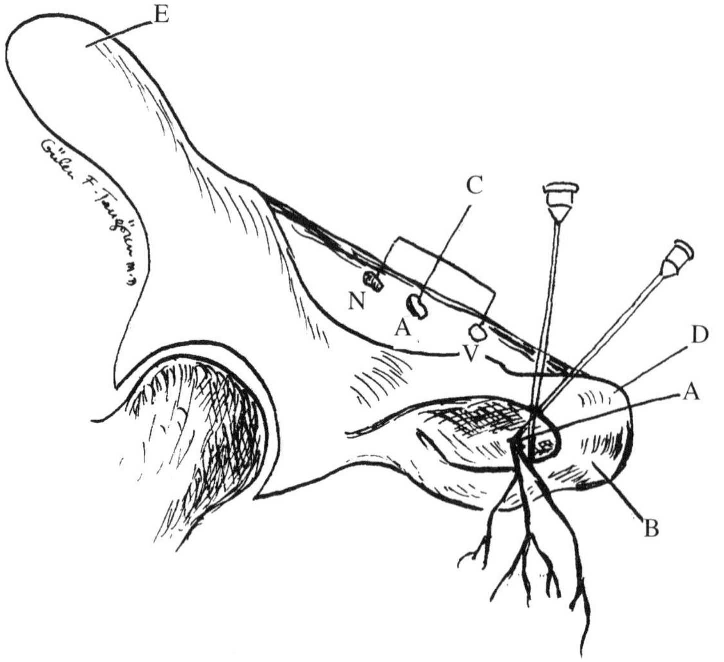

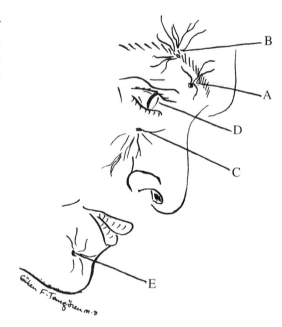

Figure 12-6. Obturator nerve block. A. Obturator nerve. B. Pubis. C. Femoral components (V = vein; A = artery; N = nerve). D. Pubic tubercle. E. Ilium.

Recommended Dose

Ten to 15 ml of 0.25% bupivacaine or 10–15 ml of 1.5% mepivacaine is recommended. In patients where an inflammatory component may exist as in radiation neuritis, 1 ml of 4% methylprednisolone may be used with the local anesthetic.

Supraorbital Nerve Block (Figure 12-7)

Indications

1. Postherpetic neuralgia of the forehead
2. Herpes zoster of the forehead (herpetic oph-thalmicus)
3. Ocular and periocular neoplasms with pain in the forehead region
4. Metastatic lesions to the cranium with pain radiating to the forehead
5. Patients with radiation neuritis pain radiating to the forehead
6. Trigeminal neuralgia (with major involvement of the ophthalmic division of the trigeminal nerve)

Figure 12-7. Supraorbital, supratrochlear, infraorbital, and submental nerve blocks. A. Supratrochlear nerve. B. Supraorbital nerve. C. Infraorbital nerve. D. Pupil. E. Submental nerve.

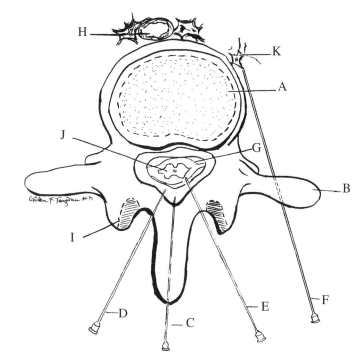

Figure 12-8. Epidural midline and lateral approach, spinal, paravertebral, and celiac plexus blocks. A. Vertebral body. B. Transverse process of vertebra. C. Needle in midline position epidural. D. Needle in lateral position epidural. E. Needle in lateral position intrathechal. F. Needle at anterolateral aspect of vertebra paravertebral. G. Dura. H. Aorta. I. Facet joint. J. Spinal cord. K. Lumbar sympathetic ganglia.

Contraindications

1. Patient refusal
2. Infections in the region of the eyebrows

Complications

1. Failure of nerve block
2. Prolonged ptosis
3. Periorbital infection
4. Trauma to the eye

Recommended Dose

Three to 4 ml of 0.25% bupivacaine or 1.5% mepivacaine is recommended.

Celiac Plexus Nerve Block (Figure 12-8)

Indications

1. Abdominal and back pain secondary to cancer of the pancreas
2. Epigastric pain secondary to cancer of the liver or stomach
3. Epigastric and back pain secondary to some lymphomas
4. Abdominal pain in gallbladder carcinoma

Contraindications

1. Patient refusal
2. Coagulopathy
3. Anticoagulant medication
4. Patients who are intravascularly depleted and extremely hypotensive preblock
5. Patients with aortic aneurysm

Complications

1. Profound sympathetic block with severe hypotension and cardiovascular collapse
2. Grand mal seizure secondary to intravascular injection
3. Prolonged motor paralysis of the lower extremity
4. Nausea and vomiting
5. Paraplegia

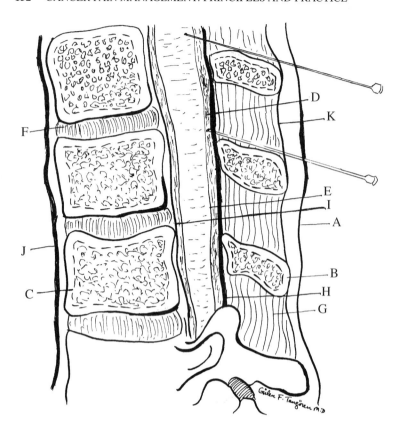

Figure 12-9. Sagittal view of lumbar vertebral bodies shown for spinal and epidural. A. Skin. B. Spinous process. C. Vertebral body. D. Epidural space. E. Dura. F. Intervertebral disk. G. Interspinous ligament. H. Ligamentum flavum. I. Posterior spinal ligament. J. Anterior spinal ligament. K. Supraspinous ligament.

Recommended Dose

The standard dose for well-hydrated adult patients is approximately 30 ml of 0.25% bupivacaine. Elderly patients or patients who are intravascularly depleted may require a decreased dose in order to prevent major hypotension secondary to sympathetic block.

Spinal and Epidural Blocks (Figure 12-9)

Indications

Spinal and epidural blocks are indicated for patients with intractable pain of the lumbosacral area, abdominal area, pelvic area, and the lower extremities secondary to direct neoplastic invasion or metastatic involvement.

Contraindications

1. Patient refusal

2. Infection at the site of the injection
3. Anticoagulant medication
4. Coagulopathy

Complications

1. Major hypotension secondary to sympathetic block
2. Neurologic sequelae including arachnoiditis and meningeal infection
3. Failure of block to work as a result of technical problems

Recommended Dose

The recommended dose for spinal and epidural blocks depends on the technique used for analgesia. The different techniques include a single-shot injection or continuous infusion. The continuous infusion may be administered by intermittent bolus injections or by a pump device or intravenous drip infusion set. Local anesthetics such as 0.125% bupivacaine are usually administered alone or with narcotic analgesic (e.g., fentanyl or morphine). The rate of infusion depends on the particular indication.

Intercostal Nerve Block (Figure 12-10)

Indications

1. Persistent chest pain following thoracotomy for pneumonectomy secondary to cancer of the lung
2. Postherpetic neuralgia affecting the thoracic chest wall
3. Herpes zoster affecting the thoracic chest wall
4. Chest pain following metastatic involvement of the ribs from other primary sites, notably carcinoma of the bronchus, thyroid, prostate, ovary, and kidney
5. Postmastectomy following surgery for breast tumor
6. Postthoracotomy pain syndrome

Contraindications

1. Patient refusal
2. Preexisting pneumothorax in either lung
3. Chronic obstructive pulmonary disease and emphysema
4. Anticoagulant therapy
5. Blood dyscrasias

Complications

1. Pneumothorax
2. Tension pneumothorax
3. Hemopneumothorax
4. Grand mal seizures (intercostal nerve blocks produce the highest plasma levels of local anesthetic of all the nerve blocks and, thus, may be associated with an unusually high incidence of grand mal seizures)

Recommended Dose

The recommended dose at each level of block is approximately 3–5 ml of 0.25% bupivacaine or 1.5% mepivacaine.

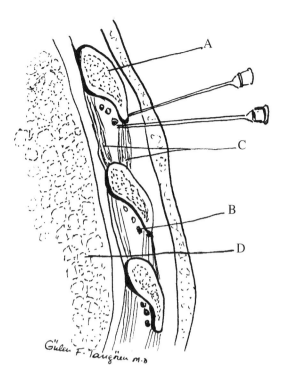

Figure 12-10. Intercostal nerve block. A. Rib. B. Intercostal nerve. C. Intercostal muscles. D. Lung parenchyma.

Caudal Epidural Block (Figure 12-11)

Indications

1. Persistent lumbosacral pain secondary to metastases to the lumbosacral vertebrae
2. Coccygeal pain secondary to tumor infiltration
3. Rectal pain in patients with carcinoma of the rectum or anus
4. Pelvic pain secondary to carcinoma of the prostate, uterus, or cervix
5. Severe coccydynia in patients with sacrococcygeal dysfunction secondary to radiation neuritis
6. Severe pelvic pain secondary to protracted constipation caused by prolonged narcotic analgesic use
7. Perineal dysesthesia secondary to high doses of dexamethasone

Contraindications

1. Patient refusal

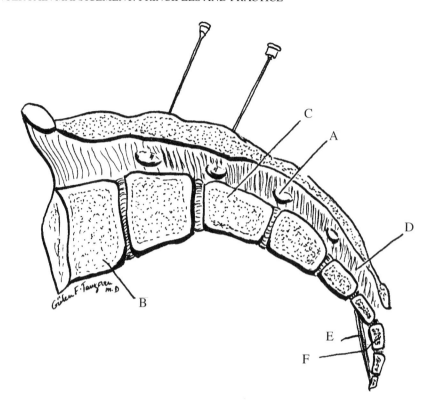

Figure 12-11. Caudal approach to epidural block. A. Sacral foramen. B. Sacral vertebra. C. Sacral canal. D. Sacral hiatus. E. Sacrococcygeal ligament. F. Coccyx.

2. Infections of the sacrococcygeal area
3. Inability of patients to lie in the prone position
4. Anticoagulation therapy

Complications

1. Inadvertent dural puncture with major cardio-vascular collapse secondary to high spinal (this complication can occur if the needle is advanced to a level more cephalad than S-2 since the dural sac ends at S-2)
2. Grand mal seizures and other neurologic signs and symptoms secondary to abnormally high blood levels of local anesthetic

Recommended Dose

The recommended dose is approximately 10–15 ml of 0.25% bupivacaine or 1.5% mepivacaine. Patients with

inflammatory components to the pain may also require 1–2 ml of 4% methylprednisolone.

Lateral Femoral Cutaneous Nerve Block (Figure 12-12)

Indications

1. Meralgia paresthetica (meralgia hyperesthetica)
2. Persistent lateral thigh pain secondary to radiation neuritis or to tumor involvement
3. Postoperative lateral thigh pain following surgery for cancer

Contraindications

1. Patient refusal
2. Anticoagulation therapy
3. Blood dyscrasias

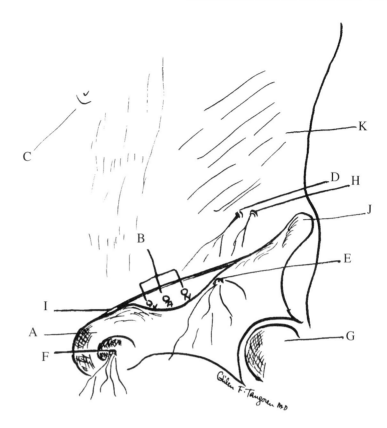

Figure 12-12. Ilioinguinal, iliohypogastric, femoral, lateral femoral cutaneous, and obturator nerve blocks. A. Pubic bone. B. Femoral components (V = vein; A = artery; N = nerve). C. Umbilicus. D. Iliohypogastric nerve. E. Lateral femoral cutaneous nerve. F. Obturator nerve. G. Femoral head. H. Ilioinguinal nerve. I. Ilioinguinal ligament. J. Anterior superior iliac crest. K. Abdominal muscles.

4. Infection in the area of the anterior superior iliac spine

Complications

1. Failure of block
2. No major complications

Recommended Dose

Ten to 15 ml of 0.25% bupivacaine or 1.5% mepivacaine may be used in patients with radiation neuritis or any other inflammatory component of the pain. In addition, 1 ml of 4% methylprednisolone may be used with a local anesthetic.

Chapter 13

Implantable Technologies: Spinal Cord Stimulation or Spinally Administered Opioids

Elliot S. Krames

In the past, there was little to alleviate chronic pain. This is because the medical community, government regulators, and the general population all believed that opioids for chronic intractable pain would most probably lead to narcotic addiction and tolerance. As a result, many neurosurgical procedures to destroy pain-generating nervous tissues were developed. However, early enthusiasm for these procedures changed to skepticism and avoidance of these procedures because of unacceptable complications. After receiving these neurodestructive procedures, many patients would incur even greater pain problems than they initially presented with. Patients and their families would often hear the same frustrating and exasperating words from their physicians: " You must learn to live with your pain; there is nothing more that I or medicine can do for you."

In addition to this lack of effective treatment for chronic pain, there was a pervasive ignorance regarding the neuropathophysiologic mechanisms causing chronic pain. Many people in the medical and psychobehavioral community believed that chronic pain represented a behavioral disorder and thus should be treated as one. The behavioral and cognitive treatment devloped in newly formed pain clinics became the basis of treating these patients who were often thought of as "crazy" and "drug seeking" by the medical community. The main thrust of treatment was to detoxify patients from their "addictive" medications, to treat them with intensive group and individual cognitive and goal-oriented behavioral therapies, and to use intensive physical rehabilitation to restore muscles deconditioned from months or years of inactivity. Because early interventions to relieve pain often failed in the long-term and because chronic pain patients would often rely solely on the health care system and not on themselves to relieve their pain, all pain interventions were thought to be counterproductive by these pain treatment facilities.

It is only in the last 25 years, with a growing scientific understanding of the neurophysiologic, neuroanatomic, and neurochemical mechanisms of pain transmission and its modulation in the peripheral and central nervous system, that newer, more technologically advanced pain treatment modalities have been clinically introduced. The use of spinal cord stimulation to control pain was first introduced in 1967 by Norman Shealy and colleagues[1] in response to the publication of the gate control theory of pain by Melzack and Wall in 1965.[2] The gate control theory (as first published, not with the benefit of later refinements) stated that painful electrochemical nociceptive information in the periphery is transmitted to the spinal cord in small diameter, unmyelinated C fibers and lightly myelinated A-delta fibers. These fibers would terminate at the substantia gelatinosa of the dorsal horn—"the gate" of the spinal cord. Likewise, sensory information such as touch or vibration, carried in large myelinated A-beta fibers, would also terminate at this gate of the spinal cord. The basic premise of this theory is that reception of "large-fiber information," such as touch or vibration would turn off or close the gate to reception of "small-fiber information." The authors theorized that the clinical result of this gate closure would be analgesia.

Shealy et al. theorized, as did Melzack and Wall, that electrical stimulation of the large A-beta fibers of the dorsal columns would antidromically inhibit reception of painful small-fiber information at the substantia gelatinosa of the dorsal horn. In fact, Shealy et al. presented the first clinical evidence for analgesia induced by electrical stimulation. Because they believed that electrical stimulation worked only at the dorsal horns of the spinal cord, they called this treatment dorsal column stimulation. Because we now know that this electrical stimulation inhibition of nociception can occur with electrical stimulation almost anywhere in the spinal cord, this term has been replaced with the more general, but accurate term, spinal cord stimulation.

Since the first clinical report on the use of spinal cord stimulation to relieve intractable pain in humans, there have been multiple reports regarding its efficacy for widely differing chronic pain states.[3–14] Since it is known that spinal cord stimulation causes vasodilatation in animal studies, clinicians have used this modality to treat clinical pain due to peripheral vascular disease in humans. In fact, in Europe, the main indication for spinal cord stimulation is peripheral vascular disease.[15–19] Spinal cord stimulation has also effectively been used to treat the pain of intractable angina.[20–22]

The differences in technology and criteria used for patient selection and trial for efficacy make it difficult to determine what is and what is not true from these published reports. However, it is clear that spinal cord stimulation has efficacy in pain states of neuropathic origins and pain emanating from ischemic origins, but not in acute pain states or pain of nociceptive origin.

The discovery of opioid receptors and endogenous opioid compounds in the spinal cord[23] provided a rationale for early attempts to deliver opioid drugs intraspinally, first in experimental animals[24, 25] and then in patients with chronic pain.[26, 27] This experience with "selective spinal analgesia"[28] appeared to offer specific benefits to some patients and was followed by trials of continuous subarachnoid opioid infusions using implanted pumps with factory preset flow rates.[29, 30] More recent reports

Table 13-1. Nociceptive Pain

Mediated at nociceptors; widely distributed in cutaneous tissue, bone, muscle, connective tissue, vessels, and viscera
Nociceptors classified as thermal, chemical, and mechanothermal
Pain often described using terms such as sharp or dull, aching, throbbing, etc.
Opioid responsive
Examples include postsurgical pain, bone pain, pain due to trauma, colicky pain, etc.

and abstracts in the U.S. literature have repeatedly documented the safety and efficacy of implanted nonprogrammable and programmable pumps for the long-term subarachnoid delivery of opioid drugs in the management of cancer pain[31–40] and nonmalignant pain.[19, 20, 22, 25, 26, 41–50] Unfortunately, because most of these studies of intraspinal opioids alone, or in combination with a local anesthetic (primarily bupivacaine) are small, retrospective, unblinded studies, there is little information available regarding the efficacy of chronic spinal infusional analgesia. Controlled, double-blind studies are needed to obtain this information.

Although there is abundant information on patient selection and efficacy of these two implantable pain treatment modalities, little information has been written regarding when it is appropriate to use one modality over the other. This chapter outlines a possible algorithm to make that decision. This suggested algorithm is based on a review of the pertinent animal data and clinical literature and also on the author's 10 years of personal clinical experience using these modalities.

Before choosing one method over the other, it is important to understand (1) that not all pain states are the same and (2) that different modalities work for differing pain syndromes. Nociceptive pain (pain mediated by nociceptors and widely distributed in the soma of the body) is often described by patients in such terms as "dull, aching, sharp, or throbbing" (Table 13-1). Examples of nociceptive pain include postsurgical pain, trauma, vertebrogenic pain, and cancer pain emanating from bone, connective tissue, and viscera. Nociceptors respond to mechanical, thermal, and chemical noxious stimuli and transduce this noxious information to electrical information, which is transmitted to the

Table 13-2. Neuropathic Pain

Elicited by damage to or pathologic changes of the peripheral or central nervous system
May be mediated by the *N*-methyl-D-aspartate receptor
Pain often described using terms analogous to electrical-
  like sensations, such as burning, tingling, shooting, electrical-like, lightning-like
May exhibit opioid resistance
Examples include postherpetic neuralgia, trigeminal neuralgia, peripheral neuropathies, traumatic peripheral neuropathies, plexopathies, reflex sympathetic dystrophy, etc.

Table 13-3. Selection Criteria for Implantable
Modalities

More conservative therapies have failed
Further surgical intervention is not indicated
No serious, untreated drug habituation
Psychological evaluation and clearance for implantation has
  been obtained
No contraindications (e.g., sepsis, coagulopathy, etc.) to
  implantation exist
Efficacy trial has been successful

central nervous system. This nociceptive pain is modulated presynaptically and postsynaptically at the dorsal horn by endogenous and exogenous opioids acting at opiate receptors. Therefore, nociceptive pain is most usually responsive to opioid therapies delivered orally, parenterally, or spinally.

Neuropathic pain, on the other hand, is not mediated by nociceptors in the periphery, but is caused by damage to the peripheral or central nervous system or by pathologic changes in neurofunctional relationships within these systems (Table 13-2). Examples of these pathologic changes include neuromata formation with spontaneous neuronal discharge, sensitization of nociceptors, central sensitization or "wind-up," abnormal sympathetic or somatic nervous system interactions, and abnormal activation of *N*-methyl-D-aspartate receptors. These pains, unlike nociceptive pain, are usually described using terms analogous to electrical-like sensations, such as "tingling, burning, shooting, and lightning-like." Examples of neuropathic pain include the monoradiculopathies, sciatica, trigeminal neuralgia, phantom limb pain, postherpetic neuralgia, causalgia, reflex sympathetic dystrophy, peripheral neuropathies, and so forth. Neuropathic pain may respond to higher than normal opioid doses, or may not respond to opioid therapy at all.[51–55]

Before deciding on the appropriate implantable modality, it is also essential to understand the specific indications for each modality and to have taken an adequate pain history from the patient. Spinal cord stimulation is used most appropriately in patients with a single unilateral focus of pain. This procedure is most appropriate because for it to be effective, the electrode array must electrically stimulate the actual level of the spinal cord where the patient complains of pain. As a result, this modal-

ity is less effective for bilateral foci of pain and not effective at all for multiple, multilevel areas of pain. Spinal cord stimulation is effective for treating neuropathic pain but ineffective for acute or nociceptive pain syndromes. An exception, however, is that spinal cord stimulation is very efficacious for pain of ischemic processes.

Although there may be syndrome-specific indications for one implantable modality over another, all implantable devices must meet the same selection criteria (Table 13-3). These criteria include (1) a psychological evaluation including a psychological interview and appropriate psychometric testing with psychological clearance for implantation, (2) failure of community-recognized and more conservative therapies, and, most importantly, (3) a successful preimplant trial showing efficacy for either spinally administered opioids or spinal cord stimulation. Invasive therapies should only be used within the context of a treatment continuum for each pain syndrome. Least invasive therapies should be used before more invasive therapies. An example of a treatment continuum used by the author is found in Table 13-4.

Once implantable pain therapy is deemed appropriate, the physician must then choose the implantable therapy most appropriate for the patient's pain. A patient with neuropathic pain and a single focus of unilateral pain should be given a spinal cord stimulation first before considering spinally administered opioids. If the spinal cord stimulation is unsuccessful, then a trial of spinally administered opioids should be considered. It is important to remember that bilateral neuropathic pain is responsive to spinal cord stimulation if the electrode array can appropriately, and concordantly, cover the patient's area of pain complaint (Figure 13-1).

Table 13-4. Pain Treatment Continuum

Over-the-counter drugs
Nonsteroidal anti-inflammatory drugs
Muscle relaxants
Physical and occupational therapies and manipulation
Rehabilitation medicine
Cognitive and behavioral therapies
Nerve blocks: diagnostic and therapeutic
Surgery
Weak opioids
Strong opioids
Spinal cord stimulation
Intraspinally administered opioids
Destructive neuroablative procedures

If a patient presents with somatic, nociceptive, opioid-responsive pain, with either single or multiple painful foci and probable spread of disease, spinally administered opioids should be used before more invasive and irreversible procedures such as neuroablative surgeries (Figure 13-2).

Patients with certain pain syndromes, such as complex regional pain syndrome, postherpetic neuralgia, failed back surgery syndrome, abdominal pain, and so forth, are classified into one treatment category or the other. For these syndromes, the indications for spinal cord stimulation and spinally administered opioids are well described in the literature. Patients with single monoradicular pains such as lumbar monoradiculopathy are the best candidates for spinal cord stimulation. Appropriate candidates for spinally administered opioids include patients with pure visceral pain responsive to opioids or patients with metastatic cancer or clear nociceptive, nonmalignant pain conditions.

On the other hand, many patients either have mixed nociceptive or neuropathic pain syndromes and may fall into "gray" zones, having pain that may respond to either one or both pain treatment modalities (Figure 13-3).

Because the long-term central nervous system effects of the chronic infusion of spinally administered opioids are still largely unknown, these patients should be initially treated with spinal cord stimulation before considering spinally administered opioids. If a trial for spinal cord stimulation fails, or if the patient develops a tolerance to the antinociceptive effects of spinal cord stimulation, a trial for spinally administered opioids should then be considered (Figure 13-4).

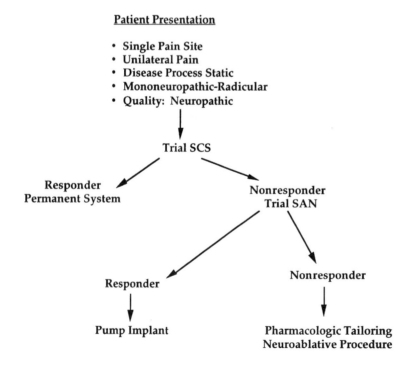

Patient Presentation

- **Single Pain Site**
- **Unilateral Pain**
- **Disease Process Static**
- **Mononeuropathic-Radicular**
- **Quality: Neuropathic**

Trial SCS

**Responder
Permanent System**

**Nonresponder
Trial SAN**

Responder

Nonresponder

Pump Implant

**Pharmacologic Tailoring
Neuroablative Procedure**

Figure 13-1. Patients presenting with pain of neuropathic origin should receive spinal cord stimulation (SCS) before spinally administered narcotics (SAN). Responders are implanted with permanent neuropulse generators or receivers. Nonresponders to this approach then undergo trials with spinally administered narcotics. Examples include monoradiculopathies, peripheral neuropathies, and plexopathies.

Figure 13-2. Patients presenting with somatic, nociceptive pain should undergo a trial with spinally administered narcotics (SAN). Responders are implanted with a spinal opioid infusion device. Nonresponders will not respond to spinal cord stimulation and thus are treated with other modalities. Examples include diffuse pain due to cancer metastases or chronic pancreatitis.

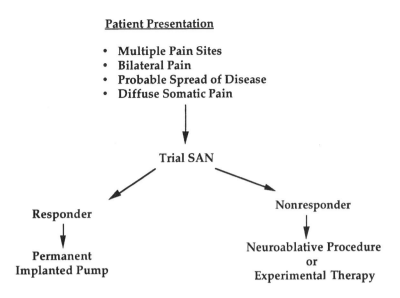

Patient Presentation

- **Multiple Pain Sites**
- **Bilateral Pain**
- **Probable Spread of Disease**
- **Diffuse Somatic Pain**

↓

Trial SAN

Responder

↓

Permanent Implanted Pump

Nonresponder

↓

Neuroablative Procedure or Experimental Therapy

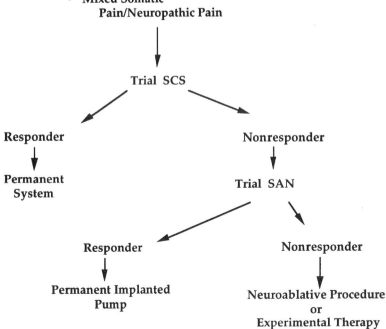

Patient Presentation

- **Bilateral Radicular Pain**
- **Disease Process Presently Static, But May Change**
- **Mononeuropathic-Radicular**
- **Mixed Somatic Pain/Neuropathic Pain**

↓

Trial SCS

Responder

↓

Permanent System

Nonresponder

↓

Trial SAN

Responder

↓

Permanent Implanted Pump

Nonresponder

↓

Neuroablative Procedure or Experimental Therapy

Figure 13-3. Patients who present with mixed nociceptive or neuropathic pain or with syndromes that may respond to either spinal cord stimulation (SCS) or spinally administered narcotics (SANs) should undergo a trial with the former first. Responders are implanted with neuropulse generators or receivers. Nonresponders next try spinally administered narcotics. Examples include chronic arachnoiditis, reflex sympathetic dystrophy, and postherpetic neuralgia.

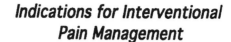

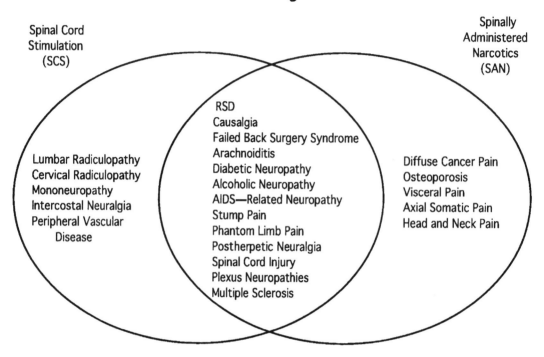

Figure 13-4. These two ellipses represent syndromes that either respond to spinal cord stimulation on the left or spinally administered narcotics on the right, respectively. The syndromes in the middle of the figure (within the overlap of the ellipses) represent a "gray zone" of syndromes that might respond to either modality or a combination of both. (RSD = reflex sympathetic dystrophy.)

This chapter has presented a decision-making tree to help the physician select the appropriate implantable technology to treat chronic nociceptive, neuropathic, and mixed nociceptive and neuropathic pain syndromes. Both spinal cord stimulation and spinally administered opioids should be used in the context of a treatment continuum, but only after failure of syndrome-specific conservative therapies. All patients for implantable pain technologies should meet the following selection criteria: absence of untreated drug habituations, psychological interview and clearance, a trial for efficacy, and absence of any surgical contraindications. Spinally administered opioids are more appropriate for opioid-responsive nociceptive pain syndromes and

spinal cord stimulation is more appropriate for mononeuropathic pain syndromes, pain of ischemic origin, and pain due to intractable angina pectoris. For patients who may actually respond to both approaches, a trial of spinal cord stimulation should be considered prior to spinally administered opioids. Spinal cord stimulation is a well-known procedure that is totally reversible, with few associated complications. Spinally administered opioids, on the other hand, is a newer procedure with scant information regarding the long-term complications of the chronic infusion of opioids into the spinal canal. Both technologies, however, should be used before considering more invasive pain treatments such as neuroablative procedures.

References

1. Shealy CN, Mortimer JT, Reswick J. Electrical inhibition of pain by stimulation of the dorsal column: Preliminary clinical reports. Anesth Anal 1967;46:489.
2. Melzack R, Wall PD. Pain mechanisms: A new theory. Science 1965;150:971.
3. Richardson RR, Siqueira EB, Cerullo LJ. Spinal epidural neurostimulation for treatment of acute and chronic intractable pain. Neurosurgery 1977;5:344.
4. Krainick JU, Thoden U, Riechert T. Pain reduction in amputees by long-term spinal cord stimulation. J Neurosurg 1980;52:346.
5. Long DM, Erikson D, Campbell J, et al. Electrical stimulation of the spinal cord and peripheral nerves for pain control: A ten year experience. Appl Neurophys 1981;44:207.
6. Ray CD, Burton CV, Lifson A. Neurostimulation as used in a large clinical practice. Appl Neurophysiol 1982;45:160.
7. Broseta J, Roldan P, Gonzalez-Dartzer J, et al. Chronic epidural dorsal column stimulation in the treatment of causalgic pain. Appl Neurophysiol 1982;45:190.
8. Siegfried J, Lazorthes Y. Long-term follow up of dorsal column stimulation in the treatment of causalgic pain. Appl Neurophysiol 1982;45:201.
9. Meglio M, Cioni B, Rossi GF. Spinal cord stimulation in management of chronic pain: A 9-year experience. J Neurosurg 1989;70:519.
10. Kumar K, Wyant GM, Ekong CEU. Epidural spinal cord stimulation for relief of chronic pain. Pain Clin 1986;1:91.
11. Spiegelmann R, Friedman WA. Spinal cord stimulation: A contemporary series. Neurosurgery 1991;28:65.
12. Barolat G, Schwartzman R, Woo R. Epidural spinal cord stimulation in the management of reflex sympathetic dystrophy. Stereotact Funct Neurosurg 1989;53:29.
13. Racz GB, McCarron RF, Talboys P. Percutaneous dorsal column stimulator for chronic pain control. Spine 1989;14:1.
14. North RB, Ewend MG, Lawton MT, et al. Failed back surgery syndrome: 5-year follow-up after spinal cord stimulator implantation. Neurosurg 1991;28:692.
15. Jacobs MJHM, Jorning PJ, Joshi SR, et al. Spinal cord electrical stimulation improves microvascular blood flow in severe limb ischaemia. Ann Surg 1988;207:179.
16. Robaina FJ, Dominguez M, Diaz M, et al. Spinal cord stimulation for relief of chronic pain in vasospastic disorders of the upper limbs Neurosurgery 1989;24:179.
17. Groth KE. Spinal cord stimulation for the treatment of peripheral vascular disease. Adv Pain Res Ther 1985;9:861.
18. Tallis RC, Illis LS, Sedgwick C, et al. Spinal cord stimulation in peripheral vascular disease. J Neurol Neurosurg Psychiatry 1983;46:478.
19. Augustinsson LE, Holm J, Carlsson CA, et al. Epidural electrical stimulation in severe limb ischemia: Evidences of pain relief, increased blood flow and a possible limb-saving effect. Ann Surg 1985;202:104.
20. Murphy DF, Giles KE. Dorsal column stimulation for pain relief from intractable angina pectoris. Med J Aust 1987;3:365.
21. Mannheimer C, Augustinsson LE, Carlsson CA, et al. Epidural spinal electrical stimulation in severe angina pectoris. Br Heart J 1988;59:56.
22. Augustinsson LE. Spinal cord stimulation in severe angina pectoris: Surgical technique, intraoperative physiology, complications, and side effects. Pace 1989;12:693.
23. Atweh SF, Kuhar MJ. Autoradiographic localization of opiate receptors in rat brain. Spinal cord and lower medulla. Brain Res 1977;124:53.
24. Yaksh TL, Rudy TA. Studies on the direct spinal action of narcotics in the production of analgesia in the rat. J Pharmacol Exp Ther 1977;202:411.
25. Yaksh TL. Analgesic actions of intrathecal opiates in cat and primates. Brain Res 1978;153:205.
26. Wang JF, Nauss LA, Thomas JE. Pain relief by intrathecally applied morphine in man. Anesthesiology 1979;50:149.
27. Behar M, Olshwang D, Magora F, Davidson JT. Epidural morphine in treatment of pain. Lancet 1979;1:527.
28. Cousins MJ, Mather LE, Glynn CJ, et al. Selective spinal analgesia. Lancet 1979;1:1141.
29. Onofrio BM, Yaksh TL, Arnold PG. Continuous low dose intrathecal morphine administration in the treatment of chronic pain of malignant origin. Mayo Clin Proc 1981;55:469.
30. Coombs DW, Saunders RL, Gaylor M, et al. Epidural narcotic infusion: Implantation technique and efficacy. Anesthesiology 1981;55:469.
31. Harbaugh RE, Coombs DW, Saunders RL. Implanted continuous epidural morphine infusion system. J Neurosurg 1981;56:803.
32. Coombs DW, Saunders RL, Gaylor, MS. Relief of continuous chronic pain by intraspinal narcotics infusion via an implanted reservoir. JAMA 1983;250:2336.
33. Krames ES, Gershow J, Glassberg A, et al. Continuous infusion of spinally administered narcotics for the relief of pain due to malignant disorders. Cancer 1985;56:696.
34. Shetter AG, Hadley MN, Wilkinson E. Administration of intraspinal morphine for the treatment of cancer pain. Neurosurgery 1986;18:740.
35. Penn RD, Paice JA. Chronic intrathecal morphine for intractable pain. J Neurosurg 1987;67:182.
36. Dennis GC, DeWitty RL. Management of intractable pain in cancer patients by implantable morphine infusion systems. J Natl Med Assoc 1987;79:939.
37. Brazenor GA. Long-term intrathecal administration of morphine: A comparison of bolus injection via reservoir with continuous infusion by implanted pump. Neurosurgery 1987;21:484.
38. Onofrio BM, Yaksh TL. Long-term pain relief produced by intrathecal infusion in 53 patients. J Neurosurg 1990;72:200.

39. Zimmerman CG, Burchiel, KM. The use of intrathecal opiates for malignant and non-malignant pain: Management of thirty-nine patients. Proc Am Pain Soc 1991;97.

40. Varga CA. Chronic administration of intraspinal local anesthetics in the treatment of malignant pain. Proc Am Pain Soc 1989;71.

41. Auld AW, Maki-Jokela A, Murdock DM. Intraspinal narcotic analgesia in the treatment of chronic pain. Spine 1984;10:777.

42. Hadley MN, Shetter AG. Intrathecal opiate administration for analgesia. Contemp Neurosurg 1986;8:1.

43. Hassenbusch SJ, Stanton-Hicks MD, Soukup J, et al. Sufentanil citrate and morphine/bupivacaine as alternative agents in chronic epidural infusions for intractable noncancer pain. Neurosurgery 1991;29:76.

44. Goodman RR. Treatment of lower extremity reflex sympathetic dystrophy with continuous intrathecal morphine infusion. Appl Neurophysiol 1987;50:425.

45. Jacobson L. Clinical note: Relief of persistent postamputation stump and phantom limb pain with intrathecal fentanyl. Pain 1989;37:317.

46. Barolat G, Schwartzman RJ, Aries L. Chronic intrathecal morphine infusion for intractable pain in reflex sympathetic dystrophy. Proc Am Cancer Pain Soc 1988;17.

47. Lamb SA, Hosobuchi Y. Intrathecal morphine sulfate for chronic benign pain delivered by implanted pump delivery systems. Proc IASP 1990;S120.

48. Krames ES, Lanning RM. Intrathecal infusion analgesia for nonmalignant pain. Proc Am Pain Soc 1991;98.

49. Burchiel KJ, Johans TJ. Management of post-herpetic neuralgia with chronic intrathecal morphine. Proc Am Pain Soc 1992;136.

50. Bedder MD, Olsen KA, Flemming BM, Brown D. Diagnostic indicators for implantable infusion pumps in non-malignant pain. Proc Am Pain Soc 1992;111.

51. Arner S, Arner B. Differential effects of epidural morphine in the treatment of cancer related pain. Acta Anaesthesiol Scand 1985;29:332.

52. Arner S, Meyerson B. Lack of analgesic effect of opioids on neuropathic and idiopathic forms of pain. Pain 1988;33:11.

53. Vecht CJ. Nociceptive nerve pain and neuropathic pain [letter]. Pain 1989;39:243.

54. Hammond DL. Do Opioids Relieve Pain? In KL Casey (ed), Pain and Central Nervous System Disease: The Central Pain Syndromes. New York: Raven, 1991;233.

55. Portenoy RK, Foley KM, Inturrisi CE. The nature of opioid responsiveness and its implications for neuropathic pain: New hypothesis derived from studies of opioid infusions. Pain 1990;43:273.

Chapter 14

Economic Outcome and Practical Efficacy of Implantable Drug Administration Systems

Benjamin W. Johnson, Jr.

Objectives

1. To define and characterize the concepts of outcome and efficacy as they relate to implantable drug administration systems (DASs) for cancer pain therapy.
2. To determine if the use of implantable DASs is justifiable in the management of cancer pain patients.
3. To stress the importance of systematic clinical studies in documenting a causal relationship between the use of implantable DASs and outcome.

Definitions

1. *Practical.* The application of knowledge to useful ends as tested by actual experience.
2. *Economic.* Pertaining to the careful management of wealth and resource; avoidance of waste by careful planning and use.
3. *Outcome.* Changes that occur in actual or potential health status after prior or concurrent health care.
4. *Efficacy.* The beneficial effects of a process of medical care as measured by the outcome achieved in a specific population of patients.

The Importance of Outcome

Outcome is a member of the classic triad of evaluators (structure, process, and outcome) regarding the quality of care. *Structure* refers to the resources available for health care intervention, whereas *process* refers to the way in which those resources are used.[1]

As Tuman points out, ". . . structure and process measures define the capability to perform, but outcome measures define the success of performance."[1] Although it is tempting to assume that satisfactory structure and process lead inevitably to a satisfactory outcome, there is evidence in the medical literature to the contrary.[2] In order for a distinct causal relationship between process and outcome to exist, validation by controlled clinical studies must be demonstrated.

Although outcome data are lacking in many areas of medicine, the field of pain medicine seems to be uniquely plagued by a lack of outcome studies in regard to the many therapeutic options available within the specialty. The most important explanation for the lack of outcome data is the subjective nature of pain itself.[3, 4] At present, there are only a few appropriately controlled clinical trials documenting the effects of implanted DASs, using outcome parameters, in cancer pain patients.[5–18] The lack of well-controlled studies correlating cost effectiveness with outcome data substantially weakens the justification for the use of these expensive devices.[19] When challenged by insurance companies, managed care organizations, consumers, legislators, health care administrators, and governmental agencies to justify the rationale of using these devices, anecdotal evidence alone is not sufficient. As Tuman notes, "The determination to cut the costs of medical care is so intense that it is not un-likely that governmental agencies will eventually fi-nance only a limited number of alternative therapies for a given medical condition based on their evalua-tion of outcome data."[1]

Appropriate economic tools are needed to evalu-ate the economic impact of the outcome of DAS im-plantation. Instruments such as cost-benefit analysis and cost-effectiveness analysis are amenable to health care economic analysis, with cost effective-ness being the most feasible.[2, 20, 21] In contrast to cost-benefit analysis, cost-effectiveness analysis rec-ognizes the difficulty (and inaccuracy) of describing cost and effectiveness in the same quantitative terms. Therefore, cost-effective analysis describes cost in monetary terms, while describing effectiveness in qualitative measures such as life-years gained, pain or symptom-free days, complications avoided, qual-ity-adjusted life-years, etc.[2] Cost-effectiveness analysis suggests that if several alternative treat-ments are equivalent in regard to efficacy that the least costly treatment should be chosen.

Therefore, if implantable DASs are to remain in the therapeutic armamentarium of the cancer pain practi-tioner, we must demonstrate their outcome-based cost effectiveness, using well-controlled clinical studies.[19]

The Challenge of Designing Appropriate Outcome Studies

The medical literature substantiates that well-controlled clinical trials are the ideal method to es-tablish a causal link between process and outcome. This ideal presents a formidable challenge when ap-plied to the DASs because the number of patients needed to satisfy sample size requirements are dif-ficult to achieve in most clinical settings. In addi-tion, the following characteristics of outcome variables must first be appreciated before designing or interpreting an outcome study.[1]

Characteristics of Outcome Variables

1. Dimension of health examined (physiologic, physical, and psychosocial)
2. Definiteness
3. Stability (over time)
4. Source of information

5. Purpose of measurement
6. Mode of data collection
7. Screening efficiency (ease of recording)
8. Timing of measurement
9. Stringency
10. Strength of causal relation to process variable
11. Reliability and validity

In addition, one should be familiar with the fac-tors affecting the validity of outcome studies.

Factors Affecting the Validity of Outcome Studies

Population Characteristics

1. Heterogeneity of severity of illness
2. Multicenter versus single-center database
3. Teaching versus nonteaching hospitals
4. Uniformity of process of care
5. Outcome definitions (specificity, uniformity, and appropriateness)

Methods of Data Collection

1. Case sampling (randomization, sequence, or se-lected cases)
2. Perspective or retrospective
3. Source of information or objectivity and data recording
4. Voluntary or compulsory reporting
5. Response rate
6. Timespan of study
7. Reliability and accuracy of data

Methods of Data Interpretation

1. Observed bias (definition of blame or errors)
2. Implicit or explicit assessment criteria
3. Presence of confounding factors
4. Strength of quality between process and outcome

Data Analysis

1. Clinically relevant effect size
2. Sample size and statistical power

3. Use of appropriate controls (where applicable)
4. Use of appropriate statistical analysis

The Measurement of Outcome

The importance of designing valid outcome studies to document the effectiveness, or lack thereof, of therapeutic interventions, should not be underestimated. The importance of *quality of life* as an outcome measure for cancer pain patients may be the best single outcome indicator.[22]

Recently, sociologists and clinicians have made significant advances toward assessing psychosocial outcome, specifically with the concept of quality of life. The reasons for this progress include the demands by legislators for justification of the benefit of additional health and social services to the public.

The assessment tools listed below can be easily adapted to the evaluation of the impact of implantable DASs on the quality of life for cancer pain patients. Although the term quality of life defies a unitary definition, most researchers agree that the following attributes must be considered:

Physical functioning
Mobility
Satisfaction with physical functioning
Depression
Anxiety
Loss of behavioral and emotional control
Physiologic well-being
Loneliness
Cognitive functioning
Family functioning
Sexual functioning
Social contacts
Role functioning
General health perceptions
Sleep
Energy or fatigue
Pain

The tests designed to assess and quantify these attributes include those listed below:

Sickness Impact Profile
Quality of Well-Being Scale
City of Hope Medical Center Quality of Life Survey

Subjective Well-Being Instrument for the Chronically Ill

The latter two instruments were specifically designed to evaluate cancer patients. Once adequate outcome measuring instruments have been decided on, the next step is to establish a cost-effectiveness ratio analysis in order to demonstrate the economic consequences of using this treatment modality.[2] This analysis attempts to assess the effect of a given intervention on the health care industry and society as a whole.

The Formation of a Cost-Effectiveness Ratio Analysis ($\Delta C/\Delta E$)

Definition: A ratio of net increase of health care costs to net effectiveness in terms of quality of life and enhanced life expectancy. The lower the value of the cost-effectiveness ratio ($\Delta C/\Delta E$), the more favorable the benefit from a given health care expenditure.

$$\Delta C = \Delta C_{Rx} + \Delta C_{se} - \Delta C_{morb} + \Delta C_{Rx\Delta LE}$$

where ΔC = net health care costs

ΔC_{Rx} = all direct medical and health care costs (hospitalization, physician time, medications, laboratory services, counseling, etc.)[19]

ΔC_{se} = all health care costs associated with iatrogenic effects[23–28]

ΔC_{morb} = savings in health care costs due to prevention or alleviaton of disease (e.g., pain, disability)

$\Delta C_{Rx\Delta LE}$ = cost of treating disease that occurred because of a patient's increased life span after interventional therapy (i.e., work injury, motor vehicle accident, etc.).

The direct health care costs of implanting DASs include the diagnostic workup, psychological assessment, purchase of equipment, surgical and operating room expenditures, diagnostic imaging, hospital room and board, and medications. The implantation of drug administration devices can cause a number of iatrogenic adverse effects, depending on the system implanted, the experience of the clinician, and the nature of the patient's disease process.

A consideration of the potential savings in health care costs from preventing or alleviating intractable cancer pain is of great importance due to the tremendous economic, social, and ethical costs of managing a cancer patient with unrelieved pain. The economic costs include lost work days by family members, unnecessary visits to the physician, hospital, and emergency room, multiple medication trials (and their potential side effects), as well as more frequent visits by home health and hospice personnel.

Social costs involve quality of life issues such as withdrawal from social contact, dysfunctional family relationships, decreased independence, increased dependence on health care providers, and restricted activities of daily living. Ethical costs include feelings of guilt and helplessness by the patient, family members, and health care providers. It is difficult to estimate these various costs because of the difficulty of assigning a discrete monetary value to intangible costs and benefits.

The factors comprising the denominator of the cost-effectiveness equation are also subject to difficulties arising from an inability to accurately "cost" intangible factors; however, the quantitative analysis provided by implementing a cost-effectiveness evaluation will help our assessment.

$$\Delta E = \Delta\gamma + \Delta\gamma_{morb} - \Delta\gamma_{se}$$

where ΔE = net health effectiveness (measured in quality-adjusted life-years)

$\Delta\gamma$ = expected number of unadjusted life-years (difference between age-specific life expectancy with and without the intervention)

$\Delta\gamma_{morb}$ = improvements in the quality-of-life years due to alleviation of morbidity

$\Delta\gamma_{se}$ = change in quality of life years due to iatrogenesis of intervention.

Note: The units of the denominator are $(QAL\gamma_s)$

$$QAL\gamma_s = \gamma_s \times \lambda_s$$

where γ_s = the number of years spent at a given health status

λ_s = health status (range 0.0–1.0, with 0.0 = mild disability and 1.0 = near death).

When calculating the savings of the prevention and alleviation of morbidity, one must remember the high cost of unrelieved pain:

1. Physiologic costs: neurophysiologic, endocrine, metabolic
2. Physical costs: disability, effects of prolonged bed rest (i.e., pulmonary embolism, osteoporosis, muscle wasting, etc.)
3. Costs to the family: lost work hours, dysfunctional relationships, loss of consortium, loss of income, etc.
4. Costs to society: increased unemployment, increased governmental transfers (i.e., Social Security, Workers Compensation), increased insurance rates, increased cost of goods and services, etc.

Because all of the costs and benefits of a given therapeutic intervention do not necessarily occur at the same time, it becomes necessary to combine present and future costs as well as benefits into comparable units by present value analysis. Although a detailed discussion of the role of present value analysis in choosing between therapeutic alternatives is beyond the scope of this presentation, one discussion is presented in the classic treatise by Weinstein and Stason.[2]

Chrubasik and Chrubasik reviewed 10 studies regarding the success rate of intrathecal opiate therapy for chronic cancer pain via a variety of DASs.[12] Of 306 cancer pain patients, 223 obtained good-to-excellent pain relief. Few, if any, of these studies address cost-effectiveness, alternative therapies, controls, or quality-of-life parameters (except for mention of less oral opioid requirements).[29] The criteria for patient selection were not standardized.

The most likely explanation for the lack of alternative treatments is that most patients receiving implantable DASs have demonstrated a lack of efficacy in regard to more conservative therapeutic alternatives.[30, 31] Therefore, using alternative therapies, or no therapy, as controls would present formidable ethical concerns and is not likely to be included in future studies. It is more likely that a study will be performed that compares the cost-effectiveness of various types of implantable DASs or various analgesic substances (i.e., peptides, opiates, etc.).[19]

Summary

In spite of the difficulty of evaluating the multitudinous complexities of outcome variables, it is imperative that we strive to develop and execute appropriate controlled outcome studies for implantable DASs in order to continue to justify their use in cancer pain patients. Although the number of well-controlled studies is few, the best observational studies seem to indicate that the economic outcome and practical efficacy of implantable DASs is favorable when compared with the high cost of unrelieved pain.[12] Meticulous, painstaking documentation of our observations coupled with the principles presented previously will enable us to continue our objective to deliver the most effective medical care to those in need.[32]

References

1. Tuman KJ. Evaluating Anesthetic Outcome. In RK Stoelting, PG Barash, TJ Gallagher (eds), Advances in Anesthesia (Vol. 8). St. Louis: Mosby, 1991;331.
2. Weinstein MC, Stason WB. Foundations of cost-effectiveness analysis for health and medical practices. N Engl J Med 1977;296:716.
3. Abram SE, Haddox JD. Chronic Pain. In DL Brown (ed), Risk and Outcome in Anesthesia (2nd ed). Philadelphia: Lippincott, 1992;488.
4. Samuelsson H, Hedner T. Pain characterization in cancer patients and the analgesic response to epidural morphine. Pain 1991;46:3.
5. Onofrio BM, Yaksh TL. Long-term pain relief produced by intrathecal morphine infusion in 53 patients. J Neurosurg 1990;72:200.
6. Schramm J, Heidhardt J, Vahle-Hinz C. Long-term pain relief and dosage pattern development in cancer pain treated by intrathecal morphine via a subcutaneous reservoir. Pain 1990;(Suppl. 5):S497.
7. Waldman SD. Implantable drug delivery systems: Practical considerations. J Pain Symptom Manage 1990;5:169.
8. Nitescu P, Appelgren L, Linder LE, et al. Epidural versus intrathecal morphine-bupivacaine: Assessment of consecutive treatments in advanced cancer pain. J Pain Symptom Manage 1990;5:18.
9. Crawford ME, Andersen HB, Augustenborg G, et al. Pain treatment on outpatient basis utilizing extradural opiates. A Danish multicentre study comprising 105 patients. Pain 1983;16:41.
10. Plummer JL, Cherry DA, Cousins MJ, et al. Long-term spinal administration of morphine in cancer and non-cancer pain: A retrospective study. Pain 1991;44:215.
11. Erdine S, Aldemir T. Long-term results of peridural morphine in 225 patients. Pain 1991;45:155.
12. Chrubasik J, Chrubasik S. Spinal Opioid Treatment for Chronic Pain: An Update. In J Chrubasik, M Cousins, E Martin (eds), Advances in Pain Therapy (Vol I). New York: Springer-Verlag, 1992;24.
13. Sjoberg M, Nitescu P, Appelgren L, et al. Long-term intrathecal morphine and bupivacaine in patients with refractory cancer pain: Results from a morphine:bupivacaine dose regimen of 0.5:4.75 mg/ml. Anesthesiology 1994;80:284.
14. Sjoberg M, Karsson PA, Nordborg C, et al. Neuropathologic findings after long-term intrathecal infusion of morphine and bupivacaine for pain treatment in cancer patients. Anesthesiology 1992;76:173.
15. Mercandante S. Intrathecal morphine and bupivacaine in advanced cancer pain patients implanted at home. J Pain Symptom Manage 1994;9:201.
16. Yaksh TL, Onofrio BM. Retrospective consideration of the dose of morphine given intrathecally by chronic infusion in 163 patients by 19 physicians. Pain 1987;31:211.
17. Findler G, Olshwang D, Hadani M. Continuous epidural morphine treatment for intractable pain in terminal cancer patients. Pain 1982;14:311.
18. Penn RD, Paice JA. Chronic intrathecal morphine for intractable pain. J Neurosurg 1987;67:182.
19. Bedder MD, Burchiel K, Larson A. Cost analysis of two implantable narcotic delivery systems. J Pain Symptom Manage 1991;6:368.
20. Johnston MV, Keith RA. Cost-benefits of medical rehabilitation: Review and critique. Arch Phys Med Rehabil 1983;64:147.
21. Robinson R. Cost-effectiveness analysis. Br Med J 1993;307:793.
22. Aaronson NA, Beckman J (eds). The Quality of Life of Cancer Patients. New York: Raven, 1987.
23. Crul BJ, Delhaas EM. Technical complications during long-term subarachnoid or epidural administration of morphine in terminally ill cancer patients: A review of 140 cases. Reg Anesth 1991;16:209.
24. Wu CL, Patt RB. Accidental overdose of systemic morphine during intended refill of intrathecal infusion device. Anesth Analg 1992;75:130.
25. Gustafsson LL, Schildt B, Jacobsen K. Adverse effects of extradural and intrathecal opiates: Report of a nationwide survey in Sweden. Br J Anaesth 1982;54:479.
26. Yaksh TL, Rudy TA. Chronic catheterization of the spinal subarachnoid space. Physiol Behav 1976;17:1031.
27. Plummer JL, Cherry DA, Cousins MJ, et al. Long-term spinal administration of morphine in cancer and non-cancer pain: A retrospective study. Pain 1991;44:215.
28. Hahn MB, Bettencourt JA, McCrea WB. In vivo sterilization of an infected long-term epidural catheter. Anesthesiology 1992;76:645.
29. Greenberg HS, Taren J, Ensminger WD, et al. Benefit from and tolerance to continuous intrathecal infusion

of morphine for intractable cancer pain. J Neurosurg 1982;57:360.

30. Waldman SD, Leak DW, Kennedy LD, et al. Intraspinal Opioid Therapy. In RB Patt (ed), Cancer Pain. Philadelphia: Lippincott, 1993;285.

31. Waldman SD, Coombs DW. Selection of implantable narcotic delivery systems. Anesth Analg 1989;68:377.

32. Jacox A, Carr DB, Payne R, et al. Management of Cancer Pain. Clinical Practice Guideline. AHCPR Publication No. 94-0592. Rockville, MD: Agency for Health Care Policy and Research, U.S. Department of Health and Human Services, Public Health Service, March 1994.

Chapter 15

Neuraxial Analgesic Blockade: Physiology, Pharmacology, and Complications

Marshall D. Bedder

Introduction

The World Health Organization (WHO) advocates the use of a three-step analgesic ladder that uses oral medication to treat increasing levels of cancer pain.[1] Oral analgesics are clinically not always effective in controlling increasing or severe cancer pain. A validation study of the WHO method for cancer pain relief revealed that the analgesic ladder proved efficacious in only 71% of the cases.[2] The remaining 29% of cases used destructive neurolytic blocks of pain pathways, all of limited duration. The American Pain Society handbook on principles of analgesic use for treatment of acute pain and cancer pain recognizes the role of intraspinal administration of opioids in cancer pain.[3] An important corollary of this treatment technique emphasized in the American Pain Society publication states ". . . the choice of drug and the particular technique must rest with a skilled team whose members are thoroughly familiar with the relative risks and benefits of the use of intraspinal opiates." Neuraxial analgesic blockade can also be considered a treatment option. The administration of spinal analgesics is part of the armamentarium of a well-prepared pain medicine practitioner. Many medications have been investigated for neuraxial analgesia, but sound clinical and histopathologic data are often lacking. This chapter focuses on clinically useful and potentially available analgesics that can further enhance the quality of life of cancer pain patients.

Opioids

Physiology: Mechanism of Action

Spinally administered opioids modulate pain transmission by direct action on specific receptors in the dorsal horn of the spinal cord. Immunoreactivity studies have shown the highest concentration of enkephalin-containing cell bodies and nerve terminals in laminae I, II, V, and X of the spinal cord.[4] Three spinal analgesic receptor systems have been identified: the mu-, delta-, and kappa-receptors (Table 15-1). The analgesic agonists mimic the effect of endogenously produced opioid peptides, whether administered systemically or spinally. The prototypical agonist drugs of mu-receptors are opiates and opioid peptides with a major proposed action on supraspinal analgesia. The delta-receptor prototypical agonists are the enkephalins, with a major action on spinal analgesia. Kappa-receptors also have a major proposed action on spinal analgesia, with the prototypical agonists being ketocyclazocine and dynorphin. Clinically correlated agonists for the mu-, delta-, and kappa-receptors, respectively, are morphine, d-Ala^2-d-Leu^5-enkephalin (DADL), and butorphanol. Within the mu-receptor population, various agonist drugs show different efficacy. A recent study of suppression of nociceptive responses by multiple spinal mu opioid agonists showed that, in order of efficacy,

Table 15-1. Spinal Opioid Analgesic Receptor Subtypes and Agonists

Subtype	Prototypic Agonist	Clinical Agonist
Mu	Opiates and opioid peptides	Morphine
Delta	Enkephalins	d-Ala^2-d-Leu^5
Kappa	Ketocyclazocine, dynorphin	Butorphanol

Table 15-2. Common Characteristics of Spinal Receptor Analgesic Systems

Action through the same family of K$^+$ receptors; mediated by Gi protein

Binding sites presynaptic and postsynaptic to small primary afferents

Agonism reduces the release of substance P from small primary afferents

Source: Adapted from M Sosnowski, TL Yaksh. Spinal administration of receptor-selective drugs as analgesics: New horizons. J Pain Symptom Manage 1990;5:204.

sufentanil equale DAG (enkephalin), with both being greater than morphine.[5]

At a receptor level, opioid spinal receptors have similar mechanisms of action shared by other types of spinal analgesic receptors[6] (Table 15-2).

There is a direct presynaptic effect on small high threshold primary afferents. Opioid agonists reduce the release of peptides (including substance P) contained in these small primary afferents. Postsynaptically, there is a decreased excitability of the neuron probably through receptor-mediated hyperpolarization. These effects are thought to occur through an increase in potassium conductance mediated by Gi protein.

Pharmacology

Clinical experience with neuraxially administered opioids has focused on morphine, methadone, hydromorphone, meperidine, fentanyl, sufentanil, and DADL. Less extensive data and anecdotal reports exist for other opioid agonists. This section discusses clinically useful pharmacologic principles for opioid agonists with proven efficacy supported by reasonable scientific foundation.

The opioid analgesic agents used most often to control cancer pain are of the mu-receptor opioid subtype. Important pharmacologic factors determining optimum clinical results include (1) lipid solubility, (2) binding affinity, and (3) equianalgesic dosing (Table 15-3). The less lipophilic a drug is, the longer it will remain present in the cerebrospinal fluid and the greater its distribution will be in the cerebrospinal fluid. Lipophilicity increases in the following order for these drugs: morphine, hydromorphone, meperidine, methadone, fentanyl, and sufentanil. Relatively segmental analgesia can be obtained with the highly lipid-soluble opioids, whereas analgesia can be provided for more distant sites with the less lipid-soluble opioids that establish more effective cerebrospinal fluid concentrations. This can be seen clinically with the use of morphine, administered in the lumbar region, to treat head and neck cancer.[7] Other effects related to the low lipid solubility seen with morphine are a slower onset of action and longer duration of CNS effects. In contrast, there will be a more rapid onset of action with the more lipid-soluble opioids and a correspondingly shorter duration of action.

Receptor binding of a particular opioid is recognized as being important in drug efficacy and in its interaction with drug lipid-solubility characteristics. A drug with a higher receptor affinity, such as sufentanil, is capable of producing a maximal effect at a lower receptor occupancy than a drug with a low receptor affinity, such as morphine. Binding affinity decreases in order for the following drugs: sufentanil, fentanyl, morphine, alfentanil, and meperidine. A high lipid solubility, high receptor affinity drug (i.e., sufentanil) has a rapid onset but, because of its increased receptor affinity, it has a longer duration of action.[8]

The differences in potency for spinal opioid agonists are due to physicochemical and pharmacokinetic differences among individual opioids. If adjustments are made for these factors by correcting for dose and route of administration, all opioids can be made equianalgesic.[9] Knowledge of these

Table 15-3. Important Clinical Properties of Spinal Opioids

Opioid	Lipid Solubility	Binding Affinity	Dose (Epidural)	Duration (hr)
Morphine	1.42	5.7	5–10 mg	6–24
Hydromorphone	11.36	—	1.0–1.5 mg	6–16
Meperidine	38.8	193.0	20–60 mg	6–8
Methadone	116	—	48 mg	6–10
Fentanyl	813	1.6	25–100 µg	2–4
Sufentanil	1,778	0.1	10–30 µg	4–6

Table 15-4. Complications of Spinal Opioids

Respiratory depression
Central nervous system effects
Nausea and vomiting
Urinary retention
Pruritus
Paradoxical pain
Hyperesthesia with allodynia
Hyperalgesia/myoclonus
Amenorrhea/arthralgia

conversion factors is extremely important in the optimal clinical use of spinal opioids. All equianalgesic tables have to be regarded as starting guidelines. Their use may not be applicable in all situations, i.e., chronic infusion patients. Incomplete cross-tolerance may require starting at approximately 50% of the equianalgesic dose of the new opioid. There is a 10 to 1 conversion factor seen clinically from epidural to intrathecal infusion.[10]

Complications

The complications associated with spinal opioids have been well documented and rely mainly on studies based on short-term or acute administration (Table 15-4).[11] These side effects include respiratory depression, CNS effects, nausea and vomiting, urinary retention, and pruritus. Tracking and separating side effects of medications from disease state is much more difficult in the cancer patient due to the frequent multisystem involvement of their disease.[12] A large nationwide survey was performed in Sweden involving over 750 patients treated for intractable cancer pain with epidural or intrathecal opioids. The average duration of treatment for epidural and intrathecal routes was 124 days (3–450) and 47 days (3–90), respectively. No case of respiratory depression was reported and pruritus and urinary retention were not reported as significant problems.[13] DuPen reported on 55 cancer patients treated with tunneled epidural catheters and morphine boluses for a total of 3,891 catheter-days of experience.[14] No respiratory depression was seen at doses as high as 560 mg in 24 hours. The only treatment-related side effect that was difficult to treat was nausea, which was intractable in nine patients (16%).

As experience increases regarding the use of neuraxial opioids for cancer pain, other complications related to long-term use or increased doses are being described. Hyperalgesia and myoclonus have been reported with the intrathecal infusion of high-dose morphine.[15] This effect can be reversed by lowering the morphine dose and by a systemic administration of benzodiazepam. There are several case reports of paradoxical pain with hyperesthesia and allodynia. Animal studies have shown a similar effect, which was not reversible with opioid antagonists.[16] Yaksh has postulated a pathophysiologic mechanism involving the disinhibition of glycinergic and GABA-ergic control systems on low-threshold afferents converging on nociceptive neurons at the spinal cord.[17]

Recent private communication and soon to be published case reports allude to an amenorrhea and arthralgia syndrome manifesting in younger women using chronic spinal infusions. There may also be an associated impotence syndrome in men using long-term intrathecal infusion. Until these reports are analyzed and verified, one must keep these potential side effects in mind as a possiblity in patients on long-term therapy.

Clinical Implications

A comprehensive review of neuraxial opioid administration was presented by Abram at the 1992 Bonica lecture.[18] This review attempted to analyze controlled studies, or where unavailable, selected studies that were thought to be reasonably well conducted. The conclusions or generalizations from that review represent the best overall synthesis of current knowledge on neuraxial opioid treatment. Those pertaining to cancer pain are listed below:

1. "There is a slow increase in mean daily opiate dose in all series, generally at a rate that doubles every few months. Some individual patients escalate their dose rapidly, particularly those in the terminal phases of their disease.
2. "There is a tendency for dose escalation to be slower with intrathecal administration systems.
3. "The escalation in dose over time tends to be slower in patients receiving continuous infusions as opposed to intermittent bolus injections.
4. "Higher doses of spinal and epidural (as well as systemic) opiates are required for neuropathic pain than for somatogenic pain. Opiate requirements for visceral pain are intermediate between neuropathic and somatic pain.
5. "Incident pain (occurring with activity) is much more difficult to control with either neuraxial or systemic narcotics than rest pain.
6. "Higher systemic opiate requirements predict higher neuraxial requirements."

When increasing doses of opioid are required to sustain adequate analgesia the following factors may have a role[19]:

1. Drug kinetics
2. Change in stimulus modality or intensity
3. Psychological variables
4. Pharmacodynamic variables

A switch from a mu-agonist to an alternative delta- or kappa-opioid agonist agent would seem to be a logical alternative for patients who are experiencing tolerance or unresponsiveness to the classic mu-ago-

nist agents. One must consider the variables listed previously in any situation of pain unresponsiveness. As is discussed later, neuropathic pain components may best be treated by the combination of an opioid and local anesthetic or by targeting different analgesic receptor systems. Reports of alternative opioid receptor agonists being used successfully for unresponsive cancer pain are limited, but there is some experience with the delta-receptor agonist DADL. An early case report documented the intrathecal administration of DADL to a patient who had become tolerant to intrathecal morphine.[20] DADL restored analgesia without respiratory depression but opioid withdrawal was not prevented. A recent series from the same group studied five cancer patients who were no longer responsive to intrathecal opioid infusions administered by implanted infusion pumps.[21] They concluded that intrathecal DADL restored analgesia in patients with nociceptive or mixed nociceptive neuropathic pain who were no longer responsive to intrathecal mu-opioid receptor ligands. DADL was not as effective in restoring analgesia in patients with neuropathic pain. The ability to change between various receptor subtype agonists may also be determined by the order in which they are administered. Studies with rats compared tolerance to levorphanol, which potently binds all three spinal analgesic opioid receptors, with morphine, which is fairly selective for mu sites.[22] Levorphanol infusions produced tolerance to both morphine and levorphanol whereas morphine infusions selectively produced tolerance to morphine. The researchers thought that the unidirectional tolerance might be due to the selectivity of morphine for mu-receptors compared with the ability of levorphanol to interact more potently with other relevant receptor subtypes. The order in which opioid agonists are administered may then become another important clinical factor in providing long-term pain control for cancer patients receiving intraspinal infusions.

Alpha-Adrenergic Agonists

Physiology: Mechanism of Action

Clonidine and Dexmedetomidine

Clonidine (CLON) and dexmedetomidine (DEX) are both alpha$_2$-adrenergic receptor agonists. The analgesic effects of intraspinal alpha$_2$-agonists are

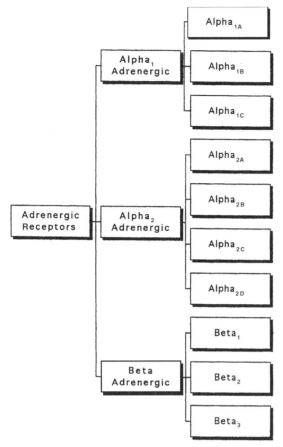

Figure 15-1. Adrenergic receptor classification. (Adapted from RG Lawhead, HS Blaxall, DB Bylund. Alpha$_{2A}$ is the predominant alpha$_2$ adrenergic receptor subtype in human spinal cord. Anesthesiology 1992;77:983.)

independent from opioid receptor activity and are secondary to stimulation of alpha$_2$-receptors at a spinal cord level. Adrenergic receptors have been traditionally divided into alpha and beta receptors. New experimental evidence suggests a classification scheme that includes three major types (Figure 15-1). The alpha$_{2A}$-adrenergic receptor subtype has been shown to be the predominant subtype in the human spinal cord.[23] Alpha$_2$-agonists appear to inhibit presynaptic afferent transmitter release from C fibers and also to have a postsynaptic effect on dorsal horn transmission.[24] CLON has been shown to have local anesthetic activity but supraclinical doses would have to be used to obtain useful peripheral nerve block.[25] This study explained the prolonged action of lidocaine in peripheral nerve block as being created by an enhancing effect of low-dose

CLON on lidocaine-evoked inhibition of C-fiber action potential.

DEX has an approximately sevenfold higher affinity for the alpha$_2$-receptor than CLON.[26] It appears that DEX is a full alpha$_2$-agonist whereas CLON is a partial agonist, with a 220 to 1 selectivity for the alpha$_2$-receptor.[26]

Pharmacology: Clinical Application

The availability of useful alternative agonists, apart from the opioids and local anesthetics, is extremely limited. These agents are not approved by the Food and Drug Administration for intraspinal administration and are often unavailable in sterile, preservative-free preparations unless under an investigational new drug protocol. This has been the case for CLON, which has been the most studied of all the alternative agonists. Many of the analgesic studies involving CLON have come from the postoperative pain management and obstetric literature.

When used for postoperative analgesia, CLON appears to provide superior analgesia compared with bupivacaine.[27] This study also showed that a combination of CLON and bupivacaine resulted in significantly better and longer duration of analgesia than single-drug treatment. A randomized double-blind study looked at the analgesic effect of the combination of epidural morphine and CLON versus epidural morphine alone in patients undergoing major abdominal surgery.[28] The epidural CLON group had improved forced vital capacity secondary to improved pain relief. Side effects were similar in both groups and the authors concluded that epidural CLON enhances the analgesic effect of epidural morphine. Side effects of epidural CLON included a decrease in heart rate and blood pressure.

The use of combination hydromorphone (Dilaudid) and CLON, delivered intrathecally by an implanted infusion pump, was described by Coombs in a patient with intractable cancer pain.[29] In this patient, who had a history of severe sensitivity to morphine, hydromorphone successfully treated the pain associated with her metastatic uterine cervical cancer. When significant tolerance to the hydromorphone developed, the addition of CLON to the infusion maintained pain control up until her death. An open-label, dose-ranging study investigated the analgesic and side effects of epidural CLON

(100–900 µg) in patients with intractable cancer pain.[30] This study was the first systematic examination of the analgesic efficacy of epidural CLON in cancer patients with intractable pain. The patients all had extensive metastases and were having increasing pain not controlled by escalating doses of systemic or epidural opioids. Epidural CLON provided effective analgesia during the trial phase in all nine patients. Following the study, seven patients were treated with combination epidural CLON and morphine infusions at home for up to 5 months with sustained analgesia. This study also reinforced the ability of epidural CLON to effectively treat neuropathic pain. Previous studies have shown the inadequacy of morphine or equivalent doses of other opioids to treat neuropathic deafferentation pain.[31] Based on opioid infusion studies, others have suggested that what we in fact may be seeing in neuropathic pain is a rightward shift of the dose-response curve to opioids.[32] Regardless of whether this phenomenon is true, the clinician is left with a group of patients who are not achieving pain relief even on escalating doses of both systemic and epidural opioids. A placebo-controlled, blinded, multicenter study of epidural CLON for intractable cancer pain showed that this therapy was particularly effective for patients with neuropathic pain.[33] Patients enrolled in the study had poor analgesia with large doses of systemic or epidural morphine or had dose-limiting side effects. Of the 85 patients, 56% treated with epidural CLON versus 5% treated with placebo had statistically significant efficacy in the treatment of their neuropathic pain. No serious or unexpected adverse events were reported.

Clearly, the alpha-adrenergic agonists hold promise for treating patients refractory to opioids or patients experiencing neuropathic pain. The immediate goal is to facilitate the approval or availability of spinal CLON in order to compassionately care for a group of patients who have few options left.

Complications

Hypotension and decrease in heart rate are seen following intraspinal injection of CLON.[28, 30] These studies also reinforced earlier observations that pre-existing hypertension may exaggerate the decrease in blood pressure following epidural injection. In-

trathecal injection produces a greater decrease in blood pressure than epidural administration.[34] The action of epidural CLON on brainstem sites and its direct inhibition of spinal preganglionic sympathetic outflow is responsible for the observed hypotensive effects.[35, 36] It appears that CLON has both direct cardiac effects and central effects, which contribute to the decrease in heart rate. Sedation effects of intraspinal CLON have been transient and not a limiting factor in long-term therapy.[30]

Peptide Analgesic Agonists

Physiology: Mechanism of Action

Somatostatin and Octreotide

Somatostatin (SST) is a tetradecapeptide that has been shown to have wide distribution from supraspinal, dorsal root ganglia, and intraspinal neurons CNS as determined by studies in rats.[37] The mechanism of action of SST is unclear but there is evidence of its role as a transmitter, modulator, and selective depressant to noxious stimuli as well as to general excitatory effects.[38] SST-mediated analgesia is not reversed by naloxone and it is suggested that SST acts in its own central receptor sites.[39] The analgesic potency of epidural SST has been shown to be similar to epidural morphine after abdominal operations and acute and chronic pain treated by spinal infusions.[39] SST is an unstable peptide for long-term infusion because it is rapidly degraded by enzymes in the CNS.[40] Because of neurotoxicity, the stable, nonenzymatically degraded analogue of SST—octreotide (Sandostatin)—is now being investigated in both animal and human studies. Octreotide is an 8-amino acid analogue with a molecular weight of 1,019 compared with a molecular weight of 1,638 for the 14-amino acid SST. The high molecular weight of these substances makes it unlikely that they could access the CNS after systemic administration.

Pharmacology: Clinical Application

Early work by Chrubasik in 1984 stimulated interest in SST as an alternative intraspinal agent in postoperative and cancer pain treatment.[41–45] This early enthusiasm was tempered by animal studies that revealed a neurotoxic effect of SST on spinal cord neurons, as seen in rat models. Intrathecal administration in rats produced antinociception, hind limb paralysis, and neuronal damage of the spinal cord in a dose-dependent manner.[37] Further studies performed on cats and mice revealed an initial excitatory response, hind leg motor dysfunction, and spinal cord histopathology. Antinociception was only seen in the mice during the period of temporary loss of hind limb motor function.[38] Follow-up primate studies were conducted with continuous infusions of octreotide into the lateral ventricles.[46] These studies found that neurologic function was unaffected, that no abnormal coordination was seen, and that brain tissue histology was within normal limits. Prior to human trials, intrathecal and intraventricular toxicity studies had been conducted at doses up to 40 µg per hour for 51 days in an intrathecal group and up to 207 days in an intraventricular toxicity study.[47] Results of the toxicity studies showed no changes in SMA-18, hematology, urinalysis, neurologic function, or spinal cord and spinal root histology. Six cancer patients with pain unrelieved by oral opioids were subsequently treated with intrathecal octreotide, 5–20 µg per hour, from 13–91 days.[47] Pain relief occurred in patients who had previously not obtained satisfactory pain relief with systemic or intrathecal opioids. Prior intravenous infusions of octreotide in five patients failed to show any analgesic effect. Intraventricular administration of octreotide has reportedly been used to treat pain in five patients with incurable cancer of the cervicofacial region.[48] Treatment involved a single daily bolus from a rechargeable subcutaneous reservoir delivering approximately 20 µg of octreotide. This preliminary report showed excellent analgesia, improvement in performance status, and well-being at much lower doses than reported with intrathecal administration. The utility of intrathecal octreotide in treating neuropathic pain is still undecided, with the limited human studies performed to date.

Complications

Complications relating to neurotoxicity of SST have been discussed (see clinical applications). Octreotide has reportedly produced sedation in both animal and humans.[49] Penn's study specifically questioned patients regarding side effects commonly seen with systemically administered SST, i.e., diarrhea, nausea, and sedation, but found no such occurrence. They did not see changes in blood glucose, blood urea nitrogen, or liver function either. These findings contrast to animal work that earlier had noted significant increases in blood glucose levels.[50] Octreotide infusion has not been shown to suppress the endogenous production of SST.[51]

Local Anesthetics

Physiology: Mechanism of Action

Major textbooks and review articles have presented the established data available on the physiology of local anesthetic (LA) action.[52, 53] Some of the newer understandings of LA action have direct relevance to neuraxial blockade for cancer pain. A summary of current data would emphasize the following information.[53] Conduction blockade by LA occurs through the inhibition of voltage-gated Na^+ channels. Inhibition of the sodium channels by LA occurs through interference with the conformational changes that underlie the activation process. LA inhibition of Na^+ currents increases with repetitive depolarizations in a process called "phasic block." Binding of LA occurs at activated and inactivated Na^+ channels. LAs prevent the conformational changes of activation and have been shown to antagonize the binding of activator agents that keep channels in an activated, open state. The site of LA binding is not precisely known, but binding sites may exist in the pore of the Na^+ channels, at the membrane–protein interface, or within the protein subunits of the channel. It is likely that LA binds to other sites, as well as Na^+ channels, during epidural and spinal anesthesia. Effects on nerve root, spinal cord, and other sites may contribute to the anesthesia and analgesia.

Recent studies on differential axial blockade in epidural and subarachnoid anesthesia have provided new data on mechanisms of action.[54] It appears that the nodes of Ranvier of small myelinated axons are neither more nor less sensitive to block by LA than the nodes of large myelinated axons in the same population. At equilibrium, in a sufficient length of nerve, the concentration of LA required for tonic block appears to be the same for all sizes in a given population. The old theory that fiber size determines sensitivity to LA is giving way to the concept that the number of nodes bathed by LA is the major determinant of clinical differential block among myelinated nerves.

Aside from full conduction blockade, LA has been used clinically for its synergistic analgesic effect when administered with neuraxial opioids. Animal studies have confirmed the synergistic antinociceptive effect of intrathecal morphine with both lidocaine and bupivacaine.[55] The combined effect of the two types of drugs was stronger than their individual effects, thus indicating that the LA potentiated morphine antinociception. Recent studies with dogs have verified a dose-dependent depression of nociceptive reflexes with bupivacaine administration.[56] There was no selectivity on the nociceptive afferent and sympathetic efferent pathways. Fentanyl enhanced spinal anesthesia with bupivacaine in a synergistic manner on the afferent pathway. There was no further inhibitory effect on the efferent sympathetic activity.

Clinical Applications

Anesthetic techniques for the management of cancer pain, including neuraxial blockade, have been well recognized as valuable adjuncts in overall treatment of properly selected patients.[57] The greatest utility appears to be the combination use of LA with opioids for long-term infusion techniques. Hogan described the addition of bupivacaine to epidural morphine infusions in 16 patients.[58] The addition of bupivacaine produced analgesia in ten patients who did not respond to epidural morphine alone. They continued the combination therapy in six of ten cases and had remission of pain in some patients that lasted even after the epidural medications were discontinued. DuPen et al. describes a larger series of 68 patients whose cancer pain became refractory to epidural opioids alone.[59] Sixty-one patients (90%) were considered treatment successes, when LA was added, with a median length of therapy from 60–120 days. This study documents the ability to provide care for these patients at home or in a chronic care facility without the need for rehospitalization. Most patients had little or no sympathetic or sensorimotor impairment,

whereas patients on higher bupivacaine infusions tolerated these side effects with minimal problems. The use of combination opioid and LA has also been applied to intrathecal administration when used for long-term therapy with implanted infusion pumps.[60] Long-term results documenting efficacy for this technique are still lacking.

New modes of LA administration may improve efficacy and provide more potent analgesia than previously possible. Twelve patients were administered an epidural aqueous suspension of N-butyl-*p*-aminobenzoate (BAB), a highly lipid-soluble cogener of benzocaine.[31] These patients had pain that was not controlled by oral and epidural opioids and radiotherapy. Repeated epidural injections of BAB were administered either through an epidural catheter or needle. All patients obtained long-lasting sensory blockade (segmental analgesia) and nine patients were able to be discharged home, where eight of nine died. Postmortem examination failed to demonstrate neurotoxicity although the outer aspect of the dura mater showed signs of focal necrosis. It is thought that long-lasting sensory block (up to 6 months) without motor block is produced by the slow release of BAB, resulting in long-lasting high concentrations in the lipids surrounding the axons of the spinal nerves.

Sustained release of drugs from biopolymer matrixes is now used with levonorgestrel (Norplant) for birth control purposes. Recent animal studies have reported prolonged regional nerve blockade with implants consisting of biocompatible polymer LA matrix that biodegrades at the site of implant.[61] Reversible sensory and motor blockade was produced for 2–6 days. Further histologic studies are being performed.

Summary

Traditional analgesic regimens, even if optimally applied, can be ineffective for controlling severe cancer pain. New research and direct clinical applications of specific spinal analgesic agonists are providing novel approaches to cancer pain management. In the future, specific selective agonists may allow us to provide complete analgesia without the fear of respiratory depression or other serious side effects. Clinical innovation combined with rigorous research will ensure the safe application of new techniques. We should continue to advocate for timely intervention in severe cancer pain and not relegate neuraxial infusions to last ditch efforts.

References

1. World Health Organization. Cancer Pain Relief. Geneva: World Health Organization, 1986.
2. Ventafridda V, Tamburini M, Caraceni A, et al. A validation study of the WHO method for cancer pain relief. Cancer 1987;59:850.
3. American Pain Society. Principles of Analgesic Use in the Treatment of Acute and Cancer Pain. Skokie, IL: American Pain Society, 1992.
4. Fields H. Pain. New York: McGraw-Hill, 1987.
5. Saeki S, Yaksh T. Suppression of nociceptive responses by spinal mu opioid agonists: Effects of stimulus intensity and agonist efficacy. Anesth Analg 1993;77:265.
6. Sosnowski M, Yaksh TL. Spinal administration of receptor-selective drugs as analgesics: New horizons. J Pain Symptom Manage 1990;5:204.
7. Andersen PE, Cohen JI, Everts EC, et al. Intrathecal narcotics for relief of pain from head and neck cancer. Arch Otolaryngol Head Neck Surg 1991;117:1277.
8. Cousins MJ, Cherry DA, Gourlay GK. Acute and Chronic Pain: Use of Spinal Opioids. In MJ Cousins, PO Bridenbaugh (eds), Neural Blockade in Clinical Anesthesia and Management of Pain (2nd ed). Philadelphia: Lippincott, 1988;955.
9. Ferrante MF. Opioids. In MF Ferrante, TR VadeBoncouer (eds), Postoperative Pain Management. New York: Churchill Livingstone, 1993;145.
10. Krames ES. Intrathecal infusional therapies for intractable pain: Patient management guidelines. J Pain Symptom Manage 1993;8:36.
11. Ready LB. Acute Postoperative Pain. In RD Miller (ed), Anesthesia (3rd ed). New York: Churchill Livingstone, 1990;2135.
12. Coyle N, Adelhardt J, Foley KM, Portenoy RK. Character of terminal illness in the advanced cancer patient: Pain and other symptoms during the last four weeks of life. J Pain Symptom Manage 1991;6:408.
13. Arner S, Rawal N, Gustafsson LL. Clinical experience of long-term treatment with epidural and intrathecal opioids: A nationwide survey. Acta Anaesthesiol Scand 1988;32:253.
14. DuPen SL, Peterson DG, Bogosian AC, et al. A new permanent exteriorized epidural catheter for narcotic self-administration to control cancer pain. Cancer 1987;59:986.
15. De Conno F, Caraceni A, Martini C, et al. Hyperalgesia and myoclonus with intrathecal infusion of high-dose morphine. Pain 1991;47:337.
16. Yaksh TL, Harty GJ, Onofrio BM. High doses of spinal morphine produce a nonopiate receptor mediated hyperesthesia: Clinical and theoretic implications. Anesthesiology 1986;64:590.
17. Yaksh TL. Behavioral and autonomic correlates of the tactile evoked allodynia produced by spinal glycine inhibition: Effects of modulatory systems and excitatory amino acids antagonists. Pain 1989;37:111.
18. Abram SE. Advances in chronic pain management since gate control. Reg Anesth 1993;18:66.
19. Yaksh TL. The spinal pharmacology of acutely and chronically administered opioids. J Pain Symptom Manage 1992;7:356.
20. Krames ES, Wilkie DJ, Gershow J. Intrathecal d-Ala^2-d-Leu^5-enkephalin (DADL) restores analgesia in a patient tolerant to intrathecal morphine sulfate. Pain 1986;24:205.
21. Krames ES, Lanning RM, Wilkie J. Does the delta opioid receptor ligand D-ala-D leu-enkephalin restore analgesia in cancer patients unresponsive to mu opioid receptor ligands? Abstract presented at the 11th American Pain Society Meeting, 1992;115.
22. Masters DB, Berde CB, Dutta SK, et al. Prolonged regional nerve blockade by controlled release of local anesthetic from a biodegradable polymer matrix. Anesthesiology 1993;79:340.
23. Lawhead RG, Blaxall HS, Bylund DB. Alpha-2A is the predomonant alpha-2 adrenergic receptor subtype in human spinal cord. Anesthesiology 1992;77:983.
24. Eisenach JC. Overview: First international symposium on alpha$_2$ adrenergic mechanisms of spinal analgesia. Reg Anesth 1993;18:i.
25. Gaumann DM, Brunet PC, Jirounek P. Clonidine enhances the effects of lidocaine on c-fiber action potential. Anesth Analg 1992;74:719.
26. Virtanen R, Savola JM, Sanno U, Nyman L. Characterization of selectivity, specificity and potency of medetomidine as an alpha$_2$ adrenoreceptor agonist. Eur J Pharmacol 1988;150:9.
27. Carabine UA, Milligan KR, Moore J. Extradural clonidine and bupivacaine for postoperative analgesia. Br J Anaesth 1992;68:132.
28. Motsch J, Graber E, Ludwig K. Addition of clonidine enhances postoperative analgesia from epidural morphine: A double-blind study. Anesthesiology 1990;73:1067.
29. Coombs DW, Saunders RL, Fratkin JD, et al. Continuous intrathecal hydromorphone and clonidine for intractable cancer pain. J Neurosurg 1986;64:890.
30. Eisenach JC, Rauck RL, Buzzanell C, Lysak SZ. Epidural clonidine analgesia for intractable cancer pain: Phase I. Anesthesiology 1989;71:647.
31. Arner S, Meyerson BA. Lack of analgesic effect of opioids on neuropathic and idiopathic forms of pain. Pain 1988;33:11.
32. Portenoy RK, Foley KM, Intrussi C. The nature of opioid responsiveness and its implications for neuropathic pain: New hypotheses derived from studies of opioid infusions. Pain 1990;43:273.
33. DuPen S, Eisenach JC, Allin D, Zaccaro D. Epidural clonidine for intractable pain. Reg Anesth 1993;18(Suppl.):23.

34. Coombs DW, Saunders RL, Lachange D, et al. Intrathecal morphine tolerance: Use of intrathecal clonidine,
DADL and intraventricular morphine. Anesthesiology
1985;62:358.
35. van Zweiten PA, Thoolen JMC, Timmermans PBMWM.
The hypotensive activity and side effects of methyldopa,
clonidine and guanfacine. Hypertension 1984;6(Suppl.
II):1128.
36. Gueyenet PG, Cabot JB. Inhibition of sympathetic preganglionic neurons by catecholamines and clonidine:
Mediation by an alpha adrenergic receptor. J Neurosci
1981;1:908.
37. Mollenholt P, Post C, Rawal N, et al. Antinociceptive
and "neurotoxic" actions of somatostatin in rat spinal
cord after intrathecal administration. Pain 1988;32:95.
38. Gaumann DM, Yaksh TL, Post C, et al. Intrathecal somatostatin in cat and mouse studies on pain, motor be-
haviour and histopathology. Anesth Analg 1989;68:623.
39. Chrubasik J. Spinal infusion of opiates and somatostatin. Acta Neurochir Suppl 1987;38:80.
40. Griffiths EC, Jeffcoate SL, Holland DL. Inactivation of
somatostatin by peptidases in different areas of the rat
brain. Acta Endocrinol 1977;85:1.
41. Chrubasik J, Meynadier J, Blond S, et al. Somatostatin:
A potent analgesic. Lancet 1984;II:1208.
42. Ackerman E, Chrubasik J, Weinstock M, Wunsch E.
Effect of intrathecal somatostatin on pain threshold in
rats. Schmerz/Pain/Douleur 1985;6:41.
43. Chrubasik J, Meynadier J, Scherpeel P. Somatostatin
versus morphine in epidural after abdominal operations.
Anesthesiology 1985;63 (Suppl.):237.
44. Chrubasik J, Meynadier J, Scherpeel P, Wunsch E. The
effect of epidural somatostatin on postoperative pain.
Anesth Analg 1985;64:1085.
45. Meynadier J, Chrubasik J, Dubar M, Wunsch E. The effect of epidural somatostatin in two terminally ill patients. Pain 1985;23:9.
46. Devulder J. Is octreotide a safe drug? Pain 1992;51:261.
47. Penn D, Paice JA, Kroin JS. Octreotide: A potent new nonopiate analgesic for intrathecal infusion. Pain 1992;49:13.
48. Candrina R, Galli G. Intraventricular octreotide for cancer pain. J Neurosurg 1992;76:336.
49. Danguir J. Intracerebroventricular infusion of somatostatin selectively increases paradoxical sleep in rats.
Brain 1986;367:26.
50. LeBlanc R, Gauthier S, Gauvin M, et al. Neurobehav-
ioral effects of intrathecal somatostatinergic treatment
in subhuman primates. Neurology 1988;38:1887.
51. Kroin JS, O'Dorisio TM, Penn RD, et al. Distribution
of a somatostatin analog after continuous intraventricular administration. Neurosurgery 1989;24:744.
52. Strichartz GR. Neural Physiology and Local Anesthetic
Action. In MJ Cousins, PO Bridenbaugh (eds), Neural
Blockade in Clinical Anesthesia and Management of
Pain (2nd ed). Philadelphia: Lippincott, 1988;25.
53. Butterworth JF, Strichartz GR. Molecular mechanisms of
local anesthesia: A review. Anesthesiology 1990;72:711.
54. Fink BR. Mechanisms of differential axial blockade in
epidural and subarachnoid anesthesia. Anesthesiology
1989;70:851.
55. Akerman B, Arwestrom E, Post C. Local anesthetics
potentiate spinal morphine antinociception. Anesth
Analg 1988;67:943.
56. Wang C, Chakrabarti MK, Phil M, Whitwam JG. Specific enhancement by fentanyl of the effects of intrathecal bupivacaine on nociceptive afferent but not on
sympathetic efferent pathways in dogs. Anesthesiology
1993;79:766.
57. Ferrer-Brechner T. Anesthetic techniques for the management of cancer pain. Cancer 1989;63:2343.
58. Hogan Q, Haddox JD, Abram S, et al. Epidural opiates
and local anesthetics for the management of cancer
pain. Pain 1991;46:271.
59. DuPen SL, Kharasch ED, Williams A, et al. Chronic
epidural bupivacaine-opioid infusion in intractable cancer pain. Pain 1992;49:293.
60. Krames ES. Intrathecal infusional therapies for intractable pain: Patient management guidelines. J Pain
Symptom Manage 1993;8:36.
61. Korsten HHM, Ackerman EW, Grouls RJE, et al. Long-
lasting epidural sensory blockade by n-butyl-p-
aminobenzoate in the terminally ill intractable cancer
pain patient. Anesthesiology 1991;75:950.

Chapter 16

Stereotactic Techniques

Sri Kantha

Radiofrequency current heat techniques for selective destruction of nervous tissue have been shown to be effective in interrupting nociceptive pathways. The use of radiofrequency current to produce therapeutic lesions has gained widespread acceptance for human stereotactic surgery. In 1968, Letcher and Goldberg[1] demonstrated in vitro the effects of radiofrequency current and heat on the peripheral nerve action potentials of smaller delta and C fibers before those of the alpha and beta fibers. The demonstration by these investigators formed the neurophysiologic basis for the therapeutic use of radiofrequency current lesions.

The history of radiofrequency energy dates back to the early 1900s. In the mid-1920s, Harvey and Cushing conducted basic research using the potential of radiofrequency power for electrosurgery.[2] In the 1950s, radiofrequency power was used to create lesions in the central nervous system. Electrodes were then developed that enabled accurate temperature monitoring, thus making the techniques more refined and safer. The thermocouple electrodes are small and accurate in measuring electrode tip temperature and impedance, and in generating radiofrequency heat.

The basic principle of radiofrequency lesions involves placement of a fine insulated electrode shaft with an uninsulated tip into the nervous tissue. If an electrical generator source is connected to this shaft, the electrical impedance of the surrounding tissue allows current to flow from the generator source into the tissue itself.[2] When current flows through the source of resistance, heat is generated as a result of that resistance.[3] When the electrode current flows through the tissue, heat is generated in the tissue itself and not the electrode tip. The tip of the electrode lies in the heated tissue, and hence absorbs heat from the tissue and eventually achieves thermal equilibrium with the entire system. At equilibrium, the temperature at the probe tip will become equal to the hottest part of the heated tissue, because the current spreads into the tissue as it leaves the tip of the electrode. As a result, the greatest density of the current will be adjacent to the tip of the electrode, and the hottest part of the lesion will be in the adjacent tissue.[3] The lesion can be controlled accurately because the size of the lesion depends on the temperature of the lesion, and the cannula tip temperature is accurately measured with thermocouple electrodes. To avoid undesirable responses, a frequency higher than 250 kc per second is used. The lesion generators currently available in the market use 500 kc per second. This frequency range allows more uniform and better circumscribed lesions. The most satisfactory way to control lesion size is to maintain a constant electrode tip temperature for 1–2 seconds.[3]

Modern radiofrequency lesion generators include the Radionics Models RFG-3B and RFG-3C (Radionics, Burlington, MA), the OWL (Diros Technology Inc., Toronto), and the F.L. Fischer N50 (Leibinger & Fischer, Irving, TX). These generators all have built-in stimulation and impedance units, in addition to generating controlled lesions via Teflon-coated needles that have exposed active tips of varying sizes to generate lesions of varying sizes.

The cannula used for radiofrequency current lesioning comes in various lengths and diameters. The thermocouple electrode is inserted through the cannula for stimulation to identify the nerve or dorsal root ganglion, followed by thermocoagulation. Then, a radiocontrast dye (preferably a water-soluble, non-ionic one) is injected into the epidural space or root sleeve to outline the dura and dorsal root ganglion. The use of dye improves the accuracy of the lesioning and thus increases safety.

Radiofrequency current for therapeutic lesions offers an important component in the management of intractable pain of both benign and malignant conditions. However, as with any surgical technique, patients must be carefully selected so that the technique performed is appropriate and therapeutically effective for the underlying pathology. In certain chronic, benign pain syndromes, destructive lesions by radiofrequency current should not be considered until conservative management has been tried and failed. Conservative management for an extended period can lead to a chronic pain state that may be refractory to interventional treatment. In chronic malignant pain syndromes, radiofrequency current therapeutic lesions may be the first line of treatment, in view of limited life expectancy and because subsequent neurologic deficits, if they occur, are better tolerated by those patients. A superior quality of life can be enjoyed by the patient, in contrast to some of the complications of currently available modalities for chronic malignant pain syndromes.

To be performed accurately and safely, clinical application of radiofrequency current lesions requires that the operator have adequate skill and a satisfactory knowledge of basic techniques in the use of the radiofrequency current lesion generator machine, and the physician must have a good knowledge of the use of radiographic fluoroscopy and an understanding of the three-dimensional anatomy of the skull and spine.

Stereotactic coagulation is used to perform dorsal root entry zone lesions, rhizotomy, percutaneous anterolateral cordotomy, gasserian ganglion selective thermocoagulation, dorsal root ganglion selective thermocoagulation of spinal nerves, hypophysectomy, mesencephalic spinothalamic tractotomy, and medial thalamotomy.

The most frequently performed procedures are shown in the following list, ranked according to frequency:

1. Dorsal root ganglion selective thermoregulation of spinal nerves and trigeminal nerve for somatic pain.
2. Thoracic and lumbar sympathectomy for visceral pain, causalgia, reflex sympathetic dystrophy secondary to cancer-causing sympathetic nervous system imbalance, and for radiation neuritis.
3. Percutaneous anterolateral cordotomy at the cervical level.

Procedures performed at the first sensory neuron level (i.e., the dorsal root ganglion selective thermocoagulation) are safe and have few neurologic deficits. Procedures performed at the second sensory neuron level (i.e., anterolateral cordotomy) do carry risk of neurologic deficits, including bowel and bladder incontinence and motor weakness. These deficits, however, can be minimized with expertise and careful monitoring during the procedure. Procedures at the third sensory neuron level (i.e., stereotactic hypophysectomy, mesencephalic spinothalamic tractotomy, medial thalamotomy) are infrequently performed and have much greater risks.

Percutaneous radiofrequency lesion of the dorsal root ganglion for the relief of pain was first described by Uematsu et al.[4] and Sluijter and Mehta.[5] Similar lesions of the gasserian ganglion are now standard treatment for the relief of trigeminal neuralgia.

Radiofrequency current heat techniques for destruction of nervous tissue have been shown to be the most effective in interrupting nociceptive pathways. Advantages of radiofrequency lesion techniques include the following items:

1. The lesion size can be effectively controlled.
2. Good monitoring of the lesion temperature can be performed with a thermocouple electrode.
3. Placement of the electrode is facilitated with electrical stimulation and impedance monitoring.
4. Most radiofrequency lesions can be performed under monitored anesthetic care (intravenous sedation with monitoring).
5. When properly performed, there is low incidence of morbidity and mortality.
6. The procedure can be repeated if needed.
7. Most procedures can be performed percutaneously.

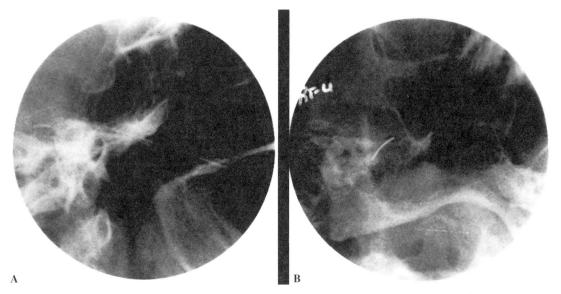

Figure 16-1. Trigeminal ganglion thermocoagulation. A. Note cannula positioned in the foramen ovale in the midpoint for second division of trigeminal nerve seen in submentovertex view. B. Cannula in the angle of clivus and petrous bone in lateral projection.

Head and Neck Pain

Pain caused by cancer is rarely confined to the distribution of the trigeminal nerve, and nearly always involves the distribution of upper cervical and lower cranial nerves. If the distribution of the trigeminal nerve is affected by cancer and severe pain follows, it is appropriate to use selective thermocoagulation of trigeminal ganglion to treat that pain syndrome.

Trigeminal ganglion selective thermocoagulation by stereotactic technique involves placing the patient in the supine position on the operating table (Figure 16-1). The C-arm fluoroscope is positioned to get a submentovertex view. With this view, the foramen ovale is visualized. A short-acting induction agent, e.g., propofol, is given intravenously. A 22-gauge, 100-mm long, Teflon-coated radiofrequency lesioning needle with a 5-mm active tip is advanced until it enters the foramen ovale. For the first division of the gasserian ganglion, the medial aspect of the foramen ovale is entered and the depth of entry is guided in a lateral projection. Once the ideal depth of the needle entry is identified in a lateral projection, stimulation is performed and needle position is further confirmed. The second division of the ganglion is entered by directing the needle to

the midpoint of the foramen ovale and again the depth is confirmed in a lateral projection. For the third division, the needle is directed to the lateral aspect of the foramen ovale and the depth guided in a lateral projection. The first division requires more depth of entry via the foramen ovale and the third division needs the least depth of entry.

In a lateral projection, the needle is advanced to the junction of the clivus and petrous bone. Free flow of cerebrospinal fluid (CSF) indicates that either the needle is in the ganglion or in the preganglionic area. This needle placement achieves better results and minimizes the chances of anesthesia dolorosa. The stylet of the needle is removed and a thermocouple probe is inserted. Stimulation is performed at 50–75 Hz and the division of the trigeminal nerve is then identified. At this point, the patient will have recovered enough from the anesthetic effects to be able to identify the stimulation and its effects. Both motor and sensory stimulation are performed so that the patient does not get any weakness of muscles of mastication. This is performed by measuring the ratio of the motor to sensory stimulation threshold. Once confirmed, thermocoagulation by radiofrequency current lesioning is performed. Before thermocoagulation,

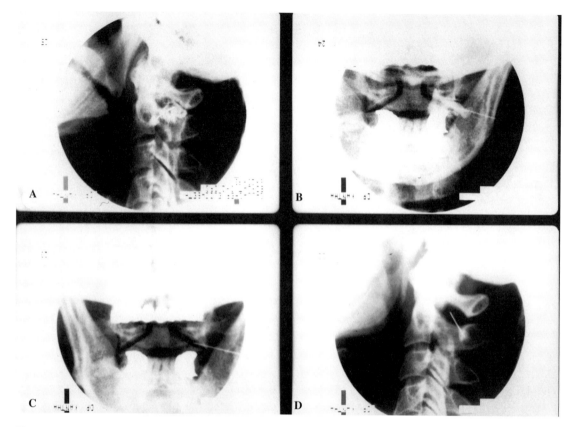

Figure 16-2. Radiofrequency cannula position for second cervical nerve dorsal root ganglion selective thermocoagulation. A. Cannula position in lateral projection of C-1 to C-2 interspace. B. Cannula position in open-mouth view. C. Cannula position after radiocontrast material is injected. D. Note radiocontrast material outlining the dura and dorsal root ganglion area in an open-mouth view.

the patient is given a brief, general anesthetic. The most commonly involved site is the mandible, and hence the mandibular division of the gasserian ganglion is the branch most commonly treated by selective thermocoagulation. Thermocoagulation should be performed in the dorsal root ganglion, the trigeminal ganglion, to prevent anesthesia dolorosa and to achieve permanent pain relief.

Involvement of a malignant lesion in the neck area including the occiput may produce pain in the neck, in addition to occipital headache and retro-orbital pain. The occipital headache may be relieved by performing radiofrequency current lesioning of the second cervical nerve dorsal root ganglion. This procedure is performed by inserting a 22-gauge, 100-mm long radiofrequency lesioning needle with a 5-mm active tip in a lateral position of the head and neck toward the interver-

tebral foramen of the first and second cervical vertebrae. The needle tip is inserted until it enters the dorsal root ganglion area, which is situated approximately halfway across the facet joint line of first and second cervical vertebrae (Figure 16-2). Correct placement is confirmed in an open-mouth fluoroscopic view projection. Radiocontrast material is injected to outline the dura and the dorsal root ganglion. During stimulation, the patient should sense paresthesia in the occiput radiating to the vertex. At this time, after confirming the placement of the needle, either the site is anesthetized with local anesthetic (1% lidocaine) and thermocoagulated, or the patient may be administered a brief general anesthesia and thermocoagulated. The author prefers giving a brief general anesthetic to avoid needle displacement while injecting the local anesthetic.

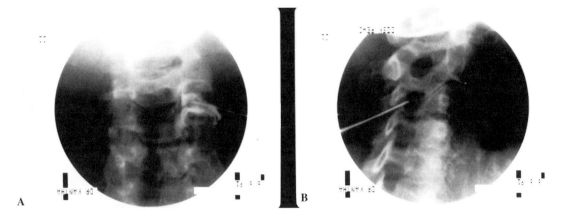

Figure 16-3. Fourth cervical nerve dorsal root ganglion selective thermocoagulation. A. Note cannula positioned in the posterior border of C-3 to C-4 intervertebral foramen and slightly caudad in oblique view. B. Cannula in place in the dorsal root ganglion outlined by dye. Dura and root sleeve are seen in the anteroposterior view.

The presence of cancer in the neck (which affects the third cervical nerve) causes pain in the suboccipital, posterior auricular, and submandibular areas, in addition to earache. In order to perform radiofrequency lesioning of the third cervical nerve dorsal root ganglion, the patient is placed supine. An oblique projection of the cervical spine is obtained using fluoroscopy. This projection will illustrate the intervertebral foramen of the second and third vertebral body. The radiofrequency lesioning cannula (22-gauge, 100-mm long with 5-mm active tip) is advanced until it approaches the dorsal and inferior aspect of the intervertebral foramen (Figure 16-3). The cannula is then further advanced in an anteroposterior direction until it enters midpoint of the facet joint. Radiocontrast material is then injected and the dura and the dorsal root ganglion are outlined. Stimulation is then performed at 50 Hz, and the patient senses paresthesia in the auricular, posterior auricular, and submandibular areas. Stimulation is performed at 2 Hz and motor fasciculation should be noted in the submandibular area and upper neck. Ideally, the motor fasciculation should be twice the voltage needed for sensory stimulation. This indicates that the cannula tip is far enough away from the motor portion of the dorsal root ganglion. Once these criteria are met and adequate dissociation between the sensory and motor supply has been demonstrated, the patient is given a brief general anesthetic and the ganglion is thermocoagulated.

A higher temperature is used in cancer pain patients than in patients with chronic benign pain. This temperature could range from 67–80°C. Cancer patients usually tolerate deafferentation pain and resultant neurologic deficits better than patients with benign pain. The duration of lesioning is approximately 120 seconds. Following the lesioning, steroids, methylprednisolone, or triamcinolone is injected locally to reduce postprocedure neuritis. The goal of thermocoagulation is to relieve the pain but also to preserve proprioception, touch, and motor function. This is achieved if meticulous detail to performing the correct technique is maintained. Patients may experience increased pain for days to a few weeks following thermocoagulation before significant relief is obtained. Patients should be warned about the increase in pain. This increase can be treated with repeated infiltration of steroids and local anesthetics at weekly intervals or with orally administered clonazepam. If severe dysesthesia is experienced, then anticonvulsants such as carbamazepine or dilantin may be used on a short-term basis.

For pain originating from the fourth to seventh cervical nerves, a similar approach, selective thermocoagulation, is used as outlined previously for the third cervical nerve dorsal root ganglion. Seventh cervical nerve dorsal root ganglion could present technical difficulties in entering the foramen. Caution should be exercised to avoid the vertebral artery, which, if inadvertently entered, can dislodge atheromatous plaque causing major neurologic complications. Stimulation parameters are similar to those for the third nerve dorsal root ganglion. Ideally, 0.4–0.8 V at 50 Hz gives paresthesia if properly positioned in the dorsal aspect of the dorsal root ganglion; motor fasciculation is noted at 1.2–1.5 V. It is desirable to administer a brief general anesthetic once needle placement is attained. However, it is important to be careful because injection of local anesthetic may displace the already correctly positioned needle, and even a millimeter shift of the needle may alter the outcome. Dorsal root ganglion lesion of the eighth cervical nerve should be avoided because of technical difficulties in entering the foramen. In addition, neurologic complications such as weakness of the small muscles of the hand may occur.

Thoracic Pain

Pain in the thoracic area originating in the chest wall, ribs, and parietal pleura is treated by selective thermocoagulation of dorsal root ganglion of the corresponding thoracic nerves. The first thoracic nerve and, in some cases, the second thoracic nerve dorsal root ganglion is thermocoagulated for involvement of the upper extremity with cancer. A modified technique is used to enter the dorsal root ganglion of the thoracic nerves to include the first thoracic nerve. The classic dorsolateral approach is hindered by the shape of the vertebra and by the proximity of the pleura. Therefore, the author prefers a dorsal approach through a drill hole made in the infrapedicle area of the corresponding vertebra. This procedure is accomplished using a 0.062-inch diameter Kirschner wire and a pneumatic drill. A lightweight pneumatic drill is preferable and provides good control while drilling. Continuous fluoroscopy is advised while the burr hole is made, and a crispy clear image on fluoroscopy helps avoid inadvertent entry of the wire into the intrathecal space, thus avoiding injury to the spinal cord. The wire is introduced percutaneously through a 12-gauge cannula until it contacts the infrapedicle area of the vertebra. The wire is connected to a pneumatic drill and a drill hole made in the infrapedicle area of the vertebral body. The wire is then guided in a lateral projection under fluoroscopy until it enters the intervertebral foramen. A "give in" sensa-

tion is felt when the wire enters the intervertebral foramen. Once the intervertebral foramen is entered, the wire is removed and a 20-gauge, 15-cm long radiofrequency lesioning needle with a 5-mm active tip is introduced. A nonionic dye is injected to outline the dura and the dorsal root ganglion area. It is preferable to outline the dura before performing thermocoagulation. This technique is used for all of the thoracic nerves so as to alleviate cancer pain, including pain due to metastases in the ribs, chest wall, and parietal pleura.

If the lung or visceral pleura is involved, the sympathetic nervous system is involved in conducting the nociceptive impulses. Stereotactic thoracic sympathectomy can then be performed to alleviate symptoms including deep-seated burning and boring pain of the chest, upper extremities, head, and neck.

Stereotactic percutaneous thermocoagulation of the upper thoracic sympathetic ganglia is a useful alternative treatment to open thoracic sympathectomy. This is performed at the T-2 to T-3 ganglia (Figure 16-4). As a result, major surgical complications associated with open surgical sympathectomy, such as pneumothorax, Horner's syndrome, intercostal artery bleeding, gustatory phenomena, and paravertebral muscle atrophy can be avoided. Pneumothorax occurs in approximately 5–10% of cases. Although this complication resolves spontaneously, the patient is nevertheless admitted overnight for observation and a check of chest radiographs. Postsympathectomy neuralgia may occur in a few cases due to thermal injury and inflammation of the intercostal nerves while inserting the needles. This neuralgia resolves spontaneously in 4–6 weeks.

The procedure involves performing a diagnostic stellate ganglion injection with 0.5% preservative-free lidocaine under fluoroscopy. The stellate ganglion is outlined using a radiocontrast dye to confirm that the injected solution is in the prevertebral fascial region and that it is not flooding the brachial plexus, thus giving a false-positive result. If symptoms resolve with the diagnostic procedure, thoracic sympathectomy will help alleviate the pain.

The procedure is performed with the patient in the prone position under local anesthesia and intravenous sedation. A 20-gauge, 15-cm long radiofrequency lesioning needle with a 10-mm active tip is inserted under direct fluoroscopy. The needle is inserted in a slightly oblique projection to the mid- to anterolateral aspect of the second and third thoracic

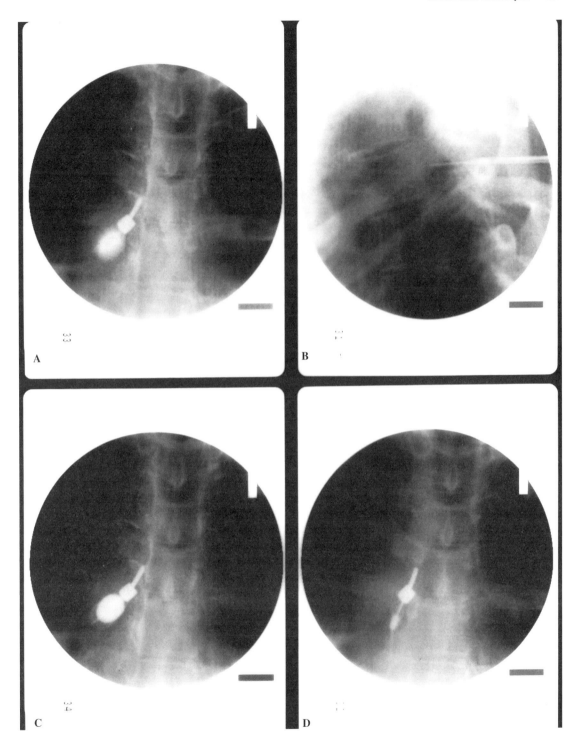

Figure 16-4. Dorsal root ganglion selective thermocoagulation of thoracic nerves. A. Twelve-gauge guide cannula in contact with dorsal surface of the vertebral body just below the pedicle. Radiocontrast dye outlines the dura. B. Lateral projection showing radiofrequency lesioning cannula in the intervertebral foramen. C, D. Thermocouple probe in place for thermocoagulation.

vertebral bodies for head, neck, and upper extremity and upper chest pain. The depth of needle insertion is guided in a lateral projection. The sympathetic chain is thermocoagulated at three sites: (1) cephalad, (2) next to the midpoint, and (3) the caudad aspect of the vertebral body. The temperature required for each site is 80°C for 120 seconds. It is preferable to perform two lesions at each level, a few millimeters apart in depth. A total of six lesions are made for each vertebral level.

Sympathetic nervous system pain involving the lower chest area is treated in a similar manner in the lower thoracic sympathetic chain.

Abdominal Pain

Pain originating from the lower abdominal viscera including descending colon, sigmoid colon, rectum, uterus, ovaries, and fallopian tubes is amenable to lumbar sympathectomy using the stereotactic technique. Pelvic pain also responds to hypogastric plexus thermocoagulation in conjunction with a lumbar sympathectomy.

In many cancer pain syndromes that involve lower abdominal viscera, pelvic viscera, and lower extremities, radiofrequency current percutaneous lumbar sympathectomy can permanently interrupt the lumbar sympathetic chain. This procedure involves less morbidity than open surgical techniques. In addition because of its relatively few complications, it is also considered less invasive than chemical interruption of the sympathetic pathways.

A thorough knowledge of the anatomy and physiology of the sympathetic nervous system is helpful in avoiding intrathecal entry of the needles, puncture of the aorta, inferior vena cava, ureters, somatic nerves of the lumbar plexus (e.g., the genitofemoral nerve), and lower abdominal viscera.

A diagnostic lumbar sympathetic ganglion blockade using a 0.5% preservative-free lidocaine should provide convincing evidence that sympathetic interruption may effectively improve the patient's symptoms. Without premedication, the patient is placed prone on a radiolucent radiographic table with a foam wedge under the lower abdomen. A single injection of 15 ml of 0.5% lidocaine is made at a point just anterior to the psoas fascia at the level of the third or fourth lumbar vertebra. Needle position is confirmed by injecting water-soluble contrast material followed by imaging in anteroposterior, oblique, and lateral planes. If the needle is in the proper fascial plane, the local anesthetic solution will spread linearly cephalad and caudad to involve the entire sympathetic chain on the injected side. If the patient's pain is satisfactorily controlled, permanent sympathectomy by radiofrequency lesioning is undertaken.

Thermocoagulation of the sympathetic chain is undertaken at the second through fifth lumbar vertebral bodies (Figure 16-5). The needle used for the procedure is a 20-gauge, 15-cm long, Teflon-coated cannula with a 10-mm active tip that will accommodate a thermocouple electrode. The percutaneous insertion of the needle should be performed using a very short-acting intravenous anesthetic (rather than local anesthetic infiltration). Subsequently, the thermocoagulation of the sympathetic chain is done under mild sedation. This will enable the patient to report any unusual or undesirable paresthesia that may occur during thermocoagulation. The patient experiences minimal discomfort during the thermocoagulation of the sympathetic chain, unless any contact is made with the somatic nerves.

The patient is placed in prone position with a foam wedge under the mid and lower abdomen so as to straighten the lumbar lordotic curve. The second to fifth vertebral bodies are identified in an oblique projection for needle entry. Once contact is made with the anterolateral aspect of the vertebral bodies, radiocontrast material is injected to outline the sympathetic chain. Ideally, the spread in a lateral projection will be linear, covering the anterior one-third of the vertebral bodies. In an anteroposterior projection, the dye will spread linearly in a cephalocaudad direction. Electrostimulation is performed to test and exclude proximity to somatic nerves. The sympathetic ganglia are then thermocoagulated at 80°C for 120 seconds with two sites at each level a few millimeters apart in depth.

The advantage of sympathetic chain thermocoagulation over surgical sympathectomy is that symptoms are ameliorated without the associated risks. Surgical sympathectomy and anesthesia may require 6–10 days of hospitalization. The procedure can be repeated with minimal morbidity, and anatomic landmarks are not lost for repeat procedures. The duration of the pain relief is comparable to surgical sympathectomy. Its advantages over chemical sympathectomy are that (1) the radiofrequency proce-

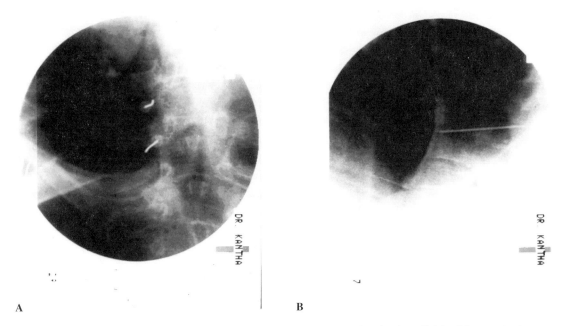

Figure 16-5. Thoracic sympathectomy at the T-2 to T-3 level. A. Anteroposterior view in a slightly oblique projection showing cannula entry sites at the T-2 to T-3 level. B. Lateral projection showing final position of needles.

dure obviates spread of neurolytic solution to the genitofemoral nerve causing neuritis, and (2) neurolytic solutions can backtrack along the communicating ramus and thus create neuritis of the third lumbar nerve, causing pain, numbness, and dysesthesia in the knee area. The neurolytic solution may also enter the dural cuff and cause weakness of lower extremities or even paraplegia. Infrequently, ureteral strictures and hypotension can also occur.

Pain in the pelvic viscera due to cancer may be in some instances treated with hypogastric plexus thermocoagulation. The plexus is approached by using 20-gauge, 15-cm long, Teflon-coated needles with a 10-mm active tip. Two needles are advanced on either side of fifth lumbar or first sacral vertebral body to about 1 cm anterior to the anterior border. Radiocontrast material is injected to outline the hypogastric plexus area followed by thermocoagulation at 80°C for 120 seconds.

Lumbar Pain

Cancer pain involving the lumbar dermatomes is treated by inserting a radiofrequency needle probe percutaneously under fluoroscopy. The needle entry site is determined by obtaining an oblique projection of the intervertebral foramen (Figure 16-6). The needle is aimed just inferior to the superior pedicle as it bounds the foramen and is advanced to enter the foramen at the same level with the medial border of the pedicle. In a lateral projection the needle tip is ideally situated in the posterior one-third of the intervertebral foramen. Once the radiocontrast dye is injected, the dura, dorsal root ganglion, and nerve root sleeve are visible. At this point, ganglion stimulation is performed at motor and sensory thresholds and the needle is further adjusted until paresthesia is obtained at approximately 0.5–0.8 V and motor stimulation at approximately 1.2–1.5 V, respectively. If more than three nerves are involved in covering the painful cancerous site, it is better to use alternative techniques such as intrathecal morphine infusion via pumps or percutaneous anterolateral cordotomy by stereotactic technique.

When it is necessary to thermocoagulate the dorsal root ganglion of the fifth lumbar nerve, a modified technique of the previously described procedure is implemented (Figure 16-7). This is due to the difficulty in negotiating entry to the dorsal as-

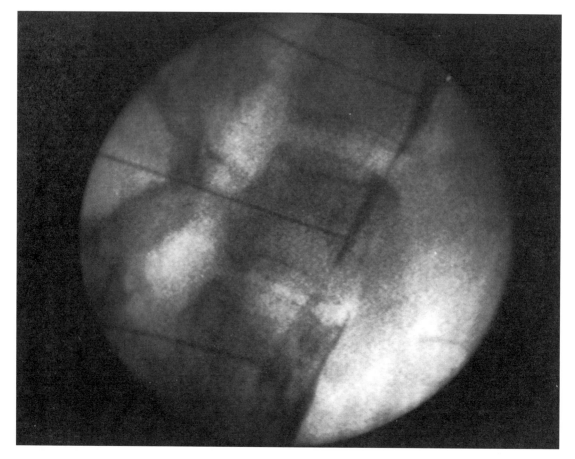

Figure 16-6. Final position of electrodes in a lateral view. Note the linear spread of the contrast medium along the antero-lateral aspect of the vertebral bodies outlining the sympathetic chain.

pect of the dorsal root ganglion of the nerve via the intervertebral foramen using the straight cannula. A 12-gauge trochar and cannula is advanced until it makes contact with the dorsal surface of the fifth vertebral body just below the pedicle. The projection of the cannula is confirmed using lateral fluoroscopy. A 0.062-inch diameter Kirschner wire is introduced using a lightweight pneumatic drill. A burr hole is made until the wire enters the dorsal aspect of the intervertebral foramen. Care is taken while drilling to sense the "give in" sensation. You should stop at this point to avoid injury to the nervous tissue by the wire. The wire is then replaced with a 20-gauge, 15-cm long, Teflon-coated radiofrequency lesioning needle with a 5-mm active tip. Once the radiocontrast dye has been injected, the dura and dorsal root ganglion are visible. Then, stimulation is performed in the motor and sensor

threshold and the dorsal aspect of the dorsal root ganglion is identified and thermocoagulated.

Sacral Pain

Cancer pain involving the sacral somatic dermatomes may be controlled by selective thermocoagulation of the corresponding sacral nerves. The dorsal root ganglia of the sacral nerves are covered by the dorsal plate of the sacral bone. It is therefore not possible to obtain a satisfactory electrode position through the sacral foramina. The electrode may end up either peripheral to the ganglion (thus causing deafferentation pain) or anterior to the ganglion (causing motor weakness). The same technique as suggested for the fifth lumbar nerve dorsal root ganglion entry is recommended for thermocoagulation

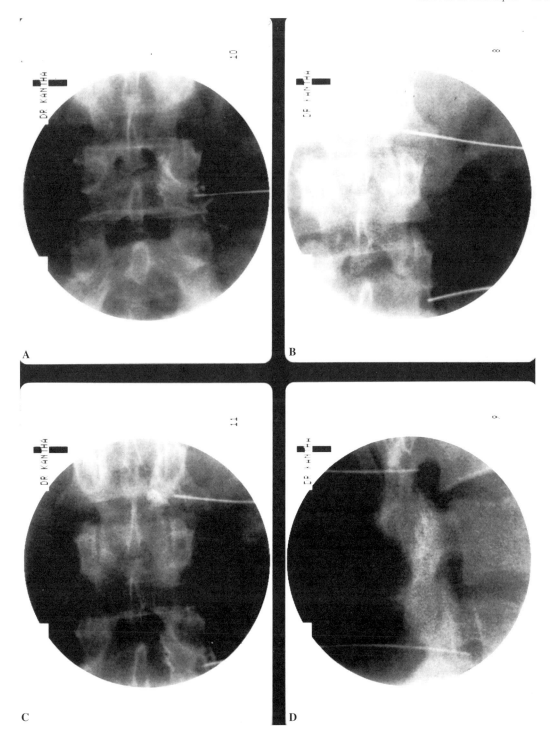

Figure 16-7. Electrode position during selective dorsal root ganglion thermocoagulation of L-2 and L-4 nerves. A. Anteroposterior view. B. Lateral view. C. Anteroposterior view. D. Lateral view.

of the sacral ganglia (Figure 16-8). The burr hole is made through the dorsal layer of the sacrum.

The dorsal root ganglion of the first sacral nerve is situated midway between the first sacral foramen and the superior border of the sacral bone, along the course of the nerve (Figure 16-9). The second sacral nerve dorsal root ganglion is situated midway between the first and second sacral foramina. The third sacral nerve dorsal root ganglion is situated in the upper border of the second sacral foramen. The fourth and fifth sacral nerve dorsal root ganglion is situated at the level of the second sacral foramen.

The coccygeal nerve is approached through the sacrococcygeal hiatus (the nerve outlined with radiocontrast dye) and thermocoagulated. Pain caused by malignant tumors in the pelvic area usually involves the third and fourth sacral nerves, and thus bilateral sacral dorsal root ganglia thermocoagulation is recommended.

Percutaneous Anterolateral Cordotomy

Interruption of the anterolateral spinothalamic tract by radiofrequency current thermocoagulation in the cervical spinal cord is a useful way to control many types of cancer pain. This technique was first described in 1963 by Mullan et al.[6] In 1965, Rosomoff et al[7] described a technique of radiofrequency lesioning at the second cervical vertebral level cordotomy using a lateral approach via the C-1 to C-2 interspace. The technique is used to treat unilateral cancer pain that involves multiple dermatomes. It is also possible to perform this procedure bilaterally if 4–6 weeks are allowed between procedures. Appropriate pulmonary function tests are recommended between procedures and in all patients with compromised respiratory functions.

The technique involves placing the patient in the supine position on the operating table, with the head immobilized by forehead cushions of a head holder. The C-arm fluoroscopy is arranged for lateral viewing. The C-1 to C-2 interspace is identified. The skin is infiltrated with 2% lidocaine at the needle entry site. Levin's cordotomy kit is recommended for this procedure. A 20-gauge, 3.5-inch spinal needle is introduced until the dura is punctured and a free flow of CSF is obtained (Figure 16-10). Three milliliters of lipiodol, oil-based contrast, is mixed with 7 ml of normal saline and 7–10 ml of air, and the mixture is emulsified in a 20-ml syringe. About 1–2 ml of this emulsion is injected rapidly so as to outline the anterior border of the spinal cord, dentate ligament, and posterior dura. A second needle, with the electrode presized by passing it through and adjusting the sizing clamp to allow for complete exposure of the noninsulated tip, is now introduced. The needle is introduced just anterior to the dentate ligament. The needle is checked in an anteroposterior projection under fluoroscopy, ideally in an open-mouth view. The thermocouple electrode is then passed through the spinal needle. An impedance monitor is then used to sense spinal cord penetration. Characteristically, impedance is 300–500 Ω when the thermocouple electrode is in the CSF and at 800–1200 Ω when it enters the spinal cord. A low- to high-frequency change of sound is audible when the monitoring probe enters the spinal cord. Final position of the electrode is determined by electrical stimulation at 75 Hz and 0.1–0.2 V. This produces paresthesia in the opposite side of the body to include the affected dermatomes. The patient may experience several other types of sensations in addition to paresthesia. These sensations include a feeling of warmness or cold blowing on the opposite side of the body. This indicates that the electrode tip is in the anterolateral spinothalamic tract. A thermal stimulation in the opposite side of the body, irrespective of paresthesia, indicates good electrode position and thermocoagulation may be performed. It is advisable to check for motor stimulation after the final electrode position is confirmed at 2 Hz and 1.0 V. No fasciculations in the opposite side of the body are a good indication that the electrode tip is in the anterolateral spinothalamic tract. Thermal lesioning is then performed at 90°C for 10 seconds. The temperature and pinprick sensation of the parts affected by cancer are checked at this time and, if inadequate, repeat thermocoagulation is performed again at 90°C for 10 seconds. The patient should be awake and alert during the procedure with the extremities of the opposite side voluntarily elevated during the thermocoagulation. If, during this period, any weakness is experienced as evidenced by sagging of the limbs, the procedure should be immediately discontinued.

Most patients with cancer pain who have had a percutaneous anterolateral cordotomy receive good quality pain relief. This procedure is recommended as the first line of treatment for progressive and ad-

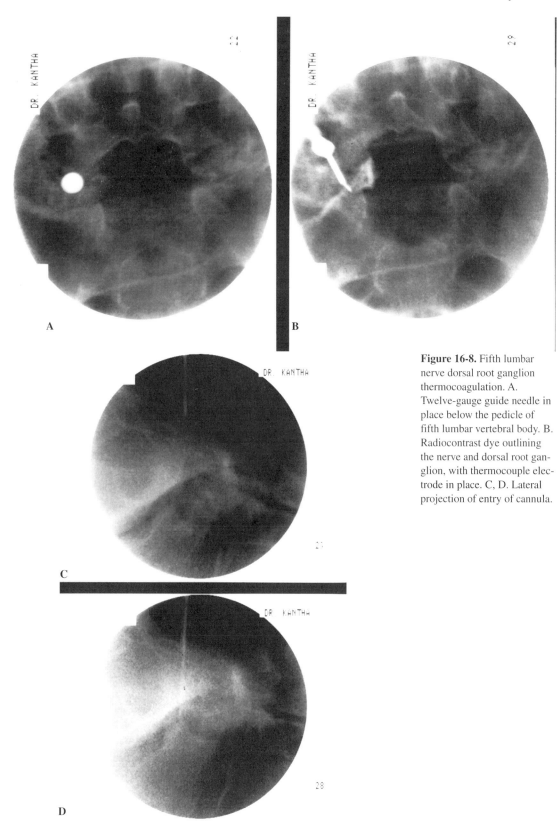

Figure 16-8. Fifth lumbar nerve dorsal root ganglion thermocoagulation. A. Twelve-gauge guide needle in place below the pedicle of fifth lumbar vertebral body. B. Radiocontrast dye outlining the nerve and dorsal root ganglion, with thermocouple electrode in place. C, D. Lateral projection of entry of cannula.

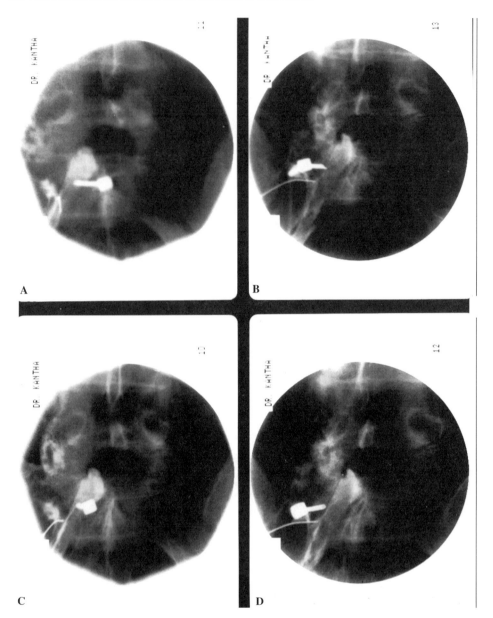

Figure 16-9. Position of the Kirschner wire during first sacral nerve dorsal root ganglion selective thermocoagulation. A. Anteroposterior view. B, C. Oblique views from symmetrical positions. D. Thermocouple probe in place.

vanced cancer affecting multiple dermatomes, including the lungs. An improved quality of life is achieved for the lifetime of the patient compared with other modalities currently available for that kind of patient. It is certainly far superior to heavy narcotic intake, which may produce unacceptable sedation and lead to poor quality of life.

Stereotactic radiofrequency, current-selective thermocoagulation to produce permanent interruption of nociceptive pathways offers an important component in the management of intractable pain of cancer. It can maintain a satisfactory quality of life for the relatively limited life span of afflicted cancer patients.

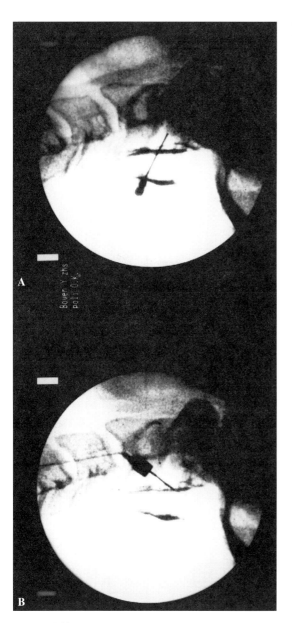

Figure 16-10. Anterolateral spinothalamic cordotomy (lateral view). A. The first needle in the intrathecal space after injecting the radiocontrast dye, lipiodol. B. The second needle with thermocouple electrode placed just above the dentate ligament. Note that lipiodol outlines the anterior surface of the spinal cord, dentate ligament, and posterior dura.

References

1. Letcher FS, Goldberg S. The effect of radiofrequency current and heat on peripheral nerve action potential in the cat. J Neurosurg 1968;29:42.
2. Cosman ER, Cosman BJ. Methods of Making Nervous System Lesions. In RH Wilkins, SS Rengachary (eds), Neurosurgery. New York: McGraw-Hill, 1984;2490.
3. Cosman ER, Nashold BS, Bendenbangh, P. Stereotactic and functional neurosurgery. Proc Soc Appl Neurophysiol 1983;46:160.
4. Uematsu S, Udvarhely GB, Benson DW, Siebens AA. Percutaneous radiofrequency rhizotomy. Surg Neurol 1974;2:319.
5. Sluijter ME, Mehta M. Treatment of Chronic Neck and Back Pain by Percutaneous Thermal Lesions. In S Lipton, J Miles (eds), Persistent Pain: Modern Methods of Treatment (Vol. 3). London: Academic Press, 1981;141.
6. Mullan S, Harper PV, Hekmatpanah J, et al. Percutaneous interruption of spinal-pain tracts by means of a strontium[90] needle. J Neurosurg 1963;20:931.
7. Rosomoff HL, Carroll F, Brown J, et al. Percutaneous radiofrequency cervical cordotomy: Technique. J Neurosurg 1965;23:639.

Chapter 17

Intraventricular Morphine: When, How, and Why?

Jacques Meynadier, Serge Blond, Jean-Claude Willer, and Daniel Le Bars

Treatments for pain have made considerable progress recently, not only because our knowledge of pain mechanisms has increased, but also because the entire medical staff (doctors, nurses, etc.) have become more aware that pain is not a necessary condition. The World Health Organization (WHO) has provided three simple steps for the relief of cancer pain. Their strategy advocates an initial administration of nonopioid analgesics (step 1), then weak opioid analgesics (step 2), and, only if these steps fail, the subsequent use of strong opioid analgesics (step 3), mainly orally administered morphine.

However, even when used correctly, oral morphine therapy has its limitations. Failures can be due to either a lack of effect or, more commonly, the side effects of the drug, e.g., nausea, vomiting, and constipation. A fourth step, based on locoregional morphine therapies, should be added to the three steps suggested by WHO. This fourth step would include lumbar intrathecal (or epidural) and intraventricular injections through catheters connected to subcutaneous injection sites.

The finding of opioid receptors in the regions surrounding the ventricles and the aqueduct prompted clinicians to use intraventricular morphine (IVM). The results were mainly positive. As early as 1964, Tsou and Jang[1] observed a profound antinociceptive effect in the rabbit after IVM use. These authors proposed that the periaqueductal gray (PAG) is one of the major supraspinal sites for the action of morphine in producing analgesia, an idea that was subsequently supported by many authors. This region contains terminals that are immunoreactive to endogenous opioids, such as beta-endorphin,[2] enkephalins,[3–5] and dynorphin,[6–8] and opioid binding sites, notably of the mu-subtype.[9–11] Intraventricular injections of small doses of morphine result in a selective activation of these opioid receptors. As a result, central receptors are activated but not peripheral receptors, thus avoiding or substantially reducing some of the peripheral effects produced by systemic administration, such as histamine liberation, the first-pass effect, hepatic glycuronoconjugation, enzymatic induction, and the effects on the gastrointestinal and urinary tracts.

Following the first publications by Leavens et al.,[12] Lobato et al.,[13] and Roquefeuil et al.,[14] IVM became a common and successfully used neurosurgical procedure for the treatment of cancer pain. From June 1983 to June 1993, we treated 203 cancer pain patients with IVM. Follow-up evaluations were performed regularly until a patient's death. This made it possible to study the advantages and difficulties associated with this method. In addition, electrophysiologic measurements of nociceptive flexion reflexes were used in some patients to investigate the possible underlying mechanisms of IVM analgesia. In these cases, experiments were approved by a local committee. According to the ethical principles of the Helsinki convention, signed informed consent was always obtained from the patients who participated in the studies.

Clinical Investigations

Selection criteria were extremely rigorous. We used IVM to treat only severe intractable chronic pain directly due to the development of the cancer, after all other possible treatments had been attempted. Life expectancy was limited to a few months. The pain was not amenable to treatment even with adjusted doses, as described by the WHO's three therapeutic stages. The pain was intractable even with oral morphine, either because of side effects or swallowing difficulties. In addition, other neurosurgical procedures (stereotactic peduncular tractotomy, selective posterior radiculectomy, dorsal root entry zone lesions) were judged insufficient, too difficult, or too dangerous. As a result of these criteria, the patients undergoing IVM were generally those suffering pain from the upper part of the body or diffusely throughout the whole body. Intrathecal morphine remained an option when the pain was located under the diaphragm and a spinothalamic cordotomy was not indicated.

Out of 203 patients, 145 (72%) were suffering pain related to bilateral or diffuse squamous cell carcinoma in the head and neck region, 34 (17%) had multifocal pain due to diffuse bony metastases, 13 (6%) exhibited extensive pain related to a Pancoast-Tobias syndrome, and 11 (5%) had miscellaneous etiologies. All had been treated previously with oral morphine (most becoming constipated), 11 (5%) receiving more than 1,000 mg, 142 (70%) receiving 500–1,000 mg, and 50 (25%) receiving less than 500 mg per day.

Before performing such a treatment, we obtained informed consent from the patients themselves, gave extensive explanations to their families, and ensured that the patients would be kept in a regular medical environment, which is an essential requirement if an efficient follow-up study is to be achieved. In this study, the mean follow-up evaluation was at 51.3 ± 33.3 days (range, 7–307 days).

The implantation of the ventricular catheter is a simple neurosurgical procedure performed under local anesthesia. A small burr hole is drilled in the right frontal bone. After hemostasis of the dura mater, a Holter ventricular catheter is inserted into the right frontal horn of the lateral ventricle. It is connected to a small reservoir placed under the scalp in which a morphine chlorhydrate solution (10 mg in 1 ml) is injected with a strictly aseptic technique. Injections must be preceded by aspiration of a few drops of cerebrospinal fluid to test the permeability of the device. In spite of the apparent simplicity of this technique, an excessive increase in its indications for use should be avoided. The dose of IVM should be determined for each individual, according to the previous dose of oral morphine and also to the pain intensity. Injections were performed immediately following implantation. The daily dose was calculated by observing the quality and duration of pain relief.

Analgesia was achieved within 5–10 minutes of IVM. The mean dose of morphine injected in the reservoir at the beginning of treatment was 0.5 ± 0.2 mg, which produced an analgesic effect for 29 ± 16 hours. At the end of treatment, just before the patient's death, the mean dose of morphine was 1.2 ± 0.6 mg, which produced an analgesic effect for 26 ± 12 hours. The lowest daily consumption seen in one patient (47-day follow-up) was 0.05 mg per day (0.2 mg injections every 96 hours) at the beginning and increasing to 0.06 mg (0.2 mg every 72 hours) at the end of treatment. The highest daily consumption seen in another patient (73-day follow-up) was 2 mg at the beginning (1 mg every 12 hours) and increasing to 5 mg per day (2.5 mg every 12 hours) at the end. Most patients (n = 153, 75%) were treated at home, with the injections into the reservoir being performed by a home nurse.

Evaluation of the analgesic effect took account of the eventual necessity to adjust the treatment with oral analgesics. Observations of the patients in their everyday life was essential: Were they confined to bed or able to gradually recover the ability to undertake some activities? The criteria to answer this question included quality of sleep, means of food intake, and nature and scope of interests.[15] Analgesia was judged excellent (total disappearance of pain and requiring no additional treatment) or good (some persistence of pain necessitating the use of nonnarcotic analgesics) for 72% and 25% of the patients, respectively. In 3% of cases, we were confronted by a stalemate situation in which the patients complained of persistent strong pain that required the use of high systemic doses of narcotic analgesics. These patients suffered from bone metastasis and, although spontaneous pain was generally well controlled by IVM, pain triggered by movement was always present. Failure in two patients was likely due to the etiology of brachial plexus pain, being both the evolution of the cancer and postradiotherapy deafferentation.

Side effects usually occurred within the first week of treatment and were less frequent than following oral morphine. Nausea and vomiting were observed in 27% of cases and were well controlled with the usual antidote. Transitory pruritus and dysphoria were noted in 10% and 19% of cases, respectively. Three patients exhibited transitory mental aberrations with agitation. Respiratory depression was observed in only two patients during the initial trial and titration period. The first was due to a mistaken dosage (a single dose of 5 mg instead of 0.5) and the second was in a patient suffering from Pancoast-Tobias syndrome with respiratory insufficiency. All of these complications were immediately reversed by naloxone.

The main complications were infections. In nine cases, ventricular meningitis due to *Staphylococcus aureus* justified local and systemic antibiotic treatment. In one case, a cutaneous infection close to the reservoir was controlled with local treatment. The only case that necessitated the removal of the device was one in which a cerebrospinal fluid fistula occurred. We never observed any case of the catheter becoming obstructed.

In summary, this study confirmed earlier reports[14–21] that IVM produced a powerful and long-lasting analgesia with a low daily consumption of morphine. The effective dose of morphine could be defined easily within 2–3 days in most patients. Tolerance phenomena were not obvious. However, in several recent cases notable for the large doses of oral morphine (> 1,000 mg per day) initially used, the effective doses were difficult to define, possibly because of a cross-tolerance between the systemic and the IVM.

IVM produced not only a satisfactory state of analgesia but also, and perhaps more importantly, an improvement in the patients' quality of life and ability to relate to their surroundings. This state was due mainly to the reduced use of all orally administered drugs, including analgesics and psychotropics.

However, a global evaluation of this therapeutic method must consider all possible means of evaluation: psychological, home care, follow-up telephone calls, and information for and from family, physicians, and nurses.

Electrophysiologic Investigations

Although our knowledge of both opioid receptors and pain mechanisms has improved recently, we still know little about the neural substrates involved in the mechanisms of morphine-induced analgesia in humans. However, one mechanism of its analgesic action is well documented. In animals, morphine is known to cause a potent depression of the transmission of nociceptive signals at the first relays in the central nervous system, i.e., in the dorsal horn of the spinal cord.[22, 23] The human spinal cord contains opioid receptors and neurons containing endogenous opioids, mainly in the most superficial layers of the gray matter. A close relationship exists in humans between a polysynaptic nociceptive flexion reflex from a knee flexor muscle (R_{III} reflex) and the sensation of pain elicited by stimulating the ipsilateral sural nerve at the ankle.[24] On the basis of studies of this reflex, a direct spinal depressive effect has been suggested as one of the main mechanisms whereby morphine produces analgesia.[25–27]

A second, indirect and complementary mechanism has been proposed to explain the analgesic properties of morphine. The drug is supposed to act at some brainstem sites, mainly the PAG, to reinforce descending inhibitory influences that are involved in modulating pain. This represents another way to depress the spinal transmission of nociceptive signals through dorsal horn neurons.[28–31] However, this idea is controversial because attempts to demonstrate that supraspinal administration of morphine decreases the activity of dorsal horn neurons have been inconclusive.[22, 32, 33]

Our patients with cancer pain provided an exceptional opportunity to evaluate the effects of IVM on R_{III} reflexes in order to test the current hypothesis that IVM reinforces descending inhibitory controls, which modulate the spinal transmission of nociceptive signals.[34] Investigations were performed on 13 of those patients suffering intractable pain from head and neck squamous cell carcinoma who were being treated with IVM (0.7–1.0 mg total dose). R_{III} reflexes in the lower limb were elicited by stimulating the ipsilateral sural nerve via a pair of needle electrodes inserted through the skin at the ankle into the retromalleolar path of the nerve. Recordings were made from the biceps femoris muscle using a pair of surface electrodes placed on the scratched and degreased skin overlying the muscle. The subjective quality (tactile or painful) and intensity of the sensation elicited by the sural nerve stimulus were estimated by the subjects on a visual scale.

The R_{III} reflexes and the associated sensations of pain elicited by sural nerve stimulation were studied before and 1–4 hours after morphine injections. In all patients, IVM relieved the clinical cancer pain. Similarly, the threshold for the experimental pain was increased from 9.04 ± 0.56 to 10.18 ± 0.89 mA. By contrast, the R_{III} reflex was not depressed but was actually slightly enhanced, with its threshold falling from 8.76 ± 0.78 to 7.43 ± 0.54 mA. These data show that IVM depresses the descending inhibitory control of nociceptive transmission at the spinal level in humans. They do not support the hypothesis that supraspinal morphine reinforces descending inhibitory controls.

Several electrophysiologic studies in animals support this assertion. For example, the depressive effects of 1–10 mg per kg administered intravenously on C fiber–evoked responses were found to be remarkably similar in intact and spinal rats.[35] The results of other studies[36, 37] are consistent with the hypothesis that morphine decreases tonic descending inhibitions. Four studies using microinjection techniques in the rat, the first two within the nucleus raphe magnus[38, 39] and the other two within the PAG,[40, 41] have shown that morphine can increase the responses evoked in dorsal horn neurons by noxious stimulation of their receptive fields. Finally, Sinclair[42] reported that perfusion of the cat ventricular system with morphine also resulted in a facilitation of dorsal horn neuronal responses to noxious stimuli, whereas the predominant effect of morphine administered within the third ventricle of the rat was a dose-related and naloxone-reversible facilitation of the C fiber–evoked responses of dorsal horn convergent neurons.[43]

The critical question regarding this problem still remains the way in which, and the circumstances during which, the descending inhibitory controls involved in pain modulation are triggered in humans. Such inhibitory processes can be activated in normal subjects: We have demonstrated that painful heterotopic conditioning stimuli inhibit the R_{III} reflex and the corresponding sensation of pain elicited by sural nerve stimulation.[44, 45] These effects were observed during and for several minutes after the conditioning procedure in normal volunteers but

disappeared in tetraplegic patients suffering from traumatic, clinically complete spinal cord transections.[46] Observations on patients with cerebral lesions[47] indicated that the brainstem is the site of a key neuronal link in the loop subserving such inhibitory effects. We concluded that a painful focus triggers descending impulses that, in turn, inhibit a spinal nociceptive flexion reflex.

The effects of a supraspinally acting dose of intravenous morphine (0.05 mg per kg) was investigated on such inhibitory processes.[48] Morphine administration resulted in a complete abolition of these inhibitions without any modification of the reflex itself (Figure 17-1). Thus, a low dose of systemic morphine completely blocked the inhibitory effects of heterotopic nociceptive conditioning stimuli on a nociceptive flexion reflex. This blockade occurred without any change in the electrophysiologic characteristics (latency, duration, and magnitude) of the R_{III} reflex itself and disappeared after subsequent naloxone administration. Thus, in humans, we are dealing with an inhibitory process sustained by a spinobulbospinal loop,[46, 47] which is blocked completely by morphine. The low dose of morphine used in this study precludes the possibility that signals emanating from upper limb nociceptors were blocked at the spinal level; indeed, a higher dose of morphine (in the 0.1–0.3 mg per kg range) is required before a direct spinal depressive effect can be observed.[25] Therefore, there must be an effect of morphine at one or more supraspinal sites.

These results are similar to those observed in the rat. Indeed, the supraspinally mediated inhibition of dorsal horn neurons by heterotopic noxious stimulation, which have been termed diffuse noxious inhibitory controls (DNIC), is blocked by morphine administered via various routes.[49] In fact, DNIC have been found to be extremely sensitive to the systemic or intracerebroventricular administration of low doses of morphine.[43, 50, 51] As previously stated, the PAG is one major supraspinal site used by morphine to produce analgesia. Further electrophysiologic data support the hypothesis that the lifting of DNIC following systemic morphine is due at least in part to binding of the drug within the PAG because of the following reasons:

1. Microinjections of morphine directly within the PAG produced a significant depression of DNIC.[40]

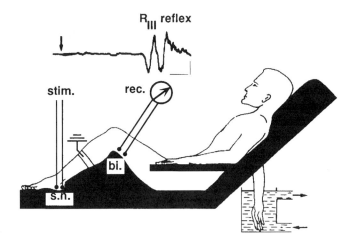

A

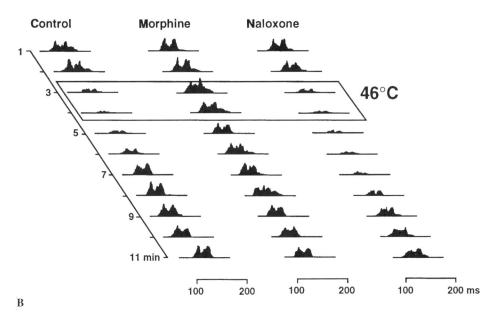

B

Figure 17-1. Example of the effects of 0.05 mg per kg of morphine and subsequent 0.006 mg per kg of naloxone intravenous injections on the inhibitions of the R_{III} reflex produced by a noxious thermal conditioning stimulus: immersion of the right hand in a 46°C waterbath for 2 minutes. A. Experimental setup used for eliciting a nociceptive reflex (R_{III}) by stimulation (stim.) of the sural nerve (s.n.) and recording (rec.) from over the left biceps femoris muscle (bi.). An example of the R_{III} reflex is shown at the top of the diagram (calibrations: horizontal, 25 ms; vertical, 100 µV). The reflex, which was evoked by juxtathreshold (1.2 times threshold) stimuli, was studied before, during, and after a 2-minute period of immersion of the right hand in a thermoregulated waterbath. B. Individual example showing the effects of the conditioning procedure on the R_{III} reflex

before (control), 15–26 minutes after morphine, and 5–16 minutes after a subsequent injection of naloxone (performed 30 minutes after the morphine injection). Each trace represents the average of ten successive full-wave rectified reflex responses recorded within a 1-minute period. The temporal evolution can be seen from back to front, with the conditioning period occurring during the third and fourth minutes (hatched areas). Note (1) that in the control situation there was a clear depression of the R_{III} reflex, both during and after the 2-minute conditioning period, (2) that the reflex was unaffected but the inhibition was blocked completely following morphine, and (3) that it recovered completely following naloxone. (Reprinted with permission from D Le Bars, T De Broucker, JC Willer. Morphine blocks pain inhibitory controls in humans. Pain 1992;48:13.)

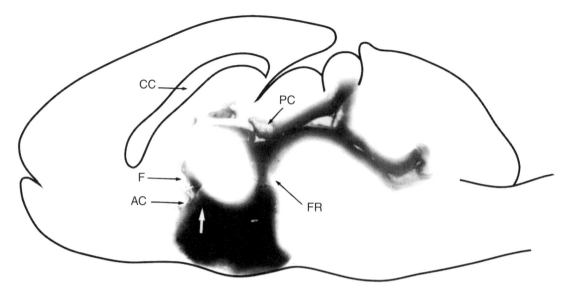

Figure 17-2. Photomontage of autoradiograms showing the maximal diffusion of 2.5 mg of morphine injected within the third ventricle of the rat. [^{3}H]Morphine (24 Ci per mmol) was microinjected into the ventricle (white arrow) over a 3-minute period; 20 minutes later, the brain was quickly removed and frozen at -50°C before being cut into sagittal sections. After 2 months of exposure, the autoradiograms revealed labeling around the ventricular system. (AC = anterior commissure; CC = corpus callosum; F = fornix; FR = fasciculus retroflexus [habenulo interpeduncular tract]; PC = posterior commissure.) Note that the diffusion (mean concentration < 50 mmol per L) was restricted to within 500 μm and was blocked by fiber tracts that appear as "ghosts" on the autoradiograms. It is interesting to compare these experimental data with our clinical observations. In humans, about 1 mg of ICVM was sufficient to elicit powerful analgesia; in this study in the rat 400-fold less was used, which is consistent with the ratio of the volumes of the respective brains. (Reprinted with permission from D Bouhassira, L Villanueva, D Le Bars. Intracerebroventricular morphine decreases descending inhibitions acting on lumbar dorsal horn neuronal activities related to pain in the rat. J Pharmacol Exp Ther 1988;247:332.)

2. DNIC were depressed in a dose-dependent fashion after microinjections of 0.6–2.5 μg of morphine within the third ventricle. In these experiments, autoradiographic controls with titrated morphine (Figure 17-2) indicated that it reached the PAG throughout its whole rostrocaudal extension.[43]

3. The effect of systemic morphine on DNIC disappeared in PAG-lesioned animals.[52]

Thus, an ever growing body of evidence in both animals and humans indicates that morphine clearly impairs descending inhibitory systems that modulate pain, at least those that are activated by nociceptive afferents.

Taking into account this decrease in descending inhibitory controls, what could be the mechanism for supraspinal morphine analgesia? This question is specifically addressed in reviews on DNIC[49] and is summarized in the following discussion.

Because convergent neurons respond to both noxious and nonnoxious stimuli, their activities in the absence of any noxious stimulation can be interpreted as a basic somatesthetic activity from which a significant nociceptive signal could not easily emerge. A local, restricted noxious stimulus induces two related phenomena at the level of the spinal cord:

1. A segmental excitation of nociceptive neurons

2. As a result of the activation of the DNIC system, a reduction in the activity of all the (other) spinal and trigeminal convergent neurons not concerned with the segmental activation

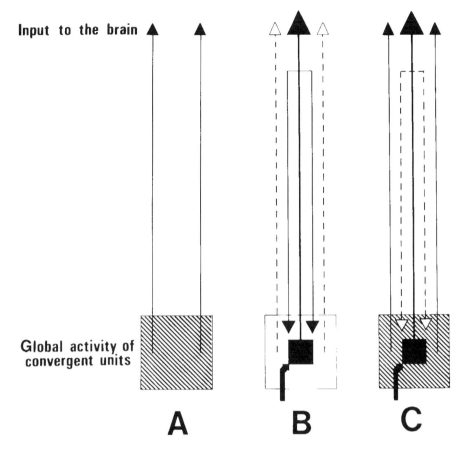

Input to the brain

Global activity of convergent units

A   **B**   **C**

Figure 17-3. Hypothetical interpretation of the global activity of all convergent neurons involved in nociception at spinal and trigeminal levels. At rest, such activity would not be negligible because of the properties of these neurons and thus a basic somatesthetic signal would be sent toward the brain (A). A nociceptive focus will activate some convergent and nociceptive specific neurons (B), which in turn will transmit an excitatory signal toward supraspinal centers. This will trigger diffuse noxious inhibitory controls (DNIC) that will inhibit those convergent neurons not directly affected by the initial stimulus and thus the background noise, which constitutes the basic somatesthetic activity, will be reduced or abolished (B). Morphine, either systemically at low doses, intracerebrally, or intraventricularly blocks DNIC and thus restores the background noise (C). (Adapted from D Le Bars, AH Dickenson, JM Besson. Opiate analgesia and descending control system. Adv Pain Res Ther 1983;5:341; D Le Bars, D Bouhassira, L Villanueva. Opioids and Diffuse Noxious Inhibitory Controls [DNIC] in the Rat. In B Bromm, JE Desmedt [eds], From Nociception to Cognition. Advances in Pain Research and Therapy [Vol. 22]. New York: Raven, 1994;517.)

The contrast signal between the excited (segmental) and the inhibited (extrasegmental) pools of neurons could indicate to higher centers that a nociceptive event was occurring. In this hypothesis, hypoalgesia could be induced by a decrease in DNIC, which would result in a restoration of the background somatesthetic activity.

The analgesia induced by IVM could result, at least in part, from a restoration of the basic somatesthetic activity of dorsal horn and trigeminal convergent neurons (Figure 17-3).

Acknowledgments

This work was supported by INSERM (Clinical Research Network), CRC AP-HP, and by la Fondation pour la Recherche Médicale. The authors are grateful to Dr. Cadden for advice in preparing the manuscript.

References

1. Tsou K, Jang CS. Studies on the site of analgesic action of morphine by intracerebral microinjection. Scientia Sinica 1964;13:1099.

2. Bloom FE, Battenberg E, Rossier J, et al. Neurones containing endorphin in rat brain exist separately from those containing enkephalin: Immunocytochemical studies. Proc Natl Acad Sci U S A 1978;75:1591.

3. Elde R, Hokfelt T, Johanson D, et al. Immunohistochemical studies using antibodies to leucine-enkephalin: Initial observations on the central nervous system of the rat. Neuroscience 1976;1:349.

4. Sar M, Stumpf WE, Miller RJ, et al. Immunohistochemical localisation of enkephalin in rat brain and spinal cord. J Comp Neurol 1978;182:17.

5. Uhl GR, Goodman RR, Kuhar MJ, et al. Immunohistochemical mapping of enkephalin containing cell bodies, fibres and nerve terminals in the brain stem of the rat. Brain Res 1979;166:75.

6. Goldstein A, Ghazarossian VE. Immunoreactive dynorphin in pituitary and brain. Proc Natl Acad Sci U S A 1980;77:6207.

7. Khachaturian H, Watson SJ, Lewis ME, et al. Dynorphin immunocytochemistry in the rat central nervous system. Peptides 1982;3:941.

8. Hollt V, Haarmann I, Boverma NNK, et al. Dynorphin-related immunoreactive peptides in rat brain and pituitary. Neurosci Lett 1980;18:149.

9. Goodman RR, Snyder SH, Kuhar MJ, et al. Differentiation of delta and mu opiate receptor localization by light microscopic autoradiography. Proc Natl Acad Sci U S A 1980;77:6239.

10. Herkenham M, Pert CB. Light microscopic localisation of brain opiate receptors: A general autoradiographic method which preserves tissue quality. J Neurosci 1982;2:1129.

11. Mansour A, Lewis ME, Khachaturian H, et al. Pharmacological and anatomical evidence of selective and opioid receptor binding in rat brain. Brain Res 1986;399:69.

12. Leavens ME, Hills CS, Cech D, et al. Intrathecal and intraventricular morphine for pain in cancer patients: Initial study. J Neurosurg 1982;56:241.

13. Lobato RD, Madrid JL, Fatela LV, et al. Intraventricular morphine for control of pain in terminal cancer patients. J Neurosurg 1983;59:627.

14. Roquefeuil B, Benezech J, Batier C, et al. Interet de l'analgésie morphinique par voie ventriculaire dans les algies rebelles neoplasiques. Neurochirurgie 1983; 29:135.

15. Bourhis A, Spitalier JM. La douleur maladie en cancérologie. Biol Med 1970;59:427.

16. Blond S, Meynadier J, Combelles-Pruvot M, et al. Indications et resultats de la morphinothérapie intracérébroventriculaire dans les algies cancereuses: À propos de 55 patients. In W Erdmann, T Oyama, MJ Pernak (eds), Pain Clinic (Vol. I). Utrecht: VNU Science Press, 1985;77.

17. Blond S, Meynadier J, Dupart T, et al. La morphinothérapie intracérébro-ventriculaire: A propos de 79 patients. Neurochirurgie 1989;35:52.

18. Blond S, Meynadier J, Eloundou, et al. La morphinothérapie intracérébro-ventriculaire: Reflexions à propos d'une expérience portant sur 111 patients. Hygiène et Médecine 1990;48:1630.

19. Lazorthes Y, Verdie JC, Caute B, et al. Intracerebroventricular Morphinotherapy for Control of Chronic Cancer Pain. In HL Fields, JM Besson (eds), Progress in Brain Research. New York: Elsevier, 1988;397.

20. Meynadier J, Blond S, Bouhassira D, et al. Opioids in Regional Techniques: Hypothesis Concerning the Mechanism of Analgesic Activity of Intra-cerebroventricular Morphine. In S Lilton, E Tunks, M Zoppi (eds), Advances in Pain Research and Therapy. New York: Raven, 1990;373.

21. Dennis GC, De Witty R. Long term intraventricular infusion of morphine for intractable pain in cancer of the head and neck. Neurosurgery 1990;26:404.

22. Duggan AW, North RA. Electrophysiology of opioids. Pharmacol Rev 1984;35:219.

23. Yaksh TL, Noueihed R. The physiology and pharmacology of spinal opiates. Annu Rev Pharmacol Toxicol 1985;25:433.

24. Willer JC. Comparative study of perceived pain and nociceptive flexion reflex in man. Pain 1977;3:69.

25. Willer JC. Studies on pain. Effects of morphine on a spinal nociceptive flexion reflex and related pain sensation in man. Brain Res 1985;331:105.

26. Willer JC, Bussel B. Evidence for a direct spinal mechanism in morphine-induced inhibition of nociceptive reflexes in humans. Brain Res 1980;187:212.

27. Willer JC, Bergeret S, Gaudy JH. Epidural morphine strongly depresses nociceptive flexion reflexes in patients with postoperative pain. Anesthesiology 1985;63:675.

28. Irwin S, Houde RW, Bennett DR, et al. The effects of morphine, methadone and meperidine on some reflex responses of spinal animals to nociceptive stimulations. J Pharmacol Exp Ther 1951;101:132.

29. Takagi H, Matsunara M, Yanai A, et al. The effects of analgesics on the spinal reflex activity of the cat. Jpn J Pharmacol 1955;4:176.

30. Mayer DJ, Price DD. Central nervous system of analgesia. Pain 1976;2:379.

31. Fields HL, Basbaum AL. Brainstem control of spinal transmission neurons. Annu Rev Physiol 1978;40:193.

32. Le Bars D, Dickenson AH, Besson JM. Opiate analgesia and descending control system. Adv Pain Res Ther 1983;5:341.

33. Advokat C. The role of descending inhibition in morphine-induced analgesia. Trends Pharmacol Sci 1988;9:330.

34. Guieu JD, Blond S, Meynadier J, et al. Intracere-

broventricular (ICV) morphine depresses descending inhibitory controls in patients with cancer pain [Abstract]. 7th World Congress on Pain, Paris, 1993;209.

35. Bars D, Guilbaud G, Chitour D, et al. Does systemic morphine increase descending inhibitory controls of dorsal horn neurons involved in nociception? Brain Res 1980;202:223.

36. Duggan AW, Griersmith BT, North RA. Morphine and supraspinal inhibition of spinal neurons: Evidence that morphine decreases tonic descending inhibition in the anaesthetized cat. Br J Pharmacol 1980;69:461.

37. Soja PJ, Sinclair JG. Spinal vs supraspinal actions of morphine on cat spinal cord multireceptive neurons. Brain Res 1983;273:1.

38. Le Bars D, Dickenson AH, Besson JM. Microinjection of morphine within nucleus raphé magnus and dorsal horn neurone activities related to nociception in the rat. Brain Res 1980;189:467.

39. Llewelyn MB, Azami J, Roberts MHT. Brainstem mechanisms of antinociception: Effects of electrical stimulation and microinjection of morphine into nucleus raphe magnus. Neuropharmacology 1987;25:727.

40. Dickenson AH, Le Bars D. Supraspinal morphine and descending inhibitions acting on the dorsal horn in the rat. J Physiol (Lond) 1987;384:81.

41. Dickenson AH, Le Bars D. Lack of evidence for increased descending inhibition on the dorsal horn of the rat following periaqueductal grey morphine microinjections. Br J Pharmacol 1987;92:271.

42. Sinclair JG. The failure of morphine to attenuate spinal cord nociceptive transmission through supraspinal actions in the cat. Gen Pharmacol 1986;17:351.

43. Bouhassira D, Villanueva L, Le Bars D. Intracerebroventricular morphine decreases descending inhibitions acting on lumbar dorsal horn neuronal activities related to pain in the rat. J Pharmacol Exp Ther 1988;247:332.

44. Willer JC, Roby A, Le Bars D. Psychophysical and electrophysiological approaches to the pain-relieving effects of heterotopic nociceptive stimuli. Brain 1984;107:1095.

45. Willer JC, De Broucker T, Le Bars D. Encoding of nociceptive thermal stimuli by diffuse noxious inhibitory controls in humans. J Neurophysiol 1989;62:1028.

46. Roby-Brami A, Bussel B, Willer JC, et al. An electrophysiological investigation into the pain relieving effects of heterotopic nociceptive stimuli: Probable involvement of a supraspinal loop. Brain 1987;110:1497.

47. De Broucker T, Cesaro P, Willer JC, et al. Diffuse noxious inhibitory controls (DNIC) in man: Involvement of the spinoreticular tract. Brain 1990;113:1223.

48. Le Bars D, De Broucker T, Willer JC. Morphine blocks pain inhibitory controls in humans. Pain 1992;48:13.

49. Le Bars D, Bouhassira D, Villanueva L. Opioids and Diffuse Noxious Inhibitory Controls (DNIC) in the Rat. In B Bromm, JE Desmedt (eds), From Nociception to Cognition. Advances in Pain Research and Therapy (Vol. 22). New York: Raven, 1994;517.

50. Bouhassira D, Villanueva L, Le Bars D. Intracerebroventricular morphine restores the basic somesthetic activity of dorsal horn convergent neurons in the rat. Eur J Pharmacol 1988;148:273.

51. Le Bars D, Chitour D, Kraus E, et al. The effect of systemic morphine upon diffuse noxious inhibitory controls (DNIC) in the rat: Evidence for a lifting of certain descending inhibitory controls of dorsal horn convergent neurons. Brain Res 1981;215:257.

52. Bouhassira D, Villanueva L, Le Bars D. Effects of systemic morphine on diffuse noxious inhibitory controls: Role of the periaqueductal grey. Eur J Pharmacol 1992;216:149.

Chapter 18

Meta-analysis on the Efficacy of Intrathecal and Epidural Opiates

Joachim Chrubasik and Sigrun Chrubasik

The discovery of opioid receptors in the spinal cord has led to the administration of opioids into the epidural or intrathecal space. This technique is an alternative method to manage intractable pain. The need for this technique is rare: only about 1% of cancer patients require spinal opioid treatment.[1, 2]

A nationwide survey in Sweden reviewing 768 patients over 124 days suggests that spinal opioid treatment is accepted as an outstanding method for the treatment of certain chronic pain states, especially those due to malignancy.[3] Unfortunately, the quality of pain relief from epidural or intrathecal opioid treatment was not recorded in these patients except in patients suffering from nonmalignant pain. Only 7 out of 13 patients reported excellent or good pain relief with long-term epidural morphine.[3] A review of the literature confirms that the success rate of spinal opioid treatment is not overwhelming. Although most patients experience at least some relief of pain, the quality of analgesia was poor in 363 out of 1,238 patients using epidural morphine or buprenorphine (Table 18-1) and 113 out of 456 patients using intrathecal morphine (Table 18-2). In light of the short mean observations of about 3 months for epidural morphine and 6 months for intrathecal morphine, the failure rate of spinal opioid treatment due to technical problems and adverse effects will be even higher with longer treatment periods. Proper patient selection with clearly defined criteria is therefore necessary so as to optimize the efficacy of spinal opioid administration in cancer patients.

Criteria for Patient Selection

Chronic pain has many origins. The pain history, which records the nature of pain, its origin, and its time pattern should clearly indicate that the patient's pain may respond to spinal opioids.[25] Many patients with neuropathic pain syndromes as well as psychogenic pain are nonnociceptive and display opioid-insensitive phenomena.[25] The best responses to spinal opioid treatment may be expected when the pain is continuous and originates from deep somatic structures. Coexisting continuous visceral pain or intermittent somatic pain originating from a pathologic fracture, for example, are less opioid-responsive. Cutaneous pain from ulcers and fistulas, and intermittent pain due to intestinal obstruction are only occasionally relieved by spinal opioids.[25] Pain characterization may, however, be difficult because nerve involvement in radiating cancer pain may only be characterized by slowly developing neuropathic lesions.[26] It may also be difficult to distinguish between visceral pain and the activation of somatic nerves close to the diseased organ.[26] When appropriate a spinal placebo administration may be useful in determining the usefulness of spinal opioids.

Main criteria for selecting the spinal mode of opioid administration[27] include opioid-sensitive pain that is not relieved by conventional treatments (e.g., surgery or oral medication) and opioid-sensitive pain of such magnitude that it totally dominates the patient's life. Spinal opioids are an alternative to sys-

Table 18-1. Number of Patients Under Epidural Morphine or Buprenorphine for Relief of Intractable Cancer Pain or Chronic Nonmalignant Pain

Number of Patients CCP/CNMP	Excellent or Adequate Pain Relief	Duration of Treatment (Mean Days)*	Reference
114/36	81	51 (7–397)	4
94/11	70	65 (7–283)	5
225/0	133	47 (7–420)	6
145/83	155	48 (7–443)	7
24/20	18/12	54/19 (6–129/3–47)	8
284/11	256/5	96/155 (1–1215)/?	9
154/0	108	? (21–501)	10
35	27/8	101 (10–333)	11

CCP = chronic cancer pain; CNMP = chronic nonmalignant pain.
*Mean (range).

Table 18-2. Number of Patients Under Intrathecal Morphine for Relief of Cancer Pain and Chronic Nonmalignant Pain

Number of Patients	Quality of Analgesia			Duration of Treatment	Reference
	Excellent	Good	Poor		
62		46	16	Initial test	12
23	19	2	2	4½ mos (12–1,500 d)	13
27	5	18	4	(1–13 mos)	14
40	27	9	4	7 mos (2–24 mos)	15
12		3	9	6 mos (up to 2 yrs)	16
35	17	11	7	5 mos	17
17		15[c]	2	147 d (6–961 d)	9
14	7	4	3	3 mos (1–23 mos)	18
		53	28	25	46 d (1–231 d)	19
		23	12	11	8 wks (1–26 wks)	20
37[b]		28[c]		231d (30–1,320d)	21
65		39	26	19 wks (4–60 wks)	22
	43[a]	28[c]	15	(within 2 years)	23
	5[a]		5	12 wks	24
	8[a]	4	4	21 mos	17

[a]Nonmalignant pain (all other malignant).
[b]Two patients had nonmalignant pain.
[c]Quality of analgesia unspecified.

temic opioids if increasing opioid dose requirement results in unacceptable side effects. Spinal opioids are an alternative to rhizotomy, cordotomy, and cerebral and spinal stimulations and may be considered when pretreatments with these techniques have been unsuccessful. The patient must consent to the spinal procedure and clearly understand the potential adverse effects and complications of spinal opioid therapy. Furthermore, the patient's physical status must allow implantation of the proposed narcotic delivery system. Coexisting psychological dysfunction, e.g., anxiety and depression, may need to be treated by pharmacologic and psychological means in addition to proceeding with spinal analgesia.

Spinal administration of opioids is contraindicated if patients suffer from opioid-insensitive pain or refuse this mode of treatment. Patients suffering from generalized sepsis, any infection at the proposed anatomic site of implantation, or patients receiving concomitant anticoagulant therapy should also be excluded from this therapeutic option.[28]

Choice of the Drug Delivery System

The costs of spinal opioid therapy in 63 patients suffering from intractable cancer pain clearly demonstrated that this mode of therapy, although expensive for long-term use (daily costs about $30), is justified because it satisfactorily alleviates pain.[29] Patients remain in better mental and physical control and need less external assistance due to the reduced opioid dose requirement. A careful choice of the drug delivery system according to the patient's life expectancy is necessary to keep the costs of treatment in a reasonable range.

Percutaneous Catheters

In short-term care of intractable pain, percutaneous catheters offer the advantages of being inexpensive and simple to insert. However, the relatively high incidence of complications with long-term use limits their use for longer treatment periods (Table 18-3). Bacterial filters connected to the spinal catheter may help prevent the introduction of infective organisms.[38]

Subcutaneous tunneling of the catheter laterally to the anterolateral chest wall or the iliac region increases the patient's comfort and prevents dislodgment of the catheter. Tunneling does not, however, influence the infection rate of percutaneous catheters,[2] as previously thought.[38] Of 100 patients treated with subcutaneous epidural catheters over an estimated mean period of 50 days, approximately 30% required more than one catheter.[39] Of 110 patients treated up to 366 days with epidural catheters, 86 patients suffered from complications. Twenty-seven of those patients had more than one complication.[30]

Implantable Reservoirs

If patients have a life expectancy of several months, the subcutaneous catheter should be connected to a subcutaneous injectable port system. The risk of infections in patients with port systems is about half that of patients with percutaneous catheters.

At present, there is a need to improve not only the catheter technology but also the portal systems so as to decrease the incidence of complications. Basic requirements for implantable reservoirs are that they should be easily palpable, easy to inject, relatively inexpensive, and able to withstand at least 1,000 injections via the skin.[38] In about 10% of implantable reservoirs, blockage of the portal system necessitates removal of the system (Table 18-3).

Externally Portable Infusion Devices

An externally worn pump can be connected to the subcutaneous catheter or to the implanted reservoir by means of a special needle inserted through the skin.[40] This produces a primarily closed circulation. The possibility of disconnecting the pump from the implanted reservoir allows the patients greater independence, e.g., unimpeded showering and greater flexibility in dressing.

A significant difference exists between the spinal infusion of opioids with constant flow rates and continuous, on-demand spinal opioid infusion. The latter offers the patient the possibilities of supplementary limited extra infusions on demand or of variation of the basal infusion rate according to the daily fluctuation in drug consumption or if tolerance develops.[40] Opioid consumption under continuous, on-demand epidural infusion is about 30% lower than under infusion with constant basal rates.[41] Furthermore, a decrease in the drug demand may be recognized, and it is occasionally possible to return to oral medication.[40]

Implantable Infusion Devices

The implantation of infusion devices is a major surgical procedure. However, implantable dosing devices, especially if programmable, are the most convenient for long-term treatment with spinal opioids. They offer a lower risk of complications than continuous opioid injection. Unfortunately, the high cost of the devices, which may only be used once, limits use of implantable dosing devices in patients with limited life expectancies. Technical

Table 18-3. Complication Rate (%) with Spinal Drug Delivery Systems in 1,512 Patients*

| | Catheter | | Port (%) | Mixed (%) |
	Percutaneous (%)	Tunneled (%)		
Number	414	431	406	326
Occlusion	53 (13)	54 (13)	40 (10)	8 (3)
Infection				
Subcutis	46 (11)	41 (10)	26 (7)	14 (5)
Major	4 (1)	15 (4)	2 (0.5)	0 (0)
Pain on injection	34 (8)	3 (1)	37 (9)	4 (2)
Dislodgment	86 (21)	12 (3)	3 (1)	28 (10)
Leakage	17 (4)	2 (0.5)	41 (10)	11 (2)
References	2, 30–32	2, 30, 33–35	2, 9, 35–37	1, 2, 6, 22

*Mean treatment period is approximately 2 months.

development is required to facilitate refilling of these devices.

Description of the Implantation Technique

The placement of the spinal catheter may be performed with the patient in the sitting, lateral, or prone position. The position should be convenient for the patient for about 15–20 minutes when placing a subcutaneous catheter, for about 30 additional minutes when a port system is implanted, and for at least 1 hour for the implantation of an infusion device. If the staff is proficient in the method, the implantation time may even be shorter and requires only minimal adjunctive narcotics or sedatives.[28]

After aseptic preparation of the skin including the tunneling site and the catheter exit site, a Tuohy needle is placed (after infiltration with local anesthetics and skin incision) into the spinal space at the desired lumbar or thoracic interspace. The catheter is then advanced through the Tuohy needle and placed several centimeters into the epidural or intrathecal space. It is sometimes easier to advance the catheter within the Tuohy needle after wetting both needle and catheter with saline.[28] After removing the Tuohy needle, a tunneling device according to the desired length is advanced in the subcutaneous tissue from the desired catheter exit site incision to the incision site of the Tuohy needle. The tunneling device is carefully withdrawn until the catheter tip is outside the skin. A subcutaneous reservoir or an implantable infusion device may then be attached to the distal end of the catheter after making a small subcutaneous pocket, and the surgical incision is closed using aseptic precautions.

Guide Prior to Implanting any Drug Delivery System

The following protocol should be considered before implanting a device for spinal opioid treatment[27]:

1. The procedure, expected goals, and potential side effects should be explained in detail to the patient and family (i.e., informed consent).
2. The opioid and its dosage should be determined.
3. The daily epidural or intrathecal opioid consumption as well as assessment parameters including subjective pain scores from the treatment, level of activity, amount of sleep, need for additional analgesics or centrally acting drugs (e.g., antidepressants), and the side effects should be recorded.

Failure to clearly demonstrate the efficacy of spinal opioids during the preimplantation trial may result in the patient being subjected to implantation of a delivery system that fails to achieve pain relief.[27]

Origin of Treatment Failure

Treatment may fail for several reasons[27]: spinal injection not made in the correct place, incorrect spinal opioid dosage or opioid-resistant pain, psychological reasons such as depression or use of pain as an attention-seeking device, and advanced tolerance to opiates or physical dependence.

Choice of the Opioid

A large discrepancy exists regarding the dose of morphine needed to produce analgesia when injected closer to the spinal cord. The epidural morphine dose requirement is about ten times lower than the intravenous morphine dose requirement,[42] but exceeds intrathecal morphine dose requirement by a factor of ten.[43, 44] Morphine is therefore an appropriate opioid for spinal treatment. The occurrence of respiratory depression due to morphine accumulation within the cerebral spinal fluid (CSF) is negligible if morphine is continuously titrated into the epidural or intrathecal space.[45]

About 30 times more meperidine than morphine is required for epidural analgesia.[42] Although its epidural dose requirement is not much lower than its intravenous dose requirement, meperidine may be used as an alternative for morphine in spinal treatment. Preservative-free morphine remains stable in plastic reservoirs for up to 60 days.[46]

Epidural methadone is only half as potent as epidural morphine.[42] Intrathecal methadone produced analgesia of inferior quality even in a dosage ten times higher than morphine.[43, 44] This finding and the fact that no methadone is saved when changing from the intravenous to the epidural route of administration due to its long terminal elimination time makes it inadvisable for spinal use.[42]

The increased risk of respiratory depression due to the dual distribution from the epidural space (via the CSF and blood) does not outweigh the benefit of spinal analgesia when short-acting fentanyl, alfentanil, buprenorphine, sufentanil, or tramadol are administered closer to the spinal cord.[42]

In order to avoid medicolegal conflicts, these opioids should not be used spinally unless it is proved that benefits outweigh the possible risks during long-term epidural or intrathecal pain treatment.[42]

Spinal coadministration of clonidine or local anesthetics may decrease spinal opioid consumption.[24, 27, 47, 48] If bupivacaine is added to the spinal opioid solution, paresthesia, motor blockade and gait impairment, or hypotension may occur.[48] The addition of bupivacaine to spinal morphine did not produce neuropathologic effects over a mean treatment time of 81 days.[49]

Adjuvant analgesic drugs (parenteral or oral) such as nonsteroidal anti-inflammatory drugs, corticosteroids, anticonvulsants, antidepressant drugs, neuroleptic drugs, antihistamines, or psychostimulants may help improve the degree of pain relief[22, 50] and to achieve adequate analgesia.

Side Effects and Complications

During long-term spinal opioid treatment, most patients have some side effects or complications. The side effects that might occur during spinal opioid treatment are either dose independent or related to the opioid dose administered. Urinary retention, pruritus, pain from bolus, transpiration, and depending on lipophilicity, sedation may occur independent of the amount of opioid administered. Dose-dependent opioid side effects include the occurrence of nausea and emesis, dysphoria, euphoria, central depression, e.g., major sedation, respiratory depression, hypotension, and constipation. The occurrence of organic hallucinosis is rare.[51] Tachyphylaxis does not necessarily occur in patients given the highest opioid dosages or having the longest duration of treatment.[3] The need for increased doses is related not only to changes in receptor sensitivity but also to changes in pain mechanism. It seems likely that disease progression may be the main factor.[52] Most patients need an increasing opioid dosage over time to control pain. A retrospective review of 163 patients by 10 physicians[53] revealed that patients suffering from pain of metastatic origin had a three- and fivefold increase over 3- and 6-month periods of intrathecal morphine, respectively. Tolerance developed more quickly with bolus intrathecal injections than with continuous intrathecal infusions.[10] Spinal drug alternatives may then be required to achieve sufficient pain relief.

Side effects and complications of spinal opioid therapy occur in more than 50% of the patients during long-term treatment.[22, 34, 47, 50, 54] Possible complications include technical failures, such as mechanical device problems, leaking reservoir, catheter disconnection, dislocation, kinking, catheter or port occlusion, infections (from local infections to meningitis) (see Table 18-3) or development of a seroma around the implanted device.[21, 22] Local skin infections at the site of the subcutaneous device with subsequent infection and colonization of the port and catheter may not necessarily predicate the removal of the system. In vivo sterilization using an antibiotic infusion has become an accepted technique together with antibiotic administration through the implanted delivery system.[55]

The most frequent complication for patients with intrathecal catheters is leak of the CSF with spinal headache. Fistulas may also occur.[22] However, spinal headache due to CSF leakage either disappears spontaneously within days or it may become severe. If conservative therapy (bed rest, analgesics) fail, the headache may be successfully treated with an epidural blood patch.[30]

Summary

Fifteen years have passed since spinal (epidural, intrathecal) opioid treatment was introduced for intractable cancer pain relief. A review of the literature reveals that the success rate of the method is far lower than previously thought. Although at least some alleviation of pain is achieved in some patients, the complication rate of the method is more than 50% and increases with the duration of treatment. The success of spinal opioid treatment is dependent on careful patient selection. The pain must be opioid-sensitive and intractable. The patient's physical and mental status should be within the normal range. Spinal opioid treatment is only an alternative to other modalities of cancer pain management and most of these other modalities are associated with side effects and complications.

Device selection is dependent on the cost ratio in relation to the patient's life expectancy. The less expensive to more expensive rank order of drug devices include percutaneous catheters (if possibly tunneled), port systems, externally portable infusion devices, and implantable infusion devices. Patient-controlled spinal analgesia with externally portable or implantable infusion devices offers independence

for the patient and relief for doctors and nursing staff. The method is preferable to intermittent spinal opioid bolus injections or infusions with constant opioid infusion rates. Morphine has been shown to be the most appropriate opioid for patient-controlled spinal analgesia because its systemic and spinal dose discrepancy is far greater than that of other opioids. In case of opioid tolerance, coadministration (spinally or systemically) of other analgesic drugs may help decrease the opioid dose requirement and increase the degree of pain relief.

References

1. Hogan Q, Haddox JD, Abram S, et al. Epidural opiates and local anesthetics for the management of cancer pain. Pain 1991;46:271.
2. Dejong PC, Kansen PJ. A comparison of epidural catheters with or without subcutaneous injection ports for treatment of cancer pain. Anesth Analg 1994;78:94.
3. Arner S, Rawal N, Gustafsson LL. Clinical experience of long-term treatment with epidural and intrathecal opioids: A nationwide survey. Acta Anaesthesiol Scand 1988;32:253.
4. Carl P, Crawford ME, Ravlo O, Bach V. Long-term treatment with epidural opiates. Anaesthesia 1986;41:32.
5. Crawford ME, Andersen HB, Augustenborg G, et al. Pain treatment on outpatient basis utilizing extradural opiates. A Danish multicentre study comprising 105 patients. Pain 1983;16:41.
6. Erdine S, Aldemir T. Long-term results of epidural morphine in 225 patients. Pain 1990;45:155.
7. Hegelun K, Nielsen FM. Pain treatment on long term basis, with extradural opiates. Acta Anaesthesiol Scand 1983;27(Suppl. 78):69.
8. Michon F, Des Mesnards VG, Girard M, et al. Analgesie peridurale morphinique de longue duree en pathologie neoplasique et vasculaire. Cahier d'Anesthesiologie 1985;33:39.
9. Plummer JL, Cherry DA, Cousins MJ, et al. Long-term spinal administration of morphine in cancer and noncancer pain: A retrospective study. Pain 1991;44:215.
10. Tryba M, Zenz M, Strumpf M. Long-term epidural catheters in terminally ill patients: A prospective study of complications in 129 patients. Anesthesiology 1990;73:A784.
11. Stamer U, Maier CH. Ambulante Epiduralanalgesie bei Tumorpatienten. Anästhesist 1992;41:288.
12. Wang JK. Intrathecal morphine for intractable pain secondary to cancer of pelvic organs. Pain 1985;21:99.
13. Brazenor GA. Long-term intrathecal administration of morphine: A comparison of bolus injection via reservoir with continuous infusion by implanted pump. Neurosurgery 1987;21:484.

14. Coombs DW, Saunders RL, Gaylor MS, et al. Relief of continuous chronic pain by intraspinal narcotic infusion via an implanted reservoir. JAMA 1983;250:2336.

15. Hernandez JLR, Padron FR, VeraReyes JA de. Administration intratecallumbar de morfina en el tratamiento del dolor del cancer avanzado. Rev Espanola Anaest Rean 1986;33:253.

16. Krames ES, Gershow J, Glassberg A, et al. Continuous infusion of spinally administered narcotics for the relief of pain due to malignant disorders. Cancer 1985;56:696.

17. Penn RD, Paice JA. Chronic intrathecal morphine for intractable pain. J Neurosurg 1987;67:182.

18. Shetter AG, Hadley MN, Wilkinson E. Administration of intraspinal morphine sulfate for the treatment of intractable cancer pain. Neurosurgery 1986;18:740.

19. Ventafridda V, Spoldi E, Caraceni A, De Conno F. Intraspinal morphine for cancer pain. Acta Anaesthesiol 1987;31(Suppl. 85):47.

20. Verdenne JB, Esteve M, Guillaume A. Injection de morphine intrathecale dans le traitement ambulatoire dela douleur neoplastique. J Chir (Paris) 1986;123:330.

21. Follet KA, Hitchon PW, Piper J, et al. Response of intractable pain to continuous intrathecal morphine: A retrospective study. Pain 1992;49:21.

22. Erdine S, Yücel A. Long-term results of intrathecal morphine in 65 patients. Pain Clin 1994;7:27.

23. Auld AW, Maki-Jokela A, Murdoch DM. Intraspinal narcotic analgesia in the treatment of chronic pain. Spine 1985;10:777.

24. Coombs DW, Saunders RL, Lachance D, et al. Intrathecal morphine tolerance: Use of intrathecal clonidine, DADL, and intraventricular morphine. Anesthesiology 1985;62:358.

25. Arner S, Arner B. Differential effects of epidural morphine in the treatment of cancer-related pain. Acta Anaesthesiol Scand 1985;29:32.

26. Samuelsson H, Hedner T. Pain characterization in cancer patients and the analgesic response to epidural morphine. Pain 1991;46:3.

27. Waldman SD. Implantable drug delivery systems: Practical considerations. J Pain Symptom Manage 1990;5:169.

28. Allen ML, Turnage G. Selection of patients for implantable intraspinal narcotic delivery systems. Anesth Analg 1986;65:883.

29. Mueller H, Lüben V, Zierski J, Hempelmann G. Long term spinal opiate treatment. Acta Anaesthesiologica Belgica 1988;39(Suppl. 2):83.

30. Crul BJP, Delhaas EM. Technical complications during long-term subarachnoid or epidural administration of morphine in terminally ill cancer patients: A review of 140 cases. Reg Anesth 1991;16:209.

31. Downing E, Busch EH, Stedman PM. Epidural morphine delivered by a percutaneous epidural catheter for outpatient treatment of cancer pain. Anesth Analg 1988;67:1159.

32. Zenz M, Piepenbrock S, Tryba M. Epidural opiates: Long-term experiences in cancer pain. Klin Wochenschr 1985;46:709.

33. DuPen SL, Peterson DG, Williams A, Bogosian AJ. Infection during chronic epidural catheterisation: Diagnosis and treatment. Anesthesiology 1990;73:905.

34. Malone BT, Beye R, Walker J. Management of pain in the terminally ill by administration of epidural narcotics. Cancer 1985;55:438.

35. Vainio A, Tigerstedt I. Opioid treatment for radiating cancer pain: Oral administration vs. epidural techniques. Acta Anaesthesiol Scand 1988;32:179.

36. Boersma FP, Noorduin H, Vanden Busche G. Epidural sufentanil for cancer pain control in outpatients. Reg Anesth 1989;14:293.

37. Findler G, Olschwang D, Hadani M. Continuous epidural morphine treatment for intractable pain in terminal cancer patients. Pain 1982;14:311.

38. Cherry DA. Drug delivery systems for epidural administration of opioids. Acta Anaesthesiol Scand 1987;31(Suppl. 85):54.

39. Carl P, Crawford ME, Ravlo O. Fixation of extradural catheters by means of subcutaneous tissue tunneling. Br J Anaesth 1984;56:1369.

40. Chrubasik J. Zur spinalen Infusion von Opiaten und Somatostatin. Verlag Hygieneplan, 637 Oberursel, 1985.

41. Jansen EC. Morphine pumps in the epidural treatment of pain. Acta Anaesthesiol Scand 1983;(Suppl. 26):68.

42. Chrubasik J, Chrubasik S, Martin E. The ideal epidural opioid—fact or fantasy. Eur J Anaesth 1993;10:79.

43. Jacobson L, Chabal C, Brody MC, et al. Intrathecal methadone and morphine for postoperative analgesia: A comparison of the efficacy, duration, and side-effects. Anesthesiology 1989;70:742.

44. Jacobson L, Chabal C, Brody MC, Ward RJ. Intrathecal methadone 5 mg and morphine 0.5 mg for postoperative analgesia: A comparison of the efficacy, duration and side-effects. Anesth Analg 1989;68:S132.

45. Chrubasik J, Chrubasik S, Mather L. Postoperative Epidural Opioids. New York: Springer-Verlag, 1993.

46. Meissner W. Formulas. In PP Raj (ed), Practical Management of Pain. Chicago: Year Book, 1986;858.

47. Laugner B, Muller A, Thiebaut JB, Farcot JM. Analgesie par site implantable pour injections intrathecales iteratives de morphine. Ann Fr Anesth Reanim 1985;4:511.

48. Sjöberg M, Nitescu P, Appelgren L, Curelaru I. Long-term intrathecal morphine and bupivacaine in patients with refractory cancer pain. Anesthesiology 1994;80:284.

49. Sjöberg M, Karlsson PA, Nordborg C, et al. Neuropathologic findings after long-term intrathecal infusion of morphine and bupivacaine for pain treatment in cancer patients. Anesthesiology 1992;76:173.

50. Cobb CA, French BN, Smith KA. Intrathecal morphine for pelvic and sacral pain caused by cancer. Surg Neurol 1984;22:63.

51. Bruera E, Schoeller T, Montejo G. Organic hallucinosis in patients receiving high doses of opiates for cancer pain. Pain 1992;48:397.

52. Collin E, Poulin P, Gauvain-Piquard A, et al. Is disease progression the major factor in morphine tolerance in cancer pain treatment? Pain 1993;55:319.

53. Yaksh TL, Onofrio BM. Retrospective consideration of the doses of morphine given intrathecally by chronic infusion in 163 patients by 10 physicians. Pain 1987;31:211.

54. Dagi TF, Chilton J, Caputy A, Won D. Long-term, intermittent percutaneous administration of epidural and intrathecal morphine for pain of malignant origin. Am Surg 1986;52:155.

55. Hahn MB, Bettencourt JA, McCrea WB. In vivo sterilization of an infected long-term epidural catheter. Anesthesiology 1992;76:645.

Chapter 19

The Role of Invasive Techniques

Jeff M. Arthur and Gabor B. Racz

Introduction

Despite increasing initiatives by the medical community and public interest groups, notably the World Health Organization (WHO), several studies evaluating cancer pain have shown that 50–70% of patients suffer needlessly.[1] In 1985, Bonica surveyed 47 published reports and revealed that 71% of patients with advanced cancer had pain as a major symptom and noted a 50% incidence of pain in patients with intermittent stage disease.[2] As recently as March 1994, Cleeland et al. reported that outpatients being treated for metastatic cancer had considerable pain but received inadequate analgesia, despite published guidelines for pain management.[3] These reports are just a few of many to show that most cancer patients do not receive effective pain management.

The invasive techniques used by many anesthesiologists to manage pain play an important role in the management of cancer pain.[4, 5] They should not be used alone and are best when used as a component of a multitherapeutic approach. This approach of course could also include multiple pharmacologic interventions, neurosurgical and neuroaugmentative procedures, physical therapy, and behavioral or psychological approaches. The multidisciplinary team approach is the most effective for treating cancer pain.

Assessment of Pain Etiology

When using invasive techniques to manage pain, it is important to know as precisely as possible the etiology and pathogenesis of the pain. In the cancer patient, pain may be related to the cancer or to many other related or unrelated conditions. For example, the pain may be due to iatrogenic causes, such as postmastectomy pain, postradiation neuritis, fibrosis, peripheral neuropathy following chemotherapy, neuroma formation, and other postsurgical scaring. However, the pain may be due to unrelated conditions such as diabetic neuropathy or other chronic painful conditions that the patient may have had prior to the tumor, such as chronic low back pain or myofascial pain. In dealing with the cancer pain patient, multiple diagnoses should always be considered, because pain is often derived from more than one etiology.[6] In addition to the initial assessment of pain, it is important to reassess the patient at regular intervals and after the initiation of any new treatment or invasive procedure. Reassessment is also important if the patient reports new pain.

Cancer can cause pain by one of many ways:

1. Obstruction or distention of a hollow viscus,
2. Invasion of nerves and blood vessels by malignancy,
3. Occlusion of blood vessels, which can lead to ischemia or swelling,
4. Inflammation, swelling, or necroses of tissue,
5. Compression of nerve roots, trunks, or plexus by invading malignancy, and
6. Compression or collapse of bony structures or invasion of bone and periosteum.[6]

Pain associated with cancer may commonly include somatic pain, which occurs as a result of nociceptors in cutaneous and deep tissues; sympathetic pain, which results from distention or chemical irritation of visceral structures or from disorders of the autonomic nervous system; or central pain, which is characterized by spontaneous burning dysesthesia, hyperpathia, and hyperalgesia in the absence of peripheral tissue damage. Central pain syndromes may result from cortical, thalamic, or spinal cord lesions.[7]

Figure 19-1 is a flow chart depicting cancer pain management from the initial assessment of pain and its causes to the various treatment modalities, including the WHO analgesic ladder and numerous other drug and nondrug modalities.[8]

The WHO ladder (see Figure 6-1) illustrates a progression in the doses and types of analgesic drugs that are effective pain management.[8] When this noninvasive approach is ineffective, alternative modalities are used, including other routes of drug administration, nerve blocks, and ablative neural surgery, as depicted in Figure 19-2.[8]

Figure 19-2 indicates that patients receiving treatments of varying degrees of invasiveness may also benefit from other modalities of treatment.[8] It should be noted, however, that the number of patients receiving these modalities, either separately or in combination, is not well documented. The estimates presented in Figure 19-2 reflect various clinical populations and may not represent all settings and populations; furthermore, they do not necessarily reflect what is optimal but only a range of current opinions.[8] As clinicians become more skilled, invasive neuroblockade procedures will be used earlier in the management of patients rather than waiting until the patients have failed all other noninvasive treatments. A good example of this current shift is reflected by the changing attitudes regarding the application of the celiac plexus block. Many authors now support using the celiac plexus block early in the treatment of pain for patients suffering from terminal pancreatic cancer.[8] Many cancer pain patients suffer many complications because of late referral, including interference with physical and mental activities, nausea, vomiting, constipation, drowsiness, mental confusion, and other side effects relating to high-dose analgesics. Early referral to a pain clinic will yield greater benefit not only by providing pain relief before depression starts, but also by allowing more precise nerve blocking before tissues are destroyed by disease or surgery.[6]

Invasive Treatment Decision Making

Invasive techniques for pain control should not be used as the primary means of control but rather concomitantly with noninvasive treatments. Nevertheless, the possibility of controlling otherwise intractable pain by the relatively brief application of local anesthetic or neurolytic agent makes neural blockade an attractive approach in some patients with cancer pain. Despite variability in published data regarding the efficacy of nerve blocks in cancer pain patients, 50–80% of patients who receive nerve blockades for cancer pain may receive some alleviation of their pain.[8] Multiple algorithms (the WHO analgesic ladder and others [Figure 19-3])[9] exist to help decide when to use a particular type of invasive therapy.

When contemplating an invasive technique, the risk to benefit ratio must be considered. One should consider not only potentially dangerous risks of the procedure itself but also the cost to patient in terms of inconvenience, recuperative time, emotional stress, physical energy required to tolerate the procedure, and the patient's ability to cooperate during the procedure. For this reason, many percutaneous "anesthetic procedures" are viewed as preferable to many neurosurgical procedures, which can be demanding on the critically ill patient.[10] The basic premise of any invasive technique should be to choose the technique with the simplest and least hazardous intervention that is associated with the highest likelihood of achieving desirable results. Although more than 70% of patients with moderate-to-severe pain will achieve adequate control of their symptoms with carefully instituted pharmacologic management, up to 30% of patients may require alternative treatment.[11–13] Many factors influence the selection of a patient for an invasive therapeutic procedure. These include the nature and severity of the symptoms, the response or lack of response to previous interventions, the patient's quality of life in relationship to his or her level of symptoms, the status of the patient's underlying disease, the patient's functional and psychosocial status (including his or her ability to cooperate), and, finally, the patient's individual preference. In addition, the practitioner's level of expertise, bias, and access to a consultant with the specialized skills and facilities to do invasive blocks will ultimately influence the patient's treatment via such techniques.

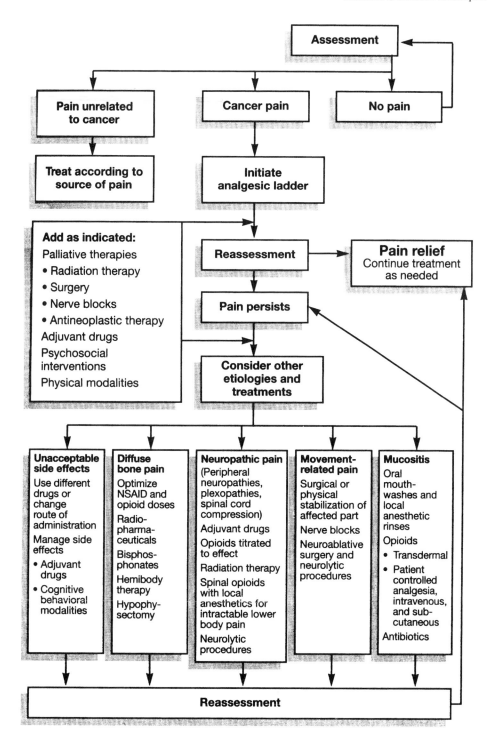

Figure 19-1. Continuing pain management in patients with cancer. (NSAID = nonsteroidal anti-inflammatory drug.) (Reprinted with permission from Cancer Pain Relief and Palliative Care: Report of a WHO Expert Committee. Geneva: World Health Organization, 1990 [Technical Report Series, No. 804; Figure 1].)

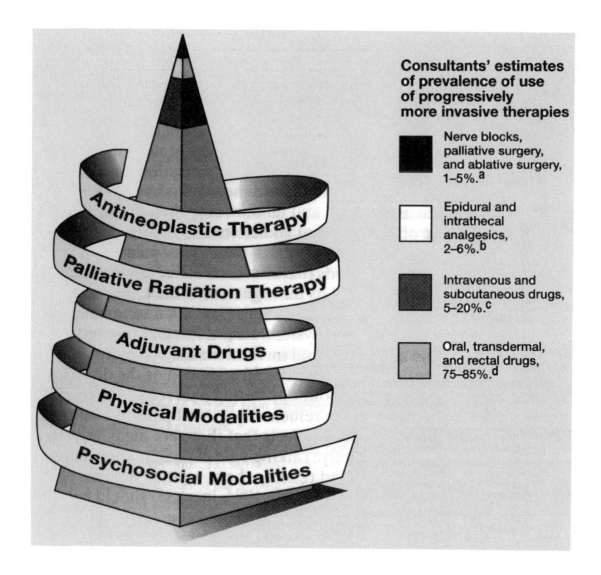

Figure 19-2. A hierarchy of pain management strategies from the least invasive (at the base) to the most invasive (at the apex). Therapies depicted on the ribbon may benefit many patients who are receiving concurrent treatments at any level of invasiveness. Estimates presented in the sidebar are based on published data and consultants' estimates for various clinical populations in industrialized nations, but may not reflect all settings and do not necessarily reflect what is optimal. [a] Hiraga, Mizuguchi, and Takeda, 1991; Portenoy, 1993; Ventafridda, Caraceni, and Gamba, 1990. [b] Hiraga, Mizuguchi, and Takeda, 1991; Ventafridda, Caraceni, and Gamba, 1990. [c] Keller, 1984; Paice, 1993; Portenoy, 1993. [d] Goisis, Gorini, Ratti et al, 1989; Hiraga, Mizuguchi, and Takeda, 1991; Scug, Zech, and Dörr, 1990; Takeda, 1986; Ventafridda, Caraceni, and Gamba, 1990; Walker, Hoskin, Hanks, et al, 1988. (Reprinted from Clinical Practice Guideline No. 9, Management of Cancer Pain. U.S. Department of Health and Human Services Public Health Service, Agency for Health Care Policy and Research, Publication No. 94-0592, 1994.)

Table 19-1. Purpose of Nerve Blocks

Diagnostic: To determine source of pain (e.g., somatic nerve versus sympathetic pathways)
Therapeutic: To treat painful conditions that respond to nerve blocks (e.g., celiac blocks for pain from pancreatic cancer)
Prognostic: To predict outcome of permanent interventions such as infusions, neurolysis, and rhizotomy
Preemptive: To prevent painful sequelae of procedures that may cause phantom limb pain or causalgia

Treatment Goals and General Considerations

Local anesthetic nerve blocks can be used for a variety of reasons. They may provide diagnostic information such as whether the pain is somatic or visceral or whether it has a sympathetic mechanism. They may provide prognostic information such as producing hypotension and changing subjective sensations, including pain relief or unpleasant numbness that might result from a planned neurodestructive procedure. These nerve blocks may also be therapeutic. Injections of local anesthetic may provide relief that outlasts its pharmacologic action, such as the prolonged benefit that may follow injection of trigger points from myofascial pain. This procedure is sufficiently simple, safe, and effective and can be accomplished by many primary care providers. Peripheral nerve blocks can also be preemptive, such as to help prevent painful sequelae, such as phantom limb pain or causalgia from limb amputation (Table 19-1).[8] The most common considerations and goals for doing nerve blocks in the cancer pain patient are as follows: (1) a patient with uncontrolled pain on treatments of oral or intravenous narcotics and other medications or (2) a patient with multiple side effects from other treatment modalities such as intractable nausea and vomiting, seizures or overwhelming sedation, with or without uncontrolled pain. By using a neuroblockade technique, the overall use of opioids and other medications may be lowered, thus allowing the patient a more functional and alert state with decreased side effects and increased quality of life and productivity. This latter characteristic is of great concern to most patients and their families, because most terminally ill patients would like to retain as much of their faculties and abilities for as long as possible. When a patient is pain-free after neurolysis or neuroblockade procedure, opioids should not be stopped abruptly; otherwise, a withdrawal syndrome may be provoked. However, in many patients who are on chronic opioids, the overall dose of opioids should be reduced in an organized and sequential manner. Without this reduction process, unacceptable sedation or other side effects may occur in the absence of their previous pain stimulation. Another consideration when contemplating neuroblockade should include the technical feasibility of the block. This would include the amount of innervated area that would need to be covered by the block, the possible complications of blocking the area (such as motor, bowel, or bladder innervation block), and the capacity to treat these complications. It is generally thought that neurolytic techniques should be reserved for localized pain, such as to a specific nerve root, dermatome, or specific sensory nerve. One exception to the localized pain rule is sympathetically mediated pain. In this situation, the patient may have widespread pain that can be interrupted by blockade of a sympathetic ganglion or plexus. Many pain syndromes that are refractory to opioid treatment are often sympathetically mediated or neuropathic in origin. In these situations, neuroblockade with local anesthetic with or without corticosteroids, or neurolysis with phenol, alcohol, or percutaneous radiofrequency thermocoagulation (RFTC) can be of significant help.

As with nonmalignant pain, the effect of the patient's psychosocial factors must be considered prior to doing any invasive techniques. This is especially true if the use of an implanted device, such as a peripheral nerve stimulator, spinal cord stimulator, or an intrathecal morphine pump, is considered.

It is not uncommon for cancer pain patients to have significantly altered blood indices as a result of their cancer treatment. Because of this, careful preblock consideration of the possibilities of infection and significant bleeding and hematoma, should be made, especially if treatment would involve neuraxial structures. In addition, because tumors may commonly metastasize to the vertebral column, consideration must be given to this fact when contemplating needle placement into tumor or areas where tumor may be involved. Tumor tis-

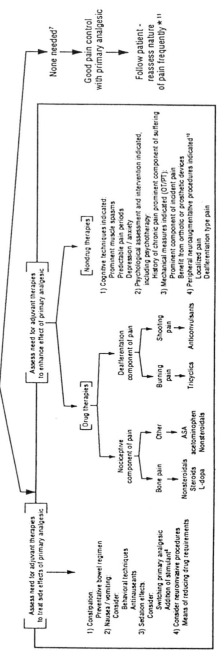

Figure 19-3. A proposed treatment algorithm for the management of cancer pain. Schema recommends treatment responses for pain of varying severity and types, drawing on the entire armamentarium of interventions available to the pain specialist. Algorithms of this type have not been rigorously tested. Due to the factors cited in the text, such algorithms only approximate the complex decision making that must be applied on an individual basis according to the specific needs of each patient. (ASA = acetylsalicylic acid; TENS = transcutaneous electrical nerve stimulation.) (Reprinted with permission from CS Cleeland, A Rotondi, T Brechner, et al. A model for the treatment of cancer pain. J Pain Symptom Manage 1986;1:209.)

Footnotes for Pain Treatment Flow Chart

1. Treat patient's pain according to indications. Monitor for recurrence of cancer.

2. Evaluate patient for antitumor therapy, or changes in current antitumor therapy.

3. The patients' treatment is selected to match their level of pain, not the etiology of the disease.

4. First try a nonsteroidal anti-inflammatory drug. Most of these drugs have ceiling effects indicating that increasing dosage will not provide additional analgesia after ceiling dose is reached. If customary dosages fail to provide adequate analgesia, try switching drugs or adding an opiate.

5. Start with titration of an opiate/nonsteroidal combination drug (eg. codeine/aspirin). The physician must be aware of reaching unacceptable side effects before analgesia occurs with these drugs. If pain continues at the maximum tolerable dose, switch to a potent opiate.

6. Administer a potent opiate. Titrate upward until dose has been reached for appropriate analgesic effects, or unacceptable side effects occur. For a patient who is not currently receiving opiates, one may try an opiate/nonsteroidal combination drug (eg. codeine/aspirin) for a brief period—typically this will only be for one or two days—to see if this will provide adequate pain control.

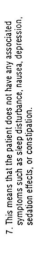
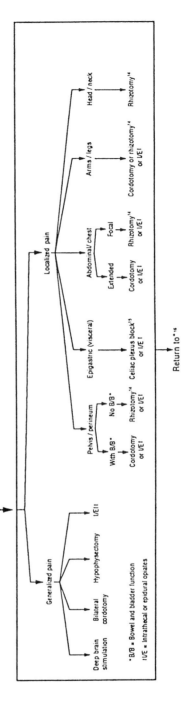

7. This means that the patient does not have any associated symptoms such as sleep disturbance, nausea, depression, sedation effects, or constipation.

8. The treatment of sedation with stimulants is still controversial and remains a subject for clinical research.

9. Other nonsteroidal anti-inflammatory drugs may also be used; however, there is no evidence of benefit from combining them.

10. This includes TENS, acupuncture, counterirritation, etc.

11. If new pain occurs, return to *assess patient's pain level* in model, where patient's pain severity is assessed.

12. Clinical evidence suggests that the new drug should be started at one-half to two-thirds the equianalgesic dose due to incomplete cross tolerance between opiate drugs. This starting dose can then be titrated upward if necessary.

13. Some of the procedures listed here may only be available at some medical centers.

14. Chemical or surgical.

15. Celiac plexus blocks have been found to be very effective in treating pain due to pancreatic cancer. It may be appropriate to use this procedure during the early stages of pain management in these cases.

16. Return in model to patient's pain level assessment after a neuroinvasive procedure has been used.

sue is often friable, bleeds easily, and heals poorly. In general, neurolytic nerve blocks are most appropriate for pain that is (1) well characterized, (2) well localized, (3) somatic or visceral in origin, and (4) is not a component of a pain syndrome characterized by multifocal "aches and pains."[10]

Patients who have vague complaints and who "feel bad all over" may be experiencing symptoms not just from their tumor pain but also from their cognitive, psychosocial, psychological, and economic situation, which may be playing a significant role in their disease state. In this clinical situation, no amount of analgesia or neurolysis will improve their pain. For this reason, it is recommended that careful psychological screening be conducted prior to any invasive technique.[10] It is common that patients usually have pain present in more than one location simultaneously.[10] Frequently, after neurolytic blockade of the dominant pain, the patient will complain of pain in some other location, which is then perceived as increased in severity.[10] However, even in patients with multiple sources of pain, the removal of the primary complaint of pain by individual nerve blockade may be of therapeutic value.

Considerations for Neurolytic Methods

Local Anesthetics Versus Neurolytic Agents

The use of local anesthetic injections for diagnostic and prognostic blocks has previously been discussed. With respect to therapeutic procedures, local anesthetics still have a useful role in the treatment of cancer pain, just as they do in the treatment of nonmalignant pain. Local anesthetics with or without steroids may be administered as a single shot, in a series through a catheter, or as an infusion epidurally. They are useful for pain of a neurogenic or inflammatory nature that is not expected to persist. Local anesthetics also have a therapeutic role in the management of the nononcologic pain syndromes that occur in patients with cancer, such as herpes zoster, postherpetic neuralgia, postthoracotomy, postmastectomy pain, myofascial pain syndromes, neuroma formation, and incisional pain. In addition, local anesthetic blocks administered in a series or in a continual epidural infusion via catheter may be useful in managing in the pain emergency to relieve pain and distress until a more accurate assessment and long-term plan can be determined.[10] One should not underestimate the use of local anesthetics with steroids for the reduction of inflammatory pain secondary to tumor. This therapeutic modality often provides relief that outlasts the duration of the local anesthetic.

Neurolytic Agents

Neurolytic blocks are most appropriate for pain that is due to specific tissue injury in terminal patients. Neurolytics, especially in the periphery, may cause neuritis and deafferentation pain. Because of this, the degree of pain severity and intractability and the predicted life expectancy one must consider when trying to determine whether a neurolytic block is warranted. As previously mentioned, the risk of the destruction of motor nerves, mixed nerves, or sphincter innervation (resulting in incontinence or bowel dysfunction) must always be considered when using permanent neurolytic agents. However, after informed consent, the patient may be willing to accept loss of function, especially if some preexisting organ dysfunction exists and the pain is extremely severe.

Perineural injections have been used therapeutically since the discovery of cocaine by Koller in 1884. The application of neurolytic substances to provide relief for patients with cancer has been practiced since 1930.[6] Interruption of pain pathways by the injection of neurolytic drugs is a well-established modality for treating chronic pain. The first reported injection of a neurolytic solution in the treatment of pain was probably by Luton,[14] who in 1863 administered subcutaneous injections of irritant substances into painful areas. Levy and Baudouin (1906) were the first to administer the injection of neurolytic agents percutaneously. Doppler, in 1925, was the first to report the use of phenol for neurolysis. The first use of phenol for subarachnoid neurolysis was reported by Maher in 1955.[6]

Phenol

Significant experience has been gained regarding the use of phenol as a single-dose subarachnoid injection for the treatment of chronic pain caused by malignancy. The destruction caused by phenol affects all nerves of the spinal cord. The histologic changes in the nerves produced by phenol are indistinguishable from those caused by alcohol (ethanol).[6] Both phenol and alcohol can result in postinjection neuritis, but there is a greater incidence after alcohol.[6] Phenol, however, has been reported to have a greater affinity for vascular than neural tissue.[15] Burkel and McPhee also found that phenol caused damage to perineural vascular tissue.[16] Phenol has also been used in the epidural space for neurolysis. Comparisons of epidural and subarachnoid injections of phenol show that no spinal cord damage was noted after epidural injection.[17] In contrast, massive neural tissue damage occurs following subarachnoid injection of phenol.[18] Blood vessels present in the areas of spinal cord destruction have shown normal morphology, illustrating the direct neurotoxic effect of phenol on the nerves rather than an effect secondary to vascular destruction.[18] Racz et al. have demonstrated that phenol does not readily pass through the dura, dural sleeve, or nerve roots, thereby exhibiting a selective neurolysis.[18] Two percent phenol does not cause tissue destruction and behaves similarly to local anesthetic. A concentration of 3% phenol produces damage equivalent to a 40% solution of alcohol.[6] Phenol tends to bind to tissue more readily than alcohol and diffuses less. Repeat injections of 6% phenol into the epidural space have been reported to be safe, and the injections have been repeated to an endpoint of 24 hours of pain relief. This is thought to produce a more thorough neurolysis through repeat application of the phenol rather than a single-shot neurolytic technique.[18] Concentrations of phenol vary in clinical use from 3–25%. Concentrations of phenol below 6% may be mixed with water or saline; however, in concentrations higher than this, phenol must be mixed with glycerin, or some other solution such as iohexol (Omnipaque) in order to prevent precipitation due to its low solubility. When mixed with glycerin, phenol solutions are hyperbaric, which has great applications when phenol is used intrathecally.[6]

Alcohol (Ethanol)

Alcohol has been used as a neurolytic drug for more than 50 years. In 1931, Dogliotti introduced alcohol injections into the subarachnoid space. In 1954, Bonica reported that of 514 cancer patients treated with alcohol, 63% had complete relief, 24% partial relief, and 13% no relief.[17] A 1966 review of alcohol neurolytic blocks showed an incidence of transient side effects as high as 10%.[19] Recently, ethanol has fallen to some disfavor other than its use for neurolysis of the celiac plexus. Reasons for its declining use include its high diffusability and solubility, which cause it to spread rapidly from the injection site, necessitating large volumes to be injected in order to produce adequate neurolysis. Because larger volumes of alcohol (than phenol) are required, the resultant neurolytic lesion is less precise.[6] Another recent hazard associated with alcohol has reportedly been a disulfiram-like effect, causing nausea, vomiting, hypotension, flushing, headache, respiratory difficulty, sweating, palpitations, chest pain, and global motor weakness.[6] Ethanol is an irritant and causes significant pain on injection. When injected into the intrathecal space, it is hypobaric and may spread significantly. Furthermore, ethanol has been reported to cause neuritis in 10% of patients when used on peripheral nerves.

Hypertonic Saline

The use of hypertonic saline for neurolytic purposes has not gained the widespread popularity of either phenol or alcohol. Ventrafridda and Spreafico used intrathecal hypertonic saline solutions in 81 patients with cancer to attempt to find optimal sodium chloride concentrations.[20] Hitchcock was the first to use intrathecal saline injection for intractable facial pain due to neoplasms.[19] Racz et al. have had good-to-excellent results by administering 10% sodium chloride solutions with local anesthetic and steroids epidurally, both for nonmalignant and malignant pain[21] (see following Case Report). This technique has been especially useful when used for movement-related pain due to neoplasms and bone metastasis to the spine. Generally, a higher osmolality results in greater neurolysis. Unfortunately, sufficient research has not been performed to define the precise mechanisms of action of hypertonic sodium chloride solutions. Clinical experience, however, shows safe use of hypertonic saline in the epidural space for prolonged pain relief without motor paralysis or neuritis. This characteristic differentiates hypertonic saline solutions from other neurolytics.[21]

Case Report

A 58-year-old man with prostate cancer with bony metastases was referred for management of back and leg pain. The back pain had been managed by epidural infusion of morphine for 1 year. The morphine provided him satisfactory pain control as long as he was immobile. On reexamination, a radiograph showed a lytic lesion on the L-5 vertebral body on the left side. A caudal epidural spring Racz catheter (Epimed International) was placed for lysis of epidural adhesions at L-5. The patient received daily injections of local anesthetic, steroid, and hypertonic saline for 3 days. This therapy produced significant pain relief that lasted for 3 months; he was even able to go fishing. The epidural morphine infusion was continued. The pain then recurred, necessitating a second epidural catheter series with local anesthetic, steroid, and hypertonic saline, which gave him pain relief until he died 3 months later.[6]

Percutaneous Radiofrequency Thermocoagulation

RFTC uses a Teflon-coated insulated needle with either a 5- or 10-mm noninsulated tip. This needle is usually of the 20-gauge size and can be inserted percutaneously. The RFTC machine will allow sensory stimulation from 50–70 Hz, and motor stimulation at 2–5 Hz to ensure proper placement of the needle on the appropriate nerve. Once this has been done, the tip of the needle can be heated with the SMK (Sluijter Mehta Kit manufactured by Radionics) thermocouple electrode. Typically, this is in the 80–90°C range for 60–90 seconds, depending on the lesion that one wishes to create. Some advantages of radiofrequency coagulation of nerves versus chemical neurolysis are listed here:

1. There is minimal risk to the patient.
2. The procedure can be performed on an outpatient basis.
3. There is a decreased incidence of neuritis compared with the use of alcohol or phenol.
4. Relatively few postoperative thromboembolic

phenomena are reported compared with alcohol or phenol.
5. The lesion is controllable and selective; typically, the lesion produced by the needle tip is the size of the needle plus approximately 1 mm in radius from the needle.
6. When used to perform sympathectomy, profound hypotension has not been reported.
7. The incidence of impotence when used to perform lumbar sympathectomies is rare.

Racz et al. have reported no serious complications in more than 500 lumbar RFTCs.[6] A possible disadvantage to RFTC is the small size of the lesion. Because of this, needle placement must be exact. There is no allowance for lack of precision or the lesion will not achieve adequate results. By the same reasoning, areas that need large coverage, such as the hypogastric plexus and the celiac plexus, are not suitable for RFTC.

Cryoneurolysis

Cryotherapy has been used for many years. The distinct advantage of cryotherapy on nerves over RFTC, phenol, or alcohol, is that there is no reported neuritis or neuroma formation after this form of neurolysis. Furthermore, cryoneurolysis is not permanent, as the nerve only undergoes wallerian degeneration and will subsequently regenerate. As with RFTC, the lesion is selective; however, it is significantly larger than the radiofrequency lesion. Typically a 14-gauge gas expansion cryoprobe will create a freeze zone lesion of approximately 6–8 mm in diameter. Most modern cryoprobes also allow for stimulation for appropriate location of motor and sensory nerves. Possible disadvantages to cryoneurolysis include:

1. The significantly large size of the cryoprobe may make insertion difficult.
2. Complexity and cost of the cryoprobe make it delicate and expensive to replace, since a slight distortion of the probe will make it inoperable.
3. The duration of this block will only last several days to weeks, as opposed to several weeks or months with RFTC, phenol, or alcohol.

Considerations for Specific Techniques and Blocks

Sympathetic Blocks

The sympathetic nervous system has a wide diversity in its anatomy from areas that are specific to areas that are generalized. As a result, appropriate selection of the proper neurolytic technique depends on the area that is to be treated. Typically, the stellate ganglion, the celiac plexus, the hypogastric plexus, and the ganglion of impar are most easily blocked by a chemical technique rather than radiofrequency or cryotechnique. This is because these sympathetic fibers tend to spread out over a large area, which makes it difficult to adequately block those areas where a discreet lesion such as that produced by a cryoprobe or RFTC needle. Typically, the stellate ganglion, hypogastric plexus, and ganglion of impar are blocked with phenol because these areas tend to need a more discrete lesion than that of celiac plexus, and to use alcohol in this area would require an extremely large volume that might destroy contiguous tissue that was not intended to be neurolysed, such as nerve innervation to the throat (i.e., the recurrent laryngeal nerve) or innervation to the bladder. The celiac plexus has been blocked with both phenol and alcohol, and, more recently, phenol has been used increasingly for this block. However, the fear of potential vascular destruction by phenol still makes ethanol the preferred neurolytic. Areas where the sympathetic nervous system have a more consistent anatomy, such as the thoracic or lumbar sympathetic chain, make it amenable to radiofrequency thermocoagulation. This is especially true in the thoracic area where extremely discrete lesions are necessary in order to avoid destruction of lung tissue and other vascular structures.

Neuraxial Neurolysis

The most frequently used methods for neuraxial neurolysis today are intrathecal alcohol, intrathecal phenol, and epidural phenol. Each technique has its own advantages and disadvantages. We compare subarachnoid phenol and subarachnoid alcohol. Subarachnoid phenol, when mixed with glycerin, is hyperbaric. Subarachnoid alcohol (95–100% alcohol) is hypobaric. Phenol does not cause pain on injection, whereas al-

cohol usually causes pain on injection. Phenol tends to produce a more discrete lesion and rapid tissue binding, whereas alcohol may spread for some distance from the site of injection and is more lipophilic. The phenol lesion can be created with slightly less volume, whereas the alcohol lesion requires more volume because of its ability to spread and dissolve lipid tissue. When placed in the subarachnoid space, the analgesic potency of alcohol tends to be more potent than that of phenol. The precise reason for this is not known, but it may be due to the greater volume of alcohol used when producing that lesion. There is a higher incidence of neuritis reported with alcohol than when compared with phenol. Phenol may have a greater affinity for vascular tissue and therefore may cause slight increase in vascular damage, although this issue is controversial.[15, 16, 18]

Epidural Neurolysis Versus Subarachnoid Neurolysis

Subarachnoid neurolysis[22] has both advantages and disadvantages when compared with the epidural technique:

1. Return of spinal fluid verifies subarachnoid needle placement, whereas localization of the epidural space must be inferred from results of epidurograms or a test dose of local anesthetic.
2. Subarachnoid neurolysis generally results in a more profound analgesia related to an increased direct contact between the drug and the target nerve roots; reinjection is rarely necessary in the acute stage of the block.
3. Subarachnoid injection is easily performed on an outpatient basis.
4. Epidural neurolysis usually requires repeated administration of phenol through indwelling catheter, which mandates inpatient hospitalization.
5. Patient positioning and gravity are relied on to control the spread of both epidural and subarachnoid phenol.[23] Control of spread is possible in both cases; however, it is postulated that the epidural spread might be slightly easier to control in that the nerve exposure can be more precisely controlled when given through the indwelling catheter than by a single injection technique.
6. The epidural technique offers the advantage of a widespread neurolysis with greater control be-

cause of the ability to reinject the patient several times over a number of days while slightly altering the patient's position for each reinjection or by altering position of the catheter.

It should be emphasized that the main advantage of epidural phenol neurolysis is its use for pain that occupies a wide dermatomal distribution or is bilateral. The main disadvantages are a shorter duration of action with a decreased intensity of analgesia when compared with subarachnoid neurolysis.[24] The major disadvantage of subarachnoid neurolysis is the possibility of permanent spinal cord damage with loss of motor, bowel, bladder, and sexual function. Studies suggest that these shortcomings may be overcome by repeated epidural administration over time through an indwelling catheter.[18, 25, 26] By careful placement of the epidural catheter and small repeated injections, the neurolytic agent tends to affect the dorsal roots while sparing the ventral motor roots. Ethanol has been used in the epidural space for neurolysis, but, in the awake patient, it produces agonizing pain unless preceded by injections of local anesthetic. This added volume local anesthetic may decrease the success rate and may also decrease the practitioner's ability to accurately pinpoint the spread of the neurolytic versus the spread of the local anesthetic. It should be noted that postinjection neuritis and neuralgia has been observed after epidural alcohol. Backache is the most common patient complaint after epidural neurolysis with either alcohol or phenol.[6]

Intraspinal Opioids

The addition of intraspinal opioids to the armamentarium of the pain specialist has significantly increased the therapeutic options available. This is especially true in the light of the development of highly sophisticated intraspinal delivery systems, such as implanted continuous and programmable delivery pumps (Table 19-2).[8] The main advantage of opioid therapy is its reversibility as compared with neurolysis and the availability of multiple simple screening measures to determine its likelihood of efficacy. Intraspinal opioids are more likely to be effective when responsiveness to opioids has already been demonstrated but treatment by opioids has been limited by systemic side effects.[10] In-

traspinal opioid therapy is generally more appropriate when the pain is of multiple origin or is widely distributed. At present, there is controversy about the selection of the most appropriate drug delivery system, scheduling of delivery, and appropriate drugs to be delivered. Currently, only morphine and baclofen have been approved for use in implanted intrathecal pumps. However, fentanyl, sufentanil, and hydromorphone have been used successfully, alone as well as with solutions of local anesthetics, (typically, bupivacaine). When neuropathic or sympathetic pain is encountered in this situation, pain relief is usually enhanced with the addition of local anesthetic to the opioid. The disadvantages of this, however, are potential for motor blockade, decreased bowel and bladder function, and a potential for "high spinal" with the associated complication of respiratory depression. The distinct advantage of intraspinal opioids is that extremely potent doses of opioid can have profound effects on the brain and spinal cord with minimal effects on other organ systems. Thus, significant side effects can be avoided.

Other Modalities

Percutaneous cordotomy is an important option for intractable pain that is unilateral and restricted to the lower half of the body.[27] Its application is most useful for pain located below the midthorax. It should be cautiously used in patients with pulmonary disease, and bilateral cordotomy should be avoided so as to minimize the risk of nocturnal respiratory failure (Ondine's curse).

Pituitary ablation is available as a possible technique of relieving pain that is due to widespread bone metastases and in patients with primary tumors that are hormonally responsive, such as breast and prostate.[27]

Strontium 89 has recently been released as a systemically injectable radionuclide specifically indicated for decreasing pain secondary to bone metastasis. Single outpatient doses have been shown to provide pain relief for an average of up to 6 months. In general, approximately 75% of patients with metastatic prostate cancer and more than 50% of patients with metastatic breast cancer obtain satisfactory pain relief.[28] However, its use for bone neoplasms is still investigational, and it is not indicated for use in patients with cancer not involving

Table 19-2. Intraspinal Drug Delivery Systems

System	Advantages	Disadvantages
Percutaneous temporary catheter	Used extensively both intra-operatively and postopera-tively. Useful when prognosis is limited (<1 mo)	Mechanical problems include catheter dislodgment, kinking, or migration
Percutaneous spring catheter	Soft tip, less chance of migra-tion. No kinking, therefore, aspiration verifies tip location. Can be sutured in place	—
Permanent silicone-rubber epidural	Catheter implantation is a minor procedure. Dislodgment and infection are less common than with temporary catheters. Can deliver bolus injections, con-tinuous infusions, or patient-controlled analgesia (with or without continuous delivery)	—
Subcutaneous implanted injection port	Increased stability, less risk of dislodgment. Can deliver bolus injections or continuous infusions (with or without patient-controlled analgesia)	Implantation more invasive than external catheters. Approved only for epidural catheter in U.S. Potential for infection increases with frequent injections
Subcutaneous reservoir	Potentially, reduced infection in comparison with external system	Difficult to access, and fibrosis may occur after repeated injection
Implanted pumps (continuous and programmable)	Potentially, decreased risk of infection	Need for more extensive operative procedure. Need for specialized, costly equipment with programmable systems

bone.[29] Its side effects may include the depression of white cell blood count (20%) and a decrease in platelet activity (30%). Repeat injections as needed can be used at intervals at not less than 90 days.[29]

Spinal Cord Stimulation

Spinal cord stimulation (SCS; previously called dorsal column stimulation) involves the placement of stimulating electrodes in the proximity of the spinal cord in the posterior epidural space. Effective SCS, like peripheral stimulation, obtunds pain by generating paresthesia over the painful region. Although many instances of success have been reported, overall results indicate a need for better patient selection.[30–32] A review of 16 series reporting on spinal stimulation for 88 patients with cancer pain shows that treatment was successful in 48% of patients.[30, 31]

An increased use of the percutaneous method of implantation may allow better patient selection and earlier clinical application at a decreased risk and cost. SCS has not emerged as an important option in patients with cancer pain.[33] Currently, it is not thought that permanent SCS technology justifies the cost of implantation of a device, as the patient may develop pain beyond the stimulating zone. However, temporary devices with percutaneous electrodes have been used, especially for visceral and pancreatic pain, with some success.[34]

Deep Brain Stimulation

Stimulation of deep brain structures is currently regarded as experimental, and the role of electrical stimulation remains controversial. However, stimulation of areas that are rich in opioid receptors (periaqueductal gray) has been shown to be effective in somatic pain syndromes,[35] whereas thalamic stimulation may be effective for neuropathic pain.[36]

Summary

The approach to the patient with cancer pain should use multiple therapeutic modalities. Therapeutic intervention may be as simple as epidural blockade with local anesthetic and steroids or a combination of modalities including implantable intrathecal pumps, neurolytic blocks, stimulating electrodes, and oral therapeutic agents. Cancer patients may not only be suffering from pain directly due to their tumor but may have many coexisting pain syndromes along with other psychosocial factors influencing their pain. With so many procedures available for the management of cancer pain, it is important for the primary physician to refer patients early in the disease process, despite the myth that neurolytic procedures should only be used as a last resort. These procedures are safe, used for nonmalignant pain syndromes, and should be offered to the patients with cancer pain early in the course of treatment. Early invasive pain treatment may allow an increased quality of life without pain, unnecessary sedation, and side effects.

> We all must die. But, if I can save him from days of torture, that is what I feel is my great and ever new privilege. Pain is a more terrible lord of mankind than even Death Himself.
>
> Albert Schweitzer[37]

References

1. Daut RL, Cleeland CS. The prevalence and severity of pain in cancer. Cancer 1982;50:1913.
2. Bonica JJ. Treatment of cancer pain: Current status and future needs. Adv Pain Res Ther 1985;9:589.
3. Cleeland CS, Gonin R, Hatfield AK, et al. Pain and its treatment in outpatients with metastatic cancer. N Engl J Med 1994;330:592.
4. Cousins MJ. Anesthetic Approaches in Cancer Pain. In KM Foley, JJ Bonica, V Ventafridda (eds), Advances in Pain Research and Therapy. New York: Raven, 1990;249.
5. Bonica JJ. Treatment of cancer pain. Current status and future needs. Semin Anesth 1985;9:589.
6. Arter OE, Racz GB. Pain management of the oncologic patient. Semin Surg Oncol 1990;6:162.
7. Patt RB, Jain S. Recent Advances in the Management of Oncologic Pain. In R Stoelting, P Barash, Gallagher (eds), Advances in Anesthesia. Chicago: Year Book, 1989;6:355.
8. Clinical Practice Guideline No. 9, Management of Cancer Pain. U.S. Department of Health and Human Services Public Health Service, Agency for Health Care Policy and Research. Publication No. 94-0592, 1994;13–15, 60, 95, 97, 223.
9. Cleeland CS, Rotondi A, Brechner T, et al. A model for the treatment of cancer pain. J Pain Symptom Manage 1:209, 1986.
10. Patt R. Cancer Pain. Philadelphia: Lippincott, 1993.
11. Ventafridda V, Tambutini M, Carceni A. A validation study of the WHO method for cancer pain relief. Cancer 1987;59:850.
12. Toscani F, Carina M. The implementation of the WHO guidelines for the treatment of advanced cancer pain in a district general hospital in Italy. Pain Clin 1989;3:37.
13. Takeda F. Preliminary report from Japan on results of field testing of WHO draft interim guidelines for relief of cancer pain. Pain Clin 1986;1:83.
14. Luton A. Etudés sur la médication substitutive. Première partie, de la substitution parenchymapeuse. Deuxieme partie de la medication substutive; son Éntendue, ses divisions. Archives Generales de Medicin, 1863;ii:57.
15. Nour-Eldin F. Preliminary report: Uptake of phenol by vascular and brain tissue. Microvasc Res 1970;2:224.
16. Burkel WE, McPhee M. Effect of phenol injection into peripheral nerve of rat: Electron microscope studies. Arch Phys Med Rehab 1970;51:391.
17. Bonica JJ. The management of pain of malignant disease with nerve blocks. Anesthesiology 1954;39:1249.
18. Racz GB, Heavner J, Haynsworth R. Repeat Epidural Phenol Injections in Chronic Pain and Spasticity. In S Lipton, J Miles (eds), Persistent Pain: Modern Methods of Treatment. London: Grune & Stratton, 1985;157.
19. Kuzucu EY, Derrick WS, Wilbur SA. Control of intractable pain with subarachnoid alcohol block. JAMA 1966;195:541.
20. Ventrafridda V, Spreafico R. Subarachnoid Saline Perfusion. In JJ Bonica (ed), Advances in Neurology. New York: Raven, 1974;477.
21. Racz GB, Heavner J, Singleton W, Carline M. Hypertonic Saline and Corticosteroids Injected Epidurally for Pain Control. In GB Racz (ed), Techniques of Neurolysis. London: Kluwer, 1989;73.
22. Racz GB, Holubec JT. Lysis of Adhesions in the Epidural Space. In GB Racz (ed), Techniques of Neurolysis. London: Kluwer, 1989;57.
23. Ferrer-Bredner J. Epidural and intrathecal phenol neurolysis for cancer pain. Anesthesiol Rev 1981;8:14.
24. Swerdlow M, Subarachnoid and extradural blocks. Adv Pain Res Ther 1979;2:325.
25. Jain S, Foley K, Thomas J, et al. Factors influencing efficacy of epidural neurolysis therapy for intractable cancer pain. Pain 1987;(Suppl. 4):S134.

26. Shibutani K, Kizelshteyn G, Allyne L, et al. Low volume intermittent lumbar epidural phenol injection for relief of cancer pain. Pain 1987;(Suppl. 4):S32.

27. Twycross RG. Relief of Pain. In CM Saunders (ed), The Management of Terminal Disease. Chicago: Year Book, 1978;65.

28. Nielsen OS, Munro AJ, Tannock IF. Bone metastases: Pathophysiology and management policy. J Clin Oncol 1991;9:509.

29. Metastrone Strontium-89 Chloride injection: An effective way to manage metastatic bone pain [Product insert]. England: Amersham International, 1993.

30. Loeser JDDD. Dorsal column and peripheral nerve stimulation of relief of cancer pain. Adv Pain Res Ther 1979;2:499.

31. Meglio M, Cioni B. Personal experience with spinal cord stimulation in chronic pain management. Appl Neurophysiol 1982;45:195.

32. Shealy CN, Mortimer JT, Reswick JB. Electrical inhibition of pain by stimulation of the dorsal columns: A preliminary report. Anesth Analg 1967;46:489.

33. Patt R. Pain Control in Oncology. In P Rubin (ed), Clinical Oncology Syllabus: A Multidisciplinary Approach for Medical Students and Physicians. Philadelphia: Saunders, 1991.

34. Racz GB, Lewis R, Laros G, Heavner JE. Electrical Stimulation Analgesia. In PP Raj (ed), Practical Management of Pain (2nd ed). St. Louis: Mosby, 1992;922.

35. Young RF, Brechner T. Electrical stimulation of the brain for relief of intractable pain due to cancer. Cancer 1986;57:1266.

36. Hosobuchi Y. Subcortical electrical stimulation control of intractable pain: Report of 122 cases. J Neurosurg 1986;64:543.

37. Quote from Schweitzer A. In Cancer Pain. A Monograph on the Management of Cancer Pain. A Report of the Expert Advisory Committee on the Management of Severe Chronic Pain in Cancer Patients, to the Honorable Monique Begin, Minister of National Health and Welfare, Canada, 1984.

Chapter 20

The Role of Neurolytic Procedures

Subhash Jain

Introduction

An estimated 440,000 people in the United States die from cancer each year. Most suffer from periods of severe chronic pain at various stages of their illness. The satisfactory management of cancer pain has been a difficult and frustrating goal for physicians for many years. Many modalities have been used in attempts to control or palliate the pain and suffering. These include narcotic and nonnarcotic medications, transcutaneous electrical nerve stimulation, physiotherapy and psychotherapy, hypnosis, acupuncture, and surgery.

Nerve blocks, including subarachnoid, epidural, and local injection of neurolytic agents, are part of an armamentarium available to the physician to treat intractable cancer pain. The initial neurolytic nerve blocks were plagued by problems of asepsis, inexperience, and difficulty in limiting the spread of the injected agent to the nerves responsible for the pain without compromising other structures. As a result, physicians long militated against these nerve blocks as viable options for chronic pain management.

Neural Blockade

Perineural injections of local anesthetics have been used therapeutically since the late nineteenth century following the development of the hollow needle by Rynd (1845) and Wood (1855) and the introduction of cocaine by Koller in 1884. The use of neurolytic substances to provide relief of pain for patients with cancer has been practiced since these techniques were popularized by Dogliotti,[1] Maher,[2] and others. Neither the methods of blockade nor the useful pharmacologic agents have undergone marked change over the intervening years. Contemporary applications of these techniques represent an advance in care insofar as (1) increased experience and the availability of additional alternatives permit more sophisticated decision making with regard to screening patients and selecting the proper procedure; (2) recognition of the problem of "total pain," and integration of anesthesia into a multidisciplinary matrix, promise improved overall results; and (3) an increase in the dissemination of knowledge, the number of skilled practitioners, and the frequency of evaluations and procedures performed translates into greater benefit to a greater number of patients.

Recent enhancements of neurolytic techniques include the application of more sophisticated techniques of radiologic guidance, such as computed tomographic (CT) assisted localization of the celiac axis. Although pituitary ablation does not involve destruction of a discrete neural pathway per se, its addition to the armamentarium of the anesthesiologist involved in cancer pain management represents a substantial advance. In addition, the epidural application of phenol is undergoing a resurgence of interest. Investigators have reported increased efficacy by using repeated instillation of dilute solutions of phenol through an indwelling catheter over several days. Techniques of neural blockade for treating cancer pain have progressed only modestly in recent years. Increased recognition of the value of these established techniques is related to a greater availability of skilled providers and improvements in the distribution of knowledge. This permits the greatest use of recent advances with enhanced opportunities to relieve pain and suffering.

General Considerations

Despite limited revision in the principles and techniques of neurolytic blocks, guidelines for their use in clinical practice are presented to define their role in the context of comprehensive cancer pain management, and by virtue of their unique utility to the anesthesiologist involved in managing cancer pain. Standard sources are recommended for the practitioner interested in technical details of individual procedures.[3, 4]

Consideration for neurolytic intervention in patients with cancer-related pain is indicated when pain symptoms cannot be controlled adequately with medications and other conservative therapy, and when life expectancy is limited. Failed conservative care exists when pain persists despite escalation of therapeutic measures or when side effects related to those measures are viewed as intolerable by the patient, family, or physician. Restrictions related to life expectancy are not rigid. Upper limits of 6–18 months have been recommended, but each case should be considered individually. At the opposite end of the spectrum, procedures may be performed up through the last days of life, particularly at the bedside, if warranted by unrelieved pain and suffering. Regardless, referring physicians should be encouraged to seek consultation early in the course of terminal disease because many techniques require patient cooperation to produce optimal results. Also, some series indicate a higher incidence of failure when pain has persisted for longer than 3–4 months.[5] Operant factors may include psychological maladaptation and isolation of targeted neural tissue by radiation fibrosis or malignant cells.

Patient Selection

Many investigators in this field believe that the injection of neurolytic agents for nerve blocks should follow strict guidelines and, in general, should be limited to the terminally ill patient suffering from cancer pain. Several reports describe better results when comparing neurolytic blocks for cancer and noncancer patients.[6]

Patients must undergo a full medical examination including a thorough history, physical examination, appropriate laboratory tests, and radiographic studies (CT scan, myelogram, etc.), before they are considered for a neurolytic block. Relative contraindications to nerve blocks in the back include a history of trauma, infection, or congenital anomalies. The presence of active infection at the block site or anticoagulant therapy are absolute contraindications to needle placement.

Once the primary diagnosis is established and the etiology of the patient's pain is understood, a comprehensive pain management plan can be designed, incorporating considerations for future problems resulting from progression of the disease.

Initially, aggressive narcotic and nonnarcotic medication should be used to relieve the pain. Fears of addiction and tolerance are appropriate, but they should not lead to the premature use of more invasive and irreversible therapies. Other modalities, such as transcutaneous electrical nerve stimulation, physical therapy, etc., can often be helpful adjuncts in controlling chronic pain. It is only after these modalities have proved unsatisfactory, either because of inadequate pain control or complications from the therapy itself (i.e., nausea, constipation, sedation, etc.), that neurolytic nerve blocks should be considered.

Neurolytic blocks should always be preceded by a temporary diagnostic block using local anesthetics. Such injections are useful in confirming the neurologic component of the pain. In addition, in many cases, various degrees of relief can be obtained from repeated blocks with local anesthetics alone.

Some cancer pain syndromes are more amenable to nerve blocks than others. These include a celiac plexus block to treat the pain of tumors of the liver, stomach, and pancreas, or paravertebral somatic blocks for patients with postthoracotomy pain. The best results often occur with patients who are blocked at an early stage of their illness.

Those patients who are extremely ill and weak or who have other medical problems that increase their risk for general anesthesia are poor candidates for surgical operations such as cordotomy. Neurolytic nerve blocks are excellent options for these patients.

In general, patients suffering from localized cancer pain, which involves visceral, somatic, traumatic, or peripheral neuralgias not primarily associated with the central neural axis, are excellent candidates for neurolytic blocks. Patients with conditions involving epidural or subarachnoid obstruction are not good candidates for block therapy.

Physiologic Considerations for a Neurolytic Block

Normal sensation is transmitted to the posterior horn of the spinal cord segment via peripheral somatic and visceral nerves. These are composed of various nerve fiber types: A fibers (further classified into alpha, beta, gamma, and delta) are myelinated fibers of various diameters (1–20 μm) and conduction velocities (12–120 m per second); B fibers are myelinated preganglionic sympathetic neurons with diameters of 1–3 μm and conduction velocities of 14 m per second; and C fibers are small unmyelinated nerves with diameters of 0.5–1.0 μm with slow conduction velocities of 1.0–1.2 m per second. Pain sensation is conveyed primarily by the A delta and C fibers. The former carry the fast, sharp-shooting pain sensations, whereas the latter carry the dull, aching, burning pains often associated with tumors.

Many investigators have demonstrated that susceptibility of nerves to instilled solutions is inversely proportional to their diameter and the presence or absence of myelin. It is therefore not surprising that differential nerve blocks are possible. One can block the sensation of pain and temperature, which is mediated by the small, thin, unmyelinated C fibers, without sacrificing the other modalities of sensation and motor control carried by the thicker, myelinated fibers. This has been demonstrated with both hypotonic and hypertonic solutions, ammonium salt mixtures, and phenol.

Neurophysiologic Aspects of Impulse Conduction

A nerve membrane is composed of a semipermeable double-thickness wall of lipid molecules with globular protein molecules interspaced throughout. Some of these proteins span the entire thickness of the membrane, creating channels that permit ions to pass through the membrane. Sodium is actively removed out of the inner axoplasm environment; potassium is pumped internally and a high sodium concentration is maintained externally. The membrane is less permeable to sodium than to potassium, thus allowing some potassium to diffuse down its concentration gradient to the outside of the cell. This generates a relative electrical imbalance of –70 to –90 mV.

Depolarization occurs when, as a result of an electrical stimulation, the membrane becomes more permeable to sodium, allowing a sudden, massive influx internally. Depolarization continues along the nerve as the impulse is carried along. This impulse propagation can be blocked by local anesthetics and neurolytic agents. Local anesthetics produce a transient block by stopping the flow of sodium through the membrane channels. This prevents depolarization from occurring. Neurolytic solutions produce a permanent block through the disruption and destruction of nerve tissue. Such a block remains until the nerve tissues regenerate.

Neurolytic Drugs

Alcohol is commercially available in 1-ml ampules as a colorless solution that can be injected readily through small-bore needles and is hypobaric with respect to cerebrospinal fluid (CSF). Depending on the site of injection and the concentration of alcohol, administration is accompanied by a variable degree of discomfort that, at its extreme, is excruciating but transient. It is generally used undiluted (absolute or 100% alcohol) and, if left exposed to the atmosphere, will be diluted by absorbed moisture. Denervation and pain relief sometimes accrue over a few days following injection. Injectable phenol requires preparation by a pharmacist. The process for this has been described by Raj.[7] Various concentrations of phenol prepared with saline, water, glycerine, and different radiologic dyes have been advocated. Phenol is relatively insoluble in water (Table 20-1), and at room temperature, concentrations in excess of 6.7% cannot be obtained without the addition of glycerine. Phenol mixed in glycerine is hyperbaric with respect to CSF but is so viscous that, even when warmed, injection is difficult through needles smaller than 20

Table 20-1. Differences Between Two Commonly Used Neurolytic Agents

	Phenol	Alcohol
Physical properties	Clear, colorless, pungent odor; poorly soluble in water; unstable at room temperature; hyperbaric relative to CSF	Clear, colorless; readily absorbs water on exposure to air; hypobaric relative to CSF; stable at room temperature
Chemical structure	Acid	Alcohol
Concentrations used	6–10%	50–100%
Equipotent neurolytic concentrations	5%	40%
Complications	Neuritis is uncommon; hepatic and cardiac toxicity in higher doses	Neuritis is common; no hepatic or cardiac toxicity at commonly used doses
Site of use (in order of preference)	Epidural	Intrathecal
	Paravertebral	Celiac ganglion
	Peripheral nerve roots	Lumbar sympathetic chain
	Intrathecal	Cranial nerves
	Cranial nerves	Paravertebral
		Epidural (low concentrations)

CSF = cerebrospinal fluid.

gauge. Shelf life is said to exceed 1 year when preparations are refrigerated and not exposed to light. Clinically, a biphasic action has been observed, characterized by an initial local anesthetic effect producing subjective warmth and numbness, which gives way to chronic denervation. Quality and extent of analgesia may fade slightly within the first 24 hours of administration. Less commonly, ammonium sulfate and chlorocresol are used to produce neurolysis. The pathologic changes that follow the administration of neurolytic drugs, and proposed mechanisms of neurolysis, have been described in the literature.[2, 8, 9]

Effects of Neurolytic Agents on Nerve Tissue

In 1961, Gallagher et al. described demyelination and degeneration of the posterior roots following subarachnoid administration of neurolytic agents.[10] In 1964, Smith et al. reported destruction and demyelination to be localized more to the dorsal root ganglia and posterior horn cells, than in the anterior roots; however, they were unable to exclude the influence of the patient's neoplasm on this finding.[8] Initial studies of the histologic effects of hypotonic and hypertonic solutions on nerves demonstrated a poor correlation between the clinical effects and histopathology. In some cases, the unmyelinated fibers were totally destroyed and no relief was appreciated, whereas in others complete relief occurred when no appreciable nerve damage was noted.[11]

The neurolytic action of alcohol is thought to occur through a dehydration action on the nerve tissue, with the extraction of cholesterol, phospholipids, and cerebrosides and the precipitation of mucoproteins. This results in sclerosis of the nerve fibers and myelin sheath destruction.[11]

Phenol acts by protein denaturation, and like ethyl alcohol, is an extremely potent neurolytic agent. Numerous investigations have demonstrated a direct relationship between phenol concentration and extended nerve destruction in resultant block.[10, 12–15] Maher et al.[16] stated in 1957 that varied phenol concentrations in glycerine (from 3.3–10.0%) produced mostly sensory blocks with subarachnoid injection of less than 5%, whereas higher concentrations created motor blockades as well. Initial observations by Iggo and Walsh,[17] later confirmed by Nathan et al.,[13] described 5% phenol in Ringer's solution or oil contrast as producing selective blocks of smaller nerve fibers. Descriptions of low phenol concentrations as having properties similar to those of local anesthetics have also been reported.[13]

Peripheral Blockade

Peripheral neurolysis has a definite, although limited, role in the management of pain of malignant origin.[18] To ensure effective analgesia, neural interruption is planned proximal to the source of irritation. In technically difficult cases, such as blockade of upper intercostal nerves (where the overlying scapula and muscle increase the risk of a pneumothorax), a more proximal paravertebral or subarachnoid blockade should be performed. Anatomic landmarks tend to be more obvious in the presence of cachexia and weight loss. Because the sensory distribution of peripheral nerves overlaps, blockade of neighboring segments is recommended. Many peripheral nerves are of mixed function. A pretherapeutic prognostic block with local anesthetic is essential to evaluate the impact of concomitant motor deficit. In performing a peripheral neurolytic block, accuracy is essential for good results and to avoid damage to nontargeted structures. This is particularly true in the cervicofacial region, where abundant neural and vascular structures are closely spaced, and more so when alcohol or phenol are used because their diffusibility in biological tissue is less than that of the local anesthetics.

Regeneration of peripheral nerves is sometimes accompanied by the development of neuritis or neuroma formation. Alcoholic neuritis is thought to be related to incomplete destruction of somatic nerves, and the incidence is less when a solid, prolonged block has been obtained.[3] Alcohol seems to have more propensity to produce local irritation than phenol, and local reaction seems to be less common in cranial nerves than in other peripheral nerves. Central nervous system maladaptation to deafferentation, as well as local phenomena, may result in burning pain that has a potential to be even more objectionable than the original complaint of pain. The threat of postablative dysesthesia is of limited consequence when life expectancy has definite limits or when intractable pain already exceeds tolerance levels.

Cranial Nerve Block

Pain related to malignant neoplasm of the head and neck poses one of the most challenging management problems to all care providers. Conventional analgesic therapy may prove inadequate, partly because of the failure of physiologic splinting, a normal coping strategy that is unavailable when pain is aggravated by relatively involuntary activities such as swallowing, eating, talking, and moving the head. Cephalic pain is rarely limited to the distribution of a single nerve because of overlapping sensory innervation (cranial nerves V, VII, IX, and X; dorsal roots of the second and third cervical nerves). Major surgical intervention introduces considerable risks of mortality and morbidity and is regarded by many neurosurgeons as a last resort. Surgery is often accompanied by prolonged hospitalization, additional functional deficit, and disfigurement, the prospects of which are poorly tolerated in the preterminal patient. When pain is intractable, nonsurgical treatment (radiotherapy, systemic and regional chemotherapy) should be aggressively pursued. If conservative measures have been exhausted, consideration should be given to analgesic methods that produce generalized effects (epidural or intraventricular narcotics, deep brain stimulation).

When pain is related to metastatic instability of the cervical spine, anterior stabilization should be considered. In a retrospective review of surgical decompression and stabilization for patients with cervical spine metastases, significant pain relief for more than 3 months was achieved in 11 of 17 patients and 5 of 11 paralyzed patients experienced significant neurologic recovery.[19]

Select patients could also benefit from blockade of the involved cranial and upper cervical nerves. When ablative blocks or surgery are being considered, local anesthetic blocks help ascertain the relative contribution of individual nerves to the painful state. Lasting pain relief is difficult to achieve with discrete nerve blocks because of sensory overlap. Also, technical difficulties may be encountered because of the tendency for tumors in these regions to erode and destroy surrounding tissue, and due to the high proportion of patients who come to treatment after surgery or radiotherapy. Oncogenic pain that is limited to the distribution of the trigeminal nerve or one of its branches may be amenable to thermal or chemical interruption of the involved nerve. When feasible, thermocoagulation may be the treatment of choice because analgesia can frequently be obtained without sensory loss. A recent analysis of a series of 21 patients treated in this fashion reported no morbidity or mortality and "very good" long-term results in more than half the patients.[20] Before a chemical block of a branch of the fifth nerve is to be undertaken, consideration should be given to the likelihood of further tumor extension and prophylactically extending the field of analgesia by blocking the gasserian ganglion.[21] Keratitis and corneal ulcer are possible complications but are of limited consequence. If extension of analgesia is necessary, consideration may be given to blocking the second and third cervical roots and the ninth and tenth cranial nerves. Bilateral block of cranial nerves IX and X should not be attempted because resulting paralysis of pharyngeal and laryngeal muscles will impair swallowing and phonation. When neural blockade is planned to eliminate pain over the occiput and neck, and there has been extensive radiotherapy, the paravertebral approach to the cervical nerves may be difficult. The epidural route should then be considered.

Sacral Nerve Block

Selective blockade of the sacral nerve roots via their dorsal foramina is a useful alternative to subarachnoid or caudal block in patients who have pain from pelvic or rectal malignant neoplasm but also have intact bowel and bladder function. Pain may be due to direct invasion, chronic infection, fistula formation, or postradiation cystitis. Diagnostic blocks of the individual sacral roots with local anesthetics performed in succession will determine the pathways involved in the transmission of pain. The second and third sacral roots are most commonly implicated in maintenance of bladder function, and unilateral predominance of innervation of detrusor reflex activity has been observed with some frequency,[22] so treatment that avoids bilateral S-2 and S-3 blocks is likely to preserve function. Of 15 patients with bladder pain (treated first with a series of prognostic local anesthetic blocks), ten were selected to receive discrete sacral nerve root blocks with 6% aqueous phenol. Seven of the ten patients experienced long-term pain relief (average, 26.5 months), and no mortality or significant morbidity was observed.[22] Good results without complications were obtained in a small series of cancer patients with perineal pain treated with injections of phenol through the fourth sacral foramen.[23]

Subarachnoid and Epidural Neurolytic Block

Several classic publications describe the techniques of these and other nerve block procedures in detail,[3, 24, 25] and the reader is encouraged to consult them to review technical aspects. The advantages of neuroaxial neurolysis are (1) a high proportion of good results in properly selected cases; (2) ease of performance with minimal requirements for equipment; (3) minimal or no requirements for hospitalization; (4) duration of pain relief that is generally adequate for the preterminal state; (5) ease of repetition when necessary; (6) suitability for aged or debilitated patients; and (7) a low complication rate when proper technique is observed.

Lytic neuroaxial block produces pain relief by chemical rhizotomy. Despite early speculation that phenol was capable of exercising selective blockade of small sensory fibers,[2] pathologic studies have demonstrated that, regardless of size, nervous fibers are affected indiscriminately by both alcohol and phenol.[8, 26] The degree and extent of sensory loss depends on the actual number of fibers destroyed rather than fiber type; this is, in turn, determined by the concentration and quantity of the neurolytic agent.[9] This relationship is supported by recent reports of higher success rates in patients with pelvic malignant neoplasms who were treated with 10% and 15% subarachnoid phenol versus a 7.5% preparation,[27] and in patients with a variety of neoplasms treated with 15% versus 10% subarachnoid phenol.[28] Controlled studies comparing the results of alcohol and phenol neurolysis are not available. Most authorities agree that neither agent offers a clear advantage, except insofar as variations in baricity relative to CSF, facilitate positioning of the patient in selected cases.[25, 29]

Dozens of reports documenting a large series of patients treated with chemical rhizolysis have appeared in the medical literature. Results are difficult to compare because of variations in patient selection, extent and type of underlying malignant neoplasms, injection techniques, and criteria for success. Swerdlow[30] has analyzed the results of 13 published series documenting the treatment of more than 2,500 patients. In 58% of patients, "good" relief was obtained, 22% achieved "fair" pain relief, and 20% had "little or no" relief. Average duration of relief is difficult to estimate but generally is regarded by authorities to be 3–4 months,[31] with a wide range of distribution. Reports of analgesia persisting longer than 1 or even 2 years are not infrequent.[30]

Chemical rhizolysis can be performed at any level up to the midcervical region. Above this level, the spread of caustic agent to medullary centers carries significant risk of cardiorespiratory collapse. Subarachnoid injections of phenol at the C-3 to C-4 interspace have been performed without complications.[5] Access to the subarachnoid and epidural spaces above the lumbar region presents a technical challenge that decreases as experience accumulates.

Cervical Block

Some investigators have reported only fair results when using subarachnoid phenol rhizolysis for brachial and upper thoracic pain,[32] a phenomenon that has also been observed after neurosurgical procedures for brachiothoracic pain.[33, 34] The aggressive growth characteristics of lesions involving the brachial plexus and chest wall may play a role. Nevertheless, in carefully selected patients, cervicothoracic subarachnoid and epidural neurolysis have been found to relieve upper extremity pain with relative success.[2, 24] These options are not considered unless pain is intractable and so severe as to render the involved limb immobile and useless. An early trial of stellate ganglion blocks is useful to exclude sympathetically mediated pain that could be permanently blocked without sacrificing function.[35, 36] When pain does not involve the whole extremity, paravertebral or more distal nerve blocks may be considered to preserve maximum function. Brachial plexus block with dilute phenol has been reported in a small number of patients as being moderately effective but introduces the risk of spread to adjacent structures and may require frequent repetition.[37] When pain is related to infiltration of the brachial plexus with tumor or radiation fibrosis, neuroaxial block with phenol or alcohol will often provide effective relief. Motor and proprioceptive deficit are anticipated, thus emphasizing the importance of careful patient selection.

Thoracic Block

Patients with radicular thoracic or upper abdominal pain are ideal candidates for discrete chemical rhizotomy because medication can be introduced distant from the major limb plexuses and the origin of nerves subserving bladder and bowel function. Intercostal muscle paresis may occur despite meticulous positioning but seldom produces increased respiratory compromise. Indeed, it is observed once splinting has been eliminated by successful neural blockade.

Lumbar Block

When using subarachnoid techniques for pain in regions subserved by the lumbar nerves, it is important to observe the rule that instillation of a neurolytic substance should be planned at the level at which the involved nerve roots exit from the spinal cord rather than their site of egress from the vertebral column. The more proximal site of injection affords greater surface area for exposure of the targeted neural tissue to the neurolytic drug,[3] and, more importantly, because the terminal portions of distal nerves are less exposed to the neurolytic agent, more discrete analgesia can be expected and the incidence of complications should be reduced. Charts indicating the relationship between the spinal column and the nerve roots as they emerge from the spinal cord[3] should be carefully checked before each procedure. By using this method, access to lumbar nerve roots is gained through dural puncture between the low thoracic vertebrae. Additional precautions undertaken to maximize efficacy and limit complications include the use of an operating room-type table that can be readily manipulated, careful attention to maintenance of patient posture, and conservative selection of dosage and rate of injection. Maximum suggested doses should be respected,[3, 38] and communication with the patient is essential to verify the desired location and extent of blockade. For safety measures, it is better to expose the patient to a repeated procedure or to inject small boluses through multiple needles than to exceed standard recommendations.[3, 38] Patients need to be told in advance that although the actual puncture and injection ordinarily produces only minimal discomfort, maintenance of optimal posture for 15–30 minutes after the neurolytic drug has been instilled may produce more discomfort.

Bowel and bladder dysfunction are the two most feared complications of neuroaxial lytic block;

however, their actual incidence and severity are low when proper technique is observed, regardless of the agent used.

Saddle Block

Perineal and pelvic pain are amenable to neuroaxial lytic blockade by several routes. A useful approach for unilateral pain involves placing the patient in a lateral position (dependency dictated by choice of agent) and injecting the neurolytic agent through a low lumbar puncture. If pain is bilateral, the procedure can be repeated after a few days with the patient's position reversed. It is not uncommon for bilateral pain to resolve significantly after a unilateral block, making a second procedure unnecessary.[39] Alternatively, a true saddle block can be used for pain that crosses the midline.[25] Hyperbaric phenol is introduced through a low lumbar puncture, and the patient is maintained in the sitting position modified by a 45-degree posterior tilt for 15–30 minutes. Recently, the injection of small volumes of dilute phenol via the caudal route has been described in a series of 26 patients with perianal pain due to malignant neoplasm.[40] Pain relief persisted for a mean of just 12.7 days, but only one complication (transient urinary retention) was described. Despite all precautions, at least temporary urinary or even anal dysfunction can be anticipated in a high proportion of these patients, these techniques should be reserved for patients with indwelling catheters or patients who are bedridden and accept the risk of additional deficit.

Subarachnoid Versus Epidural Neurolysis

Subarachnoid neurolysis offers the following potential advantages over classic epidural techniques: (1) Return of CSF verifies subarachnoid needle placement, whereas localization of the epidural space must be inferred from the results of epidurograms and test doses of local anesthetic. (2) Subarachnoid neurolysis generally results in more profound analgesia, and as a result, reinjection is required less often. This phenomenon is probably related to increased direct contact between drug and targeted nerve roots. (3) Subarachnoid injection is readily performed on an outpatient basis, or even at the bedside. Recent recommendations that epidural neurolysis be accomplished by repeated administration of phenol through an indwelling catheter mandate inpatient hospitalization. (4) Although reports indicate that gravity and position can be partially relied on to control the effect of epidural block with hyperbaric phenol,[41] these factors can be used to exert more precise control in the case of subarachnoid injection. (5) The excessive viscosity of pure phenol-glycerine preparations prevents injection through small caliber tubing. If epidural block is planned with the intention of reapplication through a catheter, then the phenol-glycerine mixture must be diluted with water, saline, or dye, thus reducing viscosity and introducing the potential for reduced control of spread. A newly designed epidural catheter made from spiral stainless steel coils coated with fluoropolymers has recently been introduced with intention of facilitating radiologic localization, aspiration, and repositioning.[42] No controlled studies have been conducted comparing epidural and subarachnoid neurolysis. The main advantage of phenol epidural neurolysis is its applicability for pain that occupies a wide distribution or is bilateral. Despite the considerations noted previously, the main disadvantages cited for classic epidural neurolysis are impressions of a shorter duration of action and inferior intensity of analgesia when compared with subarachnoid techniques.[30] Recent studies suggest that these shortcomings may be overcome by repeated administration over time through an indwelling catheter.[43–45] Epidural injection has been postulated to limit spread to dorsal nerve roots,[44] which should reduce the likelihood of motor dysfunction. Using an in vitro model, Racz et al.[45] have demonstrated that sections of canine dura apposed to reservoirs of CSF are relatively impermeable to 2.75% and 5.5% phenol in saline. Risks of meningeal irritation, postdural puncture headache, and intracranial spread are less with epidural than subarachnoid neurolysis.[30]

The most commonly recommended neurolytic agent for epidural use is still phenol. Despite reports of favorable results using alcohol,[46] its instillation in awake patients produces agonizing pain[31] unless preceded by injections of local anesthetic, which reduce predictability. Postinjection neuropathy and neuralgia have been observed after epidural alcohol.

Sympathetic Nerve Block

Local anesthetic infiltration of the sympathetic nervous outflow can be performed for diagnostic, prognostic, or therapeutic purposes. A diagnostic nerve block helps establish the relative contribution of the autonomic versus somatic nervous system to pain transmission. Response to local anesthetic blockade helps determine whether repeated local anesthetic blocks, a neurolytic block, or surgery is likely to provide prolonged relief. Finally, in carefully selected patients, a therapeutic effect may be obtained either by serial injections of a local anesthetic drug or by the injection of a neurolytic agent.

Cervicothoracic (Stellate) Ganglion Block

Repeated sympathetic nerve blocks with local anesthetic are a well-documented method of relieving the pain of reflex sympathetic dystrophy[47, 48] and may also be of value for tumor-induced sympathetic mediated pain as well. This phenomenon has been most thoroughly documented for brachiocephalic pain because carefully performed local anesthetic stellate ganglion blocks are well tolerated and practitioners are reluctant to inject neurolytic agents in the vicinity of the stellate ganglion. Neurolytic stellate ganglion block is regarded as hazardous because the cervicothoracic ganglion may be difficult to locate precisely and spread to nontargeted structures may produce severe complications due to the close proximity of major neurovascular structures. Specific risks include erosion, thrombosis or spasm of major vessels, cerebral infarction from intravascular injection, prolonged hoarseness from spread to the recurrent laryngeal nerve, upper limb dysfunction if elements of the brachial plexus are affected, and sloughing of the superficial tissues. Nevertheless, there have been anecdotal reports of stellate gangliolysis performed with up to 10 ml of 6% aqueous phenol with good results and no complications.[35] Bonica[3] reserves neurolytic stellate block for exceptional cases and then limits the injectate to either a small volume of phenol or no more than 1.5 ml of absolute alcohol. Lofstrom and Cousins[49] recommend 1–2 ml of 6% aqueous phenol in iothalamate meglumine (Conray) dye. If surgical sympathectomy is contraindicated re-quiring a neurolytic stellate block to be undertaken, the following precautions should be observed: (1) a thorough trial of local anesthetic blockade; (2) careful explanation of the procedure and its possible sequelae; (3) radiologic visualization of a characteristic spread of contrast medium[50]; (4) meticulous aspiration and needle immobilization; (5) evidence of sympathetic block following the injection of 1–2 ml of local anesthetic solution; (6) injection of 1–2 ml of dilute neurolytic preparation (3–6% phenol); and (7) flushing the needle before its removal.

Lumbar Sympathetic Block

Neurolysis of the lumbar sympathetic ganglia may be undertaken provided that trials of local anesthetic injections have been shown to provide pain relief. In the presence of malignant disease, the most common indication for lumbar sympatholysis is pelvic pain of urologic, gynecologic, or rectal origin. Other indications include lower extremity pain from lymphedema or reflex sympathetic imbalance. With simple attention to detail, risks of interference with bladder and bowel function are virtually nonexistent.

Lumbar sympathetic block, as described by Mandl in 1926 and subsequently modified,[3] is accomplished by injecting through three needles positioned with their tips anterior to the psoas muscle, at the anterolateral aspect of the bodies of the second, third, and fourth lumbar vertebrae. In keeping with Winnie's[51] concept of "plexus anesthesia," it has become common practice to substitute a single injection of a large volume of local anesthetic solution (up to 20–30 ml) through a single needle positioned in the correct fascial plane near the second lumbar vertebra. Results are comparable, and patient discomfort is reduced.[49] A recently published fluoroscopic and pathologic analysis of the relevant regional anatomy in cadavers suggests useful guidelines for the single-needle technique.[52] In a small series of patients, complications were not observed after injections of 10 ml of 10% phenol through a single needle.[53] The concern that large volumes of injectate may spread outside the correct fascial compartment to involve lumbar somatic nerves still influences most practitioners to use two or three needles when a neurolytic agent is employed.[49]

Celiac Plexus Block

Neurolytic celiac plexus block (NCPB) has received widespread attention because of its excellent potential to relieve upper abdominal and referred back pain secondary to malignant neoplasm involving structures derived from the foregut. The most common indication for celiac plexus block is pancreatic cancer, which, contrary to traditional teaching, is frequently associated with painful rather than painless jaundice. Also, NCPB is efficacious for pain associated with neoplasms involving the distal esophagus, stomach, liver and bile ducts, small bowel, proximal colon, adrenals, and kidneys. The posterior percutaneous approach, introduced by Kappis (1914) and popularized by Moore[54] and others, which uses two needles (6 inch, 20-gauge) is most commonly advocated. There has been renewed interest in using an anterior approach, as radiologists have become more experienced with this route for biopsy and drainage procedures. Ischia et al.[55] have reported on a transaortic technique that is similar to conventional approaches, except that the needle is deliberately passed through the aorta in a manner resembling the transarterial method of brachial plexus blockade. No complications occurred in 28 patients treated with this method. Pain relief was obtained in 93% of patients, and favorable patterns of dye dispersion were consistently observed. Another recent modification (described by Singler[56]) involves deliberate perforation of the diaphragmatic crura under CT guidance to ensure the spread of injectate anterior to the aorta. An underused approach is injection under direct vision by the surgeon at the time of laparotomy. At times, this may not be possible because diagnosis is made on a nonsurgical basis or because of the presence of diffuse intra-abdominal disease. By using an intraoperative injection, an 88% incidence of postoperative pain relief was reported by Flanigan and Kraft,[57] with a mean duration of 4.3 months. They recommended that when intraoperative injection is not possible, a radiolucent clip be placed in the region of the celiac axis to facilitate postoperative percutaneous localization. Surgeons need to be made aware of the potential of this maneuver to relieve postoperative suffering.

An 85–94% incidence of good-to-excellent pain relief has been obtained in several large series of patients undergoing NCPB for pain from pancreatic cancer per se[58] or a variety of intra-abdominal conditions,[59,65] although repetition is required in some patients. In a series of 136 patients,[58] analgesia was present until the time of death in 75% of cases, and in an additional 12.5% of cases pain relief was maintained for more than 50% of survival time.

The location of the celiac axis deep within the retroperitoneum near the vertebral column in close proximity to major vessels (aorta, vena cava, and their branches) and viscera (kidneys, pleura) provides the potential for devastating complications. Reported complications include pneumothorax, chylothorax, pleural effusion, convulsions, and paraplegia.[58–64] Nevertheless, the results of several large series indicate that, given sufficient attention to detail, the incidence of complications should be minimal. In a series of 136 patients, the only significant complication was pneumothorax, which occurred in two patients, neither of whom required tube thoracostomy.[58] Also, of 114 blocks performed in another group of 100 patients, the only significant complication was partial unilateral lower extremity paralysis in an obese patient who could not be positioned properly.[59] Postural hypotension and diarrhea occur frequently but are usually self-limited.

Using roentgenographic and CT controls, Moore et al.[65] studied needle trajectories and the distribution of injectate in patients and, at autopsy, in cadaveric specimens. They concluded that at the level of the inferior border of the twelfth rib, an insertion site no greater than 7.0–7.5 cm lateral to the corresponding spinous process is desirable to avoid renal puncture. Their findings also suggested that to produce optimal results: (1) two needles should be used, (2) 25 ml of solution should be injected through each needle, and (3) proper depth of insertion may slightly exceed that which has been traditionally taught. The findings of another recent cadaveric study[66] emphasize anatomic variability but suggest that superior results can be obtained by placing the left-sided needle tip at the junction of the lower and middle thirds of the first lumbar vertebral body, and the right-sided needle tip 1 cm higher. The authors also suggest that when the celiac artery can be identified, injection should be planned 0.5–1.0 cm below the origin of the artery.

The role of roentgenographic, fluoroscopic, and CT guidance is controversial. Most authors agree that when neurolytic solutions are to be injected, some form of radiographic verification is desirable from medicolegal and technical standpoints, although the possibility of a complication is still not excluded. The use of CT adds to the cost, procedure time, and logistic difficulties but provides improved documentation of the spread of injectate and relationships among needle trajectory, viscera, and vasculature. No controlled studies have compared the results of NCPB performed with and without different radiographic controls; nevertheless, our opinion is that some form of radiologic guidance is mandatory, and the use of CT guidance is highly desirable.

Superior Hypogastric Block

Intractable pelvic pain syndrome is a great challenge to the oncologist and pain physician. The etiology of pelvic pain can be due to malignancy of pelvic organ, i.e., rectum, vagina, cervix, and other pelvic organs. The pain is often somatic, visceral, or a combination of both. The pelvic organs are innervated by somatic and sympathetic fibers. With advanced pelvic malignancy, the incidence of pain can be as high as 95%. The initial pain syndrome is treated with oral medications. However, a select group of patients require neuroablative and neurolytic procedures.

The role of hypogastric plexus was described by Jain et al.[67] and Plancarte et al.[68] in 1990. Hypogastric neurolysis is indicated for only a select group of patients after other modalities have failed to relieve intractable pain.[69] The technique requires adequate support of biplanar radiologic facilities. The diagnostic and therapeutic blockades require a well-trained physician because an injury to sacral nerve fibers or hollow viscus, i.e., rectum, bladder, or ureter, can occur.

Conclusion

Chronic pain patients are often physically and emotionally drained. They are often frustrated by inadequacies of other therapeutic options and arrive with expectations of miracles. Patient selection and education is therefore essential, as there are limitations, complications, and side effects that these patients must accept prior to initiating such a block. Such preliminary discussions are also helpful in avoiding legal proceedings by an already litigious population.

Many new ways to control chronic pain are now being explored. One option is placement of an indwelling epidural catheter with an embedded subcutaneous pump or reservoir for the instillation of narcotics or local anesthetics. Another involves the surgical placement of dorsal root column nerve stimulation wire to block pain relays to the higher centers. At present, these options are available to only a small portion of the population who suffer from chronic pain.

Neurolytic nerve blocks offer an excellent option for the physician trying to control chronic pain in cancer patients. The success of these nerve blocks is mostly dependent on the patient's understanding and cooperation and the experience of the physician. With proper training and experience, physicians can use these blocks help provide pain relief.

References

1. Dogliotti AM. Traitement des syndromes douloreux de la peripherie par l'alcolisation subarachnoidienne des racines posterieures a leur emergence de la moelle epiniere. Presse Med 1931;39:1249.
2. Maher RM. Relief of pain in incurable cancer. Lancet 1955;1:18.
3. Bonica JJ. Management of Pain. Philadelphia: Lea & Febiger, 1954;672.
4. Cousins MJ, Bridenbaugh PO (eds). Neural Blockade (2nd ed). Philadelphia: Lippincott, 1988.
5. Stovner J, Endresen R. Intrathecal phenol for cancer pain. Acta Anaesth Scand 1972;16:17.
6. Wilkinson MA, Mark VH, White JC. Further experiences with intrathecal phenol for the relief of pain. J Chronic Dis 1964;13:1055.
7. Raj PP (ed). Practical Management of Pain. Chicago: Year Book, 1986;857.
8. Smith MC. Histological findings following intrathecal injections of phenol solutions for relief of pain. Br J Anaesth 1963;36:387.
9. Stewart WA, Lourie H. An experimental evaluation of the effects of subarachnoid injections of phenol-pantopaque in cats: A histological study. J Neurosurg 1963;20:64.
10. Gallagher HS, Yonezawa T, Hoy RC, Derrick WS. Subarachnoid alcohol block II: Histologic changes in the central nervous system. Am J Pathol 1961;38:679.
11. Cousins MJ, Bridenburgh PO. Neural Blockade in Clinical Anesthesia and Management of Pain. Philadelphia: Lippincott, 1980.

12. Nathan PW, Scott TG. Intrathecal phenol for intractable pain. Safety and dangers of method. Lancet 1958;1:76.

13. Nathan PW, Sears TA, Smith MC. Effects of phenol solution on the nerve roots of the cats an electrophysiological and histological study. J Neurol Sci 1965;2:7.

14. Nourj Eldin F. Preliminary report uptake of phenol by vascular and brain tissue. Microvasc Res 1970;2:224.

15. Pappo I, Visca A. Phenol rhizotomy in the treatment of cancer pain. Anesth Analg 1974;53:6.

16. Maher RM. Neurone selection in relief of pain. Further experiences with intrathecal injection. Lancet 1957;1:6.

17. Iggo A, Walsh EG. Selective block of small fibers in the spinal roots by phenol. Brain 1960;83:701.

18. Doyle D. Nerve blocks in advanced cancer. Practitioner 1982;226:539.

19. DeWald R, Bridwell KH, Prodramas C, et al. Reconstructive spinal surgery as palliation for metastatic malignancies of the spine. Spine 1985;10:21.

20. Siegfried J, Broggi G. Percutaneous thermocoagulation of the gasserian ganglion in the treatment of pain in advanced cancer. Adv Pain Res Ther 1979;2:463.

21. Madrid JL, Bonica JJ. Cranial nerve blocks. Adv Pain Res Ther 1979;2:347.

22. Simon DL, Carron H, Rowlingson JC. Treatment of bladder pain with transsacral nerve block. Anesth Analg 1983;61:46.

23. Robertson DH. Transsacral neurolytic nerve block. Br J Anaesth 1983;55:873.

24. Bonica JJ. The management of pain of malignant disease with nerve blocks. Anesthesiology 1954;15:280.

25. Swerdlow M. Intrathecal neurolysis. Anaesthesia 1978;33:733.

26. Peyton WT, Semansky EJ, Baker AB. Subarachnoid injection of alcohol for relief of intractable pain with discussion of cord changes found at autopsy. Am J Cancer 1937;30:709.

27. Ischia S, Luzzani A, Ischia A, et al. Subarachnoid neurolytic block (L5-T) and unilateral percutaneous cervical cordotomy in the treatment of pain secondary to pelvic malignant disease. Pain 1984;20:139.

28. Takagi Y, Koyama T, Yamamoto Y. Subarachnoid neurolytic block with 15% phenol glycerine in the treatment of cancer pain. Pain 1987;S4:T33.

29. Katz J. Current role of neurolytic agents. Adv Neurol 1974;4:471.

30. Swerdlow M. Subarachnoid and extradural blocks. Adv Pain Res Ther 1979;2:325.

31. Holland AJC, Youssef M. A complication of subarachnoid phenol blockade. Anaesthesia 1979;34:260.

32. Swerdlow M. Spinal and peripheral neurolysis for managing Pancoast syndrome. Adv Pain Res Ther 1982;4:135.

33. Pagni CA. Neurosurgical treatment: Status of the problem. Adv Pain Res Ther 1982;4:165.

34. White JC, Sweet WH. Pain and the Neurosurgeon: A 40-Year Experience. Springfield, IL: Thomas, 1969.

35. DeBacker LJ, Kienzle WK, Keasling HH. A study of stellate ganglion block for pain relief. Anesthesiology 1959;20:618.

36. Warfield CA, Crews DA. Use of stellate ganglion blocks in the treatment of intractable limb pain in lung cancer. Clin J Pain 1987;3:13.

37. Mullin V. Brachial plexus block with phenol for painful arm associated with Pancoast's syndrome. Anesthesiology 1980;53:431.

38. Hay RC. Subarachnoid alcohol block in the control of intractable pain. Anesth Analg 1962;41:12.

39. Watson CPN, Evans RJ. Intractable pain with cancer of the rectum. Pain Clin 1986;1:29.

40. Rohde J, Hankemeier U. Neurolytic caudal blocks for the relief of perianal cancer pain. Pain 1987;S4:T32.

41. Ferrer-Brechner T. Epidural and intrathecal phenol neurolysis for cancer pain. Anesthesiol Rev 1981;8:14.

42. Racz GB, Sabonghy M, Gintautas J. Intractable pain therapy using a new epidural catheter. JAMA 1982;24B:579.

43. Jain S, Foley K, Thomas J, et al. Factors influencing efficacy of epidural neurolysis therapy for intractable cancer pain. Pain 1987;S4:T34.

44. Shibutani K, Kizelshteyn G, Allyne L, et al. Low volume intermittent lumbar epidural phenol injection for relief of cancer pain. Pain 1987;S4:T32.

45. Racz GB, Heavner J, Haynsworth R. Repeat Epidural Phenol Injections in Chronic Pain and Spasticity. In S Lipton, J Miles (eds), Persistent Pain. New York: Grune & Stratton, 1985;157.

46. Korevaar WC, Kline MT, Donnelly CC. Thoracic epidural neurolysis using alcohol. Pain 1987;S4:T33.

47. Miller RD, Munger WL, Powell PE. Chronic Pain and Local Anesthetic Neural Blockade. In MJ Cousins, PO Bridenbaugh (eds), Neural Blockade (1st ed). Philadelphia: Lippincott, 1980;616.

48. Payne R. Clinical neuropathic pain syndromes, with special reference to causalgia and reflex sympathetic dystrophy. Clin J Pain 1986;2:59.

49. Lofstrom JB, Cousins MJ. Sympathetic Neural Blockade of Upper and Lower Extremity. In MJ Cousins, PO Bridenbaugh (eds), Neural Blockade (2nd ed). Philadelphia: Lippincott, 1988;461.

50. Carron H, Litwiller R. Stellate ganglion block. Anesth Analg 1975;54:567.

51. Winnie AP. Plexus Anesthesia. Philadelphia: Saunders, 1983.

52. Umeda S, Toshiyuki A, Hatano Y, et al. Cadaver anatomic analysis of the best site for chemical lumbar sympathectomy. Anesth Analg 1987;66:643.

53. Goucke CR, Lovegrove FTA, Finch PM. Lumbar sympathectomy: Spread of radiopharmaceuticals following a single needle technique. Br J Anaesth 1987;59:944.

54. Moore DC. Regional Block (4th ed). Springfield, IL: Thomas, 1975.

55. Ischia S, Luzzani A, Ischia A, et al. A new approach to the neurolytic block of the coeliac plexus: The transaortic technique. Pain 1983;16:333.

56. Singler RC. An improved technique for alcohol neurolysis of the celiac plexus. Anesthesiology 1982;56:137.

57. Flanigan DP, Kraft R. Continuing experience with palliative chemical splanchnicectomy. Arch Surg 1978;113:509.

58. Brown DL, Bulley CK, Quiel EC. Neurolytic celiac plexus block for pancreatic cancer pain. Anesth Analg 1987;66:869.

59. Thompson GE, Moore DC, Bridenbaugh PO, et al. Abdominal pain and alcohol celiac plexus nerve block. Anesth Analg 1977;56:1.

60. Jones J, Gough D. Coeliac plexus block with alcohol for relief of upper abdominal pain due to cancer. Ann R Coll Surg Engl 1977;59:46.

61. Benzon HT. Convulsions secondary to intravascular phenol: A hazard of celiac plexus block. Anesth Analg 1979;58:150.

62. Yoshihisa F, Takaori M. Pleural effusion after CT-guided alcohol celiac plexus block. Anesth Analg 1987;66:911.

63. Galizea EJ, Lahiri SK. Paraplegia following coeliac plexus block with phenol. Br J Anaesth 1974;46:539.

64. Fine PG, Bubela C. Chylothorax following celiac plexus block. Anesthesiology 1985;63:454.

65. Moore DC, Bush WH, Burnett LL. Celiac plexus block: A roentgenographic, anatomic study of technique and spread of solution in patients and corpses. Anesth Analg 1981;60:369.

66. Ward EM, Rorie DK, Nauss LA, et al. The celiac ganglia in man: Normal anatomic variations. Anesth Analg 1979;58:461.

67. Jain S, Kestenbaum A, Shah N, Khan Y. Hypogastric plexus block: A new technique for treatment of perineal pain. Anesth Analg 1990;70:S175.

68. Plancarte R, Amescua C, Patt RB, et al. Superior hypogastric plexus block for pelvic cancer pain. Anesthesiology 1990;73:236.

69. Deleon-Cassasola, OA, Kent E, Lema MJ, et al. Neurolytic superior hypogastric plexus block for chronic pelvic pain associated with cancer. Pain 1993;54:145.

Chapter 21

Psychological Intervention

Janice M. Livengood

It has been said that pain is no longer considered simply a nociceptive event, but rather is recognized as a psychological one involving nociception, pain perception, and pain expression.[1–11] This is particularly true for cancer pain. Psychological variables contributing to the cancer pain experience include anxiety, depression, perception of control, the meaning of pain from the patient's perspective, fear of death, and hopelessness.[1–8, 10, 12–18]

This chapter has three objectives: (1) to examine the reasons why psychological intervention should be used in the treatment of cancer pain patients; (2) to identify appropriate psychological intervention strategies; and (3) to suggest ways that psychological interventions can be effectively incorporated into the treatment process.

Use of Psychological Intervention

Because emotions are thought to play a role in the development and course of cancer,[15, 19] attention to psychological issues may, in conjunction with standard treatment for cancer, alter the course of malignancy.[15] Emotional responses and characteristics found to correlate with an undesirable course of malignancy include depression, denial, repression, defensiveness, and rigidity of beliefs.[15] Characteristics that correlate with a positive outcome include emotional resiliency, physical activity, flexibility of beliefs, strong self-concept, and social autonomy.[15] Patients with advanced cancer who received psychological intervention along with medical treatment survived twice as long as would have been expected based on the national average.[15] The goal of psychotherapy, however, is not to extend life, but to make life more meaningful.[16] In fact, the major goal is to enhance the patient's sense of personal control, or self-efficacy.

One may ask, "How can an individual's psychological state affect cancer pain, and how can psychological intervention be of help?" An individual's psychological state is known to be associated with increased *perception* of pain.[2, 14, 20] For example, the patient's perception of new pain may be interpreted as a worsening of the disease, in which case the patient may benefit from identifying and clarifying any misperceptions. Pain that the patient may perceive to indicate a new growth or tumor may, in reality, be pain caused by increased muscle tension due to excessive worry and anxiety.[21] According to Payne and Foley,[22] 10% of cancer patients have pain unrelated to the cancer or the cancer therapy. Unfortunately, patients do not always tell the physician about new pain or increased pain for many reasons including the following: (1) they want to be considered a "good patient"; (2) they are afraid they will not get attention and care if they complain; (3) they fear the pain will worsen later and their doctor will not believe them if they continue to complain; or (4) they fear that increased medication may lead to addiction. In these cases, a psychologist can help the patient learn to communicate with the physician in such a way that the physician can understand the patient's concerns and adjust treatment accordingly. In addition, the patient's improved ability to appropriately communicate his or her needs can lead to increased self-efficacy, increased self-esteem, and the feeling of being "heard" by the medical profession.

Another way the patient's perception can affect cancer pain is that the pain may be perceived as uncontrollable. This belief leads to feelings of hopelessness, helplessness, depression, and anxiety. The patient may also fear abandonment, i.e., he or she may fear that the medical staff will be unable to help and will eventually leave the patient to let him or her struggle alone. The psychologist can help the patient learn self-control techniques such as relaxation skills, diaphragmatic breathing, and appropriate self talk, all of which can help reduce muscle tension or muscle spasms; increase blood flow by decreasing sympathetic arousal; control mood states, such as anxiety and depression; and enhance self-esteem and restore a sense of control. Patients can regain a sense of self-control if they can identify and correct distorted perceptions, misinterpretations, unrealistic expectations, and irrational beliefs.[1, 2, 12, 14, 21, 23] Some examples of these misinterpretations and irrational beliefs include the following: "Pain is inevitable because I have cancer"; "I'm not going to be able to cope with my pain"; "The medical staff is not going to be able to help me reduce this pain"; or "Any new pain I experience means I'm going to die sooner." Patients can be taught to monitor their thought processes and replace irrational thoughts with more rational ones.

The incorporation of psychological intervention into cancer pain management can provide the patient with the support, knowledge, and skills necessary to restore a sense of control,[1] and to enhance effective communication between the patient and physician so that optimal care can be provided. The goal is not to eliminate pain, although the patient's pain intensity may be reduced, but to help the patient realize he or she is not helpless in dealing with the pain and to help the patient live a more effective and satisfying life.[24]

Strategies

Psychological intervention strategies include behavioral and cognitive-behavioral techniques, education, and supportive psychotherapy.[1–10, 12–18, 21–39] These strategies are most effective if applied within a systems framework.[40]

Behavioral and Cognitive Behavioral Therapy

Overt behaviors are modified in behavioral therapy; covert behaviors are modified in cognitive-behavioral therapy. Overt behaviors include physiologic pain reactions (such as muscle tension, as a response to painful stimulation), respondent pain behaviors (such as bracing, limping, guarding, grimacing, sighing), and operant pain behaviors (such as verbal complaints, temper tantrums, and inactivity).[12] Covert behaviors include cognitions, which are subjective mental phenomena such as perceptions, thoughts, images, beliefs, interpretations, and expectations.[12] Cognition (or cognitive processes) can also refer to mental activities involved in the management of situations, such as problem solving or coping.[12] The goal of behavioral and cognitive-behavioral therapy is to increase adaptive behaviors and cognitions, such as the use of coping and problem-solving skills, and to decrease maladaptive behaviors and cognitions, such as muscle tension, grimacing, and imagining catastrophes. The term *maladaptive* refers to behaviors and cognitions that increase, rather than decrease, the suffering associated with cancer and pain.[12]

Behavioral methods of intervention include self-monitoring, systematic desensitization, and contingency management.[3, 10, 23, 26, 33, 41] *Self-monitoring* is the ability to monitor one's behaviors, allowing the individual to notice his or her dysfunctional reactions and control them. *Systematic desensitization* is helpful in extinguishing anticipatory anxiety that leads to avoidant behaviors and in remobilizing inactive patients. This treatment can be applied effectively to patients' fears of painful treatment procedures. A hierarchy of anxiety-producing experiences is listed by the patient and then each is paired with relaxation until the patient no longer associates anxiety with the previously anxiety-producing experience.[1] *Contingency management* is a method to reinforce only "well" behaviors, thereby modifying dysfunctional operant pain behaviors associated with secondary gain.[12, 23]

Cognitive-behavioral therapy is a therapeutic process to help individuals modify their behaviors and feelings by altering their patterns of thought. Thus, the focus of such therapies is on monitoring and changing one's negative, erroneous thinking or negative self-statements that lead to undesirable responses. Eight styles of negative thinking include blaming, "shoulds," polarized thinking, imagining catastrophes, control fallacies, emotional reasoning, filtering, and entitlement fallacy.[42]

Blaming involves making someone or something else responsible for one's pain. Although it is a natural outgrowth of being tired, frustrated, and angry, blaming only makes a bad situation worse, because instead of taking responsibility for what is happening, the patient expects others to assume that responsibility. However, some people go too far in the other direction and focus all the blame on themselves, which is a self-defeating stance that can serve as an excuse for inactivity.[42]

"Shoulds" are the cornerstone of irrational thinking. They can be either a way to admonish oneself for not being perfect or a way of creating a set of expectations for other people to meet.[42] Examples of shoulds include, "I shouldn't have to hurt like this," or "My doctor should have been able to end my pain by now."

Polarized thinking is the process of thinking all in one way, e.g., black or white, good or bad, all or nothing. Polarized thinking assumes that things must go perfectly and often leads to damaging overgeneralizations. This thinking can be directed toward the medical profession, e.g., "If they can't cure me, then they are useless."[42]

Imagining catastrophes is the process of reacting to life situations by imagining the worst possible outcome and then reacting to these fears as though they will in fact come true. "What if" statements characterize catastrophic thinking and add greatly to anxiety levels.[42] Some examples of what ifs include, "What if I never get control of my pain," or "What if my doctor gives up on me."

Control fallacies involve seeing oneself as "externally controlled" by others, such as by the medical profession. By giving a doctor or a clinic total power over their fate, patients can make themselves helpless victims of their pain and of the system, thereby absolving themselves of any responsibility.[42]

Emotional reasoning assumes that what one feels *must* be true. If a person is frightened the pain will never stop, then he or she *believes* it will never stop. These patients let their feelings rule their reasoning ability. Although it is usually helpful to get in touch with one's feelings, *what* one feels may be quite unrealistic.[42]

Filtering involves the tendency to see one's pain through tunnel vision while filtering out any potential positive aspects. These patients make things worse than they are by focusing only on the pain and nothing else. Fears can be magnified to the point that they preoccupy an individual's awareness to the exclusion of everything else.[42]

Entitlement fallacy refers to feeling that one is "entitled" to a totally pain-free existence. This belief implies that one should not have to suffer any amount of pain or loss and leads to feeling cheated. The luxury of ignoring or taking one's body for granted is considered one's right.

Each of these processes is interrelated and can be modified through cognitive-behavioral therapy. Cognitive-behavioral techniques, in addition to self-monitoring and alteration of erroneous thought patterns, include progressive muscle relaxation, relaxation with mental imagery, autogenic training, cognitive distraction, biofeedback, and hypnosis.[23]

Progressive muscle relaxation[23, 26, 43] is an effective way for patients to learn about the amount of muscle tension in their body. It is possible for patients to walk around with clenched teeth or fists all day and not even realize it. However, usually in the evening, a tension headache or sore shoulder helps them realize what they have been doing. Progressive muscle relaxation is an active exercise in which the patient physically tenses and relaxes his or her muscles in order to learn more about the amount of tension in the body and to relieve that tension.[42] The patient is taught to recognize even slight muscle contractions so that he or she can avoid them and achieve the deepest degree of relaxation possible.[27]

Relaxation with mental imagery involves the use of distraction to control the focus of attention. Relaxation techniques are reportedly most helpful when combined with distracting or pleasant imagery.[1, 14, 23] Imagery involves using the imagination while in a relaxed state. For example, the patient can imagine himself or herself on a beach or imagine transforming the pain into a warm or cold sensation. The patient can also imagine transforming the context of pain, e.g., viewing oneself in battle with the pain on the football field instead of in a hospital bed.[23]

Autogenic training is a relaxation method used to generate feelings of heaviness and warmth in the extremities.[26, 42] It can be especially useful for cancer pain patients because there is no physical activity involved as with the physical tensing and releasing in progressive muscle relaxation. During autogenic training, the patient experiences increased blood flow and decreased respiratory rate, heart rate, and muscle tension.[26]

Cognitive distraction involves control over the focus of attention. This process can involve mental imagery, as discussed previously, or becoming engaged in a pleasurable activity to divert attention away from pain.[1, 23]

Biofeedback is the process of using special instrumentation to teach a person to control a biological response that is usually not under voluntary control.[10, 20, 37] It is a way for patients to monitor their relaxation progress. Electrodes connected to a biofeedback machine and to the patient's body give the patient and therapist "feedback" about the patient's level of tension and relaxation (electromyelographic biofeedback) or level of warmth (thermal biofeedback). According to Breitbart,[1] most cancer patients can use electromyelography and temperature biofeedback techniques to learn relaxation-assisted pain control.

Hypnosis is a state of heightened and focused concentration and thus can be used to manipulate the perception of pain.[1] Hypnosis has been shown to be efficacious in the treatment of cancer pain; however, one-third of cancer patients cannot be hypnotized, and, therefore, other techniques must be used.[1] Those patients who can be hypnotized can often alter sensations in a painful area by changing temperature sensation or experiencing tingling.[1]

The goals of cognitive-behavioral therapy are to modify patient's thoughts and feelings toward a sense of control over pain.[1, 2, 12, 23, 27] The fundamental philosophy that motivates the application of cognitive-behavioral therapy, according to Fishman and Loscalzo,[12] is that pain and suffering are not the same. Suffering refers to a conscious state of mind determined by many different influences. Although pain is one of these influences, its presence does not necessarily produce suffering.[12] Patients can limit their suffering and enjoy aspects of their personal experience by acquiring substantial control over their conscious experience and behavior.[12] According to Payne and Foley,[22] "probably the single most important advance is that these approaches [i.e., behavioral and cognitive behavioral approaches] are being integrated into the care of the patient with cancer pain." In addition to behavioral and cognitive-behavioral therapeutic techniques, educational approaches and supportive psychotherapy are helpful for managing cancer pain.

Education

Education is often part of the therapeutic process for cancer pain patients.[12, 36, 38, 44] It may include sleep education and problem-solving and communication skills training.

Sleep education is often useful for patients who, because of their pain, either have difficulty falling asleep or difficulty waking. These patients are encouraged to relax before bedtime, possibly by using some of their relaxation techniques and by allowing themselves a period of about 1 hour to relax before bedtime. They are also encouraged to adhere to a schedule for retiring nightly and rising each morning. Even if they do not sleep well the night before, they are discouraged from taking naps during the day and encouraged to arise at the same time each morning, so they will be more likely to adjust their biological clock and sleep better the following night.

Patients are instructed to use their bed only for sleeping or sexual activity. Reading, eating, and watching television in bed can condition the mind and body to expect to stay awake after one lies down. Patients are taught not to fight sleep. Tossing and turning are often associated with mental worry and are also a way of conditioning the body *not* to sleep while lying in bed. If patients find themselves tossing and turning for more than just a few minutes, they are encouraged to get up for a short period, engage in a relaxing activity, and not return to bed until they feel drowsy. Patients are asked to monitor the relaxing activity they choose should they arise during the night. One patient reported smoking several cigarettes, another drinking iced tea or coffee, and still another watching a frightening movie. Not surprisingly, none of these patients was able to easily fall asleep after these activities. In fact, patients are cautioned to avoid stimulants or stimulating activities for at least 4 hours before bedtime.

In *problem-solving skills* training, the patient is taught to monitor his or her thought processes, behaviors, and the possible outcome of those behaviors. Patients are discouraged from rationalizing, overgeneralizing, and catastrophic thinking, and encouraged, instead, to think calmly and rationally about how to solve problems. They are guided through the process of (1) identifying the problem, (2) thinking of as many solutions to the problem as possible, (3) thinking of probable outcomes if these solutions are applied, and finally (4) choosing the most effective solution(s).

The application of problem-solving skills requires effective *communication*. Because all behavior is communicative, people are always communicating, even when they are "doing nothing." Dysfunctional communication patterns include (1) blaming and criticizing; (2) mind reading, e.g., assuming others feel or think a certain way without checking with them to make sure, e.g., "My doctor doesn't think I'm going to get any better"; (3) making incomplete statements, e.g., "I'm very angry," without identifying why or at whom; (4) making statements that imply that events are unalterable, e.g., "This pain will never get any better;" and (5) overgeneralizing, e.g., "Bad things always happen to me."

Thus, communication skills are a useful adjunct to cognitive-behavioral therapy, because both involve examining one's thoughts, feelings, and subsequent ways of expressing those feelings instead of overgeneralizing and making statements that imply that events are unalterable. Therapy may involve helping the patient and family members identify problematic interaction patterns as they occur and then teaching them clearer communication skills. Some examples of these patterns include making "I" statements to avoid blaming or criticizing and talking *with* rather than *about* other family members or medical staff. This involves listening to what others have to say and asking for clarification instead of assuming one knows what the other person thinks.

Supportive Psychotherapy

Supportive psychotherapy emphasizes empathic understanding and unconditional positive regard, with the primary goal being to help patients achieve congruence between self and experience, e.g., between the ideal self and the experience of cancer.[10] Empathic understanding refers to the therapist's ability to understand the patient and to convey such understanding to him or her. Patient-centered therapists use several methods to express empathy, including nodding, eye contact, and reflection of feeling. Unconditional positive regard indicates a genuine concern and care for the patient and involves affirming the patient's worth as a person and accepting him or her without evaluation. The provision of positive regard does not require the therapist to feel posi-

tively about all of the patient's actions but rather, to avoid any overt or covert judgment of the patient's behavior. Because a judgment of any kind represents a "condition of worth," positive judgments are considered as nontherapeutic as negative judgments. Genuineness refers to honesty in communication. This does not mean that the therapist must self-disclose but only that the therapist must honestly communicate his or her feelings whenever it is appropriate to do so. The desired outcome of supportive therapy is to help the patient incorporate his or her experience (e.g., cancer) into the concept of self in order to become a more fully functioning, self-actualized person.

Systems Framework

All of the treatment modalities (behavioral, cognitive-behavioral, educational, and supportive) are most effective if applied within a systems framework.[10, 25, 34, 40, 45–51] A systems approach takes into account the patient's role(s) in his or her concentric social circles, particularly within the family system. To implement treatment modalities without considering the subsequent changes that will occur within the patient's social systems, is to provide treatment as a technician, instead of as a therapist or clinician.[2]

Once the patient's behavior is changed during the psychotherapeutic process, his or her modified behaviors will affect the homeostasis of the family system. Homeostasis refers to the tendency for any system to react toward the restoration of the status quo in the event of any change. In family systems, it refers to the tendency of any family to maintain balance in order to keep a certain equilibrium, or to ensure a relatively stable family environment. Systematic attempts are made by the family to restore equilibrium, or homeostasis, when it is threatened in any way. According to Minuchin,[52] a family is composed of more than the individual biopsychodynamics of its members—it is a system. All families are believed to have an implicit structure that determines how each member relates to one another. Boundaries are the barriers or rules that determine the amount of contact that is allowed between family members. When boundaries are overly rigid, family members are isolated from one another; when boundaries are too diffuse, family members are overly dependent. The dysfunction is the result of an inflexible family structure that prohibits the family from adapting to situational changes, e.g., cancer or chronic pain.

The therapist engages in three steps when working with the patient and his or her family: (1) The therapist joins the family in a position of leadership in order to develop a therapeutic system. Joining involves blending with the family by adopting its affect, style, and language. (2) The therapist evaluates the family's structure, including its transactional patterns, power hierarchy, subsystems, boundaries, and flexibility. Based on this evaluation, specific goals of therapy are formulated. (3) The therapist uses a number of techniques to restructure the family system, including reframing, which involves relabeling behaviors so that they can be viewed in more positive ways. Because a cancer patient's illness causes distress in other members of the family, it is important to work within the entire family system. This may begin with the initial sharing of the diagnosis of cancer.

Implementation

Physicians or other health care providers who identify signs of depression and anxiety or other needs for psychological intervention should not hesitate to refer patients to a psychologist or psychiatrist. This referral should be done in such a way as not to infer that psychological intervention is the last resort or that the patient's pain is not real.[2] The patient should also be assured that the physician has no intention of taking away needed analgesics, even if the patient achieves some success in pain reduction using behavioral control.[2] Before referral of patients to a psychologist is considered, however, physicians are often faced with the difficult task of sharing critical news with patients and their families. How does the physician deliver this type of news? Will the family be present? Does the patient want to limit how much information the physician may share with the family? Or, does the family want to protect the patient from information that may be emotionally painful but necessary?

During the delivery of the diagnosis, once the patient hears the word *cancer*, he or she may hear little more that the physician says after that point. As a result, any instructions or suggestions may need to be written and given to the patient, and then reviewed at the next office visit. Patients often equate the word cancer with death or pain. Therefore, questions are likely to include, Am I going to die? How long do I have to live? Will I experience uncontrollable pain? Will I become a physical or financial burden to my family? It is difficult to describe how physicians should respond to such challenging and difficult questions.

According to Kriesel,[7] physicians should consider three issues when delivering a diagnosis of cancer or other critical news: (1) an understanding of the patient's previous coping styles, (2) telling the truth, and (3) including the family in the diagnosis process.

Physician awareness of the patient's *previous coping style* is useful for helping predict how the patient will respond to current stress and crises. Cancer patients who complained often of financial, medical, and physical problems, and who suffered from reduced self-esteem were found to also have a higher number of emotional problems, such as anxiety and depression.[7] If the patient had been depressed in the past, depression is more likely to redevelop. The patient's and family's coping mechanisms should be incorporated into the treatment plan. Kriesel[7] suggests, for example, that the physician might respond to a desperate patient or to a family hoping for a miracle with a response like, "I wish that were possible," instead of talking about whether miracles do or do not occur.

Telling the truth is another factor to consider when delivering a diagnosis of cancer or other difficult news. Patients must be told truthfully and honestly about their condition. Patients want to find out what is likely to happen to them beforehand and also want a statement of hope, not just for a cure, but hope that they can still have pleasurable experiences in life and meet some of their goals with the support of others.[7] Sharing a diagnosis honestly involves trust. If patients sense that they are not being told the truth, this reinforces their own sense of helplessness and hopelessness and may cause them to feel betrayed by the physician.[7]

Including the family can help decrease the likelihood that crippling, dysfunctional communication will occur among family members later. Patients and family members can be encouraged to talk about questions that may later occur. The physician can also share other resources available to the family, such as psychotherapy, local cancer support groups, and hospice organizations.

Any number of responses are likely to occur from the patient and family members once news of the malignancy is delivered. There may be little or no overt reaction, or there may be uncontrollable crying that verges on the point of hysteria. In the case of uncontrollable crying, the physician can instruct the patient or family member to engage in diaphragmatic breathing. For example, patients should place one hand on their abdomen and one hand on their chest and primarily move the hand on the stomach as they inhale and exhale. Patients are instructed to inhale through the nose and exhale through the mouth, as if blowing a feather. Not only should this provide a calming distraction, but it is virtually impossible to cry uncontrollably while simultaneously breathing deeply and rhythmically. Once the patient and family have regained control and are calmer, they can be reassured by the physician that the medical staff will be with them during this experience and the patient and family will not be left to struggle alone. Relaxation techniques, such as progressive muscle relaxation and autogenic training are pragmatic strategies that the medical staff can then teach to the patient and family members. These techniques can be effectively applied when necessary without direct involvement by the psychologist or psychiatrist.

Summary

Although psychological interventions should never be considered a substitute for appropriate medical management,[2] they can be useful adjunctive treatment modalities. A major component of psychological intervention is behavioral or cognitive-behavioral therapy, along with education and supportive psychotherapy, all applied within a systems framework. The major goal of psychological intervention is not to eliminate pain or to lengthen life but instead to help the patient to regain a sense of control over managing his or her symptoms and improve his or her quality of life. In the words of the Stoic philosopher Epictetus, "Men are distracted not by things, but by the views which they take of them." Clearly, patients' perceptions of their pain will influence their feelings, actions, and ability to regain a sense of self-efficacy and meaningful quality of life.

References

1. Breitbart WS. Assessment and treatment of psychiatric syndromes in cancer pain patients: Why do we care? Cancer Pain Symposium. New York: Memorial Sloan Kettering Cancer Center, 1992;213.
2. Loscalzo M, Peyser S, Jacobsen, PB. Cognitive and behavioral approaches in adults: Why do we care? Cancer Pain Symposium. New York: Memorial Sloan Kettering Cancer Center, 1992;239.
3. Fernandez E. A classification system of cognitive coping strategies for pain. Pain 1986;26:141.
4. Driscoll CE. Pain management: Primary care. Manage Cancer Patient 1987;14:337.
5. Loscalzo M, Jacobsen PB. Practical behavioral approaches to the effective management of pain and distress. J Psychosoc Oncol 1990;8:139.
6. Foley KM. Pain syndromes in patients with cancer. Cancer Pain 1987;71:169.
7. Kriesel HT. The psychosocial aspects of malignancy. Prim Care 1987;14:271.
8. Crisson JE, Keffe FJ. The relationship of locus of control to pain coping strategies and psychological distress in chronic pain patients. Pain 1988;35:147.
9. Kinzel T. Relief of emotional symptoms in elderly patients with terminal cancer. Geriatrics 1988;43:61.
10. Cleeland CS, Tearnan BH. Behavioral Control of Cancer Pain. In AD Holzman, CD Turk (eds), Pain Management: A Handbook of Psychological Treatment Approaches. New York: Pergamon, 1986;193.
11. Kelly JF. Psychological assessment and management of pain. International Pain Symposium Update. Atlanta: Southeastern Pain Institute, Georgia Baptist Medical Center 1992;382.
12. Fishman B, Loscalzo M. Cognitive-behavioral interventions in management of cancer pain: Principles and applications. Med Clin North Am 1987;71:271.
13. Silberfarb PM. Research in adaptation to illness and psychosocial intervention: An overview. Cancer 1982;50:1921.
14. Redd WH. Cognitive and behavioral approaches for specific symptoms: Why do we care? Cancer Pain Symposium. New York: Memorial Sloan Kettering Cancer Center, 1992:267.
15. Simonton OC, Matthews-Simonton S, Sparks TF. Psychological intervention in the treatment of cancer. Psychosomatics 1980;21:226.
16. Linn MW, Linn BS, Harris R. Effects of counseling for late stage cancer patients. Cancer 1982;49:1048.
17. McCalla JL. A multidisciplinary approach to identification and remedial intervention for adverse late effects of cancer therapy. Nurs Clin North Am 1985;20:117.
18. Angarola RT, Joranson DE (eds). Pain and euthanasia: The need for alternatives. Am Pain Soc Bull 1992;2:10,17.
19. Morse RH. Pain and Emotions. In S Brena, S Chapman (eds), Management of Patients with Chronic Pain. New York: Spectrum, 1983;47.

20. Chapman SL. Relaxation, Biofeedback, and Self-hypnosis. In S Brena, S Chapman (eds), Management of Patients with Chronic Pain. New York: Spectrum, 1983;161.

21. Cleeland CS. Psychological Aspects of Pain Due to Cancer. In SE Abram (ed), Cancer Pain. Boston: Kluwer, 1989;33.

22. Payne R, Foley KM. Advances in the management of cancer pain. Cancer Treat Rep 1984;68:173.

23. Breitbart WS. Psychosocial assessment and intervention: Why do we care? Cancer Pain Symposium. New York: Memorial Sloan Kettering Cancer Center, 1992;113.

24. Turk DC, Meichenbaum D. A Cognitive-behavioral Approach to Pain Management. In PD Wall, R Melzack (eds), Textbook of Pain. New York: Churchill Livingstone, 1984;787.

25. Elliott DJ, Trief PM, Stein N. Mastery, stress, and coping in marriage among chronic pain patients. J Behav Med 1986;9:549.

26. Benson H, Pomeranz B, Kutz I. The Relaxation Response and Pain. In PD Wall, R Melzack (eds), Textbook of Pain. New York: Churchill Livingstone, 1984;817.

27. Pilowsky I. Pain and Illness Behavior: Assessment and Management. In PD Wall, R Melzack (eds), Textbook of Pain. New York: Churchill Livingstone, 1984;767.

28. Jessup BA. Biofeedback. In PD Wall, R Melzack (eds), Textbook of Pain. New York: Churchill Livingstone, 1984;776.

29. Pearce S. A review of cognitive-behavioral methods for the treatment of chronic pain. J Psychosom Res 1983;27:431.

30. Gallagher-Thomspon D, Thompson LW. Cognitive-behavioral therapy with older adults: A case example and discussion of common treatment issues [unpublished presentation], 1992.

31. Thompson LW, Gantz F, Florsheim M, et al. Cognitive-Behavioral Therapy for Affective Disorders in the Elderly. In WA Myers (ed), New Techniques in the Psychotherapy of Older Patients. Washington, DC: American Psychiatric Press, 1991;3.

32. Libo LM, Arnold GE. Relaxation practice after biofeedback therapy: A long-term follow-up study of utilization and effectiveness. Biofeedback Self Regul 1983;8:217.

33. Redd WH, Andrykowski MA. Behavioral intervention in cancer treatment: Controlling aversion reactions to chemotherapy. J Consult Clin Psychol 1982;50:1018.

34. Adams-Greenly M. Psychosocial assessment and intervention at initial diagnosis. Pediatrician 1991;18:3.

35. Redd WH. Treatment of excessive crying in a terminal cancer patient: A time-series analysis. J Behav Med 1982;5:225.

36. Jacobs C, Ross RD, Walker IM, Stockdale FE. Behavior of cancer patients: A randomized study of the effects of education and peer support groups. Am J Clin Oncol 1983;6:347.

37. Davis MW, Wilson L, Burish TG. Psychological Assessment and Treatment of Cancer Pain. In WCV Parris (ed), Contemporary Issues in Chronic Pain Management. Boston: Kluwer, 1991;271.

38. Gordon WA, Freidenbergs I, Diller L, et al. Efficacy of psychosocial intervention with cancer patients. J Consult Clin Psychol 1980;48:743.

39. Leake E. Social work: Playing a vital role in cancer pain treatment. Am Pain Soc Bull 1992;2:17.

40. Seeman J. Toward a model of positive health. Am Psychol 1989;44:1099.

41. Chapman SL. Behavior Modification. In S Brena, S Chapman (eds), Management of Patients with Chronic Pain. New York: Spectrum, 1983;145.

42. Catalano EM. The Chronic Pain Control Workbook: A Step-By-Step Guide for Coping with and Overcoming Your Pain. Oakland, CA: New Harbinger Publication, 1987.

43. Jacobsen E. Progressive Relaxation. Chicago: University of Chicago Press, 1938.

44. Derdiarian AK. Effects of information on recently diagnosed cancer patients' and spouses' satisfaction with care. Cancer Nurs 1989;12:285.

45. Pinsky JJ, Crue BL. Intensive Group Psychotherapy. In PD Wall, R Melzack (eds), Textbook of Pain. New York: Churchill Livingstone, 1984;823.

46. Jeans ME, Rowat KM. Counseling the Patient and Family. In PD Wall, R Melzack (eds), Textbook of Pain. New York: Churchill Livingstone, 1984;795.

47. Sholevar GP, Perkel R. Family systems intervention and physical illness. Gen Hosp Psychiatry 1990;12:363.

48. Holmes BC. Psychological evaluation and preparation of the patient and family. Cancer 1987;60:2021.

49. Adams-Greenly M. Psychological staging of pediatric cancer patients and their families. Cancer 1986;58:449.

50. Cassileth BR, Lusk EJ, Stouse TB, et al. A psychological analysis of cancer patients and their next-of-kin. Cancer 1985;55:72.

51. Parsonnet L, O'Hare J. A group orientation program for families of newly admitted cancer patients. Soc Work 1990;35:37.

52. Minuchin S. Families and Family Therapy. Cambridge, MA: Harvard University Press, 1974.

Chapter 22

Psychiatric and Psychological Aspects of Cancer Pain

William S. Breitbart, David K. Payne, and Steven D. Passik

Introduction

The diagnosis of cancer is a particularly frightening and stressful event that is made more distressing in part by the patient's perceptions of the disease, the prognosis, and the associated social stigma.[1] Advances in the treatment of cancer, including early detection, chemotherapy, radiotherapy, and surgery, have lead to increased life expectancy for patients who formerly would have died. Despite these improvements, however, these patients experience pain related to their cancer.[2, 3] The role of pain in the cancer experience has been termed "total pain," which denotes the influence that the experience of cancer has on the perception of pain, its psychological concomitants, and available methods of coping with cancer. The negative impact that pain has on a cancer patient's mood and coping abilities underscores the importance of investigating the role that pain has in a patient's experience with cancer.[4]

The multifactorial nature of cancer pain highlights the difficulties and challenges for clinicians. Given the relationship between psychological and physical factors, the clinician who treats the cancer patient faces complex assessment and treatment issues. A multidisciplinary approach to the management of cancer pain suggests that it is essential to recognize the importance of appropriate diagnosis and treatment of the concurrent psychological symptoms and psychiatric syndromes that accompany cancer pain.[5] This chapter reviews (1) the psychiatric, diagnostic, and treatment issues most salient in cancer pain, (2) issues of suicide, (3) the request for physician-assisted suicide, (4) euthanasia, (5) the psychiatric and psychological interventions, and (6) the diagnosis and treatment of pain related to acquired immunodeficiency syndrome (AIDS).

Multidimensional Model of Cancer Pain

The definition of pain developed by the International Association for the Study of Pain[6] states that "pain is an unpleasant sensory or emotional experience associated with actual or potential tissue damage, or described in terms of such damage." This definition reinforced the conclusion that pain is an experience that involves not only nociceptive events but also a complex psychological association of nociception, pain perception, and pain expression.[7, 8]

Recently, researchers have noted the importance of cognitive, emotional, socioenvironmental, and nociceptive aspects of cancer pain. This model points to the challenge of untangling the psychological and physical issues associated with cancer pain and also gives a framework to develop interventions designed to address the major dimensions of cancer pain.[9] Fortunately, somatically oriented interventions, which have been specially designed to alleviate cancer pain, have also been shown to reduce psychological distress. Conversely, psychosocial interventions that are aimed at relieving emotional distress have a profound impact on nociception. The ideal intervention for cancer pain patients involves a simultaneous multidisciplinary approach.[5]

Psychological Variables in Cancer Pain Patients

In the absence of pain, patients who are initially informed of the diagnosis of cancer pass through a predictable sequence of responses.[5, 10, 11] There is usually a period of shock, disbelief, or denial, which can be followed by anxiety and depression. Disturbances in sleep and appetite accompanied by pervasive thoughts about cancer may occur at the time of diagnosis and frequently reappear at salient points in the treatment process: prior to tests or surgery, at the point of relapse, at the start of treatment, and at the conclusion of treatment. These distressing emotional experiences subside for most patients, letting them return to their original state of emotional homeostasis.

There is considerable variability in the degree of psychological distress experienced by cancer patients. This is due in part to two sets of factors: medical (stage of disease, presence of pain, and the impact of specific treatments) and psychological (the patient's preexisting psychological makeup including coping abilities, emotional development, and the presence of psychiatric disorders). Although it is tempting to view the role of psychological issues as paramount in the cancer experience, most cancer patients are psychologically healthy individuals who are predictably reacting to the stressors associated with cancer and cancer treatments. In those cancer patients who do have a psychiatric disorder, more than 90% of the disorders are related to reactions to the stress of cancer or to a manifestation of the disease or the treatment.[11, 12]

Cancer pain differs with site, stage, and extent of illness. Approximately 15% of all patients without metastatic disease report significant pain.[13, 14] Sixty percent to 90% of patients with advanced disease report pain that is debilitating, and as many as 25% of patients die in pain.[2, 15–17]

Pain, either as a result of the disease or its treatment, is one of the most feared aspects of the cancer.[1, 18] Most cancer patients do not report pain until after their diagnosis,[19] and this experience of pain is in part related to the patient's fears and the meaning of cancer.

Once cancer has been diagnosed, psychological factors influence the experience and intensity of cancer pain. In the early stages of cancer, the correlation between pain intensity and disease progression is weak[20] and, consequently, pain experienced by cancer patients is likely a result of both psychological as well as physical factors. Psychological factors such as perceived control, meaning of the pain, depression, anxiety, and fear of death all appear to contribute to reports of more intense pain.[4, 21]

For many cancer patients, pain is a signal of advancing disease. Cancer patients who attribute a new pain to the progression of their disease report greater distress and interference with their activity than do those who make benign attributions concerning their pain.[13, 22] Likewise, in a population of women with metastatic breast cancer, more intense pain was experienced if it was believed that the pain heralded the progression of their disease and if they were more depressed.[22] In advanced disease, patients with high levels of emotional disturbance accept more pain.[23] Of course, those patients may have been more emotionally distressed because they had such severe uncontrolled pain. A relationship does exist between the report of pain and psychological distress. However, it is often difficult to conclude that this is always a clear unidirectional causal relationship. More likely, the relationship is interactive and quite complex.

Although psychological factors clearly exacerbate or ameliorate the cancer pain, it would be inaccurate to propose that they account for all or even a majority of the pain experience. Psychological variables have been posited to explain the lack of treatment response when other medical factors have been overlooked. The evaluation of psychological distress in patients with cancer pain should include a thorough assessment of the adequacy of pain management. Similarly, the presence of personality factors that are problematic may be exaggerated by the presence of pain and often resolve following the appropriate treatment for the patient's pain.[15, 24]

Psychiatric Disorders in Patients with Cancer-Related Pain

A multicenter study that assessed the presence of psychiatric disorders in cancer patients found that 53% of patients did not meet *Diagnostic and Statistical Manual*, 3rd edition (DSM-III) criteria for a psychiatric diagnosis (Table 22-1).[12] Of the remaining patients who did receive a psychiatric diagnosis, most (68%) met the DSM-III criteria for

Table 22-1. Rates of Diagnostic and Statistical Manual, 3rd edition, Psychiatric Disorders and Prevalence of Pain Observed in 215 Cancer Patients from Three Cancer Centers

Diagnostic Category	Number Diagnostic Class (%)	Percent of Psychiatric Diagnoses	Number with Significant Pain (%)*
Adjustment disorders	69 (32%)	68%	
Major affective disorders	13 (6%)	13%	
Organic mental disorders	8 (4%)	8%	
Personality disorders	7 (3%)	7%	
Anxiety disorders	4 (2%)	4%	
Total with psychiatric diagnosis	101 (47%)		39 (39%)
Total without psychiatric diagnosis	114 (53%)		21 (19%)
Total patient population	215 (100%)		60 (28%)

Source: Adapted from LR Deragotis, et al. The prevalence of psychiatric disorders among cancer patients. JAMA 1983;249:754.
*Score greater than 50 mm on a 100-mm visual analog scale for pain severity.

an adjustment disorder with depressed or anxious mood. An additional 13% met the criteria for a major depressive episode and the remaining 19% met the criteria for anxiety disorders, organic mental syndrome, and personality disorders. The relationship between pain and psychiatric disorder is demonstrated by noting that 39% of the patients with a psychiatric diagnosis also reported experiencing significant pain, whereas only 19% of patients without a psychiatric diagnosis reported significant pain. Adjustment disorder with depressed or anxious mood and major depression represented the majority of the diagnoses and are seen more frequently in cancer pain patients.

Patients with advanced cancer are at increased risk for pain, depression, and delirium.[25] Severe depressive symptoms are noted in 25% of all cancer patients, with the prevalence increasing to 77% in those with advanced disease. The presence of organic mental disorders (delirium) that require psychiatric intervention ranges from 25–40% and can increase to as high as 85% in patients with end-stage disease.[26] Narcotic analgesics, which are commonly used in the management of cancer pain, can cause confusional states, especially among the elderly or terminally ill patients during periods of rapid titration of dose or with high-dose infusions.[27]

Given the impact of pain on psychiatric symptoms, it is essential to reassess a patient for the presence of a psychiatric disorder following adequate treatment for pain. Not only do the psychiatric complications of cancer pain result in increased morbidity and mortality, they also affect the patient's quality of life. Although the management of specific psychiatric disorders has been reviewed in detail in *The Handbook of Psychooncology,*[28] a brief guide to the diagnosis and management of these disorders is presented in this chapter.

Anxiety and Cancer Pain

The impact that anxiety has on pain can be illustrated using three mechanisms. First, anxiety can exacerbate pain by initiating a sequence of physiologic changes that result in nociception. Stress leads to nociception through an accentuated ability by the central nervous system (CNS) to provoke muscular spasms, vasoconstriction, or visceral disturbance.[29] Second, anxiety has been shown to alter the individual's ability to perceive noxious stimuli. Patients who are anxious have a decreased ability to distinguish between harmful and innocuous stimuli.[30] High levels of physiologic arousal may cause individuals to label sensory events as pain rather than as the result of emotional distress.[31] Finally, anxiety that is evoked in a context relevant to the patient's fears, e.g., anxiety about medical procedures, will result in a greater perception of pain.

Three types of anxiety are commonly found in cancer patients regardless of the presence of pain. The first is a reactive anxiety related to the stresses of having cancer and its treatment. The second type of anxiety is a product of a medical or physiologic problem related to cancer or treatment, such as an organic anxiety disorder secondary to either uncontrolled pain or steroid administration. The third type of anxiety is that which predates the cancer experience but worsens during illness, e.g., generalized anxiety disorder or panic disorder.[32]

The presence of transient anxiety states is a common experience during the diagnosis and treatment phases of cancer. Although the severity differs from patient to patient, anxiety can (1) disrupt the patient's ability to function normally, (2) interfere with interpersonal relationships, and (3) impair the patient's ability to comprehend and adhere to medical treatments.

Although anxiety can be the result of psychological issues, the clinician must remember that the cancer patient is exposed to multiple organic agents that can result in symptoms of anxiety including uncontrolled pain, infection, metabolic abnormalities, and medications. Organic anxiety presumes that a medical factor is the etiology of the anxious symptoms. Patients receiving corticosteroids often display symptoms of anxiety and insomnia that can be treated with benzodiazepines or low-dose neuroleptics.[33] Acute pain or respiratory distress can create symptoms of anxiety that are best treated with opioids or oxygen. Patients who present with an evolving encephalopathy often exhibit signs of anxiety or restlessness. Other medical conditions resulting in symptoms of anxiety include alcohol withdrawal, hyperthyroidism, brain tumor, seizure disorder, and mitral valve prolapse. The diversity of these etiologies underscores the need for careful medical evaluation.[5, 32]

Phobias and Panic

Most individuals with panic disorder or a phobia report that the disorder predates their cancer diagnosis. However, occasionally, patients will have their first episode of panic or phobia while in a medical setting. At Memorial Sloan Kettering Cancer Center, approximately 20% of patients undergoing a magnetic resonance imaging scan develop anxiety or claustrophobia so severe that they are unable to complete the procedure.[34] These particular anxiety disorders (e.g., panic disorder, needle phobia, or claustrophobia) can interfere with medical treatment

and so require early psychological intervention. The major treatment approaches for these disorders include behavioral and pharmacologic interventions. With adequate preparation, behavioral approaches such as relaxation training, systematic desensitization, and in vivo or imaginal exposure for phobias can reduce stress. These approaches take patients days or weeks to master and are advisable if the patients are required to undergo a procedure repeatedly. If, however, immediate relief from anxiety is needed because of the urgency of the medical procedure, then benzodiazepines (e.g., alprazolam, 0.25–1.0 mg orally) are used in conjunction with emotional support therapy to help the phobic patient undergo necessary procedures.

Treatment of Anxiety Symptoms and Disorders

Alprazolam, oxazepam, and lorazepam are the drugs of first choice for anxiety symptoms. Patients with relatively mild levels of anxiety can benefit from the use of cognitive behavioral techniques such as relaxation or cognitive restructuring.[35] When time and resources permit, the optimal treatment of anxiety is a combination of pharmacologic and cognitive behavioral techniques. Other medications that are useful in managing anxiety in cancer pain patients include buspirone, antipsychotics, antihistamine, beta-blockers, and antidepressants. Although not traditionally thought of as anxiolytics, many analgesics also help reduce anxiety (Table 22-2).

Benzodiazepines

Because drug interactions and decreased clearance are often factors in treating cancer pain patients, benzodiazepines with shorter half-lives (alprazolam, lorazepam, and oxazepam) are preferred. Factors such as severity of the anxiety, the patient's physical status (respiratory and hepatic impairment), and the concurrent use of other medications (antidepressants, analgesics, and antiemetics) must be taken into account when determining the starting dosage. Dosing regimens depend on the half-life of the drug; shorter acting benzodiazepines need to be given three to four times a day, whereas

Table 22-2. Anxiolytic Medications Used in Cancer Pain Patients

Generic Name	Approximate Daily Dosage Range (mg)	Route
Benzodiazepines		
Very short acting		
Midazolam	10–60 per 24 hrs	IV, SC
Short acting		
Alprazolam	0.25–2.0 tid–qid	PO, SL
Oxazepam	10–15 tid–qid	PO
Lorazepam	0.5–2.0 tid–qid	PO, SL, IV, IM
Intermediate acting		
Chlordiazepoxide	10–50 tid–qid	PO, IM
Long acting		
Diazepam	5–10 bid–qid	PO, IM, IV, PR
Clorazepate	7.5–15.0 bid–qid	PO
Clonazepam	0.5–2.0 bid–qid	PO
Nonbenzodiazepines		
Buspirone	5–20 tid	PO
Neuroleptics		
Haloperidol	0.5–5.0 q2–12 hrs	PO, IV, SC, IM
Methotrimeprazine	10–20 q4–8 hrs	IV, SC, PO
Thioridazine	10–75 tid–qid	PO
Chlorpromazine	12.5–50.0 q4–12 hrs	PO, IM, IV
Antihistamines		
Hydroxyzine	25–50 q4–6 hrs	PO, IV, SC
Tricyclic antidepressants		
Imipramine	12.5–150.0 q12hr	PO, IM
Clomipramine	10–150 q12hr	PO

Note: Parenteral doses are generally twice as potent as oral doses; intravenous bolus injections or infusions should be administered slowly.

longer acting benzodiazepines can be administered on a twice daily schedule. Although anxiolytics can be given on an as needed basis for patients who are anxious about upcoming procedures, the most effective treatment regimen for chronic anxiety should be on an around-the-clock basis. Drowsiness, confusion, and motor incoordination are the most common side effects of benzodiazepines. The synergistic interaction of benzodiazepines with other CNS depressants should be monitored and, if problematic, the dose should be decreased or the drug should be stopped completely. It must remembered, however, that an abrupt discontinuation of benzodiazepines can precipitate a withdrawal reaction similar to alcohol withdrawal. Midazolam (Versed), an extremely short acting benzodiazepine, has been found to be effective in sedating patients prior to undergoing stressful procedures such as bone marrow aspirations, endoscopy, lumbar punc-

ture, or in critical care settings where the goal is to maintain an agitated patient on a respirator.

Clonazepam, a longer acting benzodiazepine, is useful not only for anxiety and phobic disorder, but also for depersonalization and derealization in patients with seizure disorders, brain tumors, and mild organic mental disorders. It has also been shown to be useful in patients with mood lability and as an adjuvant analgesic in patients with neuropathic pain. It may also be useful for anxious patients who experience end of dosing problems with shorter acting benzodiazepines.[36, 37]

Nonbenzodiazepine Anxiolytics

Buspirone is a nonbenzodiazepine anxiolytic that, in conjunction with psychotherapy, is effective for patients with chronic anxiety or anxiety related to adjustment disorders. The onset of anxiolytic action is delayed relative to a benzodiazepine and it is not uncommon for relief to take 5–10 days to begin. Because buspirone is not a benzodiazepine, it is not useful in preventing benzodiazepine withdrawal. The dose of buspirone is 5–20 mg three times a day.[38]

Antipsychotics such as thioridazine may be indicated for patients who are unresponsive to benzodiazepines or for treating anxiety in patients with cognitive impairment in whom benzodiazepines may worsen their organic features. Dosing can be started at low doses (10–20 mg two to three times per day) and can be increased, if necessary, up to 100 mg three times per day. Antihistamines are infrequently prescribed for anxiety because of their low efficacy; hydroxyzine can be useful for anxious patients with respiratory impairment in whom benzodiazepines are relatively contraindicated. Although benzodiazepines are useful for acute bouts of panic, long-term maintenance is better accomplished with antidepressants. Tricyclic antidepressants and monoamine oxidase inhibitors have been shown to have antipanic effects. Propranolol can be a helpful adjuvant in blocking the physiologic manifestations of anxiety in patients with panic disorder.[32]

Depression and Cancer Pain

Major depression occurs in 20–25% of all cancer patients. Its prevalence increases with the presence of pain, advancement of illness, and functional disability.[25, 39, 40] Certain types of cancer are more likely to be associated with a diagnosis of depression, e.g., patients with pancreatic cancer are more prone to develop depressive symptoms than patients with other types of intra-abdominal cancer.[41]

Given the physical symptoms associated with cancer, the criteria used to diagnose depression in the cancer population must be modified from that commonly used in a psychiatric setting dealing with the physically healthy. In the cancer population, the presence of somatic symptoms typically associated with depression, e.g., anorexia, fatigue, insomnia, and weight loss, may not be reliable indicators of depression given that they may be more reflective of the physical impact of the disease, rather than a depressive disorder. One way to increase diagnos-

tic reliability in the medically ill cancer patient is to use alternative, nonsomatic criteria—the so-called Endicott Substitution criteria.[42] Somatic criteria are thus replaced by the following nonsomatic items: tearfulness, depressed appearance, social withdrawal, decreased talkativeness, brooding, self-pity, pessimism, and lack of reactivity.[42] These criteria, in addition to the traditional psychological symptoms of depression (depressed mood, hopelessness, worthlessness, helplessness, anhedonia, and suicidal ideation), present a framework by which depression can be more accurately diagnosed.[25, 39–41] In addition, the presence of a past history of depression or a family history of depression lends credence to the diagnosis of depression.

Once the presence of depressive symptoms has been identified, coexisting organic factors must also be considered before starting treatment. Standard therapeutic approaches such as the use of corticosteroids, chemotherapeutic agents (vincristine, vinblastine, asparaginase, intrathecal methotrexate, interferon, and interleukin[30, 43–46]) whole brain radiation,[44] and amphotericin[47] have been implicated in the etiology or exacerbation of depressive symptoms in cancer patients. Likewise, the presence of CNS metastases, metabolic and endocrine complications,[48] and paraneoplastic syndromes[49] have been shown to contribute to the presence of depressive symptoms.

Treatment

Depressed cancer patients are usually treated with a combination of psychological treatments (cognitive behavioral and supportive psychotherapeutic modalities) and psychopharmacologic interventions (antidepressants and psychostimulants).[39] Psychotherapeutic approaches specifically aimed at ameliorating pain are discussed later in this chapter. Many of these same techniques have been used successfully in the management of psychological distress in cancer patients and have been applied to the treatment of depression and anxiety in patients with cancer and cancer-related pain. Psychological interventions administered in either an individual or group format have been shown to significantly reduce psychological distress and depressive symptoms in cancer patients.[50–52] Despite the utility of psychological interventions in the treatment of the depression associated with cancer and cancer-related pain, antidepressants have proven efficacy in cancer patients[53–55] and remain the intervention of choice (Table 22-3).[39]

Tricyclic Antidepressants

Tricyclic antidepressants (TCA) are the most well established of the pharmacotherapies for depressed cancer pain patients. The choice of a TCA is dependent on the profile of depressive symptoms exhibited by the patient, the concomitant medical problems, the side effect profile, and the patient's prior experience with specific antidepressants. Depressed patients who exhibit agitation or insomnia may benefit from the administration of amitriptyline or doxepin, both of which have prominent sedative effects. Patients who are receiving multiple medications with anticholinergic properties (e.g., meperidine, atropine, phenothiazines, or diphenhydramine) are at risk for developing an anticholinergic delirium with the addition of a high anticholinergic TCA. In addition, TCAs with anticholinergic effects are contraindicated for patients in whom the exacerbation of urinary retention, decreased intestinal motility, and stomatitis is to be avoided. Consequently, if an antidepressant is indicated, one should use a TCA that is relatively low in anticholinergic activity such as desipramine or nortriptyline. The initiation of treatment with a TCA should be tailored to the age and physical condition of the patient. Elderly patients or patients who are physically debilitated should initially receive low doses of a TCA such as amitriptyline (10–25 mg at bedtime) and the dose should be increased gradually by 10–25 mg every 1–2 days toward a dose of 150 mg per day or until either treatment-limiting side effects or the desired result is reached. It is quite likely that the dose required to achieve a therapeutic effect in cancer patients may be considerably lower than that required by patients who are physically healthy.[39] Nortriptyline, which has a "therapeutic window of efficacy," should be prescribed in similar fashion with serum drug levels assessed frequently to ensure that one does not overshoot this therapeutic window. The route of administration can be chosen to meet the physical demands of the patient. Amitriptyline, imipramine, and doxepin can be administered intramuscularly or rectally if patients

Table 22-3. Antidepressant Medications Used in Cancer Pain Patients

Drug	Therapeutic Daily Dosage (mg, PO)
Tricyclic antidepressants	
Amitriptyline	25–125
Doxepin	25–125
Imipramine	25–125
Desipramine	25–125
Nortriptyline	25–125
Clomipramine	25–125
Second-generation antidepressants	
Buproprion	200–450
Trazodone	150–300
Heterocyclic antidepressants	
Maprotiline	50–75
Amoxapine	100–150
Serotonin-specific reuptake inhibitors	
Fluoxetine	20
Sertraline	50–200
Paroxetine	10–40
Monoamine oxidase inhibitors	
Isocarboxazid	20–40
Phenelzine	30–60
Tranylcypromine	20–40
Psychostimulants	
Dextroamphetamine	5–30
Methylphenidate	5–30
Pemoline	37.5–150.0
Benzodiazepines	
Alprazolam	0.75–6.00
Lithium carbonate	600–1,200

Source: Adapted from MJ Massie, JC Holland. Depression and the cancer patient. J Clin Psychiatry 1990;51:12.

are unable to take medication orally.[56] Although the intravenous route of administration is not approved for use in the United States, TCAs such as amitriptyline have been administered safely intravenously by slow infusion.[10, 39]

Second-Generation Antidepressants

Patients who are unable to take TCAs because of the side effects or because there is an inadequate response to a TCA can use one of the second-generation (buproprion, trazodone), heterocyclic (maprotiline, amoxapine) or serotonin-specific reuptake inhibiting (fluoxetine, sertraline, paroxetine) antidepressants. The second-generation antidepressants are generally associated with fewer cardiac complications than the TCAs.[57] Trazodone is relatively sedating and in low doses (50–100 mg at bedtime) is particularly helpful in dealing with insomnia associated with depression. Given the association between trazodone and priapism, caution should be taken in prescribing this drug with men.[58] Although relatively new and infrequently used in a cancer population, buprorion may be considered for patients who have demonstrated a poor response to more commonly used antidepressants. It can be somewhat energizing and may therefore be useful for medically ill patients. Buprorion should be avoided, however, in patients with seizure disorders, brain tumors, or those who are malnourished.[59]

Serotonin-Specific Reuptake Inhibitors

Fluoxetine, a selective inhibitor of neuronal serotonin uptake, demonstrates fewer sedative and autonomic effects than the TCAs.[60] The energizing properties of fluoxetine have been shown to be useful in cancer patients who are persistently fatigued. The most common side effects are nausea and an initial period of anxiety, which usually diminishes following several weeks of the therapy. Anorexia or reduction in appetite is also a common side effect of fluoxetine. Although useful in treating overweight patients, this drug may not be indicated in cachectic cancer patients. In addition, although the general side effect profile of fluoxetine makes it useful for depressed cancer patients, its relatively long half-life and its active metabolite norfluoxetine can be problematic in the medically ill patient in whom the ability to clear the drug may be impaired. Two new selective serotonergic reuptake inhibitors, paroxetine and sertraline, have shorter half-lives and inactive metabolites and may therefore be more useful in a medically ill population.[61, 62]

Heterocyclic Antidepressants

The side effect profile of the heterocyclic antidepressants is similar to that of the TCAs. Amoxapine has mild dopamine-blocking activities and therefore patients who are taking other dopamine blockers (e.g., antiemetics) are at risk for developing extrapyramidal symptoms and dyskinesias.[63] Maprotiline should be avoided in

patients with brain tumors and in patients with seizures because this medication increases the incidence of seizures.[64] Although found to be effective in the treatment of both depression and as an adjuvant analgesic in Europe and Latin America, mianserin is not available in the United States.[65]

Psychostimulants

Although not traditionally thought of as antidepressants, psychostimulants have been underused medications in the armamentarium of the clinician treating the cancer patient with depression. Psychostimulants (dextroamphetamine, methylphenidate, and pemoline) have been shown to be effective antidepressants for cancer patients with and without pain, as well as for other medically ill populations.[66–70] They appear to be most effective for patients with advanced disease and pain and for those patients whose depressed mood is associated with decreased energy, psychomotor retardation, and mild cognitive impairment. Psychostimulants have been demonstrated to effect an improvement in general neuropsychological performance in the medically ill population, with attention and concentration being most affected.[67] In relatively low doses, psychostimulants can increase appetite, promote a sense of well-being, and decrease weakness and fatigue. An additional benefit of psychostimulants is that they reduce the sedation secondary to opioid analgesics and can provide adjuvant analgesia for cancer patients.[71] The appropriate dose of either dextroamphetamine or methylphenidate in cancer patients begins at a low level usually with a dose of 2.5 mg at 8 A.M. and again at noon. This is gradually increased over several days until the desired effect is achieved or treatment-limiting side effects (overstimulation, anxiety, insomnia, paranoia, confusion) intervene. Although 30 mg or less a day is often an adequate dose for cancer patients, patients occasionally require up to 60 mg per day. Patients are usually maintained on stimulants for 1–2 months, and approximately two-thirds can be withdrawn without recurrence of depressive symptoms. In those patients with recurrent depressive symptoms, the use of psychostimulants can be safely continued for up to 1 year without significant abuse problems (although tolerance can develop and dose adjustments may be necessary).

Although pharmacologically unrelated to amphetamines, pemoline is a new psychostimulant that is less potent and has little abuse potential.[66] In addition to the relative lack of abuse potential and milder sympathomimetic effects as compared with other stimulants, pemoline has the advantage of being available in a chewable form that allows it to be absorbed through the buccal mucosa, thus providing an alternate route of administration for those cancer patients who have difficulty swallowing or have intestinal obstruction. Pemoline has been demonstrated to be as effective as methylphenidate or dextroamphetamine.[72] Caution should be taken, however, in using pemoline in patients with liver impairment. In fact, liver function tests should be monitored at initiation and during treatment with this stimulant.[73] Initial dosing regimens should begin with 18.75 mg in the morning and at noon and can be titrated upward until symptom relief is achieved.

Monoamine Oxidase Inhibitors

The use of monoamine oxidase inhibitors (MAOIs) in the cancer pain population should be approached with caution. The avoidance of foods containing tyramine may only further limit the diets of cancer patients who may already have dietary and nutritional restrictions. In addition, the use of narcotic analgesics may be problematic or dangerous in patients taking MAOIs because myoclonus and delirium have been reported.[10] The use of meperidine in patients taking an MAOI is absolutely contraindicated and can lead to hyperpyrexia and cardiovascular collapse. Finally, other sympathomimetic drugs and less obvious MAOIs such as the chemotherapeutic agent procarbazine can, when combined in a patient taking an MAOI, result in a hypertensive crisis. If a patient has responded to a MAOI in the past and other antidepressants are not effective, continuance on a MAOI may be warranted but should be monitored with caution.

Lithium Carbonate

Patients who have been treated with maintenance lithium therapy can be continued on this regimen cancer treatment. It is important, however, to monitor the level of this medication especially during the preoperative and postoperative periods during which fluid and salts may be restricted and fluid

balance shifts may occur. The required maintenance dose of lithium carbonate may need to be reduced in seriously ill patients. Given the nephrotoxic effects of many chemotherapeutic agents, renal function should be carefully monitored in patients being given lithium. Although several authors have noted the ability of lithium to stimulate leukocyte production, the viability of these leukocytes has not been determined. In any event, this leukocyte stimulating effect appears to be transient.[74]

Benzodiazepines

The trazolobenzodiazepine alprazolam has been shown to be a mildly effective antidepressant as well as an anxiolytic. Alprazolam is particularly useful in cancer patients who have mixed symptoms of anxiety and depression. Alprazolam, however, is probably not adequate as the sole medication for major depression. The starting dose is 0.25 mg three times per day, although therapeutic effects may require 4–6 mg daily.[35]

Electroconvulsive Therapy

Electroconvulsive therapy may be considered in those patients whose depression includes psychotic features, who demonstrate an agitated depression, or for whom treatment with conventional antidepressants is unadvisable. The safe, effective use of electroconvulsive therapy in depressed cancer patients has been reviewed by others,[39] and this alternative may yield secondary analgesic benefits for the depressed patient with otherwise unrelieved pain.

Suicide and Cancer Pain

Uncontrolled pain is a major risk factor for suicide and suicidal ideation in cancer patients.[75–78] The public perceives cancer as an extremely painful disease relative to other medical conditions. Sixty-nine percent of the public indicated, in a public opinion survey, that cancer pain can get so bad that a person might consider suicide.[79] Physicians who work with cancer patients report that persistent or uncontrolled pain accounts for the majority of requests they receive for physician-assisted suicide or euthanasia. The vast majority of cancer suicides occur in patients with severe pain that was inadequately controlled or tolerated poorly.[75, 76] Pain plays an important role in vulnerability to suicide; however, associated psychological distress and mood disturbance seem to be essential cofactors that increase the risk of cancer suicide. Cancer patients with pain are twice as likely to suffer from a psychiatric complication (anxiety or depressive disorder) as those without pain.[12] Pain has adverse effects on a cancer patient's quality of life and sense of control. Pain interferes with a patient's ability to receive support from family and others. Cancer patients with advanced cancer and pain are especially vulnerable to suicide owing to the increased likelihood of the presence of multiple risk factors such as depression, delirium, loss of control, and hopelessness.

The role that cancer pain plays in suicidal ideation is complex. Evidence suggests that it is not merely the extent or degree of pain that plays a role in cancer-related suicidal ideation, but rather the suffering experienced as part of one's psychological reactions to cancer pain, such as depression and hopelessness. Studies at Memorial Sloan Kettering Cancer Center examined the relationship of cancer pain to suicidal ideation.[77, 80] In a series of 71 patients who had suicidal ideation with serious intent, significant pain was a factor in only 30% of cases. In striking contrast, virtually all 71 suicidal cancer patients had a psychiatric disorder (mood disturbance or organic mental disorder) at the time of evaluation.[77] We also studied cancer pain patients involved in ongoing research protocols at the Memorial Sloan Kettering Cancer Center Pain and Psychiatry Services.[80] Suicidal ideation occurred in 17% of the population, with the most patients reporting suicidal ideation without intent to act. Interestingly, in this population of cancer patients who all had significant pain (Visual Analog Scale pain intensity mean score of 5.4), suicidal ideation was not directly related to pain intensity, but rather was strongly related to the degree of depression and mood disturbance (as measured by the Beck Depression Inventory and Memorial Pain Assessment Card, Visual Analog Mood Scale). Duration of pain did not predict suicidal ideation. Pain was related to suicidal ideation indirectly in that patients' perception of poor pain relief was associated with suicidal ideation. As a result, perceptions of pain relief may have more to do with aspects of hopelessness than pain itself.

Patients who have uncontrolled pain, advanced illness, depression, delirium, helplessness, preexisting psychiatric illness, and a family suicide history are at increased risk for suicide. Early intervention should be directed at assessing mental status for the presence of delirium or confusion and appropriately treating and controlling pain and depression. Often, cancer patients believe that their continued life is a burden to their families. Therefore, the clinician should have the patient's family involved in the therapeutic management process. Although it is appropriate to intervene when medical or psychiatric factors are clearly the driving force in a suicidal patient, there are circumstances in which overly aggressive interventions may be less helpful. In patients with advanced illness, the goal should be to establish rapport, develop an alliance, and to provide management of poorly controlled symptoms as an alternative to suicide.

Delirium (Organic Mental Disorders)

The third most common psychiatric diagnosis among cancer patients is delirium. Delirium is present in approximately 15–20% of hospitalized cancer patients.[81] The incidence of delirium increases as disease progresses. Massie et al.[26] found that more than 75% of terminally ill cancer patients met criteria for a diagnosis of delirium. A recent chart review at Memorial Sloan Kettering Cancer Center revealed that 45% of patients who were receiving continuous infusion of opioids developed delirium. The etiology of delirium can be traced either to the direct effects of cancer on the CNS or to the indirect CNS effects of the disease or treatment (medications, electrolyte imbalance, failure of organ systems, infection, vascular complications, and preexisting cognitive impairment or dementia). A common error among medical and nursing staff is to conclude that the presence of the psychological symptoms associated with delirium represents a psychological disorder before adequately considering, evaluating, or eliminating possible organic etiologies.

Delirium is as an etiologically nonspecific, global cerebral dysfunction characterized by concurrent disturbances in any of a number of different functions including level of consciousness, attention, thinking, perception, emotion, memory, psychomotor behavior, and sleep–wake cycle.[82] The

Table 22-4. Medications Useful in Managing Delirium in Cancer Pain Patients

Generic Name	Approximate Daily Dosage Range (mg)	Route
Neuroleptics		
Haloperidol	0.5–5.0 q2–12 hrs	PO, IV, SC, IM
Thioridazine	10–75 q4–8 hrs	PO
Chlorpromazine	12.5–50.0 q4–12 hrs	PO, IV, IM
Methotrimeprazine	12.5–50.0 q4–8 hrs	IV, SC, PO
Benzodiazepines		
Lorazepam	0.5–2.0 q1–4 hrs	PO, IV, IM
Midazolam	30–100 per 24 hrs	IV, SC

Note: IM injections should be avoided if repeated use becomes necessary; SC infusions are generally accepted modes of drug administration in the terminally ill; parenteral doses are generally twice as potent as oral doses; and IV infusions or bolus injections should be administered slowly.

critical features that distinguish delirium from other organic mental disorders are acute and abrupt onset, presumed organic etiology, disorientation, fluctuation in the sleep–wake cycle, and a waxing and waning of symptoms. Even in patients with advanced illness, delirium is reversible. This reversibility, however, may not be true in the last 24–48 hours of life and is most likely due to the irreversible influence of multiple organ failure occurring in the final hours of life.

The treatment of delirium in patients with advanced cancer is unique; however, because the organic etiology of delirium is most often multifactorial, even if there is the determination of a distinct cause, it may not be reversible (e.g., brain metastases or hepatic failure). The diagnostic evaluation may be limited by the setting (home, hospice). With the seriously ill patient, the focus is more appropriately on the comfort of the patient and, consequently, the desired benefit of unpleasant or invasive diagnostic procedures must be weighed against their potential yield. When the clinician encounters delirium in a cancer patient, a differential diagnosis should always be made. Definitive diagnostic procedures should be pursued when a suspected factor can be easily identified and treated effectively.

Although psychopharmacologic interventions cannot replace the physiologic workup and intervention required to correct the underlying cause of the delirium, they may be helpful in managing the psychiatric manifestations of the illness that frequently interfere with treatment and endanger the well-being of the patient. Antipsychotic, neuroleptic drugs have been found useful for delirium (Table 22-4). Given the variation in sedating properties and the likelihood of producing orthostatic hypotension, neurologic side effects, and anticholinergic properties, it is important to consider the symptom constellation present in the patient and the side effect profile of the medication before choosing an appropriate antipsychotic to treat delirium.

The usual first-line treatment for delirium in the cancer patient is haloperidol. In low doses, this medication is effective in managing the agitation, hallucinations, and paranoia that frequently accompany delirium. The option of intravenous administration makes this drug attractive in treating the patient whose compliance may be compromised by confusion and therefore may be unable to take medication orally.[83] The initial dose used in cancer patients should be low (0.5–1.0 mg orally, intramuscularly, or intravenously) and the dose should be repeated (every 30–45 minutes) until symptom control is achieved. Extrapyramidal side effects are commonly associated with haloperidol. Acute akithisia, parkinsonian symptoms, and dystonia can be controlled with propranolol, lorazepam, or antiparkinsonian medications such as diphenhydramine or benztropine. A rare, but serious complication of antipsychotic medication use is neuroleptic malignant syndrome. Usually occurring after prolonged high-dose administration of neuroleptics, neuroleptic malignant syndrome is characterized by hyperthermia, increased mental confusion, leukocytosis, muscular rigidity, myoglobinuria, and high serum creatine phosphokinase. Treatment consists of the discontinuation of the neuroleptic and the use of dantrolene sodium or bromocriptine mesylate.[83] A common strategy in the management of agitated delirium is to add parenteral lorazepam to a regimen of haloperidol.[84] Lorazepam (0.5–1.0 mg every 1–2 hours orally or intravenously), along with haloperidol, may be more effective in rapidly sedating the agitated delirious patient. Despite these clinical observations, benzodiazepines alone have limited benefit for treating delirium. In a double-blind, randomized trial comparing haloperidol, chlorpromazine, and lorazepam, Breitbart et al.[56] demonstrated that lorazepam alone, in doses up to 8 mg in a 12-hour period, was ineffective in treating delirium and, in fact, contributed to worsening delirium and cognitive impairment. Both haloperidol and chlorpromazine, however, in low doses (approximately 2 mg of haloperidol equivalent every 24 hours), were highly effective in controlling the symptoms of delirium (dramatic improvement in Delirium Rating Scales scores) and improving cognitive function (dramatic improvement in Mini Mental Status Examinations scores). Perhaps the only setting in which benzodiazepines alone have an established role is in the management of delirium in the dying patient.

Psychiatric Management of Cancer Pain

Inadequate Pain Management: Assessment Issues in the Treatment of Pain

Inadequate management of cancer pain is often due an inability to properly assess pain in all its dimensions.[2, 24, 79] Rather than investigating medical factors that may result in uncontrolled pain, psychological variables are often inappropriately proposed to explain the presence or exacerbation of pain. In a recent study of physician attitudes and practices in cancer pain management, 86% of the physicians surveyed thought that most patients with pain were undermedicated. Only 51% of the physicians surveyed thought that pain control in their own practice setting was good or very good. Thirty-one percent stated that they would wait until the patient's life expectancy was 6 months or less before starting strong opioid (morphine) therapy. Physicians often underused adjuvant analgesics and undermanaged side effects of opioid analgesics. Seventy-six percent of physicians surveyed rated lack of pain assessment skills as the single most important barrier to pain management.

Finally, reluctance by patients to report pain and to take analgesics and reluctance by physicians to prescribe opioids represented significant barriers.[85]

Other causes of inadequate cancer pain management include (1) lack of knowledge of current therapeutic approaches; (2) focus on prolonging life and cure versus alleviating suffering; (3) inadequate physician–patient relationship; (4) limited expectations of patients; (5) unavailability of narcotics; (6) fear of respiratory depression; and, most importantly, (7) fear of addiction.

The fear of addiction affects both patient compliance and physician management of narcotic analgesics, thus leading to undermedication of cancer patients.[24, 86] Research into the analgesic usage patterns of cancer patients indicates that, although cancer patients on long-term opioid regimens develop tolerance and physical dependence, addiction (psychological dependence) is rare and almost never occurs in patients who do not have a preexisting substance abuse history.[14] Escalation of opioid analgesic use by cancer patients is usually due to progression of cancer or the development of tolerance. Tolerance means that a larger dose of narcotic analgesic is required to maintain an original analgesic effect. Physical dependence is characterized by the onset of signs and symptoms of withdrawal if the narcotic is suddenly stopped or a narcotic antagonist is administered. Tolerance usually occurs in association with physical dependence but does not imply psychological dependence. Psychological dependence or addiction is not equivalent to physical dependence or tolerance and is a behavioral pattern of compulsive drug use characterized by a craving for the drug and overwhelming involvement in obtaining and using it for purposes other than pain relief. A prior history of intravenous drug abuse in a cancer pain patient often leads the clinician to worry unduly. In a study of cancer pain consults, only 8 of 468 patients had a history of intravenous drug usage; none of the eight, however, had been using drugs actively in the previous year. All eight were inadequately medicated for their pain prior to pain consultation in part because of the staff's fear that the patient's drug abuse was either active or would recur. Adequate pain control was ultimately achieved in these patients by using appropriate analgesic dosages accompanied by staff education.[86]

Psychological Factors in Cancer Pain

Although psychological factors have been known to play an important role in the nonmalignant chronic pain experience, the place of psychological factors in cancer pain experience has frequently been underestimated. In part this may be the result of a set of beliefs held by both clinicians and patients alike. Turk and Fernandez[3] have identified several false assumptions that likely have an impact on how patients and clinicians view and conceptualize cancer pain.

The first false assumption is that cancer is inevitably lethal. Consequently, clinicians may think that the focus should therefore be on the eradication of the disease, and, if not possible, then somatic therapies aimed at palliation are most appropriate. It is interesting to note, however, that although almost 40% of individuals with cancer survive at least 5 years after diagnosis, this disease is more feared than heart disease, which has twice the mortality of cancer and is the leading cause of death in the United States.[85]

A second false assumption is that cancer will be extremely painful and for many individuals it is the fear of pain and death that is the most fearful aspect of cancer.[13, 18] This assumption has led physicians to expect the presence of pain, take the reports of cancer pain at face value, and treat the pain with only somatic therapies, ignoring the impact of psychological factors.[3] Although pain is prevalent in cancer, patients with specific types of cancer, e.g., lung cancer and lymphoma, report little or no pain during their disease.[63, 87]

The third false assumption is that the relationship between tissue damage and cancer pain is causal, and that a patient's subjective report of pain should be taken as an accurate assessment of the organic nature of the pain. The flaw in the assumption about a one-to-one relationship between tissue damage and cancer pain is supported by several observations. First, it has been observed that patients delayed seeking treatment for what were determined to be cancerous lesions because they did not experience pain.[88] Although pain is rarely the presenting symptom that prompts patients to seek medical attention, the increase of pain following the notification of the diagnosis of cancer is dramatic.[19, 89] Second, after diagnosis, the association between pain intensity and stage of disease is

weak.[20] Finally, tissue damage can occur in the absence of pain.[90]

Although most of the literature linking psychological variables to pain has tended to focus on nonmalignant pain, there are findings regarding psychological variables that apply to cancer pain management. The following discussion lists psychological factors that have been shown to have an impact on either cancer or nonmalignant pain.[3]

Symptom Interpretation

Individuals form subjective representations of illness and symptomatology. Accordingly, when individuals experience somatic phenomenon, they engage in an analysis of the meaning of the symptoms. When faced with an illness, individuals respond based on their private, subjective, and idiosyncratic network of beliefs and fears.[91] The result is that the idiosyncratic meaning of the symptom or illness directs the attentional capacities of the individual.

Individuals with cancer tend to become more sensitive, focus on bodily sensations, and monitor their bodies hypervigilantly. These sensations become continual reminders of the fact that they have cancer and consequently have the capacity of being interpreted as pain.[31] The meaning of cancer pain, which is different from that of chronic pain, has been shown to be a subjective signal of disease progression.[4] The continual perception of a painful stimulus coupled with the belief that this is a signal of disease progression has been shown to result in a perception of increased pain.[92] This hypervigilance and monitoring may result in patients experiencing even mild nociception as unbearable.

Self-Efficacy

The individual's appraisal of their ability to perform at a given level or to cope with a particular stressor is referred to as self-efficacy. The sense of self-efficacy has been implicated as a factor in the understanding of acute and chronic pain. People who score high on measures of self-efficacy have tolerance for pain and also show increased activation of endogenous opioids when encountering painful stimuli.[93] It has been suggested that it is the beliefs that a patient has about his or her ability to cope with a particular set of medical problems, not the patient's objective physical status, that best predict how well the individual will actually deal with the physical or psychological difficulties.[94] It appears that self-efficacy is determined in part by pain response expectations and that patients have some notion of the limitations of their ability to cope with pain. Pain response expectations appear to influence performance and associated pain behavior through their effects on efficacy expectations.

Controllability

Locus of control has been shown to be an accurate predictor of the patients's ability to deal effectively with pain. Chronic pain patients differ in the degree to which they view themselves as having control over their pain (internal control) or whether they see factors such as chance or powerful others (external control) as having control. Chronic pain patients who report high levels of internal locus of control were less likely to have pain and, when they did, they reported that the pain was not as severe as did those individuals who scored lower on internal locus of control. Conversely, patients with a strong belief in chance control (external control) had higher levels of psychological distress, felt more helpless, and were more likely to use ineffective coping strategies in dealing with pain.[95]

The perception that a noxious stimulus is controllable—either by oneself or by another—has been shown to influence the perception of pain.[96] In cancer patients, the belief that the pain is controllable is related to analgesic usage, analgesic efficacy,[97] and pain relief.[98] In the evaluation of the use of patient-controlled analgesia, those patients who had control used one-third less medication to receive a comparable level of pain relief compared with patients who were dependent on nurse-administered analgesia.[99] The control of noxious stimuli in general has been shown to enhance the patient's adjustment to pain and the instillation of control is a key component of many behavioral approaches used to help patients deal with cancer-related pain.[100]

Expectancy

It comes as no surprise that the expectation that an event will be painful increases the appraisal of the ensuing nociception as more painful.[101] It has been shown that merely using the word *pain* in instructions prior to an experiment can result in greater sensitivity to stimuli and can decrease the threshold for calling an event painful.[102]

One of the most striking demonstrations of expectancy comes from research examining the use of placebos. Beecher[103] found that when subjects were given pharmacologic placebos and were told they would be effective in alleviating a range of distressing situations (including pain, nausea, and mood) 35% of the subjects indicated symptom relief. This phenomenon has also been demonstrated in surgical interventions.[103]

Learned Helplessness

The state of feeling that in a distressing situation effective solutions are not available to eliminate or reduce the stress, is known as learned helplessness. A positive correlation exists in chronic pain patients between feelings of helplessness and psychological distress.[104] It was found that the waxing and waning of symptomatology common in chronic pain patients leads to the perception of unpredictability and thus a sense of helplessness and hopelessness.[105] Patients who viewed themselves as helpless were more prone to become depressed. It seems therefore that it is not the disease that results in depression but rather the patient's interpretation of the disease as uncontrollable. Helplessness has been shown to predict level of pain and the number of visits to the physician per year.[106] In a longitudinal study of arthritis patients, helplessness was shown at both 6 months and 2 years to be associated with changes in depression, pain, and global health ratings.[107]

Psychological Interventions with Cancer Pain Patients

The effective management of cancer-related pain must be from a multimodal perspective, involving pharmacologic, anesthetic, stimulatory, rehabilitative, and psychological approaches, often in combination. The multiple goals of psychological interventions with cancer patients are to provide support, knowledge, and continuity, as well as teaching new psychological skills that may be necessary to meet the emotional demands of cancer and cancer pain.

Supportive Psychotherapy

Psychotherapy with cancer pain patients may take several forms, such as individual, family, and group. The focus of psychotherapy with cancer pain patients and their families is to help them adapt to the fact of having cancer and its concomitant pain. The therapist may encourage the patient to draw on past strengths and previously existing coping strategies such as relaxation, cognitive coping, proper use of analgesics, assertiveness, and communication skills. It is important to recognize the role that the patient's family places in the treatment process. Important considerations for family interventions include reinforcing existing communication skills or teaching new ones and assisting with the acquisition of information essential to the understanding of the disease. The use of group therapy interventions for patients or families has been shown to help patients develop new coping strategies, gain support by sharing common experiences, and reduce pain.[50, 52]

Cognitive Behavioral Interventions for Cancer Pain

Whereas general supportive psychotherapy has been shown to be effective in the management of the distress associated with cancer, most research into the use of psychotherapy for cancer pain has been in the area of cognitive behavioral techniques (Table 22-5).

The techniques most useful for cancer pain patients include passive relaxation with mental imagery, cognitive distraction or focusing techniques, progressive muscle relaxation, biofeedback, hypnosis, and music therapy.[18, 108] These techniques are useful not only in chronic cancer-related pain but also in more acute, procedure-related pain. Cancer patients are highly motivated to learn and practice these techniques, not only because of the symptom relief associated with these methods but also for their assistance in restoring a sense of control, personal efficacy, and personal involvement in their care.

Although most cancer patients with pain are appropriate candidates for these techniques, the clinician should consider not only the intensity of the pain but also the mental clarity of the patient. Those patients with mild-to-moderate pain can expect to obtain the greatest benefit; the patient with severe

Table 22-5. Cognitive-Behavioral Techniques Used by Cancer Pain Patients

Psychoeducation
    Preparatory information
Relaxation
    Passive breathing
    Progressive muscle relaxation
Distraction
    Focusing
    Controlled mental imagery
    Cognitive distraction
    Behavioral distraction
Combined relaxation and distraction techniques
    Passive relaxation with mental imagery
    Progressive muscle relaxation with imagery
    Systematic desensitization
    Meditation
    Hypnosis
    Biofeedback
    Music therapy
Cognitive therapies
    Cognitive restructuring
Behavioral therapies
    Self-monitoring
    Modeling
    Behavioral rehearsal
    Graded task management
    Contingency management

pain will benefit less from psychological interventions unless the use of somatic therapies can lower the intensity of the pain. Patients with impaired mental status will find it difficult to exercise the focused attention necessary for these techniques.[109]

Behavioral interventions include techniques for modifying physiologic pain reactions and pain behaviors. The essential method behind these interventions is self-monitoring, which allows the patient to notice dysfunctional reactions and learn to control them. Systematic desensitization—a gradual systematic exposure to frightening or distressing situations—helps stop anticipatory anxiety that leads to avoidant behaviors and remobilize inactive patients. Graded task assignment is essentially systematic desensitization because it is applied to patients who are encouraged to take small steps gradually so as to perform activities more readily. Contingency management, which provides rewards for dealing more effectively with pain as well as becoming more active, is a method of reinforcing "well" behaviors only, thus modifying dysfunctional operant pain behaviors associated with secondary gain.[107, 110]

The objectives of cognitive techniques for pain management are to increase relaxation and to reduce the intensity and distress commonly associated with the pain. This approach, which is derived from the cognitive therapy of depression and anxiety, modifies the thoughts and beliefs that patients have about their pain, and their illness in general. By restructuring or modifying the thoughts or cognitions, patients can allow for a more rational, moderated response to their pain.[18]

Relaxation and Imagery

The reduction of muscular tension, autonomic arousal, and mental distress leads to a reduction in pain.[108] Some specific relaxation techniques include (1) passive relaxation, which focuses attention on sensations of warmth and decreased tension in various parts of the body; (2) progressive muscle relaxation, which involves active tensing and relaxing of muscles; and (3) meditation.

Passive relaxation and focused breathing direct the patient's attention toward breathing, sensations of warmth and relaxation, or on the release of muscular tension in various body parts. A script for a generic relaxation exercise using passive relaxation or focused breathing that is based on and integrates the work of Erickson,[111] Benson,[112] and others[113] follows.

> Why don't you begin by finding a comfortable position. It could be in your bed or in a chair. Slowly allow your body to relax and just let it go. I wonder if you could allow your body to become as calm as possible . . . just let it go, just imagine your body sinking into that chair or bed . . . feel free to move in any way that allows your body to find the most comfortable position possible . . . just give your body permission to relax and let go.
>
> As you focus on the sound of my voice, you may find that it feels comfortable to let your eyes close. If you like, you can let the eyelids gently cover your eyes . . . let your eyes sink back deeply into their sockets . . . that's it, just let them go, falling back gently and deeply into their sockets as your lids begin to feel heavier and heavier. As you allow your head to fall back deeply into the pillow, feeling the weight of your head sinking into the pillow as you breathe out, just breathe out, one big breath. Slowly, if you can, begin to notice your breathing. Notice the gentle rise and fall of your breathing. Can you see how

> much air you take in and how much air you let out as you breath naturally and evenly, and, with the sound of my voice, I wonder if you can begin to notice the rise and fall of your breathing, in and out, in and out, breathing in calmness and quietness, breathing out tiredness and frustration . . . that's it, let it go, breathing in a sense of well-being and warmth, breathing out fear and tension . . . breathing in and out . . . in and out . . . you can enjoy breathing in this relaxed way for as long as you need to. You notice the sense of peace you are beginning to feel as you continue to observe your even and steady breathing that is allowing you to feel gentle and calm, breathing that is allowing you to feel a sense of inner quietness, breathing relaxation in and tension out . . . in and out . . . breathing in quietness and control, breathing out tiredness and tension . . . that's it. As you continue to notice the quietness and stillness of your body, why don't you take a few quiet moments to experience this sense of calmness more fully.

During the exercise, it may be helpful for the clinician to both pace and model for the patient. This may include the physician assuming a position of relaxation, closing his or her eyes, and breathing at the same rate as the patient. If the patient becomes anxious or agitated, this can be explored verbally, and if appropriate, the exercise continued. At the end of the exercise, the clinician may increase the pace, raise the volume of his voice, and shift positions so as to indicate the termination of the exercise.

Relaxation techniques prove most useful in pain management when they are combined with a pleasant or distracting image. The use of focusing or distraction involves control over the focus of attention. Imaginative attention can be used by having the patient picture himself in a pleasant setting, such as at the beach. Mental distraction involves engaging in a mental task such as "counting sheep," whereas behavioral distraction involves keeping oneself busy as a way to avoid thinking about pain. Imagery or using one's imagination while in a relaxed state can be used to transform the sensation of pain, e.g., make it feel warmer or colder. One can also imaginatively transform the context of pain, e.g., imagine oneself in battle on a football field rather than in a hospital bed. Some patients find that they can use "dissociated somatization" in which they imagine that the painful body part is no longer part of their body.[18] It is important for the clinician to remember that no one therapy will work for all patients and that not every patient will find these techniques acceptable.

Hypnosis

Hypnosis is efficacious in the treatment of some cancer pain.[50, 51, 114] The hypnotic trance is essentially a state of heightened and focused concentration that can be used to manipulate the perception of pain. The depth of hypnotizability may determine the effectiveness as well as the strategies employed during hypnosis. One-third of cancer patients are not hypnotizable and therefore other techniques are recommended. Of the two-thirds of patients who are hypnotizable, three principles apply to the use of hypnosis for pain relief: (1) use of self-hypnosis; (2) relaxation and not fighting the pain; and (3) use of a mental filter to ease the hurt in pain.[51] Although patients may vary in their ability to use hypnotic techniques, these methods can be modified to meet the needs of each patient.

Biofeedback

Fotopoulos et al.[115] noted significant pain relief in a group of cancer patients who were taught electromyographic and electroencephalographic biofeedback-assisted relaxation. Only 2 of 17, however, were able to maintain analgesia after cessation of treatment. A lack of generalization of effect can be a problem with biofeedback techniques. Although physical condition may make a prolonged training period impossible (especially for the terminally ill), most cancer patients can use electromyographic and temperature biofeedback techniques to learn relaxation-assisted pain control.[108]

Music Therapy

Munro and Mount[73] have written extensively on the use of music therapy with cancer patients. Music can often capture the focus of attention like no other stimulus and thus help patients distract their perception of pain, while expressing themselves in meaningful ways.

Psychotropic Adjuvant Analgesics for Cancer Pain

Although the mainstay of pharmacologic intervention for cancer pain continues to be narcotic analgesics, the multifactorial nature of cancer pain suggests that psychotropic medications may help manage psychiatric disorders and supplement more traditional analgesic methods as adjuvant analgesics. These medications are not only effective in managing symptoms of anxiety, depression, insomnia, or delirium that commonly complicate the course of cancer patients with pain, but they also potentiate the analgesic effects of opioid drugs and often have innate analgesic properties of their own (Table 22-6).

Antidepressants

Antidepressants have proven utility as adjuvant analgesic agents for a wide variety of chronic pain syndromes, including cancer pain.[37, 116–118] Although all classes of antidepressants have exhibited adjuvant analgesic properties, the TCAs (amitriptyline in particular) have been the most-studied medication. Amitriptyline has been shown to be effective as an adjuvant analgesic for a number of chronic pain syndromes.[119–123] Other TCAs that have been shown to have efficacy as analgesics include imipramine,[124–126] desipramine,[118] nortriptyline,[61] clomipramine,[127, 128] and doxepin.[129]

Heterocyclic and noncyclic antidepressants such as trazodone, mianserin, maprotiline, and the newer serotonin-specific reuptake inhibitors such as fluoxetine, sertraline, and paroxetine may also prove useful as adjuvant analgesics for cancer pain. Clinical trials of the effectiveness of serotonin-specific reuptake inhibitors as analgesics, however, have been equivocal with the exception of paroxetine, which has been shown to be effective as an adjuvant analgesic for neuropathic pain.[62]

Although many antidepressants have analgesic properties, there is no definite indication that any one drug is more effective than any other. The most experience, however, has been with amitriptyline, which remains the drug of first choice. It was initially thought that a low-dose regimen was as effective as a high dose in the management of pain.[122] Recently, however, researchers have demonstrated that low doses of amitriptyline yield only a modest analgesic result,[130] whereas higher serum levels (which are associated with doses of up to 150 mg) produce more effective analgesia.[123, 124] Treatment should be initiated with 10–25 mg at bedtime and increased slowly by 10–25 mg every 2–4 days toward 150 mg, with frequent assess-

Table 22-6. Psychotropic Adjuvant Analgesic Drugs for Cancer Pain

Generic Name	Trade Name	Approximate Daily Dosage Range (mg)	Route
Tricyclic antidepressants			
Amitriptyline	Elavil	10–150	PO, IM, PR
Nortriptyline	Pamelor, Aventyl	10–150	PO
Imipramine	Tofranil	12.5–150.0	PO, IM
Desipramine	Norpramin	10–150	PO
Clomipramine	Anafranil	10–150	PO
Doxepin	Sinequan	12.5–150.0	PO, IM
Heterocyclic and noncyclic antidepressants			
Trazodone	Desyrel	25–300	PO
Maprotiline	Ludiomil	50–300	PO
Serotonin-specific reuptake inhibitors			
Paroxetine	Paxil	10–40	PO
Amine precursors			
L-Tryptophan		500–3,000	PO
Psychostimulants			
Methylphenidate	Ritalin	2.5–20.0 bid	PO
Dextroamphetamine	Dexedrine	2.5–20.0 bid	PO
Phenothiazines			
Fluphenazine	Prolixin	1–3	PO, IM
Methotrimeprazine	Levoprome	10–20 q6 hrs	IM, IV
Butyrophenones			
Haloperidol	Haldol	1–3	PO, IM, IV
Pimozide	Orap	2–6 bid	PO
Antihistamines			
Hydroxyzine	Vistaril	50 q4–6 hrs	PO, IM, IV
Steroids			
Dexamethasone	Decadron	4–16	PO, IV
Benzodiazepines			
Alprazolam	Xanax	0.25–2.0 tid	PO
Clonazepam	Klonopin	0.5–4.0 bid	PO

ments of pain and side effects until a beneficial effect is achieved. The serum levels of amitriptyline should be evaluated frequently to find the dosage required to reach the therapeutic range. The maximal effect as an adjuvant analgesic may require continuation of drug for 2–6 weeks. Both pain and depression in cancer patients respond to lower doses (25–100 mg) of antidepressant than are usually required in physically healthy patients (100–300 mg) because of impaired metabolism of these drugs. Selection of the antidepressant is dependent on the side effect profile, existing medical problems, the nature of the depressive symptoms if present, and past response to antidepressants. Se-

dating drugs like amitriptyline are helpful when insomnia complicates the presence of pain and depression of a cancer patient. The anticholinergic properties of some of these drugs should be considered. Occasionally, in patients who have limited analgesic response to TCAs, analgesia can be accomplished by adding lithium to the regimen.[131]

Psychostimulants

In addition to their utility as antidepressants in the medically ill, psychostimulants such as dextroamphetamine, methylphenidate, and pemoline also help diminish excessive sedation secondary to narcotic analgesics and are potent adjuvant analgesics.[71, 132] Treatment with dextroamphetamine or methylphenidate usually begins with a dose of 2.5 mg at 8 A.M. and at noon. This dosage is slowly increased over several days until a desired effect is achieved or side effects (overstimulation, anxiety, insomnia, paranoia, and confusion) intervene. Typically, a dose of more than 30 mg per day is not necessary; occasionally, however, patients require up to 60 mg per day. A strategy useful in treating depression associated with cancer pain is to start the patient on a stimulant and then to add a TCA after several days to help prolong and potentiate the effects of the stimulant. Pemoline, a chemically unique psychostimulant, may have similar usefulness as an antidepressant and adjuvant analgesic in cancer patients.[72] There have been no studies, however, documenting pemoline's effectiveness in potentiating the analgesic properties of opioids. Pemoline can be started at a dose of 18.75 mg in the morning and at noon, which is increased gradually over several days. Typically patients require 75 mg per day or less. Caution should be taken when using pemoline in patients with impaired liver impairment; liver function tests should be monitored periodically with longer term treatment.[133]

Neuroleptics

Methotrimeprazine, a phenothiazine, has proven utility in providing analgesia by a nonopioid mechanism. In addition to its analgesic effects, methotrimeprazine is useful as an anxiolytic and in the management of agitation and confusion in terminally ill patients. Doses range from 12.5–50 mg every 4–8 hours by either slow or continuous infusions up to 300 mg per 24 hours for most patients.[134] Fluphenazine, in combination with TCAs, helps manage neuropathic pain.[61] Haloperidol has modest clinical utility as a coanalgesic for cancer pain. Both fluphenazine and haloperidol are most commonly used in low doses (2–8 mg per day) in combination with antidepressants for neuropathic pain. The benefits of long-term use must be weighed against the risk of developing tardive dyskinesia, particularly in the young patient with good long-term prognosis. Pimozide (Orap), a butyrophenone, has been shown to be effective at doses of 4–12 mg per day as an analgesic in the management of trigeminal neuralgia.[135]

Anxiolytics

Hydroxyzine, a mild anxiolytic, has proven utility for treating anxious cancer patients with pain.[136] One hundred milligrams of hydroxyzine has analgesic activity nearly equianalgesic to 8 mg of morphine and has additive analgesic effects when combined with morphine. The addition of 25–50 mg of hydroxyzine every 4–6 hours to a regimen of opioids often helps relieve anxiety as well as providing adjuvant analgesia. Although benzodiazepines have not traditionally been considered to have analgesic properties, some authors think that their anticonvulsant properties make certain benzodiazepines useful for neuropathic pain. Alprazolam has been shown to be effective as an analgesic in cancer patients with phantom limb pain or deafferentation (neuropathic) pain.[137] Clonazepam (Klonopin) may also be useful in the management of lancinating neuropathic pains in the cancer setting, and has been reported to be an effective analgesic for patients with trigeminal neuralgia, headache, and postherpetic neuralgia.[138, 139]

Pain in Acquired Immunodeficiency Syndrome

As with cancer, pain is also a significant problem for patients with human immunodeficiency virus (HIV) infection and is associated with significant psychological and functional impairments.[126, 140] As with cancer, the importance of proper assessment and management of pain in patients with HIV infection has been underestimated. The prevalence of pain in HIV-infected individuals varies depending on stage of disease, care setting, and study methodology. Contrary to popular belief, pain is a frequently encountered syndrome in this population. Estimates of the prevalence of pain in HIV-infected individuals generally range from 40–60%, with the prevalence of pain increasing as disease progresses.[141] Thirty-eight percent of ambulatory HIV-infected patients reported significant pain in a prospective study of pain prevalence over a 2-week period.[141] Fifty percent of patients with AIDS reported pain, whereas only 25% of those with earliest stages of HIV infection had pain. A study of pain in hospitalized patients with AIDS revealed that more than 50% of patients required treatment for pain, with pain being the presenting complaint in 30% (second only to fever).[126] Schofferman and Brody[142] reported that 53% of patients with far-advanced AIDS cared for in a hospice setting had pain.

The pain syndromes reported vary, but the most common are peripheral neuropathy, abdominal pain, headaches, and Kaposi's sarcoma.[141] HIV-related peripheral neuropathy affects up to 30% of AIDS patients.[143, 144] Often, patients experience two or more kinds of pain at any given time. The etiology of the pain problems in this population are traced not only to the impact of the disease but also to the effects of pharmacologic treatments designed to slow the progression of the disease. Chemotherapy, antiviral drugs, antitubercular drugs, and colony-stimulating factors have been linked to the development of pain problems in this population. As would be expected, patients with advanced disease, low T4 cell counts, histories of multiple opportunistic infections, and greater debilitation report pain as a significant problem.

Psychological Variables

Patients with HIV disease face many stressors during the course of the illness including dependency, disability, and fear of pain and painful death. Although these concerns are universal, the level of psychological distress varies and is dependent on the level of social support, individual coping capacities, personality, and medical factors such as extent or stage of the disease. As noted earlier, the presence of psychological factors such as depression or anxiety can exacerbate pain. In a study of the impact of pain on ambulatory HIV-infected patients, depression was significantly correlated with the presence of pain. In addition to being significantly more distressed and depressed, those patients with pain were twice as likely to have suicidal ideation (40%) as those without pain (20%). HIV-infected patients with pain were more functionally impaired, and this was highly correlated to levels of pain intensity and depression. Those patients who thought that pain represented a threat to their health reported more intense pain than those who did not see pain as a threat. Patients with pain were more likely to be unemployed, disabled, and reported less social support.[86]

Psychological Interventions

Most of the interventions mentioned earlier are appropriate for the management of the patient with AIDS-related pain. However, special consideration must be given to the special needs of this population. This often involves working with nontraditional families that may consist of gay lovers, estranged spouses or parents, and fragmented or extended families. People with HIV disease may also require treatment for substance abuse. Psychiatric disorders, in particular organic mental disorders such as AIDS dementia complex, can occasionally interfere with adequate pain management in HIV-infected patients. Opiate analgesics, the mainstay of treatment for moderate-to-severe pain, may worsen dementia or cause treatment-limiting sedation, confusion, or hallucinations in patients with neurologic complications of AIDS.

Pain and Suicide

Several studies have demonstrated that, relative to the general population, men with AIDS have between a 21 and 36 times greater risk of suicide.[145] Suicidal ideation in ambulatory AIDS patients was found to be highly correlated with the presence of pain, depressed mood, and low T4 cell counts.[78] While 20% of ambulatory AIDS patients without pain reported suicidal thoughts, more than 40% of those with pain reported suicidal ideation. As with cancer pain patients, suicidal ideation in AIDS patients with pain is more likely to be related to a concomitant mood disturbance than to the intensity of the pain experienced.

Danger lies in the premature assumption that suicidal ideation or a request to hasten death in the AIDS patient represents a "rational act" unencumbered by psychiatric disturbance or uncontrolled pain or physical symptoms. Studies suggest that a significant percentage of such patients are suffering from psychiatric comorbidity related to AIDS (depression, confusional states) and poorly controlled physical symptoms including pain.[78]

Pain and Substance Abuse

Fear of addiction and concerns regarding drug abuse affect both patient compliance and physician management of narcotic analgesics and often lead to undermedication of the HIV-infected patient with pain. By relying on studies with cancer pain patients, it appears that, although tolerance and physical dependence commonly occur, chronic narcotic analgesics, addiction, i.e., physical dependence and drug abuse, are rare. More problematic, however, is the management of pain in the growing segment of HIV-infected people who are actively using drugs. In this population, concerns about drug-seeking behavior, lack of compliance with drug regimens, and the possibility of the transmission of the virus by intoxicated, disinhibited patients may lead to hesitancy among clinicians to use appropriate high doses of narcotic analgesics to control pain. Most clinicians who work with this population, however, recommend that practitioners set clear and direct limits as well as develop a collaborative relationship with patients that communicates the desire of the clinician to help manage both pain and psychological problems.

Summary

Cancer patients with pain present a challenge to the clinician. This population, which is vulnerable to psychiatric complications such as depression, anxiety, and delirium, can be treated most effectively by a comprehensive management program involving both pharmacologic and psychological approaches. Although opioid analgesics are the mainstay of the treatment for cancer-related pain, there is growing awareness that psychotropic drugs (in particular the antidepressants) are useful adjuvant analgesic agents for pain problems in this population. In addition, many of these drugs are important in the treatment of the psychiatric complications that result from cancer. The pain associated with AIDS is becoming an issue that clinicians must address. It appears that the information and techniques that have been acquired in the study of cancer-related pain may be applicable to the AIDS pain population.

References

1. Massie M, Holland J. The cancer patient and pain: Psychiatric implications and their management. J Pain Symptom Manage 1992;17:99.

2. Foley KM. The treatment of cancer pain. N Engl J Med 1985;313:845.

3. Turk D, Fernandez E. On the putative uniqueness of cancer pain: Do psychological principles apply? Behav Res Ther 1990;28:1.

4. Ahles TA, Blanchard EB, Ruckdeschel JC. The multi-dimensional nature of cancer related pain. Pain 1983;17:277.

5. Breitbart W. Psychiatric management of cancer pain. Cancer 1989;63:2336.

6. Merskey H. Psychiatry and Pain. In R Sternbach (ed), The Psychology of Pain. New York: Raven, 1986.

7. Lindblom U, Merskey H, Mumford JM, et al. Pain terms: A current list with definitions and notes on usage. Pain 1986;3:5215.

8. Melzack R, Wall PD. The Challenge of Pain. New York: Basic Books, 1983.

9. Breitbart W, Holland J. Psychiatric Aspects of Cancer Pain. In KM Foley et al. (eds), Advances in Pain Research and Therapy (Vol. 16). New York: Raven, 1990;73.

10. Breitbart W, Holland JC. Psychiatric Complications of Cancer. In MC Brain, PP Carbone (eds), Current Therapy in Hematology Oncology (Vol. 3). Toronto: Decker, 1988;268.

11. Massie MJ, Holland JC. The cancer patient with pain: Psychiatric complications and their management. Med Clin North Am 1987;71:243.

12. Derogatis LR, Morrow GR, Fetting J, et al. The prevalence of psychiatric disorders among cancer patients. JAMA 1983;249:751.

13. Daut R, Cleeland C. The prevalence and severity of pain in cancer. Cancer 1982;50:1913.

14. Kanner RM, Foley KM. Patterns of narcotic use in a cancer pain clinic. Ann NY Acad Sci 1981;362:161.

15. Cleeland C. The impact of pain on the patient with cancer. Cancer 1984;54:2635.

16. Foley KM. Pain Syndromes in Patients with Cancer. In JJ Bonica, V Ventafridda, RB Fink, et al. (eds), Advances in Pain Research and Therapy (Vol. 2). New York: Raven, 1975;59.

17. Twycross RG, Lack SA. Symptom Control in Far Advanced Cancer. Pain Relief. London: Pitman Brooks, 1983.

18. Fishman B, Loscalzo M. Cognitive-behavioral interventions in the management of cancer pain: Principles and applications. Med Clin North Am 1987;71:271.

19. Black R. The chronic pain syndrome. Surg Clin North Am 1975;55:999.

20. Greenwald H, Bonica J, Bergner, M. The prevalence of pain in four cancers. Cancer 1987;60:2563.

21. Breitbart W. Psychiatric aspects of pain and HIV disease. Focus: A Guide to AIDS Research and Counseling. 1990;5:1.

22. Spiegel D, Bloom JR. Pain in metastatic breast cancer. Cancer 1983;52:341.

23. McKegney FP, Bailey CR, Yates JW. Prediction and

management of pain in patients with advanced cancer. Gen Hosp Psychiatry 1981;3:95.

24. Marks RM, Sachar EJ. Undertreatment of medical inpatients with narcotic analgesics. Ann Intern Med 1973;78:173.

25. Bukberg J, Penman D, Holland J. Depression in hospitalized cancer patients. Psychosomatic Med 1984;43:199.

26. Massie MJ, Holland JC, Glass E. Delirium in terminally ill cancer patients. Am J Psychiatry 1983;140:1048.

27. Bruera E, MacMillan K, Kachin N, et al. The cognitive effects of the administration of narcotics. Pain 1989;39:13.

28. Holland JC, Rowland J (eds). Handbook of Psychooncology. New York: Oxford Press, 1989.

29. Bolles R, Fanselow M. A perceptual-defensive-recuperative model of fear and pain. Behav Brain Sci 1980;3:291.

30. Yang J, Wagner J, Clark W. Psychological Distress and Mood in Chronic Pain and Surgical Patients: A Sensory Decision Analysis. In JJ Bonica, U Lindblom, A Iggo (eds), Advances in Pain Research and Therapy. New York: Raven, 1983.

31. Pennebaker J. The Psychology of Physical Symptoms. New York: Springer, 1982.

32. Holland JC. Anxiety and cancer: The patient and the family. J Clin Psychiatry 1989;50:20.

33. Stiefel FC, Breitbart W, Holland JC. Corticosteroids in cancer: Neuropsychiatric complications. Cancer Invest 1989;7:479.

34. Brennan SC, Redd WH, Jacobsen PB, et al. Anxiety and panic during magnetic resonance scans. Lancet 1988;2:512.

35. Holland JC, Morrow G, Schmale A, et al. A randomized clinical trial of alprazolam versus progressive muscle relaxation in cancer patients with anxiety and depressive symptoms. J Clin Oncol 1991;9:1004.

36. Chouinard G, Young SN, Annable L. Antimanic effect of clonazepam. Biol Psychiatry 1983;18:451.

37. Walsh TD. Adjuvant Analgesic Therapy in Cancer Pain. In KM Foley, et al. (eds), Advances in Pain Research and Therapy (Vol. 16). New York: Raven, 1990;155.

38. Robinson D, Napoliello M, Schenk J. The safety and usefulness of buspirone as an anxiolytic drug in elderly versus young patients. Clin Ther 1988;10:740.

39. Massie MJ, Holland JC. Depression and the cancer patient. J Clin Psychiatry 1990;51:12.

40. Plumb MM, Holland JC. Comparative studies of psychological function in patients with advanced cancer. Psychosom Med 1977;39:264.

41. Holland JC, Hughes Korzun A, Tross S, et al. Comparative psychological disturbance in pancreatic and gastric cancer. Am J Psychiatry 1986;143:982.

42. Endicott J. Measurement of depression in patients with cancer. Cancer 1984;53:2243.

43. Adams F, Quesada JR, Gutterman JU. Neuropsychiatric manifestations of human leukocyte interferon therapy in patients with cancer. JAMA 1984;252:938.

44. DeAngelis LM, Delattre J, Posner JB. Radiation-induced dementia in patients cured of brain metastases. Neurology 1989;39:789.

45. Denicoff KD, Rubinow DR, Papa MZ, et al. The neuropsychiatric effects of treatment with interleukin-w and lymphokine-activated killer cells. Ann Intern Med 1987;107:293.

46. Holland JC, Fassanellos, Ohnuma T. Psychiatric symptoms associated with L-asparaginase administration. J Psychiatric Res 1974;10:165.

47. Weddington W. Delirium and depression associated with amphotericin B. Psychosomatics 1982;23:1076.

48. Breitbart W. Endocrine-Related Psychiatric Disorders. In J Holland, J Rowland (eds), The Handbook of Psychooncology: The Psychological Care of the Cancer Patient. New York: Oxford Press, 1989;356.

49. Posner JB. Nonmetastatic Effects of Cancer on the Nervous System. In JB Wyngaarden, LH Smith (eds), Cecil's Textbook of Medicine. Philadelphia: Saunders, 1988;1104.

50. Spiegel D, Bloom JR, Yalom ID. Group support for patients with metastatic cancer: A randomized prospective outcome study. Arch Gen Psychiatry 1981;38:527.

51. Spiegel D. The use of hypnosis in controlling cancer pain. CA Cancer J Clin 1985;4:221.

52. Spiegel D, Bloom R. Group therapy and hypnosis reduce metastatic breast carcinoma pain. Psychosom Med 1983;4:333.

53. Popkin MK, Callies AL, Mackenzie TB. The outcome of antidepressant use in the medically ill. Arch Gen Psychiatry 1985;42:1160.

54. Purohit DR, Navlakha PL, Modi RS, et al. The role of antidepressants in hospitalized cancer patients. J Assoc Physicians India 1978;26:245.

55. Rifkin A, Reardon G, Siris S, et al. Trimipramine in physical illness with depression. J Clin Psychiatry 1985;46:4.

56. Breitbart W, Platt M, Marotta R, et al. Low-dose neuroleptic treatment for AIDS delirium [abstract]. 144th Annual Meeting, American Psychiatric Association, May 11-16, 1991.

57. Glassman AH. The newer antidepressant drugs and their cardiovascular effects. Psychopharmacol Bull 1984;20:272.

58. Sher M, Krieger JN, Juergen S. Trazodone and priapism. Am J Psychiatry 1983;140:1362.

59. Peck AW, Stern WC, Watkinson C. Incidence of seizures during treatment with tricyclic antidepressant drugs and buprorion. J Clin Psychiatry 1983;44:197.

60. Cooper G. The safety of fluoxetine: An update. Br J Psychiatry 1988;153:77.

61. Gomez-Perez FJ, Rull JA, Dies H, et al. Nortriptyline and fluphenazine in the symptomatic treatment of diabetic neuropathy: A double-blind cross-over study. Pain 1985;23:395.

62. Sindrup SH, Gram LF, Brosen K, et al. The selective serotonin reuptake inhibitor paroxetine is effective in the treatment of diabetic neuropathy symptoms. Pain 1990;42:135.

63. Ayd F. Amoxapine: A new tricyclic antidepressant. Int Drug Ther Newslett 1979;14:33.

64. Lloyd AH. Practical consideration in the use of maprotiline (Ludiomil) in general practice. J Intern Med Res 1977;5:122.

65. Costa D, Mogos I, Toma T. Efficacy and safety of mianserin in the treatment of depression of women with cancer. Acta Psychiatr Scand 1985;72:85.

66. Chiarillo RJ, Cole JO. The use of psychostimulants in general psychiatry. A reconsideration. Arch Gen Psychiatry 1987;44:286.

67. Fernandez F, Adams F, Levy J, et al. Cognitive impairment due to AIDS related complex and its response to psychostimulants. Psychosomatics 1988;29:38.

68. Fisch R. Methylphenidate for medical inpatients. Int J Psychiatry Med 1985/1986;15:75.

69. Katon W, Raskind M. Treatment of depression in the medically ill elderly with methylphenidate. Am J Psychiatry 1980;137:963.

70. Kaufmann MW, Murray GB, Cassem NH. Use of psychostimulants in medically ill depressive patients. Psychosomatics 1982;23:817.

71. Bruera E, Chadwick S, Brennels C, et al. Methylphenidate associated with narcotics for the treatment of cancer pain. Cancer Treat Report 1987;71:67.

72. Breitbart W, Mermelstein H. Pemoline: An alternative psychostimulant in the management of depressive disorders in cancer patients. Psychosomatics 1992;33:352.

73. Munro SM, Mount B. Music therapy in palliative care. Can Med Assoc J 1978;119:1029.

74. Stein RS, Flexner JH, Graber SE. Lithium and granulocytopenia during induction therapy of acute myelogenous leukemia: Update of an ongoing trial. Adv Exp Med Biol 1980;127:187.

75. Bolund C. Suicide and cancer. II. Medical and care factors in suicide by cancer patients in Sweden, 1973–1976. J Psychosoc Oncol 1985;3:17.

76. Bolund C. Suicide and cancer. I. Demographic and social characteristics of cancer patients who committed suicide in Sweden, 1973–1976. J Psychosoc Oncol 1985;3:17.

77. Breitbart W. Cancer Pain and Suicide. In KM Foley, et al. (eds), Advances in Pain Research and Therapy (Vol. 16). New York: Raven, 1990;339.

78. Breitbart W. Suicide Risk and Pain in Cancer and AIDS Patients. In R Chapman, KM Foley (eds), Current Emerging Issues in Cancer Pain: Research and Practice. New York: Raven, 1993.

79. Levin DN, Cleeland CS, Dan R. Public attitudes toward cancer pain. Cancer 1985;56:2337.

80. Breitbart W. Suicide in cancer patients. Oncology 1987;1:49.

81. Posner JB. Delirium and Exogenous Metabolic Brain Disease. In PB Beeson, W McDermott, LH Wyngaarden (eds), Cecil's Textbook of Medicine. Philadelphia: Saunders, 1979;644.

82. Lipowski ZJ. Delirium (acute delusional states). JAMA 1987;285:1789.

83. Fleishmann SB, Lesko LM. Delirium and Dementia. In J Holland, J Rowland (eds), The Handbook of Psychooncology: Psychological Care of the Cancer Patient. New York: Oxford Press, 1989;342.

84. Adams F, Fernandez F, Andersson BS. Emergency pharmacotherapy of delirium in the critically ill cancer patient. Psychosomatics 1986;27:33.

85. Von Roenn J, Cleeland C, Gopnin R, et al. Physician attitudes and practice in cancer pain management. Ann Intern Med 1993;119:121.

86. Macaluso C, Weinberg D, Foley KM. Opioid abuse and misuse in a cancer pain population [abstract]. Second International Congress on Cancer Pain, New York, July 14–17, 1988.

87. Turnbull F. The nature of pain that may accompany cancer of the lung. Pain 1979;7:371.

88. Simmons C, Daland E. Cancer: Factors entering into the delay in its surgical treatment. Boston Med Surg J 1920;183:298.

89. Woodforde JM, Fielding JR. Pain and cancer. J Psychosom Res 1970;14:365.

90. Sternbach R. Congenital insensitivity to pain: A critique. Psychol Bull 60:252.

91. Cioffi, D. Beyond attentional strategies: A cognitive-perceptual model of somatic interpretation. Psychol Bull 1991;109:25.

92. Cassell E. The nature of suffering and the goals of medicine. N Engl J Med 1982;306:639.

93. Bandura A, O'Leary A, Taylor C, et al. Perceived self-efficacy and pain control: Opioid and non-opioid mechanism. J Pers Soc Psychol 1987;53:563.

94. Council J, Ahern D, Follick M, Kline C. Expectancies and functional impairment in lower back pain. Pain 1988;33:323.

95. Crisson J, Keefe F. The relationship of locus of control to pain coping strategies and psychological distress in chronic pain patients. Pain 1988;35:147.

96. Peterson C, Stunkard A. Personal control and health promotion. Soc Sci Med 1989;28:819.

97. Hill H, Kornetsky C, Flanary H, Wikler A. Effects of anxiety and morphine on discrimination of intensities of painful stimulus. J Clin Invest 1952;31:473.

98. Hijzen T, Slangen S, Van Houweligew H. Subjective, clinical, and EMG effects of biofeedback and splint treatment. J Oral Rehabil 1986;13:529.

99. Chapman C, Turner J. Psychological control of acute pain in medical settings. J Pain Symptom Manage 1986;1:9.

100. Turk D, Holzman A. Chronic Pain: Interfaces Among Physical, Psychological and Social Parameters. In A Holzman, D Turk (eds), Pain Management: A Handbook of Psychological Treatment Approaches. New York: Pergamon, 1986;1.

101. Spanos N, Radtke-Bodorik H, Ferguson J, Jones B. The effects of hypnotic susceptibility, suggestions for analgesia and utilization of cognitive strategies on the reduction of pain. J Abnorm Psychol 1979;88:282.

102. Hall K, Stride E. The varying response to pain in psychiatric disorders: A study in abnormal psychology. Br J Med Psychol 1954;27:48.

103. Beecher H. Relationship of significance of wound to the pain experience. JAMA 1956;161:1609.

104. Smith T, Peck J, Ward J. Helplessness and depression in rheumatoid arthritis. Health Psychol 1990;9:377.

105. Nicassion P, Walston K, Callahan L, et al. The measurement of helplessness in rheumatoid arthritis: The development of the arthritis helplessness index. J Rheumatol 1985;12:462.

106. Flor H, Turk D. Chronic back pain and rheumatoid arthritis: Predicting pain and disability from cognitive variables. J Behav Med 1988;11:251.

107. Stein M, Wallston K, Niccassion P, Custoe N. Correlation of clinical classification scheme for the arthritis helplessness subscale. Arthritis Rheum 1988;31:876.

108. Cleeland CS. Nonpharmacologic management of cancer pain. J Pain Symptom Manage 1987;2:523.

109. Loscalzo M, Jacobsen PB. Practical behavioral approaches to the effective management of pain and distress. J Psychosoc Oncol 1990;8:139.

110. Loprinzi CL, Ellison NM, Schaid DJ, et al. Controlled trial of megestrol acetate for the treatment of cancer anorexia and cachexia. Journal of the National Institutes of Health 1990;82:1127.

111. Erickson MH. Hypnosis in painful terminal illness. Am J Clin Hypnosis 1959;1:1117.

112. Benson H, Pomeranz B, Kutz, I. The Relaxation Response and Pain. In PD Wall, R Melzack (eds), Textbook of Pain. New York: Churchill Livingstone, 1984;817.

113. Benson H. The Relaxation Response. New York: William Morrow, 1975.

114. Barber J, Gitelson J. Cancer Pain: Psychological management using hypnosis. CA Cancer J Clin 1980;3:130.

115. Fotopoulos S, Graham C, Cook MR. Psychophysiologic Control of Cancer Pain. In JJ Bonica, V Ventafridda (eds), Advances in Pain Research and Therapy (Vol. 2). New York: Raven, 1979;231.

116. Butler S. Present Status of Tricyclic Antidepressants in Chronic Pain Therapy. In C Benedetti et al. (eds), Advances in Pain Research and Therapy (Vol. 7). New York: Raven, 1986;173.

117. France RD. The future for antidepressants: Treatment of pain. Psychopathology 1987;20:99.

118. Walsh TD. Antidepressants and chronic pain. Clin Neuropharmacol 1983;6:271.

119. Max MB, Kishore-Kumar R, Schafer SC, et al. Efficacy of desipramine in painful diabetic neuropathy: A placebo-controlled trial. Pain 1991;45:3.

120. Max MB, Culnane M, Schafer SC, et al. Amitriptyline relieves diabetic-neuropathy pain in patients with normal and depressed mood. Neurology 1987;37:589.

121. Pilowsky I, Hallett EC, Bassett DL, et al. A controlled study of amitriptyline in the treatment of chronic pain. Pain 1982;14:169.

122. Sharav Y, Singer E, Schmidt E, et al. The analgesic effect of amitriptyline on chronic facial pain. Pain 1987;31:199.

123. Watson CP, Evans RJ, Reed K, et al. Amitriptyline versus placebo in post herpetic neuralgia. Neurology 1982;32:671.

124. Langohr HD, Stohr M, Petruch F. An open and double-blind crossover study on the efficacy of clomipramine (Anafranil) in patients with painful mono-and polyneuropathies. Eur Neurol 1982;21:309.

125. Sindrup SH, Ejlertsen B, Froland A, et al. Imipramine treatment in diabetic neuropathy: Relief of subjective symptoms without changes in peripheral and autonomic nerve function. Eur J Clin Pharmacol 1989;37:151.

126. Young DF. Neurological Complications of Cancer Chemotherapy. In A Silverstein (ed), Neurological Complications of Therapy: Selected Topics. New York: Futura, 1982;57.

127. Lebovits AK, Lefkowitz M, McCarthy D, et al. The prevalence and management of pain in patients with AIDS. A review of 134 cases. Clin J Pain 1989;5:245.

128. Tiegno M, Pagnoni B, Calmi A, et al. Chlorimipramine compared to pentazocine as a unique treatment in postoperative pain. Int J Clin Pharmacol Res 1987;7:141.

129. Hammeroff SR, Cork RC, Scherer K, et al. Doxepin effects on chronic pain, depression and plasma opioids. J Clin Psychiatry 1982;2:22.

130. Zitman FG, Linssen ACG, Edelbroek PM, Stijnen T. Low dose amitriptyline in chronic pain: The gain is modest. Pain 1990;42:35.

131. Tyler MA. Treatment of the painful shoulder syndrome with amitriptyline and lithium carbonate. Can Med Assoc J 1974;111:137.

132. Bruera E, Brenneis C, Paterson AH, MacDonald RN. Use of methylphenidate as an adjuvant to narcotic analgesics in patients with advanced cancer. J Pain Symptom Manage 1989;4:3.

133. Nehra A, et al. Pemoline associated hepatic injury. Gastroenterology 1990;99:1517.

134. Oliver OJ. The use of methotrimeprazine in terminal care. Br J Clin Pract 1985;39:339.

135. Lechin F, et al. Pimozide therapy for trigeminal neuralgia. Arch Neurol 1989;9:960.

136. Beaver WT, Feise G. Comparison of the Analgesic Effects of Morphine, Hydroxyzine and Their Combination in Patients with Postoperative Pain. In JJ Bonica, Albe-Fessard (eds), Advances in Pain Research and Therapy. New York: Raven, 1976;533.

137. Fernandez F, Adams F, Holmes VF. Analgesic effect of alprazolam in patients with chronic, organic pain of malignant origin. J Clin Psychopharmacol 1987;3:167.

138. Caccia MR. Clonazepam in facial neuralgia and cluster headache: Clinical and electrophysiological study. Eur Neurol 1975;13:560.

139. Swerdlow M, Cundill JG. Anticonvulsant drugs used in the treatment of lancinating pains: A comparison. Anesthesia 1981;36:1129.

140. Patt RB. Pain management in the patient with AIDS. Stem Oncol Ann 1994;2:391.

141. Breitbart W, Passik S, Bronaugh T, et al. Pain in the ambulatory AIDS patient: Prevalence and psychosocial correlates [abstract]. 38th Annual Meeting, Academy of Psychosomatic Medicine, Atlanta, Georgia, October 17–20, 1991.

142. Schofferman J, Brody R. Pain in Far Advanced AIDS. In KM Foley (ed), Advances in Pain Research and Therapy (Vol. 16). New York: Raven, 1990;379.

143. Cornblath DR, McArthur IC. Predominantly sensory neuropathy in patients with AIDS and AIDS-related complex. Neurology 1988;38:794.

144. Parry GJ. Peripheral neuropathies associated with human immunodeficiency virus infection. Ann Neurol 1988;23(Suppl.):349.

145. Kizer K, Green M, Perkins C, et al. AIDS and suicide in California. JAMA 1988;260:1981.

Chapter 23
Cancer Pain Syndromes and Their Management

Winston C. V. Parris

Since the beginning of time, mankind has suffered from plagues and epidemics, including pneumonia, polio, diphtheria, and tuberculosis. With the advent of vaccines, antibiotics, improved anesthesia, and surgical techniques, these disease processes have been better understood and treated more effectively. The fundamental objective for clinicians is to provide relief from pain and suffering induced by these diseases. As we approach the end of the twentieth century, the two major disease entities that have significant morbidity and mortality for humans are cardiovascular disorders (including heart attacks, stroke, and hypertension) and cancer. A strategy for dealing with the former is based primarily on prevention and good health habits. Some of these principles may be applicable to cancer. Thus, adequate nutrition, exclusion of high cholesterol and saturated fatty foods, cessation of smoking, decreased stress, and the increase in physical activity have been shown to decrease significantly the incidence of cancer.[1] However, cancer is still prevalent in our society and some forms remain poorly managed. The main reasons for the poor management of cancer include inadequate knowledge of cancer and its pathogenesis and the undertreatment of cancer pain.[2] To facilitate more effective treatment of cancer pain patients, it is important to know about those pain syndromes that are typically associated with cancer, its complications, and treatment. These cancer-related pain syndromes have distinct clinical characteristics and, in some cases, there are specific therapeutic protocols recommended to treat those

patients. This chapter reviews some common cancer-related pain syndromes and their management.

Cancer pain syndromes may be broadly classified as follows:

1. Pain due to cancer and its spread
2. Pain due to cancer therapy
3. Pain due to a known noncancer-related etiology
4. Pain of unknown etiology (which may or may not be related to cancer)

Cancer pain syndromes have characteristic clinical features by virtue of their invasion of contiguous structures and by the pathophysiologic complications of that tissue invasion. The invasion of the contiguous structures produces specific signs and symptoms that may compound the original pain problem. For example, many of the symptoms associated with cancer including anorexia, dyspnea, constipation, vomiting, and xerostomia may aggravate the cancer pain. Thus, an appreciation of the unique symptomatology of the cancer-related pain syndromes is important for their management. Pain from a particular cancer-related syndrome may be due to (1) tumor invasion, (2) deterioration of the general health status of the patient, or (3) anxiety about the progression of the illness and its possible outcome.

The spread and progression of a tumor may be facilitated by direct spread to contiguous structures or by metastatic spread via blood vessels and lymphatic channels.[3] As a result, patients may experience infiltration or destruction of nerves, secondary infection, metastases to bony structures, obstruction of a hollow viscus, or stretching of the capsule of a solid organ. It is important to keep in mind that there could be more than one etiology of pain in a cancer patient and that there could be more than one pain site.[4] Thus, frequent and regular pain assessments and the flexibility of clinical judgment of the whole pain team regarding the management process contribute to effective management of cancer-related pain syndromes. In this chapter, cancer-related pain syndromes are classified as follows:

1. Pain syndromes associated with tumor invasion
   a. Tumor invasion of nerves and neural structures
   b. Tumor infiltration of bone
   c. Tumor invasion of a hollow viscus
2. Pain syndromes associated with cancer therapy
   a. Postsurgical pain syndromes
   b. Postradiation pain syndromes
   c. Postchemotherapy pain syndromes
   d. Postbiological therapy pain syndromes
3. Pain syndromes unrelated to cancer or to cancer therapy

Pain Syndromes Related to Direct Tumor Invasion

Tumor Invasion of Nerves and Neural Structures

Direct invasion of neural tissue by a progressing cancer may produce a variety of pain syndromes that may be dependent on the location of the tumor and the rate of disease progression. The following clinical syndromes may occur as a result of tumor infiltration of nerves:

1. Brachial plexopathy[5]
2. Intercostal neuropathy[6]
3. Peripheral neuropathy[7-9]
4. Cervical plexopathy[10]
5. Lumbosacral plexopathy[11]
6. Tumor infiltration of cranial, spinal, or other nerve roots[12]
7. Tumor infiltration of the epidural space
   a. Epidural spinal cord compression[13]
   b. Back pain[13]
8. Leptomeningeal metastases[14]

9. Glossopharyngeal neuralgia[15]
10. Trigeminal neuralgia[16, 17]
11. Sensory neuropathy[18]
12. Sensorimotor peripheral neuropathy[19, 20]

These pain syndromes produce pain that is referable to the anatomic region affected. Most of the symptomatology is due to direct tumor infiltration of nerves or progressive compression of neural structures. Occasionally, the neoplastic process may have some specific effect on peripheral nerves or other neural tissues.

Patients with painful peripheral neuropathy have other causes of pain besides invasion or metastatic spread. These causes may include metabolic abnormalities, such as renal dysfunction, diabetes mellitus, and hepatic dysfunction. This is not unusual because some patients may have a neoplastic process coexisting with another systemic illness.[21] In addition, many cancer patients develop hepatic and renal dysfunction that may secondarily produce nutritional deficiencies, ultimately producing painful peripheral neuropathy.[22] Some cancer pain patients develop neurotoxic complications as a result of chemotherapy. The two chemotherapeutic agents that commonly produce painful peripheral neuropathies are cisplatin and vincristine. Paraneoplastic syndromes may, on occasion, cause painful neuropathy. When this occurs, the painful neuropathy may be the initial manifestation of an underlying occult malignancy. Nutritional deficiencies (particularly vitamin B_1 and B_{12} deficiencies) may occur as a result of a neoplastic process and may ultimately produce painful peripheral neuropathies.[23] All these cancer-related pain syndromes are important to recognize because the corresponding therapeutic strategies depend primarily on the etiologic factors producing the pain syndrome.

Therapeutic options for cancer-related pain syndromes secondary to tumor infiltration of nerves include the following:

1. Initiation of the World Health Organization (WHO) recommendation using the three-step ladder for comprehensive pain management.[24] This principle uses nonsteroidal anti-inflammatory agents as a first step for mild pain. If the pain persists or increases in intensity, the second step is to introduce a mild-to-moderate opioid in conjunction

with nonopioid drugs and other analgesic adjuvants. These adjuvants include tricyclic antidepressants, e.g., nortriptyline, anticonvulsants, e.g., phenytoin, and other centrally acting drugs, e.g., carbamazepine, and antispasmodic drugs, e.g., baclofen (Lioresal). If the moderate pain persists or increases, then a strong opioid (e.g., oral morphine) is introduced with or without the concurrent use of nonopioid medications or other analgesic adjuvants. Mexilitine has been found to play a major role in the management of persistent neuropathic cancer pain.[25]

2. Selected nerve blocks[26] may be used for patients who have specific plexopathy and neuropathy along a particular anatomic distribution.

3. The dorsal root entry zone procedure[27] may be used for patients with brachial plexopathy and related neuropathic lesions.

4. Glucocorticosteroids may be useful for patients with direct invasion of major nerve groups.[28] For example, dexamethasone (6–12 mg) daily may be used to treat patients with brachial plexus pain.

5. If anxiety is believed to play a major role in the pain syndrome, diazepam or fluoxetine[29] may be used.

6. Patients with nerve invasion secondary to bony or lymph nodal metastases should receive local radiation or treatment with radioactive isotopes (e.g., strontium 89).[30] New techniques are currently being introduced to deal with some specific cancer-related pain syndromes.

Tumor Infiltration of Bone

Many people equate cancer with pain. This connection is made because of the frequency with which patients who become afflicted with cancer develop pain. The main reason for pain development in cancer patients is the frequency with which secondary deposits occur in bone as the malignancy progresses. The resulting pain is perceived as severe and does not usually respond to routine therapeutic modalities. As we begin to better understand the pathogenesis of bone pain secondary to cancer, effective therapeutic strategies may be applied and successfully implemented to treat bone pain. Although any cancer may metastasize to bony structures, the cancers that are predisposed to metastasize to bone are listed here[31]:

1. Thyroid cancer
2. Bronchogenic cancer
3. Prostate cancer
4. Breast cancer
5. Renal cancer
6. Multiple myeloma*

The bones usually involved in metastatic spread include the skull, thoracic cage, vertebral bones, and pelvis. Occasionally, bony spread may occur in the bones of the upper and lower extremities.

When metastases occur to the skull, specific syndromes may occur as a result of the strategic importance of the blood vessels and the nerves originating from or going to the brain. These specific syndromes are described later. Tumor invasion of the thoracic cage usually presents as chest pain. It is important to differentiate the chest pain caused by lung parenchymal involvement from that caused by other pulmonary disease processes. Various radiologic techniques including magnetic resonance imaging (MRI) and computed tomography (CT) along with careful physical examination may help differentiate those pain syndromes.[32] Pain affecting the vertebral bones is usually well localized and confined to the area of involvement. If there is compression of the spinal cord or involvement of selective spinal nerves and their sympathetic components, then unique pain syndromes may occur providing major therapeutic challenges. Metastases to the pelvis usually result from tumors of the large bowel, colorectal cancer, and gynecologic cancer.[33] These patients may present with low back pain, perineal pain, and pelvic pain. Because these patients usually have bladder and bowel dysfunction and possibly colostomy and urinary diversion procedures, respectively, it is appropriate to be aggressive in using neurolytic procedures to treat these patients, even though the risks of bladder and bowel complications are relatively high. Regardless of the therapeutic strategy used, it is always important to obtain adequate informed consent not only from the patient but also from the family.

When patients develop metastases to the frontal or parietal bones, the resulting pain may be minimal for some patients whereas other patients may

---

*Multiple myeloma is not a solid tumor but a hematogenous neoplasm that, by its very pathogenesis, spreads to most bones. It is included in this classification because of the severe bone pain associated with its manifestation and spread.

be asymptomatic. However, when metastases occur at the level of the base of the skull, major clinical problems may develop.[34] These clinical problems manifest as well-recognized cancer-related pain syndromes, and an understanding of the pathogenesis of each syndrome facilitates an effective therapy. The cranial bone pain syndromes that may occur are presented in the following discussion.

Sphenoidal Sinus Metastatic Involvement

When metastases invade the sphenoidal sinuses, patients present with severe bilateral frontal headache radiating to both temporal regions. The pain may radiate to the retro-orbital area and may be associated with a sensation of "water in the head" and nasal stuffiness. Unilateral or bilateral sixth nerve (abducens) palsy may occur, ultimately producing diplopia.

Jugular Foramen Syndrome

This syndrome is associated with occipital pain radiating to the ipsilateral shoulder, upper extremity, and vertex of the head. Physical examination reveals exquisite tenderness over the occipital condyle; slight movement of the head may exacerbate the pain. The jugular foramen is in close proximity to several cranial nerves and, depending on the particular nerve involved, a variety of signs and symptoms may develop in association with the previously described pain. The signs and symptoms include ptosis, dysarthria, neck and shoulder weakness, hoarseness, and dysphagia attributable to lesions of the glossopharyngeal, vagus, accessory, and hypoglossal nerves. It is not unusual for all four cranial nerves to be involved in the jugular foramen syndrome secondary to neoplastic involvement. The precise location of the lesions may be evaluated by radiologic techniques, and radioisotopic scans are very sensitive in evaluating the location and extent of bony involvement.

The pain mechanism in bony metastasis is believed to be due to liberation of prostaglandins by tumor deposits in the bone. The liberated prostaglandins cause resorption of bone around the tumor and sensitization of nerve endings to painful stimuli. These changes are similar to an inflammatory reaction in the bone, and it is clear that the amount of pain perceived is not always consistent with the size of the tumor. Thus, treatment with nonsteroidal anti-inflammatory drugs (NSAIDs) may be effective because their mechanism of action is to inhibit the cyclo-oxygenase pathway of prostaglandin synthesis from arachidonic acid.[35] Any NSAID may be used to treat bony pain in cancer patients. The author's preference is choline magnesium trisalicylate (Trilisate), 750–1,000 mg three times a day. Parenteral ketorolac tromethamine (Toradol) has also been found to be effective in managing metastatic bone pain.[36] As metastases increase, they stretch the periosteal covering of bones. Because the periosteum is well innervated, nociceptive stimuli are generated thus producing pain. Further, the stretching and eventual distortion of the bone may produce pathologic fractures. When this process occurs in the vertebral column, the affected vertebrae may collapse and the pain of vertebral collapse may be aggravated by nerve root compression. An understanding of these pain mechanisms can greatly enhance the capability to deliver effective pain relief for cancer patients.

Clivus Metastases

Tumors in the area of the clivus usually involve the inferior cranial nerves (i.e., abducens, facial, auditory, glossopharyngeal, vagus, accessory, and hypoglossal). The initial pain presentation may be unilateral but, with advance of the disease, the pain may become bilateral. The pain is associated with severe headache in the vertex area and flexion of the neck may not only initiate the headache but may also worsen it.

Orbital Pain

Primary tumors of the ocular and periocular structures may present with subsequent orbital and periorbital pain. Infrequently, there could be a metastasis in the orbital area that could produce periocular pain.

Fractures of the Odontoid Process

Neoplastic spread to the base of the skull may involve the first cervical vertebra. The osseous tissues in the odontoid process may be infiltrated with cancer, thus making them susceptible to pathologic fractures. When this occurs, pain in the back of the head and neck is usually the presenting symptom.[37] Secondary subluxation may occur with resulting brain stem or spinal cord compression. The pain in the back of the head is aggravated by neck movement and, in particular, by flexing the neck. Sensory and motor neurologic signs may develop and these signs may be associated with autonomic dysfunction. Unfortunately, if the correct diagnosis is not made, manipulations during radiography, feeding, or any other trivial activity may produce severe irreversible neurologic damage, resulting in quadriplegia or paraplegia. Thus, fractures of the odontoid process may have catastrophic effects, especially if an early diagnosis is not made and if appropriate prophylactic precautions are not taken.

Metastases to the Middle Fossa

Primary cerebral tumors may occur in the middle fossa but metastases may also occur, especially from the prostate, breast, ovary, and lung.

Metastases to the Parasagittal Region

These lesions may develop via hematogeneous spread from a variety of primary tumors and usually present with headache and major neurologic sequelae.

Treatment Strategies for Bone Pain Secondary to Cancer

Nonsteroidal Anti-inflammatory Drugs

The WHO principle regarding the use of NSAIDs for cancer pain should be given a satisfactory trial period so as to determine their possible efficacy. The precise NSAID used is immaterial. It is important to retain flexibility in changing the agent or adjusting the dose depending on drug efficacy or the onset of side effects. Cost may also be a factor in some cases. The side effects of NSAIDS are listed here:

1. Gastric irritation[38]
2. Nausea, vomiting, and massive gastrointestinal bleeding
3. Blood dyscrasia (aplastic anemia, thrombocytopenia, agranulocytosis)
4. Hepatic dysfunction (hepatitis, cholestatic jaundice, hepatic failure)
5. Renal toxicity (nephrotic syndrome, atubular necrosis)
6. Skin reactions (erythema, pruritus, Stevens-Johnson syndrome)
7. Central nervous system effects (vertigo, headache, tinnitus)
8. Idiosyncratic reactions

Radiotherapy for Solitary Metastasis in the Long Bones of the Upper and Lower Extremities

1. Many long bones metastases respond favorably to single doses of radiotherapy. However, it may be necessary in some patients to apply a series of treatments to achieve adequate efficacy.
2. Immobilization of the affected area or limb by traction, plaster, or sling can provide temporary pain relief.
3. Strong opioids may be used if NSAIDs and conservative physical measures fail.
4. Glucocorticosteroids may be useful in treating metastatic bone pain.[39] The possible mechanism of action of steroids in bone pain is by inhibition of phospholipase A_2 activity.
5. Selected nerve blocks, e.g., intercostal nerve blocks for rib metastases, obturator nerve blocks for hip pain, and sciatic nerve blocks for back pain radiating to the posterior surface of the leg may be administered in selected patients.
6. Calcitonin may be useful in managing metastatic bone pain.[40] The dose is 100 IU intravenously. Because calcitonin is usually associated with severe nausea and vomiting, it may be appropriate to use prophylactic intravenous droperidol, 0.3 mg, or benzquinamide (Emete-Con), 50 mg, to decrease these complications. In the author's experience, calcitonin has not been very effective in controlling the bone pain of metastatic disease. However, in two patients in whom it was successful, the effect was very beneficial to those patients.

Tumor Invasion of a Hollow Viscus

Tumors may invade a hollow viscus, thus producing unpleasant symptomatology (commonly, pain). The tumor may involve the covering of the viscus (e.g., pleural membranes or peritoneum). The organs usually affected include the lung, pancreas, gastrointestinal tract, and uterus. The description of the symptoms may vary with the extent of involvement of the covering of the viscus. In tumor invasion of the gastrointestinal tract, intestinal obstruction may be a presenting symptom and may be manifested by changes in bowel habit, weight loss, rectal bleeding, abdominal distention, and obstipation with constipation.

Miscellaneous Causes from Tumor Invasion

Other clinical syndromes may be associated with tumor invasion of the major blood vessels; however, the initial presentation is not pain. However, one should be vigilant about those manifestations because they may portend the imminent rapid spread of the disease with vascular implications.

Pain Syndromes Associated with Cancer Therapy

Postsurgical Pain Syndromes

When a patient develops a tumor, surgical considerations are frequently necessary and appropriate. However, the results of surgical interventions have not always been satisfactory. In fact, some patients developed serious postsurgical pain syndromes. As a result of these syndromes and increased funding for cancer research, a greater emphasis has been placed on the chemotherapeutic management of cancer. Thus, although surgery for cancer generally is decreasing, there are a few tumors (e.g., cancer of the breast, pancreas, lung, prostate, and bowel) that are considered suitable for surgical resection, especially if the diagnosis is made early. Patients with progressive and terminal lesions that are producing major symptoms by virtue of their anatomic locations may receive surgical debulking for palliation of pain. These radical procedures may have major side effects and complications, and their risks should be discussed with the patient and family prior to surgery.

There are a few postoperative pain syndromes that develop in the course of treating cancer patients surgically. Postsurgical pain syndromes in cancer patients develop almost immediately after surgery. It is important to differentiate between postsurgical pain and the recurrence of original tumor. This differentiation is important because it can have therapeutic and prognostic implications for the patients. Common postsurgical pain syndromes to be discussed are listed here:

1. Postradical neck dissection pain
2. Phantom limb pain
3. Stump pain
4. Postmastectomy pain syndrome
5. Postthoracotomy pain

Postradical Neck Resection Pain

When treated early by radical neck resection, cancers of the head and neck, notably the tongue, tonsil, pharynx, larynx, palate, and parotid may not only provide satisfactory extension of life but also possibly a cure. The two major complications associated with radical neck resection are cosmetic defects (which can be ameliorated by progressive plastic and reconstructive surgery) and postradical neck resection pain.[41] This pain results from injury to the cervical plexus, cranial nerves, and cervical sympathetics at the time of dissection. The symptoms that may be produced include dysesthesia in the area of sensory loss, acute lancinating pain in the facial and neck area, and shoulder and neck discomfort as a result of the removal of the strap muscles, scalene muscles, and sternocleidomastoid muscles. Thoracic outlet syndrome and problems with abduction of the arm may occur as a result of neuropraxia or surgical transection of the suprascapular nerve. A dramatically increased pain in patients immediately after surgery may be caused by soft tissue infection and recurrent tumor. Appropriate laboratory and biochemical investigations may help differentiate between infection and tumor recurrence. In the case of patients with recurrent tumor, follow-up radiologic assessments, especially CT scans and frequent head and neck physical examinations, would help determine if the pain is due to recurrence of the tumor.

The therapeutic options available to patients with postradical neck dissection pain include:

1. Appropriate nerve block therapy, depending on the anatomic region affected (e.g., brachial plexus infusion (with local anesthetic) via infraclavicular route, suprascapular nerve block, stel-

late ganglion block)
2. Controlled physical therapy, depending on the general condition of the patient
3. Trigger point injections
4. Consideration of the WHO three-step analgesic ladder

Phantom Limb Pain

Tumors of the lower extremity and upper extremity (e.g., rhabdomyosarcoma and osteoblastoma) may be treated by limb amputation. Phantom limb pain and other phantom limb phenomena may occur following amputation.[42] The severity of the phantom limb pain that develops after amputation appears to be related to the duration of the preamputation pain and the presence of pain on the day of the amputation. Bach et al.[43] demonstrated that preoperative lumbar epidural local anesthetic infusion prior to the amputation significantly decreased the incidence of phantom limb pain compared with those patients who did not receive preoperative epidural blockade. This concept of preemptive analgesia[44] has been widely used to decrease the incidence of phantom limb pain and phantom limb sensation in patients receiving amputations for cancer and other disease processes. Several medical interventions are recommended for phantom limb pain, including narcotic analgesics, sympathetic blockade, tricyclic antidepressants, anticonvulsant agents (e.g., dilantin), transcutaneous electrical nerve stimulation (TENS), and intravenous calcitonin. None of these therapies are consistently effective in patients with phantom limb pain.

Other types of phantom phenomena have been described following excision or resection of certain organs of the body. These phenomena have been described in the tongue, breast, penis, teeth, bowel, rectum, and bladder. The decrease in the incidence of those other regional phantom phenomena has not yet been shown to be decreased with regional block when administered prior to amputation.

Stump Pain

Stump pain may follow amputation of an extremity and is different in character from phantom phenomena. Phantom phenomena usually are perceived in the missing part of the body, whereas stump pain is usually located at the site of the surgical scar and may remain in that location for several years following amputation.[45] Generally, it is believed that stump pain is the result of the development of a neuroma at the site of nerve transection. The pain is usually exacerbated by activity and is characterized by sharp, shooting sensations. Stump pain may usually be localized by palpation. The injection of the trigger point in the scar with local anesthetics may provide significant pain relief. On the other hand, phantom limb pain is not relieved by trigger point injection.

Postmastectomy Pain Syndrome

This syndrome may occur in about 10% of the women who undergo simple or radical mastectomy.[46] The pain has the following characteristics: it is confined to the anterior chest wall, may radiate to the shoulder and posterior aspect of the upper arm, and is described as a burning sensation. In fact, patients with this syndrome may develop a frozen shoulder because of the continued flexed position in which they maintain their arm following mastectomy. Palpation of the axilla may reveal an exquisitely tender area with discrete trigger points, thus giving credence to the theory that the postmastectomy pain syndrome may be due to neuronal trauma to the intercostobrachial nerve.[47] It is important to differentiate between postmastectomy pain syndrome and pain due to tumor infiltration of the brachial plexus. Again, these two pain syndromes have different therapeutic and prognostic implications. The incidence of postmastectomy pain syndrome appears to increase in patients who develop intraoperative complications such as infection, wound dehiscence, and hematoma in the region of the scar. The routine management of postmastectomy syndrome includes the use of trigger point injections, sympathetic block, peripheral nerve blocks, infiltration of the intercostobrachial nerve, physical therapy, topical application of capsaicin (Zostrix), and infrequently, surgical exploration and excision of the neuroma causing the pain.

Postthoracotomy Pain

Postthoracotomy pain[48] usually follows the thoracotomy incision for lung resection and may be associated with rib fractures during the procedure, overstretching of the intercostal tissues by overaggressive use of a surgical instrument (rib spreader), and by operative trauma to the intercostal nerves.

Postthoracotomy pain can be treated with the following modalities: (1) intercostal nerve block series,[49] (2) interpleural analgesia,[50] (3) TENS, and (4) intravenous lidocaine infusion.[51]

Postradiation Syndromes

Radiotherapy and radiotherapeutic maneuvers have become increasingly popular in treating cancer patients. Although the techniques have improved and are definitely more tissue selective, there are still risks of radiation damage to structures contiguous to the tumor. Nerves and neural structures are susceptible to radiation injury and, thus, radiation neuritis is a common complication of radiotherapy for the treatment of cancer patients.[52] When the large neural structures are damaged, characteristic pain syndromes develop:

1. Radiation neuritis of the lumbar sacral plexus (lumbar plexopathy)[53]
2. Radiation neuritis of the brachial plexus (brachial plexopathy)[54]
3. Radiation myelopathy[55]
4. Meralgia paresthetica or hyperesthetica
5. Radiation-induced peripheral nerve tumors[56]
6. Oropharyngeal complications[57]

Oropharyngeal complications of radiation therapy were more prevalent a few decades ago. Their incidence has significantly decreased, probably as a result of improved radiation technology, increased sophistication of the doses required to obtain maximum efficacy and minimum side effects, and the use of prophylactic measures to decrease the incidence of these complications. The most common oropharyngeal complications of radiation therapy are presented here:

1. Dysphagia
2. Oropharyngeal mucositis
3. Infection
4. Osteoradionecrosis[58]
5. Trismus
6. Xerostomia
7. Dental caries

All of these complications may be treated by good oral hygiene including fluoride prophylaxis,

pre-radiation antibiotics, and good dental hygiene. These complications may all be associated with pain or have painful implications. The most disfiguring complication is osteoradionecrosis. The predisposing factors for osteoradionecrosis development include decreased blood supply to the area being treated and altered bone structure usually affecting the mandibula.[59] The mandible is more susceptible to developing osteoradionecrosis compared with the maxilla because the mandible has only one source of blood supply whereas the maxilla has several sources. Osteoradionecrosis may be asymptomatic in some cases. However, in cases where the bone is devitalized, the devitalized area may be subject to infection, which would subsequently delay healing. Complications of osteoradionecrosis secondary to radiation therapy include pathologic fracture, fistula formation with purulent drainage, mandible necrosis, and severe pain of the jaw and face. Malnutrition could ensue as a result of associated immobility of the jaw and trismus, thus decreasing the intake of food. This condition is more likely to occur in elderly patients in whom dental hygiene may be poor and whose general physical condition may be less than optimum.

Treatment modalities for osteoradionecrosis range from simple sequestration procedures to hemimandibulectomy and reconstructive flaps.[60] Other treatments include extensive dental extractions, rehabilatative oral surgery, the use of hyperbaric oxygen to promote tissue healing and to decrease tissue hypoxia, and the use of selective nerve blocks (i.e., gasserian or mandibular nerve blocks).

The lesions described previously are the result of radiation-induced inflammatory changes and subsequent fibrosis to the major nerve groups. As with postsurgical pain syndromes, it is important to differentiate between postradiation pain syndromes and the recurrence of cancer. This differentiation is facilitated by the use of MRI and CT scans. Other nerves may be traumatized by radiation depending on the site of the radiation. These pain syndromes may be localized and follow a particular anatomic distribution, or they may be generalized depending on the nerve involved. Treatment of individual pain syndromes may include selective nerve block and continuous nerve blockade, especially in those patients who obtain transient relief from single injections. The use of TENS and regularly administered (by the clock) narcotic analgesics may help manage these pain syndromes.

Postchemotherapy Pain Syndromes

Modest strides have been made in the fight against cancer. However, these strides do not allow for complacency, because the battle against cancer is far from being won. Significant progress against cancer has been made in the field of cancer prevention and the use of chemotherapy. Recently, aggressive chemotherapy has been used to treat tumors and, in some patients (e.g., leukemias), the results are very good. In many other situations, however, the results are not as good and leave much room for improvement. Unfortunately, some complications of chemotherapy may be life threatening and others may be associated with pain and significant discomfort, including those shown here:

1. Musculoskeletal pain
2. Herpes zoster
3. Postherpetic neuralgia
4. Headache
5. Oral mucositis pain
6. Peripheral neuropathy
7. Corticosteroid-associated pain syndromes
   a. Steroid pseudorheumatism
   b. Steroid-induced aseptic necrosis of the femoral or humeral heads
   c. Osteonecrosis secondary to steroids
   d. Perineal dysesthesia secondary to steroids

Musculoskeletal Pain. Many chemotherapeutic agents produce severe myalgia and arthralgia following their administration. These nonspecific pain syndromes may be disconcerting to patients and, in fact, may represent the major source of pain during chemotherapy. The agents commonly associated with musculoskeletal pain[61] include vincristine, interferon, and granulocyte macrophage colony stimulating factor. Jaw pain is frequently seen in patients receiving vincristine whereas diffuse myalgia and arthralgia are associated with the biological agents, e.g., interferon.

Herpes Zoster. Herpes zoster[62] is an acute viral illness that affects patients who are immunocompromised due to a disease process, infection process (e.g., human immunodeficiency virus), or immunosuppressant therapy. The varicella virus is present in most people from childhood as a result of chicken pox. After cessation of the widespread chicken pox varicella virus, the virus stays dormant in the neuraxis, usually in the dorsal root ganglion. Several decades later, either as a result of an infection (i.e., the AIDS virus), old age, or development of an illness associated with an immune response dysfunction, a reactivation of the virus occurs. The varicella virus then affects the contiguous dermatomes where it has been quiescent and the herpetiform rash and vesicles develop in the corresponding dermatomes. This symptomatology is classically described as herpes zoster. The location of the vesicles could be anywhere on the body. However, 50–60% of the rash occurs in the thoracic area between T-4 and T-10. The incidence of herpes zoster is approximately five times more likely to occur in cancer patients than in the general population. It is also more common in patients with active tumor than in patients who are in remission. Rusthoven et al.[63] showed the correlation between the dermatologic dissemination of herpes zoster and a particular tumor. Their data showed that gynecologic and genitourinary tumors showed a predilection for herpes zoster in the lumbar and sacral dermatomes whereas breast and lung carcinoma were commonly associated with thoracic dermatome involvement. The data also showed that the hematologic tumors (i.e., multiple myeloma, leukemias, and lymphoma) were more frequently associated with herpes zoster affecting the cervical dermatomes. This author has observed that approximately 60% of patients who present with herpes zoster and without a prior history of cancer may develop a cancer within 12 months after the presentation of herpes zoster. This leaves open the speculation that the herpes zoster may be an early manifestation of the immunologic dysfunction that would ultimately predispose to the development of the cancer. Studies are currently being performed to investigate this speculation. Herpes zoster also seems to occur twice as frequently in patients who had previously received radiotherapy, leaving the possibility that radiation is also a risk factor in the development of herpes zoster. It has been postulated that chemotherapy is a definite risk factor because several patients receiving chemotherapy develop herpes zoster approximately 1 month after completing chemotherapy.

Herpes zoster[64] is treated with acyclovir (800 mg five times a day for 5 days). Antipruritic or soothing agents (e.g., calamine lotion) may be used to dry herpetic lesions and minimize cutaneous discomfort and pruritus. Herpes zoster may be present in patients without the external evidence of the characteristic herpetiform vesicular rash. The pain is usually described as a severe burning localized pain associated with some sensory deficits. From a pathologic standpoint, the herpes zoster infection is characterized by acute and inflammatory changes occurring in the dorsal root ganglia, leading to necrosis and hemorrhage. This lesion extends peripherally, affecting the myelin of the peripheral nerves, leading to axonal degeneration. It is likely that central and peripheral factors may play a role in the development of pain. Demyelination and deafferentation changes that occur may be the result of a decreased blood supply secondary to an intense vasoconstriction that follows the sympathetic activity in the dorsal root ganglion. Thus, there may be both a vascular and neurogenic component to the initial process that may occur in herpes zoster. The fact that a vascular component is present lends credence to the suggestion that early sympathetic blocks may help decrease the incidence of postherpetic neuralgia. Although this observation has not yet been confirmed, there are many anecdotal reports to suggest that it is effective. Sympathetic blocks may produce vasodilatation, which helps decrease vasoconstriction that occurs following dorsal root ganglia irritation. Thus, the resulting vasodilatation may help minimize the ischemia to the inflamed peripheral nerves and may, consequently, decrease the amount of neuronal damage that usually occurs.

Postherpetic Neuralgia. In patients whose herpes zoster lesions have dried up and healed, there may be a residual pain in the affected dermatomes that may be much worse than the original herpes zoster pain. This pain is described as postherpetic neuralgia[65] and it is thought to result from the deafferentation and demyelination changes that occurred in the nerves as a result of the reactivation of the varicella virus. Postherpetic neuralgia may be distressing, and it has been clearly demonstrated that the longer the duration of the lesion, the more difficult it is to treat pain. Thus, early and vigorous treatment of herpes zoster is a good strategy to diminish the severity of postherpetic neuralgia. The pain of postherpetic neuralgia has been so severe that some patients have reported occasional bouts of suicidal ideation.

Effective treatment of postherpetic neuralgia has been disappointing. Sympathetic blocks are used, but their efficacy decreases in patients whose postherpetic neuralgia lesions have been present longer than 3 months. Epidural injections are no more effective than sympathetic blocks. Tricyclic antidepressants and carbamazepine have been quite useful in controlling the lancinating and burning components of the pain. Topical capsaicin has been used in patients with postherpetic neuralgia with some reports of success. The recommended concentration is 0.025%. Capsaicin depletes substance P in peripheral nerve endings of affected nerves. TENS, peripheral nerve blocks, and narcotic analgesics (3–5 mg per kg) have been used in patients who have not responded to treatment.

Headache. Headaches[66] may occur following the use of some chemotherapeutic agents and are associated with other symptoms (i.e., fever, neck stiffness, vomiting, irritability, lethargy). These symptoms may form a characteristic complex after chemotherapy. The chemotherapeutic agents commonly associated with postchemotherapy headaches include L-asparaginase and methotrexate.

Oral Mucositis Pain. Oral mucositis pain[67] occurs 2 or 3 weeks after the start of chemotherapy. The chemotherapeutic agents most commonly associated with this syndrome include etoposide, daunorubicin, 5-fluorouracil, methotrexate, doxorubicin, and bleomycin. Radiation therapy may produce oral mucositis pain but, in combination with the chemotherapeutic agents mentioned previously, a severe form may occur. This syndrome is usually seen in patients who have had bone marrow transplantation because both chemotherapy and radiation therapy are combined prior to the bone marrow transplantation procedure. These patients are usually unable to swallow as a result of inflammatory lesions of the mouth and pharynx and their food intake is decreased during that period. Aggressive nutritional support is necessary to prevent worsening of the cachexia that may follow. Infection of the oral cavity, pharynx, and esophagus may occur and may be associated with secondary hemorrhage. These regions may also be overgrown by fungal infections and viral organisms, particularly *Candida* *albicans* and herpes viruses. The treatment of oral mucositis pain is prophylactic therapy. Oral mouth rinses containing viscous local anesthetics (e.g., lidocaine), diphenhydramine elixir, and chlorhexidine may be useful. Intravenous narcotics administered using patient-controlled analgesia may be useful in managing resistant oral mucositis pain.

Peripheral Neuropathy. In addition to having a histolytic effect on the malignant cells, chemotherapeutic agents may also have deleterious effects on healthy neural tissue. The damage to the nerve cells may produce pain, paresthesia, hyperreflexia, autonomic dysfunction, and motor and sensory deficits. The drugs commonly associated with peripheral neuropathy[68] in cancer patients are the vinca alkaloids (e.g., vincristine, cisplatin, procarbazine, and, infrequently, misonidazole). The histologic lesion producing this symptomatology is demyelination and myelin degeneration of peripheral nerves. Electromyography and nerve conduction studies may be used to confirm the diagnosis. The treatment of painful neuropathy syndrome secondary to chemotherapeutic agents includes the use of tricyclic antidepressants, anticonvulsants, selective nerve blocks, TENS, and in those patients where the pain becomes severe and intractable, narcotic analgesics.

Steroid-Induced Pain Syndromes. Corticosteroids are used frequently alone or in conjunction with other chemotherapeutic agents to treat cancer patients. Under these circumstances, steroids may produce certain characteristic syndromes listed here:

1. *Steroid pseudorheumatism.*[69] This syndrome has many symptoms including myalgia with muscle tenderness at multiple sites and diffuse nonspecific arthralgia. These symptoms usually occur following withdrawal of steroid therapy. If pain is very severe and the discomfort is unbearable, treatment should include reinstitution of the steroids followed by gradual withdrawal.

2. *Aseptic necrosis of femoral and humeral joints.*[70] This syndrome may occur after continuous or intermittent steroid therapy. The pain should be investigated using bone scans or MRI. Treatment should include limiting the reduction of activity on the affected joint, and the use of NSAIDs and narcotic analgesics for pain management.

3. *Osteonecrosis secondary to steroids.*[71] This syndrome consists of bone pain associated with prolonged steroid use. Osteopenia is usually associated with this condition and it may lead to pathologic fractures. It is important, however, to differentiate between pathologic fractures secondary to osteonecrosis and pathologic fractures secondary to metastatic involvement.

4. *Perineal dysesthesia.*[13] This syndrome is associated with a severe burning sensation in the perineal area and has been reported by patients receiving large doses of dexamethasone. This dose schedule of steroids is usually given as part of a protocol for the treatment of metastatic epidural spinal cord compression. The pain may be discomforting but fortunately it is transient and does not require more than occasional intravenous narcotic analgesics. The etiology of this pain syndrome is thought to be due to the activation of "steroid receptors" located in the cutaneous tissues in the perineal area by high-dose dexamethasone.

Miscellaneous Causes. There are a few procedures associated with the treatment of cancer that produce specific pain syndromes. These should be managed aggressively and effectively. It is always unfortunate when a patient expresses complete satisfaction with a complicated procedure and even receives desired results but bitterly complains of an unpleasant experience during a minor procedure such as venipuncture. It is more unsatisfactory when that patient continues to have pain as a result of a lesion sustained during a relatively innocuous procedure such as a venipuncture. The following are a list of procedure-related pain syndromes:

1. *Pain-associated bone marrow biopsy.* Bone marrow biopsy is performed usually in the iliac crest of the pelvic bone. This pain can be minimized by adequate infiltration with local anesthetics, postbiopsy application of pressure packs to the area, and the general application of good technique.

2. *Lumbar puncture for diagnostic and therapeutic purposes.* Whenever a lumbar puncture is performed, cerebrospinal fluid loss occurs. Uncontrolled loss would produce a decrease in the cerebrospinal fluid pressure and may be associated with postlumbar puncture headache. The treatment of lumbar puncture headaches that do not respond to 24–48 hours of conservative therapy (i.e., high-volume oral and intravenous fluids, bed rest, oral and

parenteral narcotic analgesics) is the administration of an epidural blood patch.

3. *Bone biopsy.* Bone biopsies are performed several times to determine a histologic configuration of the nature of the lesion affecting a particular bone. This information is crucial to determine whether it is inflammatory or carcinogenic (primary or secondary). Bone marrow biopsies are performed frequently and may be associated with severe pain. Periosteal infiltration with local anesthetics and the infiltration of the surrounding tissue along with selected peripheral nerve blocks may go a long way in decreasing post bone biopsy pain.

Pain Syndromes Unrelated to Cancer Therapy

Cancer pain patients may develop pain that is totally unrelated to their cancer or to therapy. These patients may either be in the process of being treated or may have already been treated. The pain they develop should be investigated thoroughly. At the conclusion of that investigation, it is important to delineate the precise etiologic basis of the pain.

For those patients who may have headache, back pain, sympathetically mediated pain, abdominal pain, pelvic pain, or any other chronic pain syndrome that is clearly caused by a noncancer or a noncancer therapy-related syndrome, the treatment should proceed in the same way as if the patient did not have cancer. It is important to remember that those patients already have the stress of having had cancer and there are certain concerns that may require attention before commencing aggressive treatment for that noncancer-related pain syndrome. However, for those patients in whom the etiology is unknown or not clear, the need for continued reassessment and investigation should be emphasized so that as new symptoms develop they may be treated vigorously.

Summary

One must have a clear understanding of the nature of a particular cancer and its pathogenesis in order to effectively treat it. Because pain is a common associated feature of cancer and because many of the therapeutic strategies for cancer may produce pain, it is important to understand the specific pain syndromes associated with the treatment of cancer and specific pain syndromes associated with the cancer per se. Aggressive therapy for pain and continued reassessment of pain and of the patient's general condition represent the best approach to treating cancer-related pain syndromes.

References

1. Stjernsward J, Teoh N. The Scope of the Cancer Pain Problem. In KM Foley, JJ Bonica, V Ventafridda (eds), Proceedings of the Second International Congress on Cancer Pain. In Advances in Pain Research and Therapy (Vol. 16). New York: Raven, 1990;7.
2. World Health Organization. Cancer pain relief and palliative care. Report of a WHO expert committee, World Health Organization Technical Report Series, 804. Geneva, Switzerland: World Health Organization, 1990;1.
3. Payne R. Cancer pain: Anatomy, physiology and pharmacology. Cancer 1989;63(Suppl.):2266.
4. Twycross RG, Lack SA. Symptom Control in Far Advanced Cancer: Pain Relief. London: Pitman, 1983.
5. Kori SH, Foley KM, Posner JB. Brachial plexus lesions in patients with cancer: 100 cases. Neurology 1981;31:45.
6. Spiegel D, Bloom JR. Pain in metastatic breast cancer. Cancer 1983;52:341.
7. Vecht CJ, Hoff AM, deBoer MF. Types and causes of pain in cancer of the head and neck. Pain 1990;(Suppl. 5):S354.
8. Cornblath DR, McArthur JC. Predominantly sensory neuropathy in patients with AIDS and AIDS-related complex. Neurology 1988;38:794.
9. Cornblath DR, McArthur JC, Kennedy PGE, et al. Inflammatory demyelinating peripheral neuropathies associated with human T-cell lymphotropic virus type III infection. Ann Neurol 1987;21:32.
10. Elliott K, Foley KM. Neurologic pain syndromes in patients with cancer. Neurologic Clinics 1989;7:333.
11. Chad DA. Lumbosacral plexopathy. Semin Neurol 1987;7:97.
12. Bullit E. Intracranial tumors in patients with facial pain. J Neurosurg 1986;64:865.
13. Greenberg HS, Kim JH, Poster JB. Epidural spinal cord compression from metastatic tumor: Results with a new treatment protocol. Ann Neurol 1980;8:361.
14. Wasserstrom WR, Glass JP, Posner JB. Diagnosis and treatment of leptomeningeal metastases from solid tumors: Experience with 90 patients. Cancer 1982;49:759.
15. Sozzi G, Marotta P, Piatti L. Vagoglossopharyngeal neuralgia with syncope in the course of carcinomatous meningitis. Ital J Neurol Sci 1987;8:271.
16. DeAngeles LM, Payne R. Lymphomatous meningitis presenting as atypical cluster headache. Pain 1987;30:211.

17. Hakanson S. Trigeminal neuralgia treated by the injection of glycerol into the trigeminal cistern. Neurosurgery 1981;9:638.

18. Graus F, Elkon KB, Cordon-Cardo C, Posner JB. Sensory neuropathy and small cell lung cancer. Am J Med 1986;80:45.

19. Horwich MS, Cho L, Porro RS, Posner JB. Subacute sensory neuronopathy: A remote effect of carcinoma. Ann Neurol 1977;2:7.

20. Schold SC, Cho E-S, Somasundaram M, Posner JB. Subacute motor neuronopathy: A remote effect of lymphoma. Ann Neurol 1979;5:271.

21. Foley KM. Pain syndromes in patients with cancer. Med Clin North Am 1987;71:169.

22. Jaeckle KA, Young DF, Foley KM. The natural history of lumbosacral plexopathy in cancer. Neurology 1985;35:8.

23. Benedetti C, Bonica JJ. Cancer Pain: Basic Considerations. In C Benedetti, et al. (eds), Advances in Pain Research and Therapy (Vol. 7). New York: Raven, 1984;529.

24. Ad Hoc Committee on Cancer Pain of the American Society of Clinical Oncology. Cancer pain assessment and treatment curriculum guidelines. J Clin Oncol 1992;10:1976.

25. Personal communication. Parris WC, 1995.

26. Bonica JJ. Management of pain with regional analgesia. Postgrad Med 1984;60:897.

27. Nashold BS Jr, Ostdahl RH. Dorsal root entry zone lesions for pain relief. J Neurosurg 1979;51:59.

28. Bruera E, Roca E, Cedaro L, et al. Action of oral methylprednisolone in terminal cancer patients: A prospective randomized double-blind study. Cancer Treat Rep 1985;69:751.

29. Glassman AH. The newer antidepressant drugs and their cardiovascular effects. Psychopharmacol Bull 1984;20:272.

30. Hoefnagael CA. Radionuclide therapy revisited. Eur J Nucl Med 1991;18:408.

31. Payne R. Cancer pain, anatomy, physiology and pharmacology. Cancer 1989;63:2266.

32. Foley KM. Pain Syndromes in Patients with Cancer. In JJ Bonica, V Ventrafridda (eds), Advances in Pain Research and Therapy (Vol. 2). New York: Raven, 1979;59.

33. Portenoy RK. Gynecologic Oncology: Management of Pain. In WJ Hoskins, CA Perez, RC Young (eds), Principles and Practice of Gynecologic Oncology. Philadelphia: Lippincott, 1991;367.

34. Greenberg HS. Metastasis to the base of the skull: Clinical findings in 43 patients. Neurology 1981;31:530.

35. Portenoy RK. Pharmacologic Management of Chronic Pain. In HL Fields (ed), Pain Syndrome in Neurology (Vol. 10). London: Butterworth, 1989;260.

36. Maunuksela EL, Olkkola KT, Kokki H. Pharmacokinetics of intravenous ketorolac and its efficacy in relieving postoperative pain in children. J Pain Symptom Manage 1991;6:142.

37. Sundaresan N. Treatment of odontoid fractures in cancer patients. J Neurosurg 1981;54:187.

38. CSM Update. Nonsteroidal anti-inflammatory drugs and serious gastrointestinal adverse reactions. Br Med J 1986;292:614.

39. Stiefel FC, Breitbart WS, Holland JC. Corticosteroids in cancer: Neuropsychiatric complications. Cancer Invest 1989;7:479.

40. Fiore CE, Castorina F, Malatino LS, et al. Analgesic activity of calcitonin: Effectiveness of the epidural and subarachnoid routes in man. Int J Clin Pharmacol Res 1983;3:257.

41. Bruera E, Macdonald N. Intractable pain in patients with advanced head and neck tumors: A possible role of local infection. Cancer Treat Rep 1986;70:691.

42. Frederiks JAM. Phantom Limb and Phantom Limb Pain. In JAM Fredericks (ed), Handbook of Clinical Neurology (Vol. 1). Clinical Neuropsychology. New York: Elsevier, 1985;395.

43. Bach S, Noreng MF, Tjellden NU. Phantom limb pain in amputees during the first 12 months following limb amputation, after preoperative lumbar epidural blockade. Pain 1988;33:297.

44. Cousins MJ. Prevention of Postoperative Pain. In MR Bond, JE Charlson, CJ Woolf (eds), Pain Research and Clinical Management (Vol. 4). Proceedings of the VIth World Congress on Pain. Amsterdam: Elsevier, 1991.

45. Jensen TS, Krebs B, Neilson J, Rasmussen P. Phantom limb, phantom pain and stump pain in amputees during the first six months following limb amputation. Pain 1983;17:243.

46. Granek I, Ashikari R, Foley KM. Postmastectomy pain syndrome: Clinical and anatomical correlates. Proc ASCO 1983;3:122.

47. Vecht CJ. Post-axillary dissection in breast cancer due to lesion of the intercostobrachial nerve. Pain 1989;38:171.

48. Kanner RM, Martini N, Foley KM. Nature and incidence of post-thoracotomy pain. Proc ASCO 1982;1:152.

49. Bonica JJ. Clinical Applications of Diagnostic and Therapeutic Nerve Blocks. Springfield, IL: Thomas, 1959.

50. Reiestad F, Stromskag KE. Interpleural catheter in the management of postoperative pain. Reg Anaesth 1986;11:89.

51. Boas RA, Covino RB, Shahnarian A. Analgesic responses to intravenous lignocaine. Br J Anaesth 1982;54:501.

52. Berger PS. Neurological Complications of Radiotherapy. In A Silberstein (ed), Neurological Complications of Therapy: Selected Topics. Mount Kisco, NY: Futura, 1982;173.

53. Jaeckle KA, et al. The natural history of lumbosacral plexopathy in cancer. Neurology 1985;35:8.

54. Payne R, Foley KM. Exploration of the brachial plexus in patients with cancer. Neurology 1986;36:329.

55. Glass JP, Foley KM. Harmful Effects of Radiation. In AK Asbury, GM McKhann, WI McDonald (eds), Diseases of the Nervous System. Philadelphia: Saunders, 1986;1188.

56. Foley KM, Woodruff JM, Ellis FT. Radiation-induced malignant and atypical peripheral nerve sheath tumors.

Arch Neurol 1980;7:311.

57. Rothwell BR. Prevention and treatment of the orofacial complications of radiotherapy. J Am Dent Assoc 1987;114:316.

58. Guttenberg SA. Osteoradionecrosis of the jaw. Am J Surg 1974;127:326.

59. MacDougall JA, Evans AM, Lindsay RK. Osteoradionecrosis of the mandible and its treatment. Am J Surg 1963;106:816.

60. Moran WJ, Panje WR. The free greater omental flap for treatment of mandibular osteoradionecrosis. Arch Otolaryngol Head Neck Surg 1987;113:425.

61. Weiss HD, et al. Neurotoxicity of commonly used antineoplastic agents. N Engl J Med 1974;291:75.

62. Loeser J. Herpes Zoster and Postherpetic Neuralgia. In JJ Bonica (ed), The Management of Cancer Pain (2nd ed). Philadelphia: Lea & Febiger, 1990;257.

63. Rusthoven JJ, et al. Risk factors for varicella zoster disseminated infection among adult cancer patients with localized zoster. Cancer 1988;62:1641.

64. Portenoy RK, Duma C, Foley KM. Acute herpetic and postherpetic neuralgia: Clinical review and current management. Ann Neurol 1987;20:651.

65. Watson PN, Evans RJ. Postherpetic neuralgia: A review. Arch Neurol 1986;43:836.

66. Young DF, Posner JB. Nervous System Toxicity of Chemotherapeutic Agents. In PJ Vinken, GW Bruyn (eds), Handbook of Clinical Neurology. Amsterdam: North Holland Publishing, 1980;91.

67. Carl W. Oral and Dental Care of Patients Receiving Radiation Therapy for Tumors in and Around the Oral Cavity. In W Carl, K Saka (eds), Cancer and the Oral Cavity. Chicago: Quintessence, 1986;167.

68. Young DF, Poster JB. Nervous System Toxicity of Chemotherapeutic Agents. In PJ Vinken, GW Bruyn (eds), Handbook of Clinical Neurology (Vol. 9). Neurological Manifestations of Systemic Diseases. Amsterdam: North Holland Publishing, 1989;91.

69. Rotstein J, Good RA. Steroid pseudorheumatism. Arch Intern Med 1957;99:545.

70. Solomon L. Drug induced arthropathy and necrosis of the femoral head. J Bone Joint Surg 1973;55:246.

71. Ihde DC, DeVita VT. Osteonecrosis of the femoral head in patients treated with intermittent combination chemotherapy (including corticosteroids). Cancer 1975;36:1585.

Chapter 24

Orofacial Pain Management in Patients with Cancer and Human Immunodeficiency Virus

Robert C. Adler

Oral pain related to oral cancer can have serious consequences for the cancer pain patient, including an inability to speak, eat, or swallow, hastened morbidity, decreased quality of life, and compromised treatment. As devastasting as this type of pain can be for the cancer pain patient, one would assume that it would receive adequate attention in the literature. However, a review of the literature revealed only a few mentions of pain related to oral cancer, and these offerings were usually part of a discussion of routine postoperative care. Even less information was available for pain related to human immunodeficiency virus (HIV). Therefore, this chapter addresses this problem and suggests some treatment modalities.

The causes of oral cancer pain include primary lesions of the oral cavity, viral and bacterial invasion, and as a secondary effect from metastases and treatment of oral cancer and head and neck cancer. The pain may be from the stimulation of the mucosal and submucosal sensory nerve endings. In addition, recent experience has shown that, with few exceptions, oral pain from HIV is similar to that of cancer.

General Treatment Considerations

Oral pain symptoms occur from trigeminal involvement, as a result of secondary effects from treatment and from brief exacerbations of opportunistic infections. The symptoms are usually responsive to treatment, provided that all of the causative factors have been carefully identified. Accurate diagnosis is critical because the etiology of the pain can be so varied and masked. For example, dental pain may be from underlying caries and thus require a simple restoration. However, there may be a deeper neuropathic problem requiring membrane-stabilizing medications and opioids. Therefore, the clinician must carefully evaluate the tumor location and invasion pattern.

Ulcerations and invasion from viral, fungal, and bacterial sources can be managed with various topical rinses containing anesthetics, corticosteroids, and antibiotics. For example, pain from ulcerative fungal lesions can be treated with an oral rinse mixture of 4% lidocaine and diphenhydramine (while the fungal component is being treated with a nystatin rinse or fluconazole). Other anesthetic agents often used include 1% dibucaine, dyclonine, 6% cocaine, and 1% tetracaine. Herpetic viral infections must be treated with acyclovir (ganciclovir for cytomegalovirus) and anesthetic rinses.

Necrotizing ulcerative periodontitis causes pain that is described as a deep, throbbing ache. The interproximal tissue becomes ulcerated and can cause rapid pocket formation with loss of bony tooth support. Treatment consists of a mixture of 0.2% chlorhexidine gluconate and 250 mg of tetracycline applied to the lesions four times daily for 1 week. Necrotizing stomatitis is similar but can extend into the adjacent soft tissues. It can be treated by combining tetracycline and a glucocorticosteroid in a gel medium.

Because the oral mucosa is highly susceptible to painful ulcerations, the use of systemic medications causing anticholinergic effects such as xerostomia must be carefully balanced with frequent water or artificial saliva rinses in order to minimize this complication.

Patients with HIV disease can experience ulcerative aphthous lesions that tend to be larger, deeper, and more chronic. Treatment can include topical clobetasol (0.05%), 5 mg of prednisone, or Mile's ointment (tetracycline, nystatin, and hydrocortisone), all of which can be used for up to 2 weeks with good results. When patients are so compromised that anesthetic rinses and corticosteroids cannot be used, an alternative treatment is inhalation of 200 mg beclomethasone diproprionate twice daily for 1 week, then once daily.[1]

It is important that no rinse mixture contain more than a trace amount of alcohol because this will exacerbate mucosal pain. The neutral medium should be deionized water, whenever possible.

Long-acting opioids are needed for later stages of disease and during persistent or recurrent oral infection, especially when the oropharynx is involved. Liquid morphine sulfate preparations without alcohol provide the best pain relief without the complication of mucosal irritation.

Epidermoid Cancer

This condition is usually located in the mandibular gingiva and alveolar process. It commonly affects the elderly. The pain remains local and is primarily from acute ulceration and periosteum invasion.[2, 3] Treatment is limited to adhesive topical anesthetics until the lesion is excised.

Primary Tumors

Primary infiltration tumors rapidly invade the fascial planes, display early multifocal ulcerations, and are quite painful. The pain is more diffuse and generally follows the invasion pattern. Some of the painful tumors (ranked in order of highest pain intensity) include adenocystic carcinoma, adenocarcinoma, pleomorphic adenoma, and mucoepidermoid

tumors.[4–6] In addition to local treatment for the acute ulcerations, long-acting opioids provide the best pain control because pain often becomes a chronic problem.

Paranasal Sinuses

Unfortunately, cancer of the paranasal sinuses is usually diagnosed only after it has been present for some time in the retropharyngeal and cervical nodes. Cancer of the maxillary antrum often first presents as palatal erosion and pain, loosened maxillary teeth, and pain in the alveolar ridge. Other signs and symptoms include nasal swelling, frontal headache, facial pain and numbness, and contracture (trismus) of the medial pterygoid muscle. The sphenopalatine nerve may be involved if there is palatal anesthesia. Treatment for the pain symptoms includes long-acting opioids, and either baclofen or carbamazepine for the neuropathic component. Owing to the late presentation of this disease, the trismus is almost always permanent.

Surgical Intervention

Resection techniques often leave significant areas of granulation tissue, muscle scarring and pulling, and neuropathic pain, particularly from mandibular erosion around the mental nerve. The least pain-producing surgical technique is one that allows primary closure but this type of technique is possible only if tissue pulling or tension is not a factor.[7]

Transcutaneous Resection

This procedure requires a disarticulation of the temporomandibular joint, which often causes a synovitis and temporalis muscle division from the coronoid process leading to contracture (trismus). Other muscles that can become involved are the masseter and medial pterygoid. The joint inflammation and trismus are characterized by a marked limited movement and sharp pain radiating from the affected structures and attachments. Physical medicine procedures consisting of spray and stretch, mechanically assisted stretching, and therapeutic exercise will help reduce the trismus and increase a pain-free range of motion. Brief use of an anti-inflammatory agent will help control some of the pain and inflammation that are unavoidably caused by the treatment. If there are no tumor cells in the area, ultrasound as a deep heat technique to the temporomandibular joint will substantially decrease the capsular inflammation and improve function. However, beyond the limited active treatment, the patient must be encouraged to continue an aggressive home stretching program to avoid new scar formation and a permanent loss of jaw opening.[8]

Transoral Resection

This procedure does not seem to reduce the incidence of trismus, but can lower the chance of joint inflammation if attention is given to the type of mouth gag used to maintain jaw opening during surgery. Except for the physical medicine techniques previously mentioned, acute postoperative medication is usually all that is required to control the pain symptoms.

Radiation Therapy

Most head and neck cancer patients receive radiation therapy, with the usual dosage between 40 and 75 Gy over a 5- to 7-week period. The most common adverse effects occur within the salivary glands, intraoral mucosa, lymphatics, alveolar bone, teeth, and gingiva.

Salivary Glands

Degenerative changes such as atrophy and fibrosis cause a shift in salinity and associated lowering of the pH.[9, 10] A diffuse topical pain occurs that is adequately managed with oral anesthetic rinses. These rinses need to be applied every few hours or before and after each meal. The pain intensity will lessen to the point of only occasionally needing to use the rinse.

Xerostomia begins from a few hours to 3 weeks after the start of radiation therapy.[11] Artificial saliva is available in aerosol and liquid form and must be applied on a regular basis in order to minimize a burning sensation that develops along the dry mucosa. A concomitant shift in the oral flora can cause an increase in *Candida albicans,* leading to painful ulcerations and depapillation of the tongue.[12] Antifungal mouth rinses usually resolve this problem relatively quickly, except in HIV-infected patients where chronicity is fairly common. It is important to avoid alcohol and not to use medications that require oral dissolution because these agents abrade the mucosa and thus facilitate ulcerative lesions.

Mucosa

The buccal mucosa is vulnerable to trismus. The mucous membrane closely approximates the facial muscles, especially the masseter and buccinator, often resulting in early invasion of these muscles. Irradiated tumor often leaves a significant amount of granulation and scar tissue, thus causing a highly treatment-resistant contracture. Therapeutic stretching is mandatory and will require a significant commitment by the patient to perform these exercises at least six times per day. Due to tumor cell proximity, ultrasound cannot be used and so local anesthetic (0.25% procaine) is injected into the muscle attachments so that more aggressive stretching can occur with only minimal pain. Though the pain symptoms will be reduced, some contracture will be permanent.

Mucositis begins 1–2 weeks after starting radiation therapy (approximately 20–25 Gy), and presents as a diffuse inflammation occasionally covered by a grayish pseudomembrane. Rapid cell turnover is why the mucosa is very sensitive to radiation therapy.[13] The pain is usually described as intense and burning, particularly after eating or after a rapid intraoral temperature change.[14] Secondary infection by candidiasis or hairy leukoplakia causes a deeper burning pain. Many of the pain symptoms can be adequately controlled by beginning antimicrobial rinses prior to radiation therapy, and supplementing anesthetic rinses during therapy. Generally after approximately 50 Gy, the mucositis will subside, but there is no clear explanation for this phenomenon.

HIV patients will experience a particularly painful mucositis during radiation therapy of Kaposi's sarcoma.[15] Oral anesthetic rinses adequately control the pain. The pain intensity can be reduced further if antibacterial rinses are used prior to starting radiation therapy.

Lymphatics

Although fibrosis and obstruction do occur, we do not know the factors that affect their incidence or the precise mechanism for these changes. Lymphedema results in discomfort around the affected area but treatment is usually not required because the problem is self-limited and is controlled by other coincident analgesics. Some of our patients have reported additional relief by applying hot packs to the affected areas.

Osteoradionecrosis

Radiation necrosis is a problem that often does not develop for months or years after therapy. It is characterized by pathologic fracture, spontaneously exposed bone, periodontal defects, and nonhealing wounds. The pain is described as deep and dull without a radiating pattern.[16, 17, 18] Nonsteroidal anti-inflammatory agents and adjunctive opioid analgesics will control the pain until the necrotic area is treated. However, this problem can result in chronic pain most commonly experienced during mastication. Therefore, pain medications and a softer diet may be necessary on a long-term basis.

Gingiva and Teeth

A secondary periodontal inflammation and alveolar recession develops early during radiation therapy.[19] Periodontal rinses (0.12% chlorhexidine gluconate) and meticulous oral hygiene can control this problem without further complications. Radiation caries and pulp degeneration will cause dental pain that is relieved by appropriate dental restorative interventions.

Chemotherapy

Tissue changes (mucositis and bacterial or viral invasion) from chemotherapy are similar to those from radiation therapy. The chemical agent itself can cause changes in the mucosa, or the change will be secondary to myelosuppression. Mucositis will occur within 7 days of therapy initiation and generally presents as sporadic ulcerations.[20]

An important precaution is to avoid diagnosing herpetic lesions as a cytotoxic mucositis or bacterial infection due to the fact that the treatment regimens for the pain symptoms differ. Fortunately, anesthetic rinses, acyclovir, and acute analgesics provide adequate pain control until the chemotherapy is complete and the pain subsides.[21, 22]

A special diffuse facial pain can develop from use of vincristine and is often misdiagnosed as common myofascitis, which leads to the use of physical medicine procedures without any meaningful treatment outcome. Although the precise mechanism of this pain is not known, analgesics and patient reassurance are the only treatments required.

HIV patients experience xerostomia from the use of zidovudine and foscarnet. Artificial saliva and saliva-stimulating agents (sour candy, pilocarpine, etc.) greatly reduce the burning pain. Nonspecific ulcerations can occur with these medications as well as with interferon and zalcitabine. Anesthetic rinses provide adequate relief until the medications are decreased or stopped.[23]

Bone Marrow Transplantation

Tissue changes (mainly mucositis and xerostomia) are similar to those from radiation therapy and chemotherapy. Complications can occur after preconditioning with chemotherapy and radiation (erythema and ulcerations), immunosuppression (aphthous lesions, mucositis, and xerostomia), and graft-versus-host disease prevention (erythema and mucositis). The painful erythema and severe generalized aphthous lesions develop in the mouth and oropharynx, and persist about 6–10 days. However, the most painful changes occur during immunosuppression for control of graft-versus-host disease, especially when administering cyclosporin and methotrexate.

Symptoms usually start to appear approximately 3 weeks after transplantation. Proactive use of antiviral medication and antifungal rinses (three to four times daily) significantly reduces the oral symptoms.

Metastatic Lesions

A metastatic lesion to the jaw often presents with the following signs: a neuropathy of the mental nerve or mandibular division of the trigeminal nerve, pain, gingival inflammation, spontaneous fracture, and loosened teeth. Often, these signs and symptoms are the first evidence of malignancy. The most frequent primary sites are breast, kidney, lung, prostate, and thyroid. Any patient presenting with a mental neuropathy without a history of cancer should be screened with panoramic radiography and bone scans.[24, 25]

The most common sign is mental neuropathy arising from a regional lymphadenopathy compression or ramus metastases and presents as ipsilateral numbness to the chin, lip, anterior teeth, and adjacent gingiva.[26, 27] The pain is described as burning or prickly and is localized around the affected site. However, when the third division is involved, the symptoms are considerably more diffuse.

The pain symptoms must be treated just like any other neuropathic problem. Fortunately, the pain intensity is mild to moderate and thus baclofen alone, or in combination with carbamazepine, usually provides sufficient relief with minimal side effects.

Dietary Factors

Oral pain can severely compromise nutritional intake. Insufficient vitamin B_2 and folate levels manifest as a painful red tongue, angular cheilitis, and gingival ulcerations. Therefore, it is imperative to quickly recognize and control the cause and symptoms of painful lesions. Anesthetic rinses and liquid antacid coatings taken before meals will allow a reasonably comfortable dietary intake.

Conclusion

Oral pain from cancer and HIV infection is a serious, debilitating, and often overlooked problem that can lead to nutritional deficiencies, an inability to take oral medications, and an overall decline in the quality of life. Most oral pain symptoms can be successfully treated once the etiologic factors are clearly identified.

References

1. Chapnick EK, Graydon JD, Lutwick LI. Treatment of human immunodeficiency virus associated with oral aphthous ulcers with inhaled steroids. NY State J Med 1992;92:221.

2. Gorlin RJ, Chaudhry AP, Pindborg JJ. Odontogenic tumors. Classification, histopathology, and clinical behavior in man and domesticated animals. Cancer 1961;14:73.

3. Cady B, Catlin D. Epidermoid carcinoma of the gum: A 20 year survey. Cancer 1969;23:551.

4. Conley J. Concepts in Head and Neck Surgery. New York: Grune & Stratton, 1970;257.

5. Gray JM, Hendrix RC, French AJ. Mucoepidermoid tumors of salivary glands. Cancer 1963;16;183.

6. Spiro RH, Huvos AG, Strong EW. Adenocarcinoma of salivary origin: Clinicopathologic study of 204 patients. Am J Surg 1982;144:423.

7. McGregor IA, McGregor FM. Cancer of the Face and Mouth: Pathology and Management for Surgeons. New York: Churchill Livingstone, 1986;5.

8. Lefall LD Jr. Head and neck cancer. An interview. Cancer 1971;21:288.

9. Driezen S, Brown LR, Handler S. Radiation induced xerostomia in cancer patients: Effect on salivary and serum electrolytes. Cancer 1976;38:273.

10. Moore MJ. The effect of radiation on connective tissue. Otolaryngol Clin North Am 1984;17:389.

11. Mossman KL. Quantitative radiation dose-response relationships for normal tissues in man. Radiat Res 1983;95:392.

12. Brown LR, Dreizen S, Handler S. Effect of radiation-induced xerostomia on human flora. J Dent Res 1975;54:740.

13. Beumer J, Curtis T, Harrison R. Radiation therapy of the oral cavity: Sequelae and management, Part I. Head Neck Surg 1979;1:301.

14. Rubin RI, Doku HC. Therapeutic radiology: The modalities and their effect on oral tissues. J Am Dent Assoc 1976;92:731.

15. Cooper JS, Fried PR. Toxicity of oral radiotherapy in patients with acquired immunodeficiency syndrome. Arch Otolaryngol Head Neck Surg 1987;113:327.

16. Bedwinek JM, Chavoski LJ, Fletcher GH, et al. Osteonecrosis in patients treated with definitive radiotherapy for squamous cell carcinomas of the oral cavity and naso- and oropharynx. Radiology 1976;119:665.

17. Dodson WS. Irradiation osteomyelitis of the jaw. J Oral Surg 1962;20:467.

18. Larson DL, Lindberg RD, Lane E, et al. Major complications of radiotherapy in cancer of the oral cavity and oropharynx: A ten year retrospective study. Am J Surg 1983;146:531.

19. Silverman S, Chierici, G. Radiation therapy of oral carcinoma. I. Effects of oral tissue management of the periodontium. J Periodont 1965;36:478.

20. Million RR, Cassisi NJ. Chemotherapy—General Principles. In WE Ross (ed), Management of Head and Neck Cancer: A Multidisciplinary Approach. Philadelphia: Lippincott, 1984.

21. Moles B. Dental management of the cancer patient.

AAOMS Surg Update 1992;2.

22. Scully C, Laskaris G, Pindborg J, et al. Oral manifestations of HIV infection and their management. I. More common lesions. Oral Surg 1991;71:158.

23. Glick M. Oral pain. PAACNOTES 1993;6:226.

24. Castigliano SG, Rominger CJ. Metastatic malignancy of the jaws. Am J Surg 1954;87:496.

25. Roistacher SL. Numbness: A significant finding. Oral Surg 1973;36:22.

26. Massey EW, Moore J, Schold SC. Mental neuropathy from systemic cancer. Neurology 1981;31:1277.

27. Harris CP, Baringer JR. The numb chin in metastatic cancer. West J Med 1991;155:528.

Chapter 25
Chest Pain

George A. Mensah

Introduction

The presentation of chest pain in an adult patient is often associated with significant anxiety in both the patient and physician. This reaction is especially true in developed countries where chest pain is a common symptom of heart disease, the leading cause of death and disability in the Western Hemisphere. In the United States, for example, heart disease caused about 720,000 deaths in 1991, more than one-third of all deaths in that year alone.[1, 2] It is therefore not surprising that the initial evaluation of the patient with chest pain is often geared toward the exclusion of life-threatening heart disease, especially ischemic heart disease.

In the patient with known or suspected cancer, however, chest pain may be caused by a variety of etiologies other than ischemic heart disease. This chapter briefly discusses the following topics: (1) the importance of excluding chest pain of ischemic origin; (2) the relevance of coronary artery disease in patients with cancer; (3) the spectrum of nonischemic pain of cardiac origin as well as noncardiac chest pain in the cancer patient; (4) the mechanisms of chest pain; (5) the importance of the clinical history in the differential diagnosis; (6) the diagnostic evaluation in different chest pain syndromes; and (7) an overview of the therapeutic strategy.

Mechanisms of Chest Pain and the Diagnostic Evaluation

Chapter 4 provides a detailed discussion of pain mechanisms and their relevance to cancer. However, it is important in this section to focus briefly on the pathophysiology of chest pain in particular. This is a useful starting point for the subsequent discussion of the clinical approach to chest pain in the cancer patient and the diagnostic evaluation. In this regard, the innervation of the heart and structures of the chest as well as the characteristics of relevant receptors and neurotransmitters play important roles in helping us understand the complexities of chest pain.

The chest contains more than just the heart. The thoracic vertebrae, ribs, sternum, esophagus, trachea, bronchi, lungs, pleura, and the great arteries and veins are all structures within the chest that may be a source of pain. The precision with which the brain localizes pain to the correct structure and the accuracy with which a patient describes this pain are all, to a great extent, a function of nociceptor density in the relevant structure, characteristics of the nerve fibers carrying the afferent information, and the cortical somatosensory map. These parameters differ for the different structures in the chest and therefore help in the differential diagnosis of chest pain.

The heart, like other viscera, has nociceptors that are less densely packed than in skin, muscle, or fascia. These nociceptors are the terminal branches of small, unmyelinated C fibers. The esophagus is similarly less densely populated with nociceptors. The great vessels in the chest, which may be the origin of chest pain, have a greater density of nociceptors than either the heart or esophagus. The remaining chest structures including the chest muscles, overlying skin, ligaments, costosternal and costochondral cartilage, and the parietal pleura have a greater density of nociceptors than structures previously mentioned. On the other hand, the visceral pericardium, inner surfaces of the parietal pericardium, lung parenchyma, and visceral pleura do not have nociceptors and thus may not be the source of chest pain.

Visceral afferent fibers from the myocardium and structures within the heart form the cardiac plexus and travel along the middle and inferior cervical nerves and the upper five thoracic rami to enter the central nervous system (CNS). The afferent fibers from the right-sided cardiac chambers travel in the right-sided nerves, whereas afferents from the pulmonary veins, interatrial and interventricular septa, and left-sided chambers travel through the left-sided nerves. Visceral afferents from the ascending aorta, aortic arch, and pulmonary arteries also travel the same route described for the heart and enter the CNS at the same thoracic levels. The descending thoracic aorta sends visceral afferents via the third through eighth thoracic rami.

The inferior cervical sympathetic nerves and the vagus nerve carry visceral afferents from the upper esophagus whereas the thoracic cardiac sympathetic nerves and stellate ganglion carry afferents from the lower esophagus. Nociceptors in the tracheobronchial tree send afferents to the T-3 to T-5 level of the CNS and are carried in the sympathetic plexus and vagus nerve. Somatic afferent fibers from the parietal pleura, parietal pericardium, ribs, and intercostal muscles travel in the brachial plexus, intercostal nerves, and phrenic nerves. Finally, the skin overlying the chest wall sends somatic afferents via the supraclavicular and intercostal nerves.

One obvious pattern is that multiple structures in different parts of the chest send afferent "traffic" via the same cord segment and that individual structures may have afferent fibers entering the CNS at many spinal cord levels. This pattern in part explains the phenomenon of referred pain, where noxious stimuli originating in one structure arrive in the CNS and are incorrectly interpreted and localized to another structure. In addition, pathologic processes involving a particular nerve root and leading to noxious stimulation of the associated nerve may lead to incorrect localization of the pain to the structure subserved by that nerve. For example, tumor involvement and compression of the C-6 nerve root may cause pain that is localized to the chest because somatic afferents from the pectoral muscles enter the CNS at C-5 to T-1 cord segments.

The exact mechanism by which nociceptors in the chest structures are activated to cause chest pain is not completely understood. In patients with cancer, for example, primary or metastatic tumor involvement of chest structures may lead to mechanical stimulation (distention, stretching, tearing), chemical irritation (local production and release of bradykinin, histamine, serotonin, prostaglandins), or simply generalized inflammatory reaction. Edmeads and Billings[4] have suggested that the presence of inflammation in any structure drastically lowers the pain threshold, thereby rendering normally innocuous stimuli painful. Ischemia, which is independent of the presence of tumor, may also lead to nociceptor stimulation. The potential chemical mediators in this latter setting may be bradykinin, substance P, L-glutamate, prostaglandins, adenosine triphosphate, calcitonin gene-related peptide, or even hydrogen and potassium ions.[5] Kambam et al.[6] found significant differences in substance P–like immunoreactivity, acetylcholinesterase activity, and total protein content of pericardial fluid in patients with angina pectoris compared with those without angina pectoris. More likely, a combination of chemical mediators including substance P, bradykinin, serotonin, histamine, adenosine, and prostaglandins may act synergistically to produce chest pain.[7]

Clinical Approach to Chest Pain in the Adult Patient with Cancer

The three broad categories of chest pain in the cancer patient are shown in Table 25-1. If pain is of direct cardiac origin, both ischemic and nonischemic etiologies may be responsible and occasionally may coexist. The former may include the entire spectrum of ischemic syndromes from chronic stable angina pectoris to myocardial infarction. Nonischemic car-

Table 25-1. A Clinical Approach to Chest Pain in Cancer Patients

Chest pain of ischemic origin
  Stable angina pectoris
  Prinzmetal's angina
  Unstable angina
  Acute myocardial infarction
  Tumor-related angina pectoris
    Extrinsic compression of coronaries
    Tumor emboli to coronaries
    Chemotherapy-induced ischemia
Nonischemia pain of cardiac or vascular origin
  Myocardial metastases
  Pericardial metastases
  Infectious pericarditis
  Myocarditis
  Aortic stenosis
  Aortic insufficiency
  Aortic dissection
  Hypertrophic cardiomyopathy
  Mitral valve prolapse
  Mitral stenosis
  Dressler's syndrome
  Postpericardiotomy syndrome
  Pulmonary emboli
  Pulmonary hypertension
Chest pain of noncardiac origin
  Large lung tumors
  Pancoast's syndrome
  Mediastinal masses
  Pleural metastases
  Pleurisy
  Tracheobronchitis
  Pneumothorax
  Mediastinitis
  Mediastinal emphysema
  Nerve root compression syndromes
  Thoracic outlet syndrome
  Vertebral and rib fractures
  Postmastectomy syndrome
  Xiphoidalgia
  Costochondritis
  Postherpetic neuralgia
  Mondor's disease
  Gastrointestinal disorders

diac etiologies include primary or metastatic tumor infiltration of cardiac structures. When pain is of noncardiac thoracic origin in a cancer patient, the etiology may be inflammation or tumor involvement of mediastinal and other thoracic structures. The preceding discussion on mechanisms makes it clear that the exact pathophysiologic basis for chest pain in these different etiologic categories is not completely understood. Fortunately, the clinical setting in which chest pain occurs, the character and duration of pain episodes, relation to exertion, rest, respiration or body positioning, and the mode of relief, all aid in the correct diagnosis. Although every effort should be made to relieve pain, it is equally important to establish the diagnosis so that appropriate interventions may be undertaken to address the cause of chest pain.

Chest Pain of Ischemic Origin

There are at least three primary reasons why it is imperative to exclude cardiac ischemia in the adult cancer patient presenting with chest pain. First, the optimal management of angina pectoris is distinctly different from other etiologies of chest pain. The mainstay of therapy includes nitrates, calcium channel antagonists, beta-adrenergic blockers, antiplatelet agents, and therapeutic interventions to reduce cardiac work and abolish myocardial ischemia. When angina pectoris persists in the setting of optimal drug therapy, mechanical revascularization with percutaneous transluminal balloon angioplasty or coronary artery bypass surgery is indicated; therefore, referral for coronary arteriography is necessary. Second, angina pectoris may be a symptom or marker of significant underlying coronary artery disease with a prognosis that may be worse than that of the patient's cancer. Third, in a cancer patient for whom a diagnostic or therapeutic procedure under general anesthesia is anticipated, an undiagnosed and untreated cardiac ischemia may predispose to increased perioperative cardiovascular morbidity and mortality. For these reasons, the first priority in patient workup is to exclude chest pain of ischemic origin.

The clinical history should elicit the coronary risk profile and establish the pretest likelihood of coronary artery disease. A high-risk profile includes men over age 55 years, postmenopausal women, and patients who have chronic hypertension, hyperlipidemia, diabetes mellitus, smoke cigarettes, a strong family history of early coronary events, and left ventricular hypertrophy on either electrocardiography or echocardiography.

The next objective is to establish whether the chest pain is typical or atypical for cardiac ischemia. Ischemic chest pain is most often described not as a pain but as a pressure, tightness, squeezing, or aching chest discomfort. It is poorly localized and imprecisely described with the patient often using a clenched fist pressed against the chest (Levine's sign). The discomfort may radiate to either arm, neck, or jaw, and may be associated with dyspnea and diaphoresis. The pain of stable angina pectoris is often predictable, provoked by physical or emotional stress, short-lived (typically less than 30 minutes), and relieved by rest or relaxation. It rarely persists longer than 30 minutes. Chest pain that persists incessantly for days at a time is unlikely to be ischemic. Myocardial infarction results when true ischemic chest pain persists beyond 30 minutes and often for several hours. By definition, angina pectoris that is of new onset, occurs at rest, or has increased in frequency or severity, is unstable, and requires urgent referral for evaluation and treatment.

Chest pain that has none of the previously mentioned characteristics, lasts only seconds, improves with physical exercise, can be precisely located on the chest wall, or is elicited on manual palpation of the chest is unlikely to be of ischemic etiology and is thus labeled atypical chest pain. The combination of an individual's coronary risk profile and characteristics of the chest pain is often adequate to provide a good assessment of the pretest likelihood of having coronary disease.

The physical examination, biochemistry and hematology tests, chest roentgenography, and resting electrocardiography may all be normal and thus not very helpful in the differential diagnosis. The presence of significant anemia can lead to ischemic chest pain even in the absence of coronary atherosclerosis. The resting echocardiogram is useful for assessing global left ventricular function, regional wall motion abnormalities, and excluding other cardiac causes of chest pain. When the resting echocardiogram is normal, it does not exclude ischemic chest pain. In this setting, several diagnostic tests can be performed to elicit inducible ischemia. A standard treadmill exercise tolerance test is ideal when the baseline electrocardiogram is normal and the patient can walk on a treadmill. When the baseline electrocardiogram is abnormal, an exercise test can be coupled with thallium scintigraphy or radionuclide ventriculography. In patients who cannot exercise, pharmacologic stress (using adenosine, dobutamine, or dipyridamole) can be performed in conjunction with radionuclide ventriculography, thallium scintigraphy, or echocardiography. In a patient with unstable angina pectoris or typical angina at rest, coronary arteriography is preferable without a preceding exercise or pharmacologic stress test.

Angina is said to be stable when there has been no temporal change in the frequency or severity of chest pain episodes and when it does not occur at rest. By definition, new-onset angina or angina at rest is considered unstable. However, recent advances in coronary artery disease research have shown that the characteristics of the underlying stenosis or plaque are different in stable versus unstable angina. Prinzmetal's angina (also known as variable angina) is also ischemic but the large epicardial coronary arteries have no fixed obstruction. The characteristic abnormality in Prinzmetal's angina is coronary vasospasm associated with electrocardiographic ST-segment elevation. Episodes of chest pain may be provoked by exertion, emotional stress, a cold environment, and also spontaneously at rest.

Myocardial infarction has the worst prognosis of the ischemic syndromes discussed. Symptoms associated with the chest discomfort may include marked dyspnea, diaphoresis, nausea, and a sense of impending doom. In some patients, the chest pain may be associated with pain in the jaw, teeth, neck, arms, and epigastrium. Characteristic electrocardiographic changes include ST-segment elevation and peaking of the T wave. Reciprocal ST-segment depression may be present in electrocardiographic leads opposite the site of infarction. The absence of a pleuritic component and the character of the pain help differentiate acute infarction from pericarditis. Electrocardiographic changes may be subtle (or even absent) in some patients; therefore, greater emphasis should be placed on the clinical history. Some patients experience the evolution of electrocardiographic changes rapidly, with Q waves developing within 3–4 hours after symptom onset, whereas this onset may be much delayed in other patients.

Cancer and Chemotherapy-Related Ischemic Pain

When chest pain is proved to be of ischemic origin in a cancer patient, coincidental atherosclerotic coronary artery disease must be entertained as the likely cause because there is no evidence that cancer predisposes to coronary atherosclerosis.[8, 9] When conventional risk factors for coronary atherosclerosis are conspicuously absent, other explanations for coronary ischemia should be investigated. These latter etiologies include tumor emboli to coronary arteries, extrinsic compression of coronaries secondary to tumor infiltration, tumor-related coagulation abnormalities, and treatment-related coronary artery dysfunction.[10–18] The most common etiologies are extrinsic coronary compression and tumor emboli to the coronaries, both of which account for 60% and 35% of tumor-related chest pain or myocardial infarction, respectively.[11, 12] If patients without coronary risk factors develop angina or myocardial infarction for the first time during cancer treatment, the role of the chemotherapeutic agent should be examined. Several cases of ischemic chest pain or myocardial infarction have been reported during monotherapy with 5-fluorouracil, daunomycin, cyclophosphamide, or vincristine,[19-23] combination chemotherapy,[24, 25] or the combination of chemotherapy and radiation treatment.[18, 26] Proposed mechanisms underlying this association include coronary vasospasm, vasculitis, fibrosis, and accelerated atherogenesis.[12]

Nonischemic Chest Pain of Cardiac or Vascular Origin

Primary or metastatic tumor infiltration of the pericardium, myocardium, heart valves, and great vessels may lead to nonischemic cardiac pain in the cancer patient. More commonly, nonischemic chest pain of cardiac origin may be the result of nonneoplastic disease or disorder of these cardiovascular structures. This latter group of disorders comprises pericarditis, myocarditis, aortic stenosis or insufficiency, aortic dissection, mitral valve prolapse, mitral stenosis, pulmonary emboli, and pulmonary hypertension. The recognition and appropriate diagnosis of these two groups (neoplastic and nonneoplastic) of etiologies is important because their therapeutic management and overall prognosis are quite different. This section discusses the epidemiology and clinical characteristics of these causes of nonischemic chest pain of cardiac and vascular origin.

Although primary cardiac tumors are rare, metastatic infiltration of the heart and pericardium is not and may be 20–25 times more prevalent in autopsy series.[27] The majority of these metastases do not cause chest pain; however, some characteristically do. Chest pain and dyspnea are the leading symptoms when leukemic cells infiltrate the myocardium.[28] Less commonly, chest pain and associated friction rub may be the only manifestation of pericardial involvement. Myocardial infiltration with angiosarcoma also commonly causes chest pain.[29] Early clinical recognition of these complications in the cancer patient is important because the hemodynamic compromise from myocardial and pericardial involvement has an acute prognosis that may be worse than the primary disease.

The physical examination including cardiac auscultation may be normal. The presence of a pericardial friction rub may be a useful clue to the presence of pericardial involvement with tumor. Autopsy studies have showed that 10–25% of patients with established cancer have pericardial involvement with metastases or abnormalities related to cancer treatment.[30] The electrocardiogram may show PR-segment depression or ST-segment elevation in multiple leads when pericardial involvement leads to significant pericarditis.[31] However, sinus tachycardia may be the only finding in this setting. The echocardiogram is particularly useful in the diagnosis of pericardial involvement.[32] Computed tomography (CT) and magnetic resonance imaging (MRI) are helpful in establishing primary or metastatic pericardial disease. In cancer patients who have undergone extensive radiation treatment, it may not be possible to differentiate the effects of radiation from neoplastic pericardial involvement. In this case, pericardiocentesis with biopsy may be necessary.[33] When extensive tumor infiltration of the myocardium is present, electrocardiographic changes are noted and may be profound.[34] The echocardiogram, CT, and MRI are all useful diagnostic tools.

Nonischemic chest pain of cardiac or vascular origin is commonly not directly related to the underlying cancer. Pericarditis, for example, may be of viral, tuberculous, bacterial, or fungal etiology.[35] It may, however, be secondary to cancer treatment such as radiation or chemotherapy.[36–38] As previously noted, the visceral pericardium has no nociceptors and thus is unlikely to be the origin of pain in pericarditis. The diaphragmatic parietal pericardium sends afferent fibers to the CNS through the phrenic nerve; thus, referred pain to the left shoulder may be seen. Typically, the reported pain is sharp, stabbing, and aggravated by deep inspiration or by lying down. Some relief is obtained by shallow breaths, sitting upright, or leaning forward. The physical examination may be normal except for shallow, tachypneic breaths or the presence of a pericardial friction rub. Routine laboratory tests may show nonspecific markers of inflammation such as leukocytosis or elevated erythrocyte sedimentation rate. Bacterial and viral cultures as well as serial serologies are often not useful in the clinical management of individual patients. The electrocardiogram may show PR- and ST-segment abnormalities. The echocardiogram is typically normal unless associated pericardial effusion or marked pericardial thickening is present.

Acute myocarditis, which is commonly of infectious etiology,[39] may be the cause of chest pain or chest discomfort in the patient with cancer. Chest pain is often the most common symptom in acute myocarditis[40] and may be indistinguishable from the pain of pericarditis in up to 40% of patients. Less frequently, the reported chest pain may be similar in quality to that of typical angina. A history of antecedent viral illness is an important clue that may be elicited in most patients. A clinical review of systems will often show the presence of fever, fatigue, myalgias, and dyspnea. In up to one-third of patients, the physical examination will reveal a pericardial rub reflecting myopericarditis. Laboratory abnormalities may include elevated erythrocyte sedimentation rate, leukocytosis, serum creatinine kinase MB isoenzyme elevation, and electrocardiographic changes consisting of new Q waves and ST-segment shifts.[41] Echocardiography may show a dilated heart with depressed function and pericardial effusion when myopericarditis is present. The presence of a nondilated heart does not exclude this diagnosis. Serious complications may include pericardial tamponade or cardiogenic shock requiring intra-aortic balloon counterpulsation.[41] In most patients, however, the prognosis is not so grim. Less than one-third of patients develop cardiomegaly and even fewer develop overt heart failure.[40] Maisch et al.[42] showed that after a mean follow-up of 4.5 years in 85 patients with myocarditis or perimyocarditis that 55% of patients

improved, 35% were completely symptom free, and only 15% died. Recurrent and chronic forms were more likely in patients with associated pericarditis and effusions. Persistently elevated titers of antimyolemmal and antisarcolemmal antibodies were associated with unfavorable prognosis.[42]

Disorders of the aortic valve as well as the aortic root, arch, and ascending and descending segments of the thoracic aorta may all cause chest pain. Both aortic valve stenosis and insufficiency may present with chest pain. When chest pain is seen in the setting of aortic stenosis, the prognosis is poor, often with average survival less than 3 years.[43] Although most patients with aortic stenosis are pain free at rest, chest pain develops during exertion in more than two-thirds. The characteristics of the reported pain are often indistinguishable from typical angina. Chest pain may also be a symptom of aortic insufficiency; dyspnea is more common, however. Dissection involving any segment of the thoracic aorta may present as severe excruciating chest pain with very abrupt onset. Characteristically, the pain is described as severe, "tearing," "ripping," or "stabbing" and is associated with a sense of impending doom. The pain is commonly located in the anterior chest or in the back between the shoulder blades. The physical examination in these disorders may show characteristic murmurs of aortic valve disease. Concomitant decrease in volume and delayed upstroke of the carotid pulse and a decreased pulse pressure may be present in aortic stenosis while bounding pulses and widened pulse pressure are found in aortic insufficiency. When aortic dissection causes disruption of normal aortic cusp coaptation, aortic insufficiency results with a typical diastolic murmur heard in up to 25% of patients. Hypertension or hypotension, pulse deficits, and evidence of hypoperfusion may all be present. The chest roentgenogram may show a widened mediastinum or displaced aortic intima. Electrocardiographic changes may simulate acute myocardial ischemia or infarction if the dissection involves the coronary arteries. Echocardiography, especially using the transesophageal approach, is both sensitive and specific for evaluation of aortic dissection. MRI, CT, and aortography all have a high diagnostic yield.

Mitral valve prolapse syndrome and, less commonly, mitral stenosis may also present with chest pain. Although rarely indistinguishable from true angina pectoris, the chest pain in mitral valve prolapse is commonly atypical.[44, 45] When chest pain is seen in the setting of mitral stenosis, it is often indistinguishable from angina pectoris.[46] The physical examination will reveal the characteristic diastolic murmurs of mitral stenosis but may be normal in the patients with mitral valve prolapse except for the presence of midsystolic clicks and late systolic murmurs with typical responses to maneuvers. The electrocardiogram and chest roentgenograms may all be normal. Echocardiography, however, may demonstrate billowing of the mitral leaflets across the plane of the mitral annulus or late systolic displacement of the posterior leaflet.[45]

Finally, pulmonary emboli and pulmonary hypertension are important cardiovascular causes of chest pain in the patient with cancer. Cancer patients may be at increased risk for recurrent pulmonary emboli and pulmonary hypertension if the underlying cancer is associated with hypercoagulability and venous thromboembolism. The clinical history and physical findings depend on the size of the embolus.[47] Davies has stated that a large embolus that impacts the major arteries causes a sudden onset, deep, crushing visceral pain whereas small peripherally located emboli cause localized, pleuritic chest pain that is frequently associated with hemoptysis.[47] The clinical history of predisposing risk factors is particularly useful. The physical examination may reveal the presence of tachycardia, tachypnea, and pleural friction rub. Calf tenderness and evidence of deep vein thrombosis or thrombophlebitis are commonly absent. The alveolar arterial oxygen gradient may be normal or increased but the arterial oxygen tension is often lower than 80 mm Hg when the patient breathes room air. In up to 15% of patients, the arterial oxygen tension may be normal. The electrocardiogram commonly shows sinus tachycardia. An acute QRS axis shift to the right or otherwise unexplained right ventricular strain pattern may indicate pulmonary embolus. The echocardiogram may show acutely dilated right ventricle with impaired systolic function if a large pulmonary embolus is present. Large ventilation-perfusion mismatches in the setting of a clinical history consistent with pulmonary embolus give a high likelihood for the diagnosis. Pulmonary arteriography is the reference diagnostic standard, however.

Recurrent pulmonary emboli may lead to pulmonary hypertension, which can cause chest pain often indistinguishable from angina pectoris or the pain in primary pulmonary hypertension. Unlike typical angina pectoris, however, the pain in pulmonary hypertension does not radiate to the arms or jaws and is more responsive to oxygen administration than to nitroglycerin. The physical examination may reveal cyanosis and tachypnea as well as a parasternal heave on precordial palpation. The pulmonary component of the second heard sound is often increased. The electrocardiogram shows right axis deviation, right ventricular strain, and evidence of right ventricular hypertrophy. The chest roentgenogram may show a large main pulmonary artery and its central branches with relatively small peripheral branches.

Chest Pain of Noncardiac Origin

Primary or metastatic tumor involvement of the extracardiac, intrathoracic tissues may lead to a variety of noncardiac chest pain syndromes. This condition is important to exclude in the patient with established cancer. A variety of infectious, toxic, and nonneoplastic conditions also commonly lead to noncardiac chest pain. A brief synopsis of these conditions is given in this section.

The lung parenchyma and visceral pleura contain no pain receptors; however, the trachea, bronchi, lobar and segmental bronchi, parietal pleura, and the main pulmonary artery and its large branches have nociceptors. Primary tumors of the lung that are limited to the lung parenchyma therefore do not cause chest pain. Larger tumors may cause chest pain by mass effect on surrounding structures, mediastinal invasion, or because they cause stretching of the parietal pleura. It is not uncommon that pain arising from the lung itself may be referred to the larger airways or to the pulmonary artery. Marino et al.[48] studied 164 patients with nonmetastatic lung cancer and found that 40% had chest pain. The pain was typically deep, and referred to the chest anteriorly or posteriorly with good correlation between location of the pain and documented site of the tumor.[48]

Superior sulcus tumors are unique because of the characteristic pain syndrome they evoke (Pancoast's syndrome). These lesions are typically squamous cell tumors with early invasion of surrounding structures including bone, chest wall, pleura, tracheal plexus, and the cervical sympathetic chain. The degree of pain produced is often disproportional to the size of the mass. The pain may be localized to the shoulder, anterior chest, and scapular area and may radiate down the left arm. Medial extension and invasion of the sympathetic plexus at C-8 to T-1 may result in associated ipsilateral Horner's syndrome (ptosis, enophthalmos, and miosis). The clinical history and physical examination are designed to elicit the characteristic deficits mentioned previously. The electrocardiogram is often not revealing. The chest roentgenogram, CT, and MRI are useful for demonstrating the presence of the mass. Nonradiographic diagnostic tools include fiberoptic bronchoscopy, mediastinoscopy, and sputum cytology.

Inflammatory processes involving the parietal pleura may lead to pleuritic chest pain. Typically, the pain starts abruptly, is unilateral, and can be severe. The pain is characteristically sharp, knife-like, and aggravated by respirations and coughing. There may be small associated pleural effusion. Viral and bacterial infections are important in the differential diagnosis. Neoplastic involvement should be excluded in patients with known cancer. Metastatic adenocarcinoma and mesothelioma commonly have associated bloody pleural effusion. Acute onset, unilateral pleuritic pain associated with dyspnea often suggests pneumothorax or pulmonary embolus. When these symptoms develop over weeks in the setting of constitutional symptoms, they are more likely to be due to tuberculous, malignancy, or connective tissue disorders. The physical examination may be normal or reveal a localized pleural rub. The electrocardiogram commonly shows sinus tachycardia. The chest roentgenogram may show pleural effusion or the culprit lesion if it is a malignancy or pneumothorax.

Tumor, infection, inflammation, or air in the mediastinum may be the cause of noncardiac chest pain. In the case of mediastinal air or emphysema, the pain is often sudden and located in the anterior chest usually behind the sternum. It may radiate to the neck or shoulders reflecting the direction of further emphysema. The pain can be severe and is aggravated by deep breathing or by lying down. The characteristic, loud "crunching" sound (Hamman's sign) is heard on auscultation. Tumors and cysts in the mediastinum may also be the cause of dull, aching, poorly described chest pain. Lymphomas typically occur in any of the three (anterior, middle, and posterior) mediastinal compartments. Other masses are more frequently seen in only one compartment. Symptoms associated with the chest pain depend on which mediastinal structures are compressed. Neurogenic tumors of the posterior mediastinum may also cause nerve root compression and related chest and back pain. Roentgenography, CT, and MRI are used to exclude the presence of these lesions.

Disorders of the cervical or thoracic spine may be the source of referred chest pain. Posterolateral herniation of a cervical disc with nerve root compression leads to pain referred to the chest and arms depending on the level of the herniation. The pain is typically "sharp," "piercing," or "shooting" and is aggravated by neck and upper body movement, coughing, straining, or sneezing. Occasionally, the pain may be dull, aching, and described as a "tightness" or "pressure" resembling angina pectoris. Unlike typical angina pectoris, the pain in cervical and thoracic spine herniation can be reproduced by deep palpation of the posterior trigger points. Signs and symptoms of cord compression are usually not seen unless there is posterior herniation. Physical examination and roentgenography will demonstrate the presence of disc abnormalities. Alternatively, tumor compression of cervical and thoracic nerve roots may produce similar symptoms. A related cause of chest pain is thoracic outlet obstruction in which compression of the brachial plexus or brachial artery results in anterior chest pain with radiation to the arms. Specific maneuvers such as Adson's or hyperabduction tests are useful in differentiating this disorder from the other etiologies of chest pain.[49]

Chest pain that presents in contiguous dermatomal pattern most likely represents infection or reactivation of the varicella zoster virus. Patients with hematopoietic or lymphoreticular malignancies and patients with solid tumors who receive aggressive chemotherapy and radiation treatment are at increased risk.[50–52] Vesicles are initially not present and may lag by several days to weeks. The pain is typically unilateral in the T-2 to L-2 distribution and is described as sharp and burning and may be severe. Bilateral dermatomal presentation is uncommon except in severely immunocompromised patients. Laboratory tests are usually not helpful. Postherpetic neuralgia is thought to be present when the pain persists for several months or years after the acute herpetic lesions have subsided.

Various disorders of the ribs, vertebrae, costochondral and costosternal articulations, chest muscles, and the skin overlying the chest wall may lead to chest pain. Both traumatic and pathologic fractures of the ribs and vertebrae can cause severe, sharp, lancinating chest pain. The pain is often worsened by coughing, deep breathing, and movement. Point tenderness over the culprit lesion differentiates this pain from cardiac or pleuritic pain. Roentgenograms may show the fractured rib or vertebra. Inflammation of the upper costochondral junctions and tender swelling of the costosternal joints also cause chest pain that is aggravated by deep breathing or exertion.[53] Local tenderness is characteristically present and differentiates this pain from cardiac pain. A related swelling and tenderness involving the xiphoid process may cause anterior chest pain xiphoidalgia. The pain in xiphoidalgia is intermittent and often radiates to the precordium as well as the epigastrium.[3] Bonica has suggested that pathology in the xiphoid process produces widespread pain because of its innervation from the phrenic nerves and the T-4 to T-7 intercostal nerves.[3] Superficial thrombophlebitis of the anterior lateral chest wall (Mondor's disease) is uncommon but may be seen in the setting of chest wall trauma or breast surgery. Physical examination reveals a palpable, painful cord. Mild eosinophilia is noted but otherwise the laboratory tests are not helpful.[3]

Although discussed last, gastrointestinal disorders are not the least important cause of noncardiac chest pain. The esophagus, for example, can be the source of significant chest discomfort that may be difficult to distinguish from myocardial ischemia pain. Visceral afferent fibers from pain sensitive receptors in the upper and middle segments of the esophagus travel in the inferior cervical sympathetic nerves and the vagus nerve. Esophageal spasm, distension, or excessive contractions lead to activation of these receptors and the sensation of midsternal or retrosternal squeezing, tightness, or pressure. Stimulation of nociceptors in the lower one-third of the esophagus typically causes a burning sensation. In addition to differences in the quality of pain that is sensed, patients can often reliably locate the site of the discomfort to which part of the esophagus that may have the lesion. Occasionally, the associated characteristics of the pain help identify it as being of esophageal etiology. For example, when the chest pain is reproduced always during swallowing, during or after meals, and with recumbency, an esophageal etiology is highly suspect. The physical examination is usually normal. The electrocardiogram and chest roentgenogram do not help in the diagnosis. A barium swallow radiography often will show the culprit lesion. Focal or diffuse esophageal inflammation can cause retrosternal chest pain but may not be evident on barium radiography. Fiberoptic endoscopy is particularly useful in establishing the diagnosis. Repeated episodes of acute esophageal inflammations lead to chronic esophagitis. The chest discomfort in esophageal reflux disease is commonly described as a heartburn. The underlying mechanism may be direct activation of pain receptors by the change in pH or by associated esophageal spasm. Relief of symptoms (presumably cessation of spasm) after administration of nitrates can lead to the erroneous diagnosis of typical angina pectoris. It is not surprising that the prevalence of esophageal reflux or spasm was 50% in one study of patients who carried a diagnosis of angina pectoris but had normal coronary arteriogram.[54]

Peptic ulcer disease may present as an epigastric burning, frank pain, or dull ache in the lower chest. Unlike angina pectoris, however, it characteristically does not respond to oxygen administration or nitrates and it often improves postprandially. Biliary tract disorders may also present with epigastric or lower chest pain. Physical examination may show tenderness in the right upper quadrant and may be associated with laboratory abnormalities of biliary function.

Therapeutic Strategies

This section emphasizes three aspects of the therapeutic strategy: (1) reassurance of the patient; (2) expedient control of pain even when the exact cause is unknown; and (3) a diligent search for the specific etiology in order to provide targeted treatment. A detailed discussion of the treatment of specific etiologies of chest pain can be found in several excellent reference sources.[55, 56]

Reassurance of the patient with chest pain is an essential component of the therapeutic strategy. As previously noted, chest pain is often associated with significant anxiety and fear of impending death or disability. This heightened state of adrenergic activity can lead to significant increases in heart rate, blood pressure, and overall cardiac work and even myocardial ischemia; profound enough changes to confound correct diagnosis of the chest pain. Reassurance helps relieve anxiety in the patient and remove the superimposed excessive sympathetic drive. Once the patient is reassured, every effort should be made to control pain even when the exact etiology is unknown. Often, the response to different therapeutic interventions may help in the diagnostic workup. For example, chest pain that is relieved after one or two sublingual nitroglycerin tablets is likely to be from ischemia or esophageal spasm rather than pericarditis.

When chest pain is suspected to be of ischemic origin, the patient should be evaluated to determine whether symptoms are stable or unstable. Patients with unstable symptoms (new onset or recent change in the frequency or severity of chest pain) should be referred for immediate in-hospital observation. The mainstays of treatment for these patients include supplemental oxygen, nitroglycerin, intravenous heparin, aspirin, beta-adrenergic antagonists, and thrombolytic therapy (when acute thrombosis is suspected). A consultation with a cardiologist is highly recommended. In patients with stable symptoms, oral or topical nitroglycerin may be initiated while awaiting elective cardiovascular evaluation. In both groups of patients, it is important that blood pressure be controlled (if there is a history of hypertension) and predisposing factors (physical exercise, emotional stress, alcohol use) be discussed and minimized.

When nonischemic chest pain is of valvular origin, treatment often depends on the valve involved. Chest pain associated with mitral valve prolapse may respond to beta-blocker therapy whereas chest pain related to aortic stenosis or mitral stenosis requires mechanical intervention (valvuloplasty or valve replacement). In the cancer patient, the risk of the anticipated valve surgery must be weighed against the expected prognosis of the underlying cancer. When surgical risk is considered prohibitive, palliative percutaneous valvuloplasty (especially in aortic stenosis) may be considered. Chest pain in the setting of aortic dissection is a medical emergency and should be treated with systemic analgesics. However, it should be treated first with a beta-adrenergic blocker to reduce blood pressure level and the rate of pressure increase within the aorta. Additional antihypertensives such as nitroprusside, alphamethyldopa, or reserpine may then be added. Immediate surgical evaluation should be obtained. Pericarditis and myocarditis may respond to nonsteroidal anti-inflammatory agents or systemic steroid administration. Definitive treatment of purulent pericarditis is debridement and systemic antibiotics. Systemic anticoagulation with intravenous heparin is the treatment of choice when pulmonary emboli are suspected.

Noncardiac chest pain in the cancer patient with established large lung tumor, mediastinal mass, or metastatic disease to the pleura, ribs, and vertebrae often presents significant challenges for pain control. The combination of several therapeutic modalities such as surgical resection, radiation therapy, chemotherapy, and hormone treatment provides optimal management. Additional pain treatment modalities including pharmacologic, psychological, chemical, neurostimulation, and neurosurgical procedures have been discussed elsewhere in this text. A similar multimodality strategy is also adopted when pain results from tumor infiltration or metastases causing plexopathy and nerve root compression syndromes. Pancoast's syndrome can be effectively treated with narcotic and nonsteroidal anti-inflammatory agents. Often, the combination of these agents with or without tricyclic antidepressants can be very effective.[57] Percutaneous cordotomy has also been effective in severe pain of Pancoast's syndrome.[58]

Postmastectomy pain syndrome can be effectively treated with nonopioid analgesics with or without tricyclic antidepressants. The use of local anesthetics in intercostal nerve or segmental epidural block can also be effective when pharmacologic therapy alone fails. Physical therapy and transcutaneous nerve stimulation techniques provide additional pain control modalities.[58] Postherpetic neuralgia responds to carbamazepine combined with tricyclic agents. Finally, a variety of "gastrointestinal cocktails" containing antacids, anticholinergic drugs, and viscous lidocaine may provide acute relief when epigastric discomfort masquerades as chest pain. Definitive treatment with antacids, histamine blockers or cholinergic medication should be based on specific diagnosis of the gastrointestinal disorder.

References

1. National Center for Health Statistics. Health, United States, 1993. Hyattsville, MD: Public Health Service, 1994.

2. Anonymous. Mortality patterns: United States, 1991. MMWR 1993;42:891, 897.

3. Bonica JJ. General Considerations of Pain in the Chest. In JJ Bonica (ed), The Management of Pain. Malvern, PA: Lea & Febiger, 1990;959.

4. Edmeads J, Billings RF. Neurological and Psychological Aspects of Chest Pain. In DL Levene (ed), Chest Pain. Philadelphia: Lea & Febiger, 1977.

5. Cross SA. Pathophysiology of pain. Mayo Clin Proc 1994;69:375.

6. Kambam JR, Merrill W, Parris W, et al. Substance P, acetylcholinesterase, and beta-endorphin levels in the plasma and pericardial fluid of patients with and without angina pectoris. J Lab Clin Med 1990;116:707.

7. Meller ST, Gebhart GF. A critical review of the afferent pathways and the potential chemical mediators involved in cardiac pain. Neuroscience 1992;48:501.

8. Juhl S. Cancer and atherosclerosis. II. Applicability of postmortem statistics in the study of the negative correlation. Acta Pathol Microbiol Scand 1957;41:99.

9. Parrish HM, Goldner JC, Silberg SL. Coronary atherosclerosis and cancer in women. Arch Intern Med 1966;117:639.

10. Frumin H, O'Donnell L, Derin NZ, et al. Two-dimensional echocardiographic detection and diagnostic features of tricuspid papillary fibroelastoma. J Am Coll Cardiol 1983;2:1016.

11. Ackerman DM, Hyma BA, Edwards WD. Malignant neoplastic emboli to the coronary arteries. Report of two cases and review of the literature. Hum Pathol 1987;18:955.

12. Kopelson G, Herwig KJ. The etiologies of coronary artery disease in cancer patients. Int J Radiat Oncol Biol Phys 1978;4:895.

13. Favre-Gilley J, Michel D, Tommasi M. Venous, arterial, and endocardiac multiple thrombosis with consumption coagulopathy and cryofibrinogen due to ovarian carcinoma: Temporary improvement with heparin. Thromb Hemostat 1975;34:566.

14. Sack GH, Levin J, Bell WR. Trousseau's syndrome and other manifestations of chronic disseminated coagulopathy in patients with neoplasms: Clinical, pathophysiologic and therapeutic features. Medicine 1977;56:1.

15. Studdy P, Willoughby JMT. Non-bacterial thrombotic endocarditis in early cancer. Br Med J 1976;1:752.

16. Fayemi AO, Deppisch LM. Coronary embolism and myocardial infarction associated with nonbacterial thrombotic endocarditis. Am J Clin Pathol 1977;68:393.

17. Stevenson DL, Mikhailidis DP, Gillett OS. Cardiotoxicity of 5-fluorouracil. Lancet 1977;2:406.

18. Schechter JP, Jones SE, Jackson RA. Myocardial infarction in a 27-year-old-woman: Possible complication of treatment with VP-16-213 (NSC-141540), mediastinal irradiation, or both. Cancer Treat Rep 1975;59:887.

19. Baker WP, Dainer P, Lester WM. Ischemic chest pain after 5-fluorouracil therapy for cancer. Am J Cardiol 1986;57:497.

20. Von Hoff DD, Rozencweig M, Layard M, et al. Daunomycin-induced cardiotoxicity in children and adults. Acta Med Scand 1977;62:200.

21. Mandel EM, Lewinski U, Djaldetti M. Vincristine-induced myocardial infarction. Cancer 1975;30:1979.

22. Buckner CD, Rudolph RH, Fefer A. High-dose cyclophosphamide therapy for malignant disease. Cancer 1972;29:357.

23. Somers G, Abramow M, Wittek M, Naets JP. Myocardial infarction: A complication of vincristine treatment? Lancet 1976;2:690.

24. Lee KH, Lee JS, Kim SH. Electrocardiographic changes simulating acute myocardial infarction or ischemia associated with combination chemotherapy with etoposide, cisplatin, and 5-fluorouracil. Korean J Intern Med 1990;5:112.

25. Anonymous. Case records of the Massachusetts General Hospital (case 50-1970). N Engl J Med 1970;283:587.

26. Weinstein P, Greenwald ES, Grossman J. Unusual cardiac reaction to chemotherapy following mediastinal irradiation in a patient with Hodgkin's disease. Am J Med 1976;60:152.

27. Davies MJ. Tumors of the Heart and Pericardium. In A Pomerance, MJ Davies (eds), The Pathology of the Heart. London: Blackwell, 1975;413.

28. Roberts WC, Bodey GP, Wertlake PT. The heart in acute leukemia. A study of 420 autopsy cases. Am J Cardiol 1968;21:388.

29. Glancy DL, Morales JB, Roberts WC. Angiosarcoma of the heart. Am J Cardiol 1968;21:413.

30. Kralstein J, Frishman W. Malignant pericardial disease: Diagnosis and treatment. Am Heart J 1987;113:785.

31. Spodick DH. Diagnostic electrocardiographic sequences in acute pericarditis. Significance of PR segment and PR vector changes. Circulation 1973;48:575.

32. Kutalek SP, Panidis IP, Kotler M. Metastatic tumors of the heart detected by two-dimensional echocardiography. Am Heart J 1985;109:343.

33. Posner MR, Cohen GI, Skarin AT. Pericardial disease in patients with cancer. The differentiation of malignant from idiopathic and radiation-induced pericarditis. Am J Med 1981;71:407.

34. Hartman RB, Clark PI, Schulman P. Pronounced and prolonged ST segment elevation. A pathognomonic sign of tumor invasion of the heart. Arch Intern Med 1982;142:1917.

35. Fowler NO, Manitsas GT. Infectious pericarditis. Prog Cardiovasc Dis 1973;16:323.

36. Martin RG, Ruckdeschel JC, Chang P, et al. Radiation related pericarditis. Am J Cardiol 1975;35:216.

37. Hancock EW. Subacute effusive-constrictive pericarditis. Circulation 1971;43:183.

38. Harrison DT, Sanders LA. Pericarditis in a case of early daunorubicin cardiomyopathy. Ann Intern Med 1976;85:339.

39. Olinde KD, O'Connell JB. Inflammatory heart disease: Pathogenesis, clinical manifestations, and treatment of myocarditis. Annu Rev Med 1994;45:481.

40. Heikkila J, Karjalainen J. Evaluation of mild acute infectious myocarditis. Br Med J 1982;47:381.

41. Dec GW Jr, Waldman H, Southern J, et al. Viral myocarditis mimicking acute myocardial infarction. J Am Coll Cardiol 1992;20:85.

42. Maisch B, Outzen H, Roth D, et al. Prognostic determinants in conventionally treated myocarditis and perimyocarditis: Focus on antimyolemmal antibodies. Eur Heart J 1991;12(Suppl. D):81.

43. Ross JJ, Braunwald E. Aortic stenosis. Circulation 1968;38:61.

44. Alpert MA, Mukerji V, Sabeti M, et al. Mitral valve prolapse, panic disorder, and chest pain. Med Clin North Am 1991;75:1119.

45. Devereux RB, Kramer-Fox R, Kligfield P. Mitral valve prolapse: Causes, clinical manifestations, and management. Ann Intern Med 1989;111:305.

46. Wood P. An appreciation of mitral stenosis. Br Med J 1954;1:1051, 1113.

47. Levene DL, Davies GM, Saibil FG. Chest Pain Arising from Intrathoracic Structures. In DL Levene (ed), Chest Pain: An Integrated Diagnostic Approach. Philadelphia: Lea & Febiger, 1977;23.

48. Marino C, Zoppi M, Morelli F, et al. Pain in early cancer of the lungs. Pain 1986;27:57.

49. McGough EC, Pearce MB, Byrne JP. Management of thoracic outlet syndrome. J Thorac Cardiovasc Surg 1979;77:169.

50. Weller TH. Varicella and herpes zoster: Changing concepts of the natural history, control, and importance of a not-so-benign virus (second of two parts). N Engl J Med 1983;309:1434.

51. Feld R, Evans WK, DeBoer G. Herpes zoster in patients with small-cell carcinoma of the lung receiving combined modality treatment. Ann Intern Med 1980;93:282.

52. Huberman M, Fossieck BE Jr, Bunn PA Jr, et al. Herpes zoster and small cell bronchogenic carcinoma. Am J Med 1980;63:214.

53. Wolf E, Stern S. Costosternal syndromes: Its frequency and importance in differential diagnosis of coronary heart disease. Arch Intern Med 1976;136:189.

54. DeMeester TR, O'Sullivan GC, Bermudez A. Esophageal function in patients with angina-type chest pain and normal coronary angiograms. Ann Surg 1982;196:488.

55. Schlant RC, Alexander RW (eds). The Heart: Arteries and Veins. New York: McGraw-Hill, 1994.

56. Braunwald E (ed). Heart Disease: A Textbook of Cardiovascular Medicine. Philadelphia: Saunders, 1992.

57. Bonica JJ. Chest Pain Related to Cancer. In JJ Bonica (ed), The Management of Pain. Malvern, PA: Lea & Febiger, 1990;1083.

58. De Conno F, Spanzerla E, Ventafridda V. Analgesic Drugs. In JJ Bonica, V Ventafridda, CA Pagni (eds), Advances in Pain Research and Therapy (Vol. 4). New York: Raven, 1982;125.

Chapter 26

Management of Cancer Pain in Children

Gail E. Rasmussen and Joseph D. Tobias

Introduction

Recent increases in the survival of children with cancer attests to successful advances in chemotherapeutic regimens and supportive care. With such successes and prolongation of survival (whether in remission or not) issues of pain control have become increasingly important. Although increases in the intensity of chemotherapeutic regimens are directly responsible for the increased survival, these regimens are often highly toxic and contribute significantly to the etiology of pain and the production of adverse effects such as mucositis, drug-induced neuropathy, and radiation dermatitis.

Although much of the knowledge of the treatment of adult cancer pain may be applied to children, significant differences do exist. Most important, the spectrum of malignancies and, therefore, the disease-related pain states are different in children. While the primary malignancies in adults are solid tumors (colon, breast, and lung cancer), those in children are primarily hematologic such as acute lymphocytic leukemia, and the solid tumors are generally either primary lesions of the central nervous system (CNS) or sarcomas. A second confounding factor is the difficulty in assessing pediatric pain, regardless of the etiology. Although most adult studies rely on self-report scales for evaluating pain, these measures are often not applicable in preverbal children. Therefore, the treatment of pediatric cancer pain requires not only an understanding of normal childhood development, but also experience with methods and tools of pain assessment in

children. Finally, dosing guidelines and adverse effects related to opioids and other pharmacologic agents used to treat childhood pain may be different than those used in adults.

With such caveats in mind, a more comprehensive approach to the treatment of cancer pain in children is possible. When dealing with the pediatric cancer patient, it may be easiest to treat the pain based on its etiology. Based on this method, cancer-related pain may be divided into the following categories: (1) acute disease or treatment-related pain (seen at the initial presentation and relapse or due to the toxic effects of chemotherapeutic agents), (2) procedure-related pain, (3) postoperative pain, and (4) chronic pain usually seen in the terminal stages of the disease. This chapter discusses the management strategies and pharmacologic agents used in the treatment of pain as related to these four broad categories.

Acute Disease and Treatment-Related Pain

Acute disease and treatment-related pain are particularly important in pediatric cancer pain management. There appears to be a predominance of treatment-related pain in pediatric patients, as opposed to cancer-related pain in adults. One study classifies pediatric cancer pain as therapy related (52%), cancer related (24%), and pain unrelated to malignancy (24%).[1] The pediatric cancer patient associates pain more with the multiple procedures and chemotherapy regimens than with the malignancy itself. This may reflect the higher predominance of hematologic malignancies in pediatrics as opposed to solid tumors in adults.

Pain assessment in children is difficult and more complex than the use of self-reporting in adults. Children are less adept at explaining the nature and quality of their pain. In addition, the more debilitated they become the less they report pain to avoid interventions (e.g. needle sticks) that may be painful in and of themselves. Visual analog scales (VAS) may be used in older children to delineate pain effectively. In the preverbal child, assessment may be even more difficult and one must look for behavioral or physiologic changes that may indicate pain. These behavioral changes include decreased activity or interest in environment, persistent crying, abnormal gait, and physiologic changes that may include changes in heart rate, respiratory rate, sweating, and flushing.

Other important factors in pediatric pain assessment are the role and perceptions of the parents or caregiver. They may be able to detect subtle changes in a child's behavior because of their familiarity with the child. Their input may be vital to the ability of health care providers to establish reasonable expectations and develop a successful treatment regimen. There are those parents, however, who can be quite difficult and demanding, even to the point of obstructing care for their child. They may be manifesting their own frustrations in dealing with a child with cancer, particularly one who is suffering from pain.

It is important to try and delineate the etiology of the pain in order to treat it appropriately. For instance, a tumor can cause severe pain from direct compression on a nerve or nerve root. Treatment of this cancer with chemotherapy or radiation therapy can further contribute to an overall pain state by causing nausea, vomiting, or mucositis. The multiple etiologies of cancer pain in children are summarized in Table 26-1.

Pain that is related to the treatment of the tumor varies not only in the type of tumor but in the therapeutic modalities used to treat it. The predominant forms of treatment for children are chemotherapy and radiation therapy, each of which has its own associated causes for pain.

The most frequent source of pain from chemotherapy appears to be mucositis. It is most commonly associated with the anthracycline chemotherapy

Table 26-1. Etiologies of Pediatric Cancer Pain

Contributions from malignancy itself
  Bony metastasis
  Nerve or nerve root compression
  Tumor invasion of muscle or soft tissue
  Hollow viscus obstruction
  Elevated intracranial pressure causing headaches
Contributions from treatment of cancer (both chemotherapy
    and radiation therapy)
  Mucous membrane ulceration (mucositis, stomatitis)
  Radiation dermatitis or burns
  Nausea and vomiting
  Herpes zoster
  Secondary infections (e.g., diarrhea, pneumonia)
Contributions from opioid analgesics used in treatment
  Nausea and vomiting
  Severe constipation
  Urinary retention
Contributions from other forms of treatment
  Postdural puncture headache
  Bony pain after bone marrow aspirates
  Peripheral neuropathies, such as drug-induced pain,
    phantom limb pain
  Frequent venipunctures for blood drawing or insertion
    of intravenous cannulae
  Postoperative pain

agents (daunorubicin and doxorubicin) and may be seen less frequently with bleomycin and dactinomycin.[2] The mucositis is usually in the oropharyngeal area but may spread to the esophagus. Aside from the pain associated with oral mucositis, the patient may have difficulty eating and swallowing medications, thus requiring alternative medication delivery routes and enteral nutrition. Another commonly used chemotherapeutic agent in pediatric patients is vincristine, which is associated with a peripheral neuropathy in the hands and feet that may be refractory to high doses of narcotics.

Furthermore, radiation therapy may lead to mucositis but also can cause dermatitis and radiation burns that may become secondarily infected in a compromised, neutropenic patient. When radiation is used to treat a soft tissue tumor that is highly invasive in surrounding tissues, a painful neuropathy may develop most likely from direct radiation effects of an involved nerve. It may also exacerbate the peripheral neuropathy induced from the tumor or from chemotherapy.[2] The peripheral neuropathies are associated with a burning, dysesthetic type of pain that is often unresponsive to treatment with narcotic analgesics and may require adjuvant agents such as antidepressants or anticonvulsants.

When less potent agents are efficacious, it is not appropriate to initiate treatment of cancer pain with the most powerful medications available. The World Health Organization (WHO) has devised an analgesic ladder for cancer pain management.[3] This stepwise approach advocates starting with non-steroidal anti-inflammatory drugs (NSAIDs) and proceeding to the most potent opioid analgesics and adjuvant medications (including antidepressants, anticonvulsants, and antispasmodics). It is important to initiate this stepwise approach because the disease may progress and the pain may escalate from its initial presentation. It is also important to differentiate anxiety about treatment or procedures from the actual pain that they produce or that is produced by the tumor. Pain management in pediatric cancer patients usually requires continual adjustments in type of medication, route of delivery, time intervals, and addition of adjuvants to achieve a reasonable level of pain control. Often, a regimen that works well may, over time, begin to become less effective and may need stronger agents. In many patients, certain medications are used to the extent that they are being given in such large doses that their side effects become prohibitive and overshadow their analgesic properties. In these cases, an alternative medication may be needed or another medication added so that the side effects are minimized.

Parents play a key role in fine-tuning their child's analgesic regimen and they must be counseled as to reasonable expectations for pain control. It is not always possible to render a child "pain free," and parents need to understand what options are available and the time necessary for medications to reach their effective levels. It is not easy to adjust doses of analgesics or the time intervals at which they are received and expect immediate effects. A few days may pass before the desired level of pain control is achieved. Parents who give up on a new medication or a medication change after one dose may be negatively affecting the child and thus complicating reasonable assessment.

There are no standard regimens of medications for pediatric cancer pain. Pain management must be individualized to the particular child and the combination of drugs that works best for the particular situation. Health care providers must remember that there is no set dose for an analgesic. There are dosing guidelines, but often in cancer pain management these doses are far exceeded. The proper dose is that dose that controls the pain and minimizes excessive side effects. In the later stages of terminal illness, pediatric patients often require what seem to be staggering doses of opioids with little depressant effects on respiration. Despite these high doses, patients may still complain of pain. A tolerance to narcotic analgesics clearly develops over time, requiring escalating doses of medication to achieve a similar level of pain control. However, what we think is a high narcotic dose may be needed by the child to control the pain. Many health care professionals and parents fear drug addiction and thus withhold medications from children once a certain dose has been reached. Addiction has a negative connotation with aspects of both psychological and physiologic dependence on exogenous substances and abuse potential. In a child with painful bony metastasis who requires increasing narcotic doses to achieve a reasonable level of comfort, such narcotic tolerance should not be labeled as addiction. This child may have excruciating pain and may be dependent on the narcotics to perform simple functions such as sitting up or walking. This should not be considered drug addiction. On the other hand, during periods in the child's cancer course when the pain is not as acute or severe, it may be prudent to taper the child's narcotic regimen to prevent withdrawal symptoms.

One consideration for any child started on opioid analgesics is the associated problem of constipation. This side effect is of particular concern in patients who need opioids regularly. If not treated properly, constipation can become severe and ultimately require surgical intervention secondary to bowel obstruction. Thus, these patients require stool softeners and drugs to enhance bowel motility so as to counteract the constipation from opioid use.

Next, we discuss specific agents used to treat pediatric cancer pain including nonopioid analgesics, narcotic analgesics, adjuvants, and sedatives (Table 26-2).

Nonopioid Analgesics

The three main nonopioid analgesics available are aspirin, acetaminophen, and NSAIDs. These anal-

Table 26-2. Drug Spectrum Used for Cancer Pain

Nonopioid analgesics
    Acetylsalicylic acid
    Choline magnesium salicylate
    Acetaminophen
Nonsteroidal anti-inflammatory drugs
    Ibuprofen
    Ketorolac
    Indomethacin
Combinations
    Acetaminophen + oxycodone (Percocet)
    Acetaminophen + codeine (Tylenol No. 3)
Weak opioids
    Codeine
    Propoxyphene (oxycodone)
Strong opioids
    Morphine
    Fentanyl
    Sufentanil
    Alfentanil
    Hydromorphone
    Methadone
    Meperidine
Longer acting oral opioids
    MS Contin
    Roxanol
Infusions
    Morphine (0.04–0.07 mg/kg/hr)
    Fentanyl (0.5 µg/kg/hr and 5–15 µg rescue)
Psychostimulants
    Methylphenidate
    Dextroamphetamine
Tricyclic antidepressants
    Amitriptyline
Corticosteroids
    Dexamethasone
    Prednisone
    Hydrocortisone
Neuroleptics
    Droperidol
    Haloperidol
Benzodiazepines
    Lorazepam
    Diazepam
    Midazolam
Sedative/sleep aid
    Chloral hydrate
Antihistamines
    Diphenhydramine
    Hydroxyzine
Bowel motility/stool softeners
    Docusate sodium (Colace)
    Bisacodyl (Dulcolax)
    Senna (Senekot)
Local anesthesia
    Lidocaine
    Bupivacaine
    Chlorprocaine
    Tetracaine

gesics are the most widely prescribed analgesics and are the first-line drugs used to treat pain symptoms. They are generally well tolerated and have minimal side effects in terms of mentation, respiratory depression, and decreased bowel motility.

Aspirin (aminosalicylic acid) is widely prescribed for its analgesic and anti-inflammatory properties. It may not be the best choice for the cancer patient because in higher doses it can cause gastric mucosal irritation and, ultimately, gastrointestinal ulceration and bleeding. This is obviously not optimal in patients with poor oral intake, and who are anemic and neutropenic. The coated aspirins (choline salicylate and magnesium trisalicylate) have less gastric irritation and less alteration of platelet function.[4] They also have the added benefit of 12-hour dosing versus 6–8 hours for regular aspirin.

Acetaminophen is not only an analgesic but is also an antipyretic agent. It has minimal gastric irritation associated with it and is well tolerated. It also is used with weak narcotics such as codeine or oxycodone to treat more intense pain because it can potentiate the effects of these narcotics.[5] Such combinations are often used to treat postoperative pain once oral intake has been resumed.

The most recent addition to the nonopioid analgesic category has been NSAIDs, which have superior qualities for treating bony pain and pain of inflammatory origin. Bony pain includes not only bony metastasis but also bone pain after bone marrow aspiration or orthopedic surgical procedures. The major NSAIDs available are ibuprofen, indomethacin, and, most recently, ketorolac. Because these medications cause gastric mucosal irritation, it is recommended that they be taken with meals. In addition, their effects on platelet function limit their use in cancer patients. Ketorolac may be given by an intramuscular route, and a parenteral route is soon to be approved. The benefits of the administration route of this drug may be seen in patients who are unable to take oral medications. Ketorolac has been found to have synergistic effects with narcotics and to have a superior level of pain relief in the acute setting.

Narcotics

Narcotics are some of the most potent drugs in the armamentarium of medications used to control pain. However, due to their potency, they also have serious adverse effects that must be taken into consideration before their use. Narcotics are the mainstay of treatment for patients with debilitating chronic pain and patients in the terminal stages of malignancy. Patients who are taking such medications on a chronic basis and in high doses may experience many troublesome side effects. Likewise, patients receiving narcotics after an operative procedure or during a course of chemotherapy may also experience undesirable side effects. These side effects can range from pruritus and urinary retention to confusion, sedation, and respiratory depression. Thus, every patient on a narcotic regimen must be monitored for such side effects.

Weaker opioids such as codeine and oxycodone are often prescribed in combination with acetaminophen as described previously. Codeine is usually prescribed at doses ranging from 0.5–1.0 mg per kg orally every 4–6 hours as needed. If the doses are increased above this level, there is little increase in analgesic effect but an increase in adverse effects. Codeine can be given orally, intramuscularly, and intravenously; the oral route is the most common, however.

The weak opioid category also contains mixed agonist-antagonist agents such as pentazocine, butorphanol, and nalbuphine. These agents are often used to treat milder pain that may not be treated with an oral medication. In patients who have been receiving opioids on a chronic basis, mixed agonist-antagonist agents are contraindicated because they can cause dysphoria and lead to withdrawal symptoms. The most predominant side effects from these drugs are psychometric effects. As a result, the use of mixed agonist-antagonist agents is questionable and limited for cancer pain, particularly in pediatric patients. Most cancer patients will need narcotics at some point and the mixed agonist-antagonists can further compound the issue of pain control.

There are many stronger opioid agents for pain management. Morphine has the longest record of use and is commonly used for long-term care. Two newer agents (fentanyl and sufentanil) are 100 and 1,000 times as potent as morphine, respectively, but also have a higher potential for adverse side effects, particularly respiratory depression. The use of these agents in pediatric patients has been predominantly for intraoperative and postoperative pain management. Fentanyl can be given by the intravenous,

transmucosal, and transdermal routes and in epidural infusions.

Morphine can be given orally, intramuscularly, intrathecally, and intravenously. It also has the added advantage that it is compatible in the intravenous form with most other drugs, except barbiturates and phenytoin.[6] It can be given as an intravenous bolus, as a continuous infusion, or in a combination of the two in a patient-controlled analgesia (PCA) pump. It has also been used successfully as a subcutaneous infusion (0.04–0.07 mg per kg per hour) for the management of acute pain in patients with sickle cell crises and those who have poor intravenous access.[7–8]

Another medication that is similar to morphine but is eight times as potent is hydromorphone (Dilaudid). It can be given orally or intravenously. It is often tolerated by those patients who cannot use full-dose morphine because of severe pruritus.

Generally, meperidine (Demerol) is no longer used in pediatric patients. It causes not only more sedation than morphine but its metabolite, normeperidine, can accumulate in the CNS. As it accumulates, normeperidine can cause CNS irritability and, ultimately, seizures, particularly in patients with renal compromise. Meperidine had been used more commonly in the past for postoperative pain control as an intramuscular injection combined with hydroxyzine and in the treatment of sickle cell crisis. Because the intramuscular route is not commonly used in pediatric neutropenic patients, meperidine is being used less.

Adjuvant and Sedative Agents

Adjuvant agents are used in an analgesic regimen, usually in combination with narcotics, to treat specific types of pain or side effects. These medications are generally added to an analgesic regimen in the step 3 phase of the WHO analgesic ladder when the less potent agents have become ineffective. They are added when a stronger combination of drugs is needed to control the pain. Step 3 medications are generally reserved for those patients requiring pain control on a chronic basis and patients in the terminal stages of their diseases. This group of agents includes tricyclic antidepressants, anticonvulsants, corticosteroids, benzodiazepines, neuroleptics, psychostimulants, antihistamines, and sedatives.

Tricyclic Antidepressants

Tricyclic antidepressants are an important addition to an analgesic regimen. When taken in doses that are lower than those needed for antidepressant effects, they are effective in treating neuropathic pain and help improve sleep–wake cycles. Neuropathic pain may be due to the peripheral neuropathy caused by repeated doses of vincristine or direct tumor compression. The effectiveness of tricyclic antidepressants in treating neuropathic pain is thought to be due to their ability to increase CNS serotonin levels,[2] a crucial neurotransmitter in pain modulation. They are commonly given at night to minimize the undesirable anticholinergic side effects, such as xerostomia and blurred vision. Amitriptyline in doses of 0.5–1.5 mg per kg at night is the most commonly used drug in this group.

Anticonvulsants

Like the antidepressants, anticonvulsants have effects on pain modulation at doses lower than those necessary for their primary anticonvulsant properties. It is thought that anticonvulsants alter neuronal excitability in the CNS and thus alter central pain pathways. They are used to treat neuropathic pain described as lancinating or stabbing that is not relieved by narcotics. The two primary anticonvulsants are phenytoin (Dilantin) and carbamazepine (Tegretol). Carbamazepine is also used to treat trigeminal neuralgia. Both medications can help treat the pain of postherpetic neuralgia and direct tumor infiltration into a nerve. Their levels must be closely monitored in patients with alterations in hepatic or renal metabolism. Patients also must be carefully observed for signs of toxicity including excessive sedation or dysphoria.

Corticosteroids

Corticosteroids are used in situations where there may be incapacitating pain from increased intracranial pressure or spinal cord compression from tumor or metastasis. Dexamethasone is most commonly used due to is superior penetration into these areas[9] (an initial dose of 10–15 mg per m^2 and then 4–10 mg per m^2 every 6 hours).

Benzodiazepines

Benzodiazepines are commonly used for their sedative capabilities and for their ability to relieve muscle spasm. When used in conjunction with narcotics, they may enhance sedation, thus reducing the level of narcotic required. Benzodiazepines will be discussed more fully in the section on procedure-related pain.

Neuroleptics and Phenothiazines

These agents are useful for treating the nausea and vomiting that are common in cancer patients. They are also used in the management of the combative and confused child. Prior to this use, however, other causes of the confusion must be ruled out including hypoxia, drug toxicity, or metabolic derangements (e.g., hypoglycemia). The phenothiazines (e.g., haloperidol) may actually potentiate narcotic analgesia and thus provide a tranquilizing effect on the patient in extreme pain.[10] These medications must be used with caution in children owing to an increased incidence of associated oculogyric crises[2] and may require the concomitant use of diphenhydramine. If no noticeable response is seen to these medications once a therapeutic level has been received after 3 weeks of treatment, a response is then highly unlikely.

Psychostimulants

Methylphenidate and dextroamphetamine are the two most commonly used psychostimulants. They are used in patients receiving large doses of narcotics to counter excessive sedation and drowsiness and to help normalize a patient's sleep–wake cycle.[11]

Antihistamines

Diphenhydramine and hydroxyzine are the two most commonly used antihistamines. They can have additive effects with narcotics and are also used to treat narcotic-associated pruritus, for their mild antiemetic and sedative effects. Diphenhydramine is often prescribed at night to help maintain a normal sleep–wake cycle.

Sedatives

Sedatives are often needed in a patient with extreme pain who becomes agitated and restless. However, they must be used cautiously because their effects may become additive with the high doses of narcotics a patient has been receiving. Chloral hydrate is a sedative pharmacologically similar to barbiturates; however, it does not cause a decrease in central respiratory drive. It is metabolized to trichloroethanol and must be used carefully in patients with derangements of hepatic function. The metabolite may accumulate and cause excessive sedation or paradoxic agitation. Many of the other adjuvant drugs discussed previously also contain sedative properties and may thus be used for both their effects on pain control and the additive sedative effects.

Procedure-Related Pain

Invasive procedures such as frequent blood drawing, bone marrow aspirates, and lumbar punctures are common in the treatment of pediatric malignancies. Such procedures are required to assess the efficacy of chemotherapeutic regimens and to deliver chemotherapeutic agents (intrathecal medications). Although these procedures may be infrequently used with solid tumors, weekly lumbar punctures may be necessary in patients with hematologic malignancies with CNS involvement. These invasive procedures are distressing for both the patient and the parents who frequently remain in the room in an attempt to comfort and support their child. In fact, many patients and parents perceive these procedures to be worse than the disease itself.[12, 13] Despite such concerns, it is only recently that interest has increased regarding the control of procedure-related pain. The approach to procedure-related pain may include both pharmacologic and nonpharmacologic options.

Nonpharmacologic options are used to decrease distress and anxiety and to improve a child's ability to cooperate with the procedures. Although these methods are frequently successful, especially in dealing with preprocedure anxiety, their use may be time consuming and may require access to psychologists and other trained personnel. Although these facilities may be readily available at larger institu-

tions, the lack of personnel may limit their use in smaller hospitals.

Preparation is the most common nonpharmacologic intervention that can be used by psychologists and nonpsychologists alike. Even without formal training in nonpharmacologic techniques of sedation and relaxation, a simple explanation to the patient of the sequence of events and what is to be expected will often help relieve some components of procedure-related distress. Such an effect relates to the theory that unexpected or unpredicted stress (fear of the unknown) is more difficult to deal with than predictable or known anxiety.[14] Preparation may include an explanation of the planned procedure, viewing videotapes, handling the equipment involved, or even letting the child perform the procedure on a doll. A key component of such preparation is also allowing time for the child and parents to ask questions and to express their fears. Other nonpharmacologic techniques include hypnosis, behavior therapy, and cognitive behavioral interaction. Although these techniques are often highly successful, pharmacologic intervention may still be required, especially during painful procedures.

Prior to using any sedative and analgesic regimen, precautions must be taken to ensure patient safety. Although most medications used for sedation are generally safe and effective, adverse cardiorespiratory effects may be seen and therefore the equipment and personnel to deal with such problems should be readily available. Such complications tend to be more common in younger patients, especially infants.[15] The risk of such problems has lead the American Academy of Pediatrics[16] to issue strict sedation guidelines for personnel and monitoring.

Although these guidelines differentiate conscious sedation and deep sedation from general anesthesia, it should be remembered that the boundaries between these states often overlap. Thus, the use of any sedative agent can result in loss of airway protective reflexes or apnea.[17] When protective reflexes are lost, vomiting and aspiration of gastric contents may occur. Therefore, prior to sedation, an evaluation of oral intake is mandatory. For elective procedures, a period of nothing per mouth based on the patient's age is recommended prior to sedation. The range is generally 6–8 hours for solid foods and 2–3 hours for clear liquids. For emergency situations, the risks of aspiration must be weighed against the benefits of the procedure requiring sedation. A delay in initiating the procedure should be considered in patients with a history of recent oral intake or other factors that increase the risk of aspiration, including altered level of consciousness, obesity, and conditions or medications that alter bowel motility.

During sedation, there should be ready access to resuscitation equipment including an oxygen supply source, proper-size resuscitation (ambu) bag and mask, suction apparatus, airway management equipment (laryngoscope, endotracheal tubes, oral airways), and resuscitation drugs. In addition, one member of the health care team should be trained in pediatric basic life support and airway management. Further training in pediatric advanced life support is recommended.

In addition to access to resuscitation equipment, proper monitoring is mandatory during sedation. One member of the team should be solely responsible for administering sedative agents and for monitoring the patient. Recommendations for monitoring include continuous electrocardiography and noninvasive blood pressure monitoring with blood pressure checked and recorded every 5 minutes throughout the procedure. Because hypoxemia is the greatest risk during the use of sedation, supplemental oxygen should be delivered to all patients until the effects of sedation have dissipated. Continuous pulse oximetry has revolutionized intraoperative monitoring during anesthesia and its use during sedation may increase the detection of hypoxemia. Because hypoxemia is a relatively late sign of inadequate ventilation, other measures of ventilation including a precordial stethoscope and end-tidal carbon dioxide monitoring should be considered. These latter two devices are recommended but are not mandatory during sedation.

Once the proper preparation has been made, the next important step is the choice of agent and route of delivery. The ideal agent for sedation should provide amnesia and analgesia, have options for route of delivery, work rapidly, dissipate rapidly, be inexpensive, and have little effect on cardiorespiratory function. No currently available agent meets all of these criteria. Therefore, each agent should be considered in the context of its advantages and disadvantages. The ideal drug is dependent on the environment in which it is used, the patient on which it is to be used, and the person responsible for its administration.

Inhalational Anesthetic Agents

The inhalational anesthetic agents (isoflurane, enflurane, halothane) have been used for years to provide amnesia and analgesia during surgical procedures. Their benefits include a rapid onset and offset of action and ease of titratability. Fisher et al. have presented their experience with inhalational anesthetic agents for sedation during invasive oncologic procedures.[18] Their technique involved inhalation induction with the children wearing their street clothes and having their parents present. After the procedure, the children emerged from anesthesia in the same setting. Of the agents available, halothane was found to be the most favorable, with fewest complications such as laryngospasm, coughing, or breath holding. Despite their success, such a program requires an available operating room or procedure room and an anesthesiologist. Both of these requirements can be difficult to arrange and increase patient costs. These issues may limit the feasibility of such programs.

Nitrous Oxide

Nitrous oxide is commonly used in dental offices to provide sedation during minor procedures. Nitrous oxide meets many of the desirable characteristics for the ultimate sedative agent, including a rapid onset of action. Owing to its relative insolubility in blood with a low blood-gas partition coefficient, nitrous oxide reaches a steady state alveolar concentration in 5–10 minutes. In addition, it is relatively easy and inexpensive to use, and, most importantly, its effects dissipate rapidly once it is discontinued. Although its delivery in the operating room is via an anesthesia machine in varying concentrations mixed with oxygen, its use outside of an operating room is best accomplished by fixed mixtures from single tanks. These are readily available from several manufacturers as a 50% nitrous oxide and 50% oxygen mixture (Entonox). This lessens the need for specialized equipment for delivery.

Unfortunately, pollution of the environment is a real concern with nitrous oxide. Specialized scavenging devices are needed to prevent environmental pollution. Such concerns are important because there are studies that document deleterious effects of prolonged exposure of health care workers to nitrous oxide, including reduced fertility with an increased risk of spontaneous abortion[19] and chronic myeloneuropathy.[20] Owing to its potential to be abused, certain precautions are required in storing nitrous oxide, which may add to logistical problems owing to the size of the tanks.

In addition to its effects on health care workers, repeated or prolonged exposure may also negatively affect the cancer patient. Acute exposure may cause alterations in cardiorespiratory function. Although nitrous oxide generally has little or no effect on cardiac function in patients with normal cardiac function, decreases in both cardiac output and blood pressure may occur in patients with myocardial dysfunction.[21] The effects on pulmonary artery pressure are also somewhat controversial; however, some researchers report significant increases during nitrous oxide administration.[22] Administration is also contraindicated in patients with altered mental status or respiratory failure.

The more serious effects of prolonged exposure including bone marrow suppression, megaloblastic anemia, alterations in white cell function and motility, and chronic myelopathy.[22–26] The effects on white cell numbers and chronic neurological dysfunction are related to nitrous oxide's inhibitory effects on vitamin B_{12} metabolism specifically altering function of the enzyme methionine synthetase. Additional concerns include alterations in cerebral blood flow and intracranial pressure. Due to these limitations, prolonged use of nitrous oxide is not recommended, although it may have some role in sedation during brief invasive procedures. However, it must only be used by persons trained in its administration and with the proper monitoring because the delivery of a hypoxic gas mixture is possible with improper use or malfunction of the equipment.

Benzodiazepines

Because of the concerns and constraints associated with inhalational agents, parenterally administered medications remain the mainstay of sedation for procedures. In many institutions, benzodiazepines are the most commonly used drugs for sedation. However, it must be remembered that they provide only amnesia and have no inherent analgesic properties.[27] Therefore, narcotics may need to be added to the regimen when painful procedures are being performed. Three benzodiazepines are commonly used for sedation: lorazepam, diazepam, and midazolam. Of the three, the duration of action of midazolam is shortest (15–20 minutes) and as such, the duration of sedation does not greatly exceed the anticipated duration of the procedure. Several studies have documented the efficacy of midazolam in doses of 0.1–0.2 mg per kg for sedation during bone marrow aspirates and lumbar punctures.[28, 29] Diazepam is diluted in propylene glycol, which can cause irritation and pain during peripheral intravenous administration and on intramuscular injection. Midazolam, on the other hand, is water soluble and pain on injection, even through a peripheral intravenous infusion, is usually not a problem. As stated previously, route of administration may also be considered when choosing an agent for sedation. Although many pediatric patients have permanent indwelling central lines, some patients will not have chronic intravenous access. In such patients, an intravenous infusion may be considered to be an invasion equal to the invasive procedure itself. As such, the need for intravenous access may limit the benefit of sedation. In such cases, nonintravenous routes of administration are needed. Several options for route of administration exist with midazolam, including rectal,[30] oral,[31] intranasal,[32] and sublingual.[33] Although midazolam is primarily used as a premedicant for the operating room, these new nonparenteral routes may increase its use.

A few minor modifications are required when using alternate routes of delivery for midazolam. For oral administration, the intravenous preparation (5 mg per ml concentration) is given in a dose of 0.5–0.7 mg per kg. This increased dose is required as a result of limited oral bioavailability and first-pass hepatic metabolism. Because the intravenous preparation contains benzyl alcohol as a preservative, the solution is usually mixed in a beverage or elixir to mask its bitter taste. We have found some success in mixing midazolam in acetaminophen (Tylenol) elixir (cherry flavor). The onset of action is 20–30 minutes. Benzyl alcohol may also cause problems with intranasal administration because it irritates the nasal mucosa. For nasal administration, 0.2–0.4 mg per kg of the 5 mg per ml solution is administered via a tuberculin syringe (needle removed) into one nostril. It is often best to allow the parents to administer the medication. Karl et al. demonstrated equal efficacy of sublingual route with decreased crying when compared with intranasal administration.[33] One advantage of the transmucosal routes (nasal and sublingual) as compared with oral administration is a slight increase in the onset of action (10–15 minutes).

Ketamine

Ketamine is a phencyclidine derivative first described for clinical anesthesia by Domino et al. in 1965.[34] It produces a state of dissociative anesthesia with a presumed mechanism as an electrophysiologic break between the limbic and thalamoneocortical systems.[35] Although initially used to induce general anesthesia, it also has shown efficacy for intraoperative anesthesia[36, 37] and postoperative sedation.[38–40] Unlike benzodiazepines, ketamine provides both amnesia and analgesia, with minimal effects on cardiorespiratory function. It also has the advantage of several routes of administration (intravenous, intramuscular, and oral).

Ketamine produces a dose-related increase in heart rate and blood pressure. Although the exact mechanisms accounting for this phenomenon have not been clearly delineated, it is thought to be mediated through the sympathetic nervous system and the release of endogenous catecholamines.[41, 42] Evidence for this mechanism has been offered by Chernow et al. who demonstrated increased urine, plasma, and cerebrospinal fluid epinephrine levels following ketamine administration.[42] This indirect sympathomimetic effect generally overshadows ketamine's direct negative inotropic properties. However, unstable patients may become hypotensive following ketamine administration.[43–45] In these patients, ketamine's direct negative inotropic properties are believed to predominate because chronic illness either depletes endogenous catecholamine stores or because sympathetic stimulation is already maximal.

An important issue in the use of ketamine in children with congenital heart disease is its possible effects on pulmonary vascular resistance (PVR). Increased PVR has been reported in adults and avoidance of ketamine has been recommended in patients with pulmonary hypertension.[46, 47] Further analysis has attributed the alterations in PVR to changes in respiratory function. Earlier studies were performed in spontaneously breathing patients without consideration for alterations in $PaCO_2$. Morray et al. found statistically significant increases in pulmonary artery pressure (20.6–22.8 mm Hg) and PVR during cardiac catheterization in spontaneously breathing patients after ketamine administration.[46] In contrast, Hickey et al. found no change in PVR in intubated infants with minimal ventilatory support (4 breaths per minute and FIO_2 of 0.4).[47] Pending further studies, ketamine should be used cautiously in patients with pulmonary hypertension and elevated PVR, especially during spontaneous ventilation.

Respiratory function is generally well maintained during sedation with ketamine. Mankikian et al. demonstrated that functional residual capacity, minute ventilation, and tidal volume were unchanged following ketamine administration.[48] Ketamine improves pulmonary compliance and relieves bronchospasm.[49] These effects have also been attributed to the release of endogenous catecholamines, because they can be blocked by the administration of beta-adrenergic antagonists.[50] Although ventilation is generally well maintained, elevations in $PaCO_2$ and a shift to the right of the CO_2 response curve may occur.[51]

Ketamine increases salivary and bronchial gland secretion through stimulation of central cholinergic receptors. Therefore, the concomitant administration of an antisialagogue such as atropine or glycopyrrolate is recommended. Controversy exists over ketamine's effects on protective airway reflexes. Although clinical use and experimental studies suggest that these reflexes are maintained, aspiration has been reported following ketamine administration.[52] Therefore, as with any sedative agent, it must be used cautiously in patients at risk for aspiration of gastric contents.

Ketamine may also increase intracranial pressure and therefore should be avoided in patients at risk for intracranial hypertension.[53] Alterations in intracranial pressure are a consequence of cerebral vasodilatation, mediated directly through central cholinergic receptors, and not secondary to alterations in cerebral metabolic rate or changes in $PaCO_2$.[54–56]

The one adverse effect that may keep ketamine from being classified as the ideal sedative agent is its capacity to cause emergence phenomena or hallucinations. Emergence phenomena are more common in older patients, are dose-related, and their incidence can be decreased by the preadministration of a benzodiazepine.[58] We have found that the administration of a benzodiazepine (usually midazolam, 0.10–0.15 mg per kg) 5 minutes prior to the administration of ketamine to be almost 100% effective in eliminating emergence phenomena. Emergence reactions have been postulated to be the result of ketamine's depression of auditory and visual relay in the inferior colliculus and the medial geniculate nucleus. This effect may lead to misinterpretation of visual and auditory stimuli.

For practical use, ketamine is generally administered in intermittent, intravenous bolus doses of 0.25–0.50 mg per kg every 2–3 minutes until the desired level of sedation is achieved. Total doses of 2–4 mg per kg are generally sufficient for brief procedures. Higher doses may be needed in patients repeatedly exposed to ketamine. Although the majority of experience is with its intravenous administration, recent clinical studies have documented its use by both oral[58] and nasal administration.[59] As with midazolam, higher doses are needed when these nonparenteral routes are used due to first-pass metabolism and limited bioavailability.

Propofol

Propofol (Diprivan) is a newer sedative-hypnotic intravenous anesthetic agent that is chemically unrelated to barbiturates and other commonly used anesthetic induction agents.[60] Rapid recovery and a lack of postoperative nausea and vomiting have increased its popularity in outpatient surgery. Owing to its rapid onset of action and quick recovery time following discontinuation, it has also become a popular agent for sedation of adult patients in the intensive care unit.[61, 62] These same properties have led to its use outside the operating room during invasive procedures and when a motionless patient is required for radiologic imaging. It has been used with increasing frequency to sedate children for painful procedures and has the advantage of minimal effects of nausea and vomiting. However, it may cause pain or irritation when administered through a small peripheral intravenous line and may need to have the coadministration of lidocaine (10 mg lidocaine in 10 ml of propofol) to reduce this effect.

However, with this increased use has also come an increased awareness of potential adverse effects. Like the barbiturates, propofol may be associated with hemodynamic instability attributed to its negative inotropic properties.[63] Although well tolerated in patients with adequate cardiac reserve, its use in hemodynamically unstable patients is not recommended. Additionally, several reports have described unusual neurologic manifestations following its use, including opisthotonic posturing, myoclonic twitching, and convulsions.[64–66] One report also describes seizures in two patients who were sedated with propofol for bone marrow biopsies.[67]

No clear explanation has been offered for the neurologic manifestations associated with propofol administration. It has been suggested that it may be related to antagonistic effects at the glycine receptor. Regardless of the mechanism of these neurologic effects, their occurrence may lessen the enthusiasm of many proponents of this agent and certainly its use may be contraindicated in patients at risk for seizures.

Barbiturates

Barbiturates are one of the oldest class of agents still being used for sedation and induction agents of general anesthesia. Although small doses produce sleep and amnesia, larger doses may blunt respiratory drive and lead to cardiovascular instability. Cardiovascular actions include both a negative inotropic effect and peripheral vasodilation. Although their cardiodepressant effects are well tolerated in patients with normal function, the rapid administration of these agents to patients with poor cardiac contractility can lead to significant decreases in cardiac output and blood pressure.

The different agents are most easily classified according to duration of activity. Short-acting agents include methohexital, pentothal, and thiamylal and longer acting agents include pentobarbital. These agents are usually used by intravenous bolus administration for brief procedures such as endotracheal intubation. Intramuscular or rectal administration may be used when longer sedation is required such as that needed during radiologic imaging. These agents have no intrinsic analgesic properties and are not recommended as the sole sedative agent for painful procedures.

Opioids

In addition to their use for providing postoperative analgesia, opioids are frequently used to provide analgesia and sedation during invasive procedures. Most importantly it should be remembered that they provide analgesia, but not amnesia. A study comparing fentanyl with midazolam for invasive procedures found that both the patients and the parents preferred midazolam.[28] The authors postulated that the patient population (generally children 2–8 years of age) preferred midazolam and the subsequent amnesia for the procedure rather than analgesia alone provided by the fentanyl. Although this study showed the element of amnesia to be of importance in pediatric procedures, there is no reason that the two agents cannot be combined, midazolam to provide amnesia and fentanyl to provide analgesia.

When choosing an opioid for sedation, one should consider the duration of the intended procedure. Because most procedures last only 10–15 minutes, narcotics with longer half-lives such as meperidine and morphine should not be used. The synthetic opioids (alfentanil, fentanyl, and sufentanil) have very brief durations of action and therefore the effects do not greatly outlast the procedure. When considering which synthetic agent to use, the potency of sufentanil (8–10 times greater than fentanyl and 1,000 times greater than morphine) makes it a difficult and dangerous agent to titrate for sedation; therefore, we prefer fentanyl and alfentanil, which are less potent. Due to cost considerations, fentanyl seems to be the best choice. When using midazolam and fentanyl, we generally administer midazolam in a dose of 0.15 mg per kg (maximum, 5 mg) over 5–10 minutes. Following this administration, fentanyl (intravenous boluses of 0.5–1.0 μg per kg) is titrated as needed every 3 minutes until the desired level of analgesia and sedation is achieved.

In patients without intravenous access, alternative routes of delivery for fentanyl are being investigated. Preliminary experience suggests that both the intranasal and sublingual routes may be effective. Additionally, oral transmucosal fentanyl citrate or the fentanyl lollipop has recently been introduced. The transdermal route (fentanyl patch) has also been developed, although it is not recommended for children under 12 years of age. Future studies are needed to exactly define the efficacy and safety of these alternative routes of delivery.

Miscellaneous Agents

Several other agents or combinations of agents have been used with varying degrees of success. These include the phenothiazine, butyrophenones, antihistamines (diphenhydramine), and chloral hydrate. The first two classes of agents are considered the major tranquilizers. Although most commonly used for their antiemetic or antipsychotic properties, these agents may also provide adequate sedation. Their use in combination with other agents (i.e., DPT: meperidine hydorchloride [Demerol], promethazine hydrochloride [Phenergan], and chlorpromazine hydrochloride [Thorazine]) may result in prolonged sedation and increased risk of respiratory depression, thereby further emphasizing the need for vigilant monitoring when such agents are used.[68] Aside from its CNS and respiratory effects, phenothiazine may also decrease arterial pressure through peripheral alpha-blockade.

Adjuncts to Sedation

In addition to sedation, topical anesthesia of the skin and subcutaneous tissues can greatly alleviate much of the discomfort associated with procedures. Several different local anesthetics are available for this purpose. The important consideration is not the anesthetic itself, but the way in which it is administered. We start the administration with a 30-gauge needle and inject the medication slowly. Because of their low pH, most local anesthetics cause discomfort on injection. Aside from injecting slowly, it has been suggested that the use of a local anesthetic with a more physiologic pH such as chloroprocaine may cause less discomfort than lidocaine. Furthermore, the addition of a small amount of sodium bicarbonate (0.1 mEq for every 10 ml) may also alleviate some of the discomfort.

When using local anesthetics, one must always be aware of the volume injected and their concentration. Inadvertent injection of excessive amounts may lead to toxicity of the cardiovascular system and CNS. In most instances, 0.5% lidocaine is the concentration used for local infiltration. Lidocaine should be limited to 5 mg per kg, whereas doses of bupivacaine should not exceed 2.5–3.0 mg per kg. Although achieving toxic doses from local infiltration is unlikely in older patients, it may be more likely in infants. For example, the maximum amount of 0.5% lidocaine that can be used in a 4-kg infant would be only 4 ml.

Aside from local anesthetics, a topical cream, EMLA, has recently been introduced by Astra Pharmaceuticals.[69, 70] The cream is a eutectic mixture of lidocaine and prilocaine. When applied to the skin for 60 minutes, anesthesia of the epidermis is achieved. Longer application times (2 hours) may provide anesthesia of even deeper cutaneous tissues. The cream can be applied over an anticipated intravenous site, lumbar puncture site, or over the procedure site. When placed over the procedure site, infiltration with local anesthetics into the deeper subcutaneous tissues is still recommended. However, the cream alleviates the discomfort associated with the initial injection of local anesthetic and allows the slow infiltration of deeper structures. The cream may also be used over subcutaneous ports of Broviac catheters prior to needle insertion to access the line. We have found success using oral midazolam to provide anxiolysis and sedation combined with topical EMLA cream followed by infiltration with local anesthetic to provide analgesia for many procedures.

Adverse effects of the cream are uncommon and generally include only local erythema and pallor, which resolve in 1–2 hours after removal. The only theoretical risk of the cream is the absorption of prilocaine and the formation of methemoglobinemia. There has been one report of methemoglobinemia in a patient who was also receiving sulfa drugs, which reportedly produce methemoglobinemia. Therefore, the cream is not recommended for children receiving other drugs that may lead to the formation of methemoglobin. In addition, because neonates have a limited capability to convert methemoglobin back to hemoglobin, the cream is not recommended for use in infants less than 2 months of age. Despite this, it has been successfully and safely used to alleviate the pain associated with neonatal circumcision.[72]

Acute Postoperative Pain

Many advances have been made in understanding, identifying, and treating postoperative pain in children. It was once generally accepted that children tolerated pain well, seldom required narcotic anal-

gesic agents, and adults.[3, 4] How these concep experience terations rate, bloo sponse to pain borns.[71] The physio of and response to pain a.

The issues of pain contro itarian implications. Anand et al. h a postsurgical stress response in infan cardiac surgery.[73] The stress response is ch ized by a metabolic, hormonal, and cardiorespi tory response to surgical trauma with the liberation of catecholamines, cortisol, glucagon, and other catabolic hormones. Additional work has demonstrated that this response is most severe in infants with the highest mortality.[74] In fact, Anand et al. have recently demonstrated differences in mortality following cardiac surgery in infants, depending on the intraoperative and postoperative analgesic techniques employed.[74, 75] Although issues of postoperative mortality and morbidity may not be pertinent following minor surgical procedures, adequate analgesia may significantly affect the postoperative course by allowing earlier postoperative ambulation, thereby limiting the risks of adverse cardiorespiratory sequelae and possibly earlier hospital discharge. All of these factors lead to a quicker return to the normal activities of daily life.

As previously mentioned the WHO has developed a three-step ladder of medications[3] to use for cancer pain that includes NSAIDs for mild pain (step 1) and progresses to the use of potent intravenous narcotics such as morphine for severe pain (step 3). A similar approach is possible for postoperative pain.

Mild pain (i.e., minor musculoskeletal trauma or pain following outpatient surgery) can be effectively treated with oral narcotic agents, NSAIDs, or a combination of the two. For such indications, oral preparations combining either acetaminophen or acetylsalicylic acid with a narcotic (codeine or oxycodone) are generally effective. These are available in either liquid or tablet forms. Initial dosing regimens should be based on the narcotic component of the compound and include 1 mg per kg for codeine and 0.15 mg per kg for oxycodone, both administered at 3- to 4-hour intervals as needed. When

needed, preparations that include
ic compound (codeine or oxycodone)
d separately because dose escalations
recommended initial starting dose can
xcessive doses of either the acetylsalicylic
he acetaminophen component.

ddition to providing analgesia when used
e, NSAIDs may also be used in conjunction
h intravenous narcotics to treat severe pain. In
his setting, the benefit of the NSAIDs is that they
decrease the total amount of narcotic used and may
therefore limit adverse effects related to narcotics
such as ileus and sedation. Although their use in the
postoperative setting had been limited by the need
for oral administration, two agents are available for
administration: indomethacin and ketorolac tromethamine. Only the latter medication is available
for parenteral use in the United States and has recently been approved for use in pediatric patients.
Maunuksela et al. found that the continuous intravenous administration of indomethacin improved
analgesia and diminished narcotic requirements following surgery in children[76] whereas Watcha et al.
demonstrated the efficacy of ketorolac for postoperative analgesia in children.[77]

Adverse effects of NSAIDs relate to their effects
on prostaglandin synthesis at sites away from the
inflammatory process. The most important effects
for cancer patients are their effects on platelet aggregation, which lead to an increased bleeding time.
Although such effects are generally minimal without clinical effects in normal patients, this may not
be the case in patients with qualitative or quantitative defects of platelet function. Decreased synthesis of prostaglandins of the E series leads to
decreased renal blood flow and glomerular filtration. Although alterations in renal function are uncommon in euvolemic patients, patients with
preexisting renal dysfunction or hypovolemia may
be prone to developing alterations in renal function.
Therefore, these agents should be used cautiously
in such patients.

Despite advances with the use of nonnarcotic
analgesic agents in children, the mainstay for postoperative pain remains narcotic analgesic agents.
When narcotic analgesic agents are administered,
three choices must be made (1) the route of administration, (2) the narcotic to be used, and (3) the
method of administration (continuous versus intermittent). Although intravenous administration is

generally chosen for the immediate postoperative
period, circumstances arise that may require the use
of alternative routes of delivery including oral,
transmucosal (nasal, buccal, rectal), transdermal,
subcutaneous, intramuscular, and spinal (intrathecal or epidural).

Aside from the management of pain related to
chronic disease, the oral administration of narcotics
is generally not the optimal way to deal with severe
postoperative pain. Several problems complicate
oral administration in the immediate postoperative
period including nausea, vomiting, and alterations
in gastrointestinal motility. Intramuscular administration is not recommended due to variability in absorption and erratic efficacy, especially when
compared with intravenous administration.[78] Intramuscular administration should be used sparingly
as children may deny the existence of pain to avoid
a "shot." The intramuscular route should also be
avoided in the thrombocytopenic cancer patient.

Despite limited experience with its use for postoperative pain, subcutaneous administration of narcotics has found widespread use and efficacy for
pain related to the terminal stages of malignancies
when oral administration has failed.[79, 80] In addition to providing analgesia, such techniques eliminate the need for chronic intravascular access and
can be taught to the parents to use at home. This
technique may be an alternative to intramuscular
administration when intravenous access becomes
difficult. For this purpose, a small-gauge butterfly
needle (23- or 25-gauge) is inserted subcutaneously
and left in place. A continuous infusion of morphine (0.01–0.02 mg per kg per hour) will generally provide adequate analgesia. Although most
narcotics may be used subcutaneously, clinical experience suggests that methadone may be an unacceptable choice due to a high incidence of local
tissue reaction and cellulitis.[81]

The transmucosal delivery of narcotics has also
been successfully used in several situations. The rectal administration of narcotic analgesic agents is
widely used in terminally ill patients,[82] whereas the
administration of synthetic narcotics (sufentanil and
fentanyl) across the nasal and oral mucosa has been
used to premedicate children prior to anesthetic induction and to treat procedure-related pain.[83–85]
Striebel et al. have demonstrated the efficacy of intranasal fentanyl for postoperative analgesia.[86] When
compared with intravenous administration, they

found that intranasal fentanyl provides equally effective analgesia with a comparable onset of action and concluded that it was suitable for postoperative analgesia. Further studies are needed to define the efficacy and dosing of such techniques in children.

Another alternative mode of narcotic delivery that has been recently introduced is the transdermal application of fentanyl. Although its efficacy has been demonstrated in adults,[87–89] experience in children is still relatively anecdotal.[90] The transdermal delivery system allows the continuous administration of fentanyl at four different doses (25, 50, 75, or 100 µg per hour). Following application, steady-state serum concentrations are achieved in 8–12 hours and last for 72 hours with a single patch.[91] The major disadvantages are that analgesic serum levels may not be reached for up to 12 hours following patch application and that the currently available dosing choices make dose titration difficult, thereby limiting its use in smaller patients. Despite these limitations, we have found that this delivery system may have some applications for children.[90, 91]

The second decision in the use of narcotic analgesic agents is the narcotic to be administered. Although route of administration has been systematically evaluated by several different investigators, there appears to be little information concerning the optimal narcotic for postoperative analgesia. In the patient with compromised cardiovascular status, either fentanyl or sufentanil may be advantageous because of their relative cardiovascular stability and beneficial effects on pulmonary vascular resistance. However, due to their short plasma half-lives, these agents need to be administered by a continuous infusion to maintain plasma concentrations adequate to provide analgesia. In patients with stable cardiovascular dynamics, morphine is an acceptable and much cheaper alternative. With adequate cardiovascular function and intravascular volume status, the minimal vasodilatory properties of morphine are well tolerated. In addition, morphine's plasma half-life is longer than either fentanyl or sufentanil and therefore analgesia can be achieved with intermittent bolus dosing. However, continuous infusion techniques (see following discussion) may provide superior analgesia to conventional on-demand intermittent dosing regimens.

Alternatives to morphine include hydromorphone (Dilaudid), meperidine (Demerol), and methadone

(Dolobid). Hydromorphone may be used when adverse effects related to histamine release such as pruritus occur with morphine.[92] In such cases, an equipotent dose of hydromorphone should be administered. This can be derived by considering the potency ratio of the two narcotics with hydromorphone (five to seven times as potent as morphine).

Another effective, although less frequently used narcotic, is methadone. Its major advantage is a long plasma half-life of 12–24 hours.[93] As such, a continuous infusion or PCA techniques (see following discussion) are not required to provide prolonged, uninterrupted analgesia. Gourlay et al. evaluated the efficacy of a single 20-mg intraoperative dose of methadone following major surgery in adults.[94] Half of the patients required only acetaminophen for analgesia in the postoperative course and those patients who did require supplemental narcotic analgesic agents were, on average, 17 hours into the postoperative course. Berde et al. evaluated the efficacy of methadone compared with morphine in children aged 3–7 years.[95] Children who received methadone had lower pain scores and required fewer doses of supplemental narcotic analgesia agents over the ensuing 36 hours.

Meperidine, on the other hand, appears to be a relatively poor choice for postoperative analgesia. Although sedation is most common, several other CNS effects occur with meperidine including dysphoria, agitation, and seizures.[96] In older children and adults, the dysphoric response may be manifested by complaints of "not feeling well" and restlessness, whereas agitation and uncontrollable crying may be the only manifestation in the younger child or infant. The CNS toxicity of meperidine is due to the accumulation of normeperidine from the N-demethylation of the parent compound. Normeperidine has a long half-life (15–20 hours) and is primarily excreted in the urine. Toxic levels are more common in the presence of renal insufficiency, the coadministration of phenobarbital or other agents that increase hepatic microsomal enzymes, and with the administration of large doses. Vetter has recently compared the analgesic efficacy of meperidine with morphine administered by PCA to children.[97] His prospective, randomized study in 50 children found improved analgesia in those children receiving morphine when compared with meperidine.

The third and perhaps most important choice in the administration of narcotic analgesic agents is the mode of delivery. Options include on-demand dosing, fixed interval dosing, continuous infusion, PCA, or a combination of these options. The problem with on-demand dosing is that health care providers may withhold doses due to unfounded fears of addiction or adverse effects. Additionally, a significant amount of time can elapse from the initial complaint of pain until medication is actually administered and takes effect. Therefore, alternative modes of delivery have been developed to improve analgesia.

Prior to the advent of PCA, the continuous infusion of narcotics supplemented with intermittent intravenous bolus doses provided the optimal level of analgesia. Although studies are limited in children, adult studies suggest that a continuous narcotic infusion provides superior analgesia and fewer adverse effects than either on-demand or fixed interval dosing.[78]

Another alternative delivery method that has been used with great success is PCA. This method allows patients to administer a preset amount of narcotic at predetermined intervals. Although the technique requires an awake, cooperative patient, its advantages include improved analgesia with decreased total narcotic use. Recent experience in the pediatric population suggests that children as young as 6–8 years of age are able to effectively use the device.[98–100]

When available, PCA appears to be the best method to deliver intravenous narcotics. Following a loading dose (intraoperatively or in the recovery room) of morphine titrated to provide analgesia, the device is set to allow the patient to deliver 0.015–0.030 mg per kg every 6–10 minutes as needed. The device may also be set to deliver a continuous background infusion of narcotic. Recent studies in adults suggest that the background infusion does not improve analgesia and may increase the incidence of adverse effects.[101, 102]

An understanding by clinicians of the pharmacokinetic principles and appropriate use of narcotics will facilitate effective analgesia for the majority of children. However, unfounded fears of adverse effects and addiction still limit the use of narcotic analgesic agents. Such fears appear to be unfounded because narcotic addiction is exceedingly rare in patients receiving narcotic analgesic agents for postoperative pain control.[103] Physical dependence does occur with prolonged narcotic administration.[104] Although physical dependence is extremely uncommon when narcotics are used for 3–7 days to control postoperative pain, certain situations arise in which prolonged narcotic therapy is necessary.

The occurrence of tolerance and physical dependency should not cause the clinician to limit the use of narcotics in children, but rather to emphasize the need to slowly taper narcotic administration in patients who have received narcotics for a prolonged period (longer than 2 weeks). We have reported our experience with the use of oral methadone to facilitate weaning from intravenous narcotic administration.[105] The advantage of methadone is that its oral bioavailability (50–60%) allows oral administration in the place of intravenous administration. This approach obviates the need for intravenous access and may also allow outpatient tapering of methadone doses.[106]

More common adverse effects other than fears of addiction may interfere with the delivery of effective analgesia. Although respiratory depression following narcotic administration is rare, certain patient populations are at risk, such as patients with underlying cardiorespiratory problems, neonates, and the former preterm infant. In such patients, the initial dose of narcotic should be one-third to one-half the usual dose. These doses may be gradually increased as needed to provide effective analgesia. Close perioperative monitoring with continuous pulse oximetry may also be indicated in certain patients. Consultation with pain specialists or anesthesiologists may also be helpful because regional anesthesia techniques (see following discussion) may provide superior analgesia and avoid the need for parenteral narcotics.

Regional Anesthetic Techniques

Although parenteral narcotics are the most commonly chosen postoperative analgesic regimen, regional anesthetic techniques may provide more effective postoperative analgesia, encourage earlier ambulation, and prevent pulmonary dysfunction while avoiding the risks of respiratory depression due to parenteral narcotics. The regional anesthetic techniques that exist for pain relief include epidural, spinal, and peripheral nerve blockade. They are being used with increasing frequency in the pediatric population.

Epidural analgesia remains the most commonly used regional anesthetic technique. The epidural space lies between the dura mater and the ligamentum flavum and extends from the base of the skull to the sacrococcygeal membrane. Although the epidural space may be entered anywhere along the spinal axis, a lumbar or caudal approach is generally used for procedures involving the lower extremities or abdomen, particularly in pediatric patients.

Several medications can be used for epidural analgesia, but current clinical practice usually uses a combination of local anesthetic and an opioid. Local anesthetics such as lidocaine and bupivacaine produce analgesia through their effects on the spinal cord, dorsal root ganglia, and spinal nerve roots. In addition to sensory blockade, these agents also cause some degree of sympathetic and motor blockade. Sympathetic blockade may lead to hypotension due to venous pooling and decreased preload. However, both cardiac output and blood pressure are generally well maintained after epidural blockade in children.[107] Motor blockade from the epidural administration of local anesthetics may lead to weakness in various motor groups supplied by nerve roots at the level of insertion. Therefore, assistance may be required during ambulation. The use of dilute solutions of local anesthetic (bupivacaine 0.0625–0.125%) limits the incidence of motor blockade while providing adequate postoperative analgesia. In addition, the local anesthetic bupivacaine provides relative sparing of motor as opposed to sensory neurons.

Epidural opioids provide selective analgesia without affecting sympathetic or motor function. Analgesia results from the binding of opioids with receptors in the dorsal horn of the spinal cord. These receptors modulate the synapse between the first-order (sensory) neuron and the second-order neuron as they synapse in the spinal cord. Epidural narcotics may cause respiratory depression, which may be related to either systemic absorption of the drug from the epidural space or cephalad spread of the narcotic within the cerebrospinal fluid to central respiratory centers. The latter event is more common with hydrophilic narcotics such as morphine and less likely with the lipophilic narcotics such as fentanyl or meperidine.[108] Regardless of the etiology, respiratory depression related to epidural narcotics can be reversed with naloxone. No other parenteral narcotics should be given to the patient who receives epidural or spinal narcotics because there is an increased risk of respiratory depression and even respiratory arrest.

There are several types of technique (one-shot versus continuous infusion) and the choice of drugs for epidural anesthesia. The final decision will be based on the type of surgery and the expected magnitude of postoperative pain. For outpatient procedures, a single caudal epidural injection of local anesthetic at the completion of the surgery prior to emergence from general anesthesia provides 6–8 hours of postoperative analgesia. When more extensive procedures are performed that necessitate inpatient admission, the placement of a catheter into the epidural space allows for either repeated dosing or a continuous infusion. For such procedures, we generally use a continuous infusion that consists of a combination of a narcotic (fentanyl) with a local anesthetic (bupivacaine).[109, 110] These techniques are applicable in patients as small as 2–3 kg.

Another method to provide prolonged analgesia without the need for catheter placement and a continuous infusion is the use of spinal (intrathecal or epidural) morphine. Owing to its hydrophilic nature, morphine's analgesic effects last 12–24 hours following a single administration. However, the risk of respiratory depression also exists for this period of time and therefore close monitoring of respiratory status is required.

The intrathecal administration of local anesthetic may be used to provide intraoperative anesthesia in infants and children,[111] whereas the intrathecal administration of morphine provides prolonged (up to 24 hours) periods of postoperative analgesia and limits the need for supplemental agents.[112] Owing to the continuous cephalad movement of cerebrospinal fluid, lumbar intrathecal morphine may be used to provide analgesia following surgical procedures of the head and neck.[112]

Adverse effects related to epidural anesthesia can be grouped into two categories: those related to catheter placement and those related to drug administration. Placement problems include bleeding, dural puncture, and infection. The epidural space contains numerous blood vessels, and uncontrolled bleeding can result in an epidural hematoma with compromised perfusion to the spinal cord leading to paralysis. Therefore, epidural anesthesia is contraindicated in patients with either qualitative or quantitative bleeding disorders (i.e., partial thromboplastin to partial thromboplastin time greater than 1.5 times control or a platelet count less than 100,000 per ml). Dural puncture may lead to a spinal headache that may require 5–7 days to resolve. Conservative treatment with bed rest is indicated due to the often self-limited nature of this complication.[113]

Adverse effects related to drug administration may be separated into those related to local anesthetics and those related to narcotics. The most severe complications related to local anesthetics are inadvertent intrathecal or intravascular injection. Inadvertent intrathecal injection results in total spinal blockade with respiratory muscle paralysis requiring airway management. This risk is present only with the large bolus doses that are administered immediately following catheter placement and dissipate within 4–8 hours. Intravascular injection of toxic doses of local anesthetics can result in toxicity of the cardiovascular system and CNS including seizures, hypotension, arrhythmias, and cardiovascular collapse. Inadvertent intravascular injection is detected and, it is hoped, prevented by using a test dose with epinephrine, which serves as a marker of intravascular injection.

Additional minor adverse effects related to epidural narcotics include pruritus, urinary retention, and nausea and vomiting. Symptomatic treatment with antipruritic agents (diphenhydramine) and antiemetics is generally effective when these adverse effects are noted. If severe and unresponsive to conservative measures, these adverse effects may be controlled with a low-dose intravenous infusion of naloxone. Reversal of these adverse effects can be accomplished with naloxone without reversing analgesia. Some practitioners employ naloxone infusion prophylactically when neuraxial opioids are being used to avoid the development of these side effects.

Peripheral Nerve Blockade

The administration of local anesthetic at selected points may be used to interrupt nerve impulse transmission and prevent postoperative pain. With the relatively long-acting agent, bupivacaine, postoperative analgesia may last up to 8 hours while placement of a catheter into the neurovascular bundle allows the use of continuous infusion techniques. A catheter may be placed into the axillary sheath for the upper extremity or in the femoral sheath for the lower extremity.

The lower extremity is supplied by two separate plexuses with anterior innervation supplied by the lumbar plexus and posterior supply by the sacral plexus. Several different approaches allow the selective blockade of these plexuses and the individual nerves branching from them.

The femoral nerve provides sensory innervation to the anterior aspect of the thigh and the periosteum of the femur. The nerve is blocked as it passes lateral to the femoral artery at the inguinal crease. A modification of this technique (the three-in-one block) is performed by holding distal pressure during injection of the local anesthetic. With this maneuver, the local anesthetic may spread up the femoral sheath and block both the obturator and lateral femoral cutaneous nerves, leading to anesthesia of the leg above the knee.

Once again, as with local infiltration, monitoring the concentration and amount of local anesthetic used is required. Regardless of the site chosen (peripheral or central blockade), the dose of anesthetic agent should be based on the patient's weight to avoid systemic toxicity. The dose should be limited to 2.5–3.0 mg per kg for bupivacaine and 5–7 mg per kg for lidocaine.

Chronic Pain Management

In the terminal stages of malignancy, pain management becomes of paramount importance. The desired goal of providing adequate analgesia to a terminal patient while avoiding excessive sedation and adverse medication side effects can be quite challenging. Chronic pain differs from acute pain in that it is ongoing and continuous with no distinct end point. Much of chronic pain management is done either in the patient's home or in a hospice where monitoring may not be available.

The fact that a terminal patient may not be in a hospital puts certain constraints on the patient's pain regimen. It must be tailored not only to the child's needs but also to those of the family or caregiver. The medication regimen must be as uncomplicated as possible so that the schedule can be reasonably followed by the family. Thus, dosing schedules are important because most patients are usually receiving several different medications. A schedule that has a patient receiving a different medication every 2–3 hours may be too burdensome on the family or caregiver and nearly impossible depending on the social structure of the home environment. Often it is easiest to attempt to plan dosing schedules with meal times, especially since certain medications are better tolerated when taken with food (e.g., NSAIDs). Most dosing schedules include a "rescue" dose of medication that the family member can deliver or the child can take if the pain escalates to an unbearable point between scheduled doses. For instance, when beginning on an oral regimen with the long-acting oral morphine (MS Contin) there may be a rescue dose of oral morphine elixir every 2–3 hours between the MS Contin doses to relieve breakthrough pain.

In addition to dosing patterns, the route of medication administration is also important in the chronic pain patient. The family member or caregiver may need to become facile with administering medications via a gastrostomy tube or indwelling catheter device such as a Broviac catheter. This becomes especially important as the patient becomes more debilitated and when the oral route for medication is not an option. The delivery of pain medications also requires the need to recognize adverse side effects and steps to reduce them.

The medications a child receives in the terminal stages of cancer must balance pain relief and the attempt to maintain a near normal sleep–wake cycle and allow the child to resume as many day-to-day activities as possible. While at home, the child may have increased interaction with other siblings who often have limited access to the sick child who is in the hospital. The home environment may also help de-emphasize the illness and treatment that have preoccupied the child's life in the hospital and help socialize a withdrawn child. It is often difficult to achieve these desired effects. Usually, several different regimens must be tried and continuously adjusted for each child's specific needs before the most optimal regimen is found. In the latter stages of cancer, most patients have already tried numerous different medications and due to the chronicity of treatment may have large requirements for pain medicine. The development of tolerance to analgesics requires continued dosage adjustments and often use of a combination of agents (i.e., narcotics and adjuvant drugs). Opioids are the mainstay of the analgesic regimen for chronic management and it is especially important to remember in the pediatric cancer patient that there is no set optimal or maximal dose of narcotics. The right dose is that dose individualized to

the patient and one that controls pain and minimizes side effects. Lack of pain control is the most common reason for hospital readmission in these patients[113] and a source of frustration for families and health professionals alike.

Drugs that have versatility in terms of route of delivery and dosing intervals are very important in chronic pain management. Morphine and methadone exhibit such versatility and warrant further discussion.

Morphine can be given by virtually any route and has the longest record of use for pain control. There are now two oral preparations that can be dosed on a 12-hour basis with a 3 to 1 oral-to-parenteral conversion. MS Contin (Purdue-Frederick, Norwalk, CT) is a controlled release tablet that has become the backbone for chronic pain management. Recently, a morphine sulfate intensified oral solution called Roxanol (Roxane Laboratories, Columbus, OH) has been introduced. Its concentration is 20 mg per ml in a liquid dropper form, which decreases the volume of medication per dose and increases palatability. It becomes an important addition to pain control in more debilitated patients who have difficulty swallowing pills because the dropper form can be trickled into the back of the throat and absorbed efficiently in patients with severe mucositis. When beginning these medications, it may take two to three doses before adequate blood levels are achieved and thus a shorter acting dose of morphine elixir is prescribed as rescue for breakthrough pain.

In cases of severe compromise, morphine may be given as subcutaneous injections or as a continuous subcutaneous infusion when a terminal patient continues to have pain and is compromised enough so that the oral and intravenous routes are not available. A subcutaneous infusion of morphine can be used (0.04–0.07 mg per kg per hour).[78] This technique is also valuable for use outside of the hospital setting because it can be taught to the parents or caregivers. The subcutaneous sites are most commonly located on the lower abdomen or upper thigh to minimize interference with movement.

In pediatric cancer patients there has been an increase in the insertion of indwelling intravenous access devices (either Hickman, Broviac, or port-a-caths) to obviate the need for numerous intravenous starts and needle sticks for blood drawing. Thus, these indwelling devices allow pain control via an intravenous route in the compromised, debilitated terminal patient. There has been an increase in home morphine infusions and, more recently, in PCA for patients out of the hospital. These options are more labor intensive in terms of teaching, dosing, maintenance, and observation for adverse effects. But, they may allow patients who do not adhere well to an oral pain regimen to go home. For PCA devices, we advocate that a basal infusion not be used to prevent the possibility of severe respiratory depression in the nonmonitored home environment. One important point is to teach both the patient and parents how to properly use the pump. Parents must be taught to resist pushing the button for the patient and increase the risk of excessive sedation and potential complications. Those patients who are sent home on PCA are patients with a large narcotic requirement and thus their narcotic needs must be evaluated and converted to an equianalgesic PCA regimen. The PCA regimen that has sustained the patient with minimal side effects while in the hospital is usually the same one used at home. For patients on home PCA, a visiting nurse is usually required to assess daily usage of the pump and evaluation of pain control and side effects. Fentanyl has also been used as an infusion and with PCA but has self-limiting respiratory depression associated with it and is used less often than morphine.

Methadone is the other narcotic that can be dosed orally on a 12-hour schedule and is useful for patients out of the hospital setting. It is a valuable alternative for those patients who demonstrate a true morphine allergy or who experience pruritus with the higher doses of morphine. It has perhaps less sedation and euphoria associated with it than morphine and may be given as 0.1–0.2 mg per kg every 8–12 hours. It again has versatility in that it can be given not only orally but subcutaneously, epidurally, and intravenously. Methadone may have a negative stigma attached to it because it is the maintenance medication for many recovering drug addicts. The reason it works so well in this situation is its 12-hourly oral dosing to prevent withdrawal symptoms from those patients with narcotic dependence. These negative associations should not prevent its use for the chronic cancer pain pa-

tient. Often in patients in which morphine, at large doses, no longer provides adequate pain control, an equipotent regimen of methadone can provide suitable analgesia (Table 26-3).

The changes in cancer treatment modalities have brought increased survival, particularly in pediatric cancers and thus pain management regimens may also reflect this increased survival. It is particularly important that pediatric cancer patients have flexibility to receive treatment in the more familiar home environment.[114] Chronic pain management is then necessary to allow the child to return home and for the terminal child to continue treatment outside of the acute hospital setting. A multidisciplinary management team is important in allowing this transition. There has been work in Great Britain with hospice care for terminally ill children.[115] Its utility is increased in a high maintenance patient, and for giving a family respite from the labor intensive care of their ill child rather than simply readmitting the child to the hospital. Continued work in this realm is clearly needed to provide optimal care for the terminally ill child.

The effective management of pediatric cancer pain is challenging to the health care professional. It requires not only an understanding of pediatric malignancies and their painful manifestations but also the ability to assess the type and intensity of pain in this population. The health care professional must also be adept at combining the various therapeutic modalities, whether it is using analgesics or regional anesthetic techniques to optimize each individual child's pain control. Many institutions now use a multidisciplinary pain management team to best manage these complex parameters. An important point to consider in cancer pain control is that it is not static. Therapy must be continuously assessed and adapted to meet changes in a patient's condition. From the diagnosis of cancer through to the terminal stages of disease there are different needs that must be met, and we as health care professionals must continuously strive to improve our ability to recognize and treat the spectrum of cancer pain that is present in the pediatric population.

Table 26-3. Administrative Routes and Dosages for Morphine and Methadone

	Morphine	Methadone
MS Contin	0.3–0.6 mg q12h PO	0.1–0.2 mg/kg q6–12h PO
Roxanol		
MS Elixir	0.3–0.5 mg/kg q3–4h PO	0.2 mg/kg q4h SQ
Infusion	0.4–0.7 mg/kg/hr	0.1 mg/kg q6–12h IV
PCA	Total dose per hour: 0.05–0.1 mg/kg/hr	
	Background infusion: one-fourth hourly dose	
	PCA bolus dose: total hourly dose	
	divided at 8–10 minute intervals1[116]	

PCA = patient-controlled analgesia.

References

1. Elliott SC, Miser AW, Dose AM, et al. Epidemiologic features of pain in pediatric cancer patients: A co-operative community-based study. Clin J Pain 1991;7:263.
2. Miser AW, Miser JS. The treatment of cancer pain in children. Pediatr Clin North Am 1989;36:979.
3. Cancer Pain Relief. Geneva: World Health Organization, 1986.
4. Danesh BJ, Saniabadi AR, Russell RI, Lowe GA. Therapeutic potential of choline magnesium salicylate as an alternative to aspirin for patients with bleeding tendencies. Scott Med J 1987;33:167.
5. Yaster M, Deshpande JK. Management of pediatric pain with opioid analgesics. J Pediatr 1988;113:421.
6. Shannon M, Berde CB. Pharmacologic management of pain in children and adolescents. Pediatr Clin North Am 1989;36:855.
7. Swafford LI, Allan D. Pain relief in the pediatric patient. Med Clin North Am 1968;52:131.
8. Mather L, Mackie J. The incidence of postoperative pain in children. Pain 1983;15:271.
9. Balis FM, Lester CM, Chraisos GP, et al. Differences in cerebrospinal fluid penetration of corticosteroids: Possible relationship to the prevention of meningeal leukemias. J Clin Oncol 1987;5:202.
10. Maltie AA, Cavenar JO, Sullivan JL, et al. Analgesia and haloperidol: A hypothesis. J Clin Psychiatry 1979;40:323.
11. Bruera E, Chadwick S, Brenneis C, et al. Methylphenidate associated with narcotics for the treatment of cancer pain. Cancer Treat Rep 1987;71:67.
12. Hilgard J, LeBaron S. Relief of anxiety and pain in children with cancer: Quantitative measures and qualitative clinical observation in a flexible approach. Int J Clin Exp Hypn 1982;30:417.
13. Zeltzer LK, LeBaron S. Hypnotic and non-hypnotic techniques for reduction of pain and anxiety during painful procedures in children and adolescents with cancer. J Pediatr 1982;101:1032.
14. Siegel LJ. Preparation of children for hospitalization: A selected review of the research literature. J Pediatr Psychol 1976;1:26.
15. Mitchell AA, Louik C, Lacouture P, et al. Risks to children from computed tomographic scan premedication. JAMA 1982;246:2385.
16. Guidelines for monitoring and management of pediatric patients during and after sedation for diagnostic and therapeutic procedures. Pediatrics 1992;89:1110.
17. Yaster M, Nichols DG, Deshpande JK, Wetzel RC. Midazolam-fentanyl intravenous sedation in children: Case report of respiratory arrest. Pediatrics 1990;86:464.
18. Fisher DM, Robinson S, Brett CM, et al. Comparison of enflurane, halothane, and isoflurane for outpatient pediatric anesthesia. Anesthesiology 1985;63:647.
19. Rowland AS, Baird DD, Weinberg CR, et al. Reduced fertility among women employed as dental assistants exposed to high levels of nitrous oxide. N Engl J Med 1992;327:993.
20. Layzer RB. Myeloneuropathy after prolonged exposure to nitrous oxide. Lancet 1978;ii:1227.
21. Eisele JH, Smith NT. Cardiovascular effects of 40% nitrous oxide in man. Anesth Analg 1972;51:956.
22. Schulte-Sasse U, Hess W, Tarnow J. Pulmonary vascular responses to nitrous oxide in patients with normal and high pulmonary vascular resistance. Anesthesiology 1982;57:9.
23. Suzuki KS, Konno M, Kirikae T, et al. Effects of prolonged nitrous oxide exposure on hemopoietic stem cells in splenectomized mice. Anesth Analg 1990;71:389.
24. Schilling RF. Is nitrous oxide a dangerous anesthetic for vitamin B12-deficient subjects? JAMA 1986;255:1605.
25. Koblin DD, Tomerson BW, Waldman FM, et al. Effect of nitrous oxide on folate and vitamin B_{12} metabolism in patients. Anesth Analg 1990;71:610.
26. Nunn JF, O'Morain C. Nitrous oxide decreases motility of human neutrophils in vitro. Anesthesiology 1982;56:45.
27. Rosland JH, Hole K. 1,4-Benzodiazepines antagonize opiate-induced antinociception in mice. Anesth Analg 1990;71:242.

28. Sandler ES, Weyman C, Conner K, et al. Midazolam versus fentanyl as premedication for painful procedures in children with cancer. Pediatrics 1992;89:613.

29. Friedman AG, Mulhern RK, Fairclough D, et al. Midazolam premedication for pediatric bone marrow aspiration and lumbar puncture. Med Pediatr Oncol 1991;19:499.

30. Beebe DS, Belani KG, Chang P, et al. Effectiveness of preoperative sedation with rectal midazolam, ketamine, or their combination in young children. Anesth Analg 1992;75:880.

31. McMillian CO, Spahr-Schopfer IA, Sikich N, et al. Premedication of children with oral midazolam. Can J Anaesth 1992;39:545.

32. Theroux MC, West DW, Corddry DH, et al. Efficacy of intranasal midazolam in facilitating suturing of lacerations in preschool children in the emergency department. Pediatrics 1993;91:624.

33. Karl HW, Rosenberger JL, Larach MG, Ruffle JM. Transmucosal administration of midazolam for premedication of pediatric patients. Anesthesiology 1993;78:885.

34. Domino EF, Chodoff P, Corssen G. Pharmacologic effects of CI-581: A new dissociative anesthetic in man. Clin Pharmacol Ther 1965;6:279.

35. Corssen G, Miyasaka M, Domino EF. Changing concepts in pain control during surgery: Dissociative anesthesia with CI-581. Anesth Analg 1968;47:746.

36. Jastak JT, Goretta C. Ketamine as a continuous drip anesthesia for outpatients. Anesth Analg 1973;52:341.

37. Rees DI, Howell ML. Ketamine-atracurium by continuous infusion as the sole anesthetic for pulmonary surgery. Anesth Analg 1986;65:860.

38. Clausen L, Sinclair DM, Van Hasselt CH. Intravenous ketamine for postoperative analgesia. S Afr Med J 1975;49:1437.

39. Ito Y, Ichivanagi I. Postoperative pain relief with ketamine infusion. Anaesthesia 1974;29:222.

40. Sheref SE. Ketamine and bronchospasm. Anaesthesia 1985;40:701.

41. Saegusa K, Furukawa Y, Ogiwara Y. Pharmacologic analysis of ketamine-induced cardiac actions in isolated, blood-perfused canine atria. J Cardiovasc Pharmacol 1986;8:414.

42. Chernow B, Laker R, Creuss D, et al. Plasma, urine, and cerebrospinal fluid catecholamine concentrations during and after ketamine sedation. Crit Care Med 1982;10:600.

43. Wayman K, Shoemaker WC, Lippmann M. Cardiovascular effects of anesthetic induction with ketamine. Anesth Analg 1980;59:355.

44. Spotoft H, Korshin JD, Sorensen MB, et al. The cardiovascular effects of ketamine used for induction of anesthesia in patients with valvular heart disease. Can Anaesth Soc J 1979;26:463.

45. Gooding JM, Dimick AR, Travakoli M, et al. A physiologic analysis of cardiopulmonary responses to ketamine anesthesia in non-cardiac patients. Anesth Analg 1977;56:813.

46. Morray JP, Lynn AM, Stamm SJ, et al. Hemodynamic effects of ketamine in children with congenital heart disease. Anesth Analg 1984;63:895.

47. Hickey PR, Hansen DD, Cramolini GM, et al. Pulmonary and systemic hemodynamic responses to ketamine in infants with normal and elevated pulmonary vascular resistance. Anesthesiology 1985;62:287.

48. Mankikian B, Cantineau JP, Sartene R, et al. Ventilatory and chest wall mechanics during ketamine anesthesia in humans. Anesthesiology 1986;65:492.

49. Hirshman CA, Downes H, Farbood A, Bergman NA. Ketamine block of bronchospasm in experimental canine asthma. Br J Anaesth 1979;51:713.

50. Bourke DL, Malit LA, Smith TC. Respiratory interactions of ketamine and morphine. Anesthesiology 1987;66:153.

51. Lanning CF, Harmel MH. Ketamine anesthesia. Annu Rev Med 1975;26:137.

52. Taylor PA, Towey RM. Depression of laryngeal reflexes during ketamine administration. Br Med J 1971;2:688.

53. Shapiro HM, Wyte SR, Harris AB. Ketamine anesthesia in patients with intracranial pathology. Br J Anaesth 1972;44:1200.

54. Gardner AE, Dannemiller FJ, Dean D. Intracranial cerebrospinal fluid pressure in man during ketamine anesthesia. Anesth Analg 1972:51:741.

55. Reicher D, Bhalla P, Rubinstein EH. Cholinergic cerebral vasodilator effects of ketamine in rabbits. Stroke 1987;18:445.

56. Oren RE, Rasool NA, Rubinstein EH. Effect of ketamine on cerebral cortical blood flow and metabolism in rabbits. Stroke 1987;18:445.

57. White PR, Way WL, Trevor AJ. Ketamine: Its pharmacology and therapeutic uses. Anesthesiology 1982;56:119.

58. Tobias JD, Phipps S, Smith B, Mulhern RK. Oral ketamine premedication to alleviate the distress of invasive procedures in pediatric oncology patients. Pediatrics 1992;90:537.

59. Weksler N, Ovadia L, Muati G, Stav A. Nasal ketamine for pediatric premedication. Can J Anaesth 1993;40:119.

60. Sebel PS, Lowdon JD. Propofol: A new intravenous anesthetic. Anesthesiology 1989;71:260.

61. Harris CE, Grounds RM, Murray AM, et al. Propofol for long-term sedation in the intensive care unit. A comparison with papaverum and midazolam. Anaesthesia 1990;45:366.

62. Beller JP, Pottecher T, Lugnier A, et al. Prolonged sedation with propofol in ICU patients: Recovery and blood concentration changes during periodic interruptions infusions. Br J Anaesth 1988;61:583.

63. Brussel T, Theissen JL, Vigfusson G, et al. Hemodynamic and cardiodynamic effects of propofol and etomidate: Negative inotropic properties of propofol. Anesth Analg 1989;69:35.

64. Trotter C, Serpell MG. Neurological sequelae in children after prolonged propofol infusions. Anaesthesia 1992;47:340.

65. Saunders PRI, Harris MNE. Opisthotonic posturing and other unusual neurological sequelae after outpatient anesthesia. Anaesthesia 1992;47:552.

66. Collier C, Kelly K. Propofol and convulsions: The evidence mounts. Anaesth Intensive Care 1991;19:573.

67. Finley GA, MacManus B, Sampson SE, et al. Delayed seizures following sedation with propofol. Can J Anaesth 1993;40:863.

68. Nahata MC, Clotz MA, Krogg EA. Adverse effects of meperidine, promethazine, and chlorpromazine for sedation in pediatric patients. Clin Pediatr 1985;24:558.

69. Benini F, Johnston C, Faucher D, et al. Topical anesthesia during circumcision in newborn infants. JAMA 1993;270:850.

70. Halperin DL, Koren G, Attias D, et al. Topical skin anesthesia for venous, subcutaneous drug reservoir and lumbar punctures in children. Pediatrics 1989;84:281.

71. Merskey H. On the development of pain. Headache 1970;10:116.

72. Maxwell LG, Yaster M, Wetzel RC, et al. Penile nerve block for newborn circumcision. Obstet Gynecol 1987;70:415.

73. Anand KJS, Hansen DD, Hickey PR. Hormonal-metabolic stress responses in neonates undergoing cardiac surgery. Anesthesiology 1990;73:661.

74. Anand KJS, Hickey PR. Halothane-morphine compared with high-dose sufentanil for anesthesia and postoperative analgesia in neonatal cardiac surgery. N Engl J Med 1992;326:1.

75. Anand KJS, Sippel WG, Aynsley-Green A. A randomized trial of fentanyl anesthesia in preterm babies undergoing surgery: Effects on the stress response. Lancet 1987;1:243.

76. Maunuksela EL, Olkkola KT, Korpela R. Does prophylactic intravenous infusion of indomethacin improve the management of postoperative pain in children? Can J Anaesth 1988;35:123.

77. Watcha MF, Jones MB, Lagueruela R, et al. Comparison of ketorolac and morphine as adjuvants during pediatric surgery. Anesthesiology 1992;76:368.

78. Rutter PC, Murphy F, Dudley HAF. Morphine: Controlled trial of different methods of administration for postoperative pain relief. Br Med J 1980;280:12.

79. Miser AW, Davis DM, Hughes CS, et al. Continuous subcutaneous infusion of morphine in children with cancer. Am J Dis Child 1983;137:383.

80. Storey P, Hill HH, St. Louis RH, et al. Subcutaneous infusions for control of cancer symptoms. J Pain Symptom Manage 1990;5:33.

81. Bruera E, Fainsinger R, Moore M, et al. Local toxicity with subcutaneous methadone. Pain 1991;45:141.

82. Cole L, Hanniing CD. Review of the rectal use of opioids. J Pain Symptom Manage 1990;5:118.

83. Ashburn MA, Streisand JB, Tarver SD, et al. Oral transmucosal fentanyl citrate for premedication in paediatric outpatients. Can J Anaesth 1990;37:857.

84. Goldstein-Dresner MC, Davis PJ, Kretchman E, et al. Double-blind comparison of oral transmucosal fentanyl citrate with oral meperidine, diazepam, and atropine as preanesthetic medication in children with congenital heart disease. Anesthesiology 1991;74:28.

85. Henderson JM, Brodsky DA, Fisher DM, et al. Preinduction of anesthesia in pediatric patients with nasally administered sufentanil. Anesthesiology 1988;68:671.

86. Striebel HW, Koenigs D, Kramer J. Postoperative pain management by intranasal demand-adapted fentanyl titration. Anesthesiology 1992;77:281.

87. Holley FR, van Steenis C. Postoperative analgesia with fentanyl: Pharmacokinetics and pharmacodynamics at constant intravenous and transdermal delivery. Br J Anaesth 1989;63:56.

88. Miser AW, Narang PK, Dothage JA, et al. Transdermal fentanyl for pain control in patients with cancer. Pain 1989;37:15.

89. Payne R. Experience with transdermal fentanyl in advanced cancer pain. Eur J Pain 1990;11:98.

90. Tobias JD. Transdermal fentanyl: Applications and indications in the pediatric patient. Am J Pain Manage 1992;2:30.

91. Duthie DJR, Rowbotham DJ, Wyld R, et al. Plasma fentanyl concentrations during transdermal delivery of fentanyl in surgical patients. Br J Anaesth 1988;60:614.

92. Rosow CE, Moss J, Philbin DM, et al. Histamine release during morphine and fentanyl anesthesia. Anesthesiology 1982;56:93.

93. Gourlay GK, Wilson PR, Glynn CJ. Pharmacodynamics and pharmacokinetics of methadone during the perioperative period. Anesthesiology 1982;57:458.

94. Gourlay GK, Wilson PR, Lamberty J. A double-blinded comparison of morphine and methadone in postoperative pain control. Anesthesiology 1986;64:322.

95. Berde CB, Beyer JE, Bournaki MC, et al. Comparison of morphine and methadone for prevention of postoperative pain in children. J Pediatr 1991;119:136.

96. Shochet RB, Murray GB. Neuropsychiatric toxicity of meperidine. J Intensive Care Med 1988;3:246.

97. Vetter TR. Pediatric patient-controlled analgesia with morphine versus meperidine. J Pain Symptom Manage 1992;7:204.

98. Berde CB, Lehn BM, Yee JD, et al. Patient-controlled analgesia in children and adolescents: A randomized, prospective comparison with intramuscular administration of morphine for postoperative analgesia. J Pediatr 1991;118:460.

99. Gaukroger PB, Omkins DP, Van Der Walt JH. Patient-controlled analgesia in children. Anaesth Intens Care 1989;17:264.

100. Lawrie SC, Forbes DW, Akhtar TM, et al. Patient-controlled analgesia in children. Anaesthesia 1990;46:1074.

101. Parker RK, Holtman B, White PF. Patient-controlled analgesia: Does a concurrent opioid infusion improve pain management after surgery. JAMA 1991;266:1947.

102. Parker RK, Holtman B, White PF. Effects of a night-time opioid infusion with PCA therapy on patient comfort and analgesic requirements after abdominal hysterectomy. Anesthesiology 1992;76:362.

103. Porter J, Jick J. Addiction rare in patients treated with narcotics [letter]. N Engl J Med 1980;302:123.

104. Arnold JH, Truog RD, Orav EJ, et al. Tolerance and dependence in neonates sedated with fentanyl during extracorporeal membrane oxygenation. Anesthesiology 1990;73:1136.

105. Tobias JD, Schleien CS, Haun SE. Methadone as treatment for iatrogenic narcotic dependency in pediatric intensive care unit patients. Crit Care Med 1991;18:1292.

106. Tobias JD, Desphpande JK, Gregory DF. Outpatient therapy of iatrogenic drug dependency following prolonged sedation in the pediatric intensive care unit. Intern Care Med 1994;20:504.

107. Payen D, Ecoffey C, Carli P, et al. Pulsed Doppler ascending aortic, carotid, brachial, and femoral artery blood flows during caudal anesthesia in infants. Anesthesiology 1987;67:681.

108. Etches RC, Sandler AN, Daley MD. Respiratory depression and spinal opioids. Can J Anaesth 1989;36:165.

109. Tobias JD, Oakes L, Rao B. Continuous epidural anesthesia for postoperative analgesia in the pediatric oncology patient. Am J Pediatr Hematol Oncol 1992;14:216.

110. Tobias JD, Lowe S, O'Dell N, Holcomb GW III. Thoracic epidural anaesthesia in infants and children. Can J Anaesth 1993;40:879.

111. Tobias JD, Flanagan J. Regional anesthesia in the preterm neonate. Clin Pediatr 1992;31:668.

112. Tobias JD, Deshpande JK, Wetzel RC, et al. Postoperative analgesia: Use of intrathecal morphine in children. Clin Pediatr 1990;29:44.

113. Tobias JD. Postdural puncture headache in children: Etiology and treatment. Clin Pediatr 1994;33:110.

114. Goldman A, Feret J, Bartollotta C, Weisman SJ. Pain in Terminal Illness (Home Care). In NL Schechter, CB Berde, M Yaster (eds), Pain in Infants, Children and Adolescents. Baltimore: William & Wilkins, 1993.

115. Goldman A, Beardsmore S, Hunt J. Palliative care for children with cancer: Home, hospital or hospice? Arch Dis Child 1990;65:641.

116. Bell C, Hughes CW, Oh TH. The Pediatric Anesthesia Handbook. St. Louis: Mosby, 1991.

Chapter 27

Management of Pain Due to Herpes Zoster and Postherpetic Neuralgia

P. Prithvi Raj

Herpes zoster, commonly known as *shingles*, is an acute infectious disease caused by a herpes zoster virus belonging to the DNA group of viruses. It primarily affects the posterior spinal root ganglion of the spinal nerves.[1] The term *herpes zoster* is derived from the Greek; *herpes* means "to creep" and *zoster* refers to a belt. Shingles is an Anglican form of the Latin word *cingulus* or the French word *chingle,* both meaning a belt or girdle. Herpes zoster appropriately describes the girdle-like vesicular eruption of the disease in the trunk. *Varicella* is a French term for variola (smallpox), because varicella was originally considered to be a lesser form of smallpox. The term *chickenpox* is probably derived from the similarity of the size of the lesions to a seed-producing plant called "pois chiche" by the French and anglicized to chickpea and later chickenpox.

Incidence

The incidence is approximately 125 per 100,000 per year in the general population. There does not appear to be a seasonal variation, and both sexes are equally affected. Age is a major factor in both the incidence of herpes zoster and in the development of postherpetic neuralgia (PHN). The disease is less common in early childhood, relatively constant between 20 and 50 years of age, then increases sharply in later decades.[1] Incidence in octogenarians is 5–10 in 1,000, whereas children have an incidence of 0.5 in 1,000 (Figure 27-1).[2] The reason for this increase with age is not clear but immunocompromise may be an explanation.[3] Less well understood is the observation that PHN develops almost exclusively in patients over the age of 50 years. The incidence of PHN ranges from 15–70%,[4–7] with most patients being in their sixth to ninth decades.[3] Herpes zoster may be triggered by surgery or trauma, irradiation and other immunosuppressive agents, arsenic, malignancies, or diseases such as tuberculosis, syphilis, and malaria. A distinction may be made between idiopathic zoster and secondary herpes zoster, which occurs as a result of inflammation, neoplasm, or injury directly to the cranial or peripheral nerve. Secondary zoster may be more frequently recurrent, clears more rapidly, and perhaps results in less scarring and pigmentation, although these differences may not be valid.[8]

Herpes zoster is more common and severe in immunosuppressed patients, especially in patients with Hodgkin's lymphoma, non-Hodgkin's lymphoma, or chronic lymphocytic leukemia, in patients receiving irradiation or chemotherapy (for cancer or after transplantation), or in patients with lupus erythematosus.[9–11] Recently, herpes zoster has become a major problem after radiochemotherapy and bone marrow transplantation, correlating with depressed cell-mediated immunity.[12] Patients deficient in T-lymphocyte macrophage–mediated immune defenses are more susceptible to the spread of virus beyond the ganglion nerve-dermatome unit. In such patients, visceral and nervous system complications represent a major threat.[13]

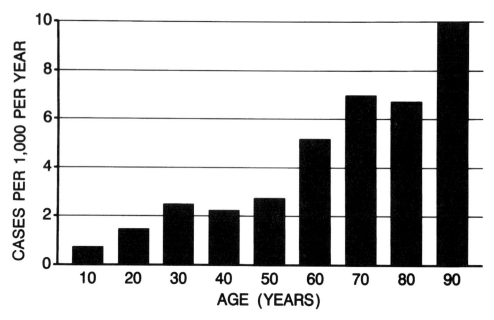

Figure 27-1. Incidence of herpes zoster with age. (Reprinted with permission from JD Loeser. Review article: Herpes zoster and postherpetic neuralgia. Pain 1986;25:149.)

Acute Herpes Zoster

Clinical Manifestations and Course

The development and course of herpes zoster depends on the virus and the host. It can progress in three stages, with virus and host factors interacting at each stage (Table 27-1).

Location of Lesions

The lesions appear in thoracic dermatomes in more than 50% of patients; in the trigeminal distribution in 3–20% of patients; the ophthalmic division in 75% of patients. Lumbar and cervical eruptions occur in 10–20% of patients, with a sacral distribution being much less common. With advancing age, the incidence of trigeminal (ophthalmic) zoster increases and that of spinal zoster declines. Bilateral zoster occurs in less than 1% of patients. Recurrent

zoster has been reported in 1–8% of patients; approximately one-half of the recurrences are at the site of the previous eruption (Table 27-2).

Signs and Symptoms

Acute herpes zoster typically presents acutely with pain, parasthesiae, and dysesthesiae in the dermatomal distribution of one or more affected posterior root ganglia. The pain may be accompanied by systemic symptoms such as fever, malaise, headache, nausea, stiff neck, and regional or diffuse adenopathy. These symptoms are present in 5% of the patients and do not seem to be correlated with the likelihood of any complications, including PHN. At first, the pain is usually mild but may increase in intensity over the succeeding days. It has variously been described as sharp, shooting, dull, aching, or burning. A vesicular eruption usually appears within 4–5 days but may appear earlier.

Table 27-1. Stages of Herpes Zoster

Stage I	Viral replication
	Loss of immune surveillance
Stage II	Clinical syndrome (acute herpes zoster)
	Viral effect on ganglion nerve-dermatome
	Antiviral immune response by the body
	Cytolysin from virus and host inflammatory reaction
Stage III	Sequelae of herpes zoster
	Central nervous system and visceral spread
	Antiviral immune response

Source: Reprinted with permission from RW Price. Herpes zoster: An approach to systemic therapy. Med Clin North Am 1982;66:1105.

Table 27-2. Site and Incidence of Acute Herpes Zoster

Site of Herpes Zoster	Incidence (Percentage)
Thoracic	50
Face (ophthalmic)	3–20
Cervical	10–20
Bilateral	< 1
Recurrent	1–8
Recurrent at the site of previous herpes zoster	50

The initial presentation is localized erythema and swelling, followed by red papules that progress through vesicles, blebs, pustules, and then crust over within 2–3 weeks. Characteristically, the lesions are unilateral in a dermatomal distribution. In mild cases, the skin lesions appear in only part of the dermatome but a thorough examination reveals that the sensation of the entire segment is affected. In more severe cases, the entire segment is involved, the blebs are larger and tend to coalesce, the burning discomfort is continuous, and any movement or change in tension of the skin will precipitate sharp, burning pain.

In most cases, during the third week, the erythema begins to resolve. The blebs dry up and become wrinkled and the sharp pain begins to recede. By the fifth week, scales of the encrusting blebs begin to fall off, leaving irregularly shaped pink scars. These scars gradually retract, producing the characteristic pocks devoid of pigment. The hyperesthesia and hyperalgesia may remain for a longer period of time but will resolve gradually over the ensuing months and the patient will become asymptomatic.

Differential Diagnosis

The diagnosis of herpes zoster is usually difficult to make in the pre-eruptive stage. Once the lesions appear, the clinical features are characteristic and the diagnosis is easy.

Prior to eruption, herpes zoster is often mistaken for other pain-causing conditions such as coronary disease, pleurisy, pleurodynia, costochondritis (Tiet- ze's syndrome), pericarditis, cholecystitis, neural disease, acute and subacute abdominal conditions, appendicitis, collapsed intervertebral disk, neuropathies, myofascial pains, and so forth.

Pathophysiology of Nociception

Although pathologic changes have been demonstrated in both herpes zoster and PHN, the mechanisms by which they produce the respective pain syndromes are poorly understood. In acute herpes zoster, activation of nociceptive primary afferents by direct viral attack, and secondary inflammatory changes in skin, nerve, posterior root ganglion, nerve roots, leptomeninges, and the spinal cord are reasonable explanations of the pain in most patients (Figures 27-2 and 27-3). The pathophysiology of PHN is more obscure and may involve both peripheral and central mechanisms. The observation of preferential loss of large nerve fibers has led to the hypothesis that impairment of segmental pain-modulating systems may play a role; as modeled in the gate control theory of pain, diminished large-fiber function may allow increased transmission of nociceptive information through the dorsal horn of the spinal cord (Figure 27-4).[14] Recently, it has been postulated that dysesthetic pain in peripheral nerve lesions may be due to damaged or regenerating nociceptive afferent fibers, and aching or stabbing pain may relate to the activation of nociceptive nervi nervorum, primary afferent fibers investing the nerve trunk itself.[15] These mechanisms may be important in PHN because it has been suggested that they are

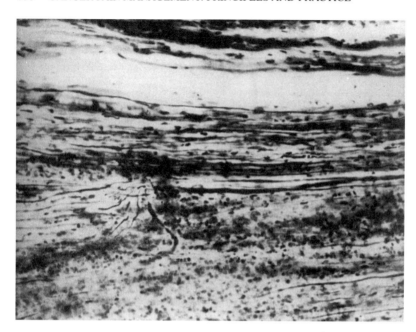

Figure 27-2. Sensory peripheral nerve showing pleomorphism, edema, and hemorrhage due to neuritis caused by herpes zoster.

Figure 27-3. Postmortem histopathologic structure of spinal ganglion in a 67-year-old patient suffering with post-herpetic neuralgia for 5 years before death.

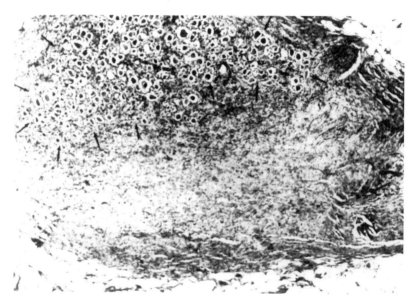

the reason why proximal deafferenting procedures such as neurectomy, spinothalamic tractotomy, or thalamotomy fail to provide sustained relief of pain. The pain of PHN is typically described as continuous aching, itching, or burning, often with superimposed severe lancinating pains that are precipitated by touching or moving the involved area. The region becomes hyperesthetic and there is frequently exquisite tenderness around vesicles that can worsen as ulceration and secondary infection occur.[16]

Treatment Goals

The goals of treatment are an early resolution of the acute disease and prevention of PHN. The earlier the treatment for herpes zoster is started, the less likely that the patient will develop PHN.[17–19]

In attempting to answer the question as to whether treating acute herpes zoster prevents PHN, Pernak reported on a prospective randomized large study of 1,011 patients.[20] She divided her patients

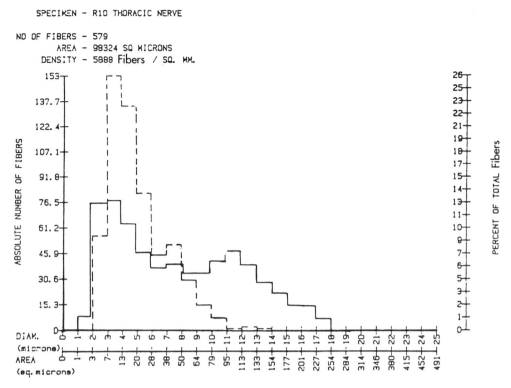

Figure 27-4. The figure shows a decrease in large fibers and proportionately higher number of small C fibers in postherpetic neuralgia patients with pain.

in four groups according to the location of the lesions (333 patients with trigeminal neuralgia and 678 patients with lesions located on the trunk). Methylprednisolone (80 mg) was injected on the gasserian ganglion for trigeminal neuralgia while 80–160 mg of methylprednisolone with 0.5% of lidocaine was injected epidurally at appropriate epidural locations. Excellent pain relief was obtained in 997 patients. Fourteen patients developed PHN. All 14 of them had persistent acute herpes zoster pain for 3 weeks. Pernak concluded that the regional application of corticosteroids is effective in pain relief and preventing PHN.

Prevention

Prevention of herpes zoster includes preventing establishment of latent infection, preventing viral neuronal reactivation, and ensuring adequate immune surveillance to maintain the reactivated virus at a subclinical level. At this time, however, none of these approaches appear to be practical. The first goal to prevent the infection is closest to being accomplished but still remains remote. Recent studies indicate that varicella in immunosuppressed children can be prevented by a live attenuated varicella zoster virus (VZV) vaccine.[21] In patients with latent VZV infection neither active nor passive immunization is likely to reduce the subsequent incidence of zoster.[22] In immunosuppressed patients, both impaired capacity to react to specific antigenic stimulation and loss of nonspecific immune effector mechanisms may contribute to development of zoster and not be effected by active immunization.

Therapeutic Approach

In immunocompetent patients, the segmental infection is stopped by intrinsic host defenses. This intrinsic host defense is inadequate in immunodeficient patients. Terminating viral replication and spread is the major way to prevent tissue injury. In fact, the

Table 27-3. Systemic Treatment Modalities for Acute Herpes Zoster

Antiviral therapy
  Viral DNA polymerase dependent
    Vidarabine
  Viral thymidine kinase dependent
    Acyclovir
    E-5-(2-bromovinyl)-2'-deoxyuridine (BVDU)
    2'-fluoro-5-ido-l-ß-1-arabinosylcytosine (FIAC)
    Interferon
Anti-inflammatory
  Corticosteroids

Source: Reprinted with permission from RW Price. Herpes zoster: An approach to systemic therapy. Med Clin North Am 1982;66:1105.

organ damage is principally related to the direct effect of viral parasitism with attendant cytolysis. Host immune and inflammatory responses also contribute significantly to tissue injury. It is this consideration that provides the basis for the use of anti-inflammatory agents.

Treatment Modalities

Antiviral Therapies

Considerable progress has been made in recent years in the use of antiviral agents (Table 27-3).[23] Within the last decade, truly effective systemic antiviral therapy for VZV infections has been introduced. Table 27-4 lists several antivirals and tentatively classifies them according to their mechanisms of action. The first medication to be shown to be truly effective after systemic administration was vidarabine. Although the mechanism of action of the drug is not precisely established, its selective activity may involve an effect on virus-coded DNA polymerase.[24] This drug is incorporated into both viral and cellular DNA. The efficacy of vidarabine in immunosuppressed patients with acute herpes zoster has now been well established.[25] When administered early in the course of infection (within the first 72 hours after the onset of rash), the drug reduced spread of the rash over the primary dermatome, accelerated healing, and prevented both cutaneous dissemination and visceral complications compared with placebo. A decrease in the duration of acute pain and PHN was also suggested. Acute drug toxicity was minimal and

included jitteriness and hallucinations, nausea and vomiting, and subclinical abnormalities in liver enzymes. In immunosuppressed patients, vidarabine therefore appears to be both effective and safe. Its major drawbacks are potential short- and long-term toxicity, and the need for intravenous infusion (a dose of 10 mg per kg by continuous 12-hour infusion for 5 days is recommended), which requires concomitant hospitalization.

A second class of antiviral drugs has been introduced recently. Drugs in this group share a mechanism of action that depends on the expression of viral thymidine kinase (TK) within infected cells. Of these, acyclovir has been investigated most extensively.[26–29] Other antivirals with a similar mechanism of action include E-5-(2-bromovinyl)-2'-deoxyuridine and (2'-fluoro-5-idi-1-ß-1)-arabinosylcytosine.[30, 31] These drugs are currently being investigated and appear to be even more potent antivirals than acyclovir. These drugs actually exploit two virus-coded enzymes in their selective antiviral effect: viral TK and DNA polymerase. Acyclovir is selectively phosphorylated by viral TK, and its triphosphate derivative in turn selectively inhibits viral DNA polymerase, thereby preventing the synthesis and replication of viral DNA. This two-step mechanism of action ensures the drug's selectivity and underlies its apparent low toxicity for uninfected cells. Potential advantages of acyclovir include its apparent selectivity and potency, its lack of acute toxicity, and the benefits of oral administration.

Neumann and Chung retrospectively documented the effect of intravenous acyclovir treatment of acute herpes zoster on the incidence of PHN.[32] Eighteen patients were administered intravenous acyclovir to treat acute herpes zoster. The mean interval from onset of lesion to commencement of treatment was 13.5 days. The mean dose was 7.8 mg per kg administered on 2 consecutive days. The overall incidence between 44 and 89 years was 28%. However, 56% of the patients also received steroids systemically or regionally. This makes it difficult to interpret correctly the real effect of acyclovir on the incidence of PHN.

Anti-inflammatory Agents

Although the effects of corticosteroid therapy on herpes zoster are still unclear, preliminary reports

Table 27-4. Various Systemic Drugs Used for the Treatment of Acute Herpes Zoster and Postherpetic Neuralgia

	Dose	Efficacy	Side Effects
Antiepileptic and tricyclic drugs			
Amitriptyline[61, 70]	25 mg/day	Moderate pain relief	Weight gain, palpitations, dry mouth
Desipramine[71]	167 mg/day	Moderate pain relief	Drowsiness
Carbamazepine[72]	600–800 mg/day	Good pain relief	Drowsiness, dizziness, diplopia, tremors
Dephenyl-hydantoin[70]	300–400 mg/day		
GABA-nergic drugs			
Baclofen[72]	60–80 mg/day	Fair pain relief: synergism with carbamazepine and phenytoin	Drowsiness, vomiting
Purine nucleotide			
Adenosine monophosphate[55]	Intramuscularly three times a week for four weeks	Decreased virus shedding; 88% pain relief	None
Central nervous system stimulant			
Amantadine hydrochloride[74]	One capsule twice daily	Shorter duration of pain than placebo	Minimal
Antifungal/antibiotic			
Griseofulvin[75] Methisoprinol	125 mg qid	Combination was effective in reducing pain	Transient headache, nausea
Phenothiazines			
Chlorprothixene[76]	25 mg qid	Satisfactory pain relief	Lethargy

are encouraging. Gelfand found that patients treated with oral cortisone reported dramatic relief of pain in less than 2 days.[33] Appleman reported equally good pain relief in his patients within approximately the same time period with intradermal or intravenous corticotropin.[34] Elliot obtained excellent results treating patients with severely painful zoster with high doses of prednisone. The average duration of pain following early prednisone therapy was 3.5 days, whereas pain averaged 3.5 weeks in untreated controls.[35] These studies, however, involved only a small number of patients with few or no controls. Eaglstein et al. found that oral corticosteroids did not shorten the course of the infection or affect pain during the first 2 weeks, but did shorten the duration of PHN. Best results are obtained when treatment is started early in the course of the disease.[11] Inflammation and scarring are reduced with use of the anti-inflammatory agents. In spite of the unclear effects of corticosteroid therapy on herpes zoster,

they have been extensively used to treat this infection.[19] A double-blind, placebo-controlled study of oral triamcinolone in 34 patients with acute herpes zoster revealed analgesic efficacy without effect on lesion healing time. In patients over 60 years old, only 30% of those receiving the steroid had pain beyond 2 months compared with 73% of the control group. Treatment with steroids therefore appears to accelerate resolution of the pain.

The role of anti-inflammatory drugs in acute herpes zoster remains controversial. If host responses contribute significantly to tissue injury, then attenuation of these responses may be beneficial. Unfortunately, those host defenses that cause tissue injury may be largely inseparable from those that eliminate or prevent the spread of infection. At this point, dissociation of protective from harmful host responses to the virus has not been clearly demonstrated. On the other hand, in the immunocompetent patient, a vigorous antiviral response is only mildly altered by steroids. Similarly, in the face of potent antiviral coverage, even in the immunosuppressed patient, reduction of the inflammatory response may eventually prove safe and have a salutary effect. These are important issues for future investigation. This issue has been addressed for PHN. Two controlled trials have suggested that a course of systemic steroids during the acute phase of zoster is capable of preventing PHN.[11, 12] Both studies used immunologically normal older patients, and in neither were untoward complications of steroid therapy, including dissemination of infection, detected.

In a meta-analysis of the four well-controlled clinical studies conducted by Lycka, the results indicated a statistically significant decrease in proportions were effected at 6 and 12 weeks compared with usual incidences.[36] Standard difference scores were −2.0559 and −4.1442, respectively. At 24 weeks, no differences were detectable between placebo and corticosteroid treated groups (SD = 0.6603; $P > 0.05$). Side effects of the treatment were rare and mild, affecting only 2.5% of patients. No patients had dissemination of disease. Systemic corticosteroid treatment decreases the proportion of patients affected by PHN, especially when the pain begins 6–12 weeks after the acute event.

Steroids are usually used within the first 10 days and continued for as long as 3 weeks. Prednisone is usually the agent of choice. It may be given orally in doses of 60 mg per day the first week, 30 mg per day the second week, and 15 mg per day the third week.

Steroids have also been administered by subcutaneous injection under affected skin, with and without a local anesthetic. Enthusiastic reports of large numbers of patients claim 80–100% success in treating acute herpes zoster, with a rapid resolution of pain and diminished incidence of PHN. These are anecdotal reports and the experience of others has been less enthusiastic.

Systemic Analgesics and Adjuvant Agents

Analgesics. Analgesics are important adjunctive therapy to antidepressants. Analgesic drugs may be categorized as nonaddictive, moderately addictive, or strongly addictive agents.[37] Selecting the optimal agent for a specific patient involves considering a variety of factors including quality, intensity, dura-

tion, and distribution of pain.

Nonnarcotic, nonaddictive drugs are useful for mild pain. Acetylsalicylic acid and acetaminophen are effective and have a low incidence of side effects. However, they are not effective for severe pain.

Codeine, propoxyphene, pentazocine, and oxycodone are examples of moderately addictive drugs. The incidence of addiction is relatively low (except for oxycodone [Percodan]), but dependence may occur with any of them. They are good analgesic agents, but they sometimes produce adverse side effects such as constipation.

When used properly, strongly addictive narcotics are effective for severe refractory pain. However, they provide relief in varying degrees. In acute herpes zoster, strong medication may be needed to control severe pain. Because the acute stage is short, strongly addictive drugs may be used for a limited time. In such cases, the narcotic is tapered off as treatment decreases the degree of pain. When pain is at a level that can be controlled by nonnarcotic drugs, the narcotics should be discontinued. The assessment of the degree of pain is based on both objective and subjective findings as a means of preventing addiction. Examples of strongly addictive drugs are morphine, hydromorphone, and meperidine.

Antidepressants and Tranquilizers. Antidepressants are believed to have two mechanisms of action: They can relieve pain and they can relieve depression. Tricyclic drugs are known to block serotonin reuptake. They would, therefore, be expected to enhance the action of this neurotransmitter at synapses, and such enhancement can produce analgesia in laboratory animals. One mechanism active in the central pain states is that of some defect in the transmission system (the neuraxis, specifically), a deficit in serotonin.[38]

There is a strong consensus among clinical investigators that centrally active antidepressants deserve a trial for any patient who is not obtaining relief of pain, whether depressed or not. Tricyclics and anxiolytics are commonly given together because, although depression is not common in acute herpes zoster, many patients experience anxiety along with severe pain. The most widely used combination is amitriptyline (Elavil) and fluphenazine (Prolixin).

In addition to their antidepressant and analgesic properties, tricyclics are also sedatives. Elavil and doxepin (Sinequan) may correct the sleep disturbance, frequent awakening, and early morning awakening that are common in severe chronic pain states (see Table 27-4).

Adverse side effects of tricyclic antidepressants include hypotension or hypertension, tachycardia, arrhythmias, drowsiness, confusion, disorientation, dry mouth, blurred vision, increased intraocular pressure, urinary retention, and constipation.

Vitamins and Minerals. It is thought that the host-immune system is incompetent during the acute outbreak. As a result, vitamins, minerals, and improved general nutrition may help improve the immunologic system or make available a missing element.

Nerve Blocks

Repeated administration of local anesthetics at various sites along the segmental pathway affected by herpes zoster has been advocated widely for the pain management. Rosenak in 1938 was the first to report good results with procaine sympathetic or somatic blocks.[39] In an uncontrolled group of patients, these agents were injected subcutaneously under affected skin as somatic blocks in the epidural space around the peripheral nerve in the paravertebral space and as sympathetic blocks. In all cases, although the number of patients was usually small and the period of follow-up brief, the reported effects on pain were extraordinarily good.

Local Infiltration

In a large group of patients, Epstein used subcutaneous injections of 0.2% triamcinolone in normal saline under the areas of eruption and the sites of pain and itching. He obtained excellent results of nearly 100%, and the development of PHN was reduced to 2%. This study suggests that subcutaneous injections of steroids and local anesthetics offer an effective treatment with many benefits for acute herpes zoster patients, including no significant complications, a simple and inexpensive technique, and a fairly predictable response to treatment.[40, 41] Our own experience with this technique corroborates these results.

Somatic Nerve Blocks. Because nerve root involvement is suspected in acute herpes zoster, somatic nerve blocks have been used to treat it. These blocks can include brachial plexus, paravertebral,

intercostal, and sciatic blocks. Regrettably, they have been found to be of limited value in the acute phase and of no value in the PHN stage.

Sympathetic Nerve Blocks. As understanding of the pathology of herpes zoster progressed, attention was directed toward the sympathetic ganglia. Sympathetic blocks have been performed to relieve the vasospasm that was thought to cause the pain and nerve damage. Evidence suggests that sympathetic blockade performed during the acute phase of herpes zoster can help the immediate pain problem, often dramatically. Of greater value, however, is the possibility that it can prevent the development of PHN. Although the evidence for this is less clear, it is probably a worthwhile prophylactic measure that should be used as early as possible.

Trigeminal herpes zoster has been treated with bupivacaine in a block of the ipsilateral stellate ganglion. Dramatic and lasting relief of dysesthesia was obtained in about 77% of patients. Some discomfort and paresthesia of the affected area persisted for several weeks in about 22%. Pain recurred after initial relief in about 22%. Vesicular skin lesions dried more quickly than in untreated patients. Transient side effects included hoarseness, paresis of the ipsilateral arm, and paresis of the hemidiaphragm. The investigators were unable to make any conclusions because of the informality of the study, but believe that these preliminary results justify further investigation.[42]

Published experience has been greater with sympathetic blockade.[42–48] In two large uncontrolled surveys, pain relief occurred in 85–90% of patients treated within 2 weeks of onset with either a paraspinal block for PHN below the head or with a stellate ganglion block for cranial herpes zoster.[43, 45] One to four blocks usually provided relief. The success rate dropped to 40% in patients treated 2 weeks or more after onset. The incidence of PHN was less than reported in epidemiologic surveys of untreated patients, suggesting that sympathetic blockade is effective in preventing this complication. Another study found no reduction in the incidence of PHN in a group of patients treated with a variety of anesthetic techniques. Thus, although the weight of anecdotal evidence suggests that sympathetic blockade is an effective measure for the treatment of pain early in the courses of herpes zoster, the reports of its use remain empirical until controlled studies of this and other anesthetic techniques are done. Lipton reports that in a controlled series of 15 patients with trigeminal neuralgia, stellate ganglion block dramatically diminished the pain in the acute phase.[42]

Epidural Blocks. Epidural blocks using local anesthetic have been successful in acute herpes zoster. The duration of infection is shorter, the lesions dry faster, and pain is relieved. In a small study examining patients with herpes zoster of 7 weeks or less duration, Perkins and Hanlon obtained 70–100% immediate relief, 90–100% relief 24 hours after treatment, and 100% relief in a 1- to 5-month follow-up. There was no subsequent report of PHN. Their studies suggested that local anesthetic alone was effective and that the inclusion of corticosteroids did not increase benefits.[49]

Spinal Blocks. Subarachnoid blocks are not usually indicated because they are not as specific as epidural blocks. A patient who has had a laminectomy in the affected area would be an exception.

Neurolytic Blocks. Neurolytic blocks are not indicated in acute herpes zoster.

Efficacy of Nerve Blocks

In a prospective study, Berger and Perkins compared the efficacy of epidural methylprednisolone alone or combined with lidocaine for treatment of PHN.[50] Group I (13 patients) received 160 mg of methylprednisolone, whereas group II (13 patients) received in addition to 160 mg of methylprednisolone, 10–20 ml of 1% lidocaine with epinephrine (1 to 200,000). If pain persisted after the first block, the block was repeated within 1 week. Significant relief occurred in both groups. In group I, 10 of 13 patients had 75% relief after one block, and 90% relief after the second block. In group II, 8 of 13 patients had 75% pain relief after the first block, but 9 patients required a second block. Patient relief persisted for 1 month at which time the study was terminated. They concluded that both techniques were effective in relieving PHN pain.

Miscellaneous Techniques

Topical Applications. Following a report on the usefulness of chloroform-aspirin for PHN, clinicians are actively pursuing, albeit anecdotally, various topical applications for their usefulness.[50–52] In one study, Morimoto et al. compared indomethacin stupe with chloroform-aspirin for efficacy in PHN.[53] They concluded that indomethacin stupe was superior to chloroform-aspirin for effectiveness and ease of use.

De Beneditio et al. have studied the effects of topically applied acetylsalicylic acid and ethyl ether for acute herpes zoster and PHN.[54] The method consists of crushing 750–1,500 mg of acetylsalicylic acid to a fine powder, adding 20–30 ml of ethyl ether, and then stirring the mixture until it has a uniform cloudiness. The emulsion is daubed onto the painful hyperpathic cutaneous areas. In their study, De Beneditio et al. found that of 15 patients with acute herpes zoster and 10 patients with PHN, excellent pain relief was obtained in 73% of acute cases and 50% in PHN. They recommended this method for acute herpes zoster and also as an alternative for PHN.

Topical capsaicin has been advocated for PHN.[51, 52] Drake et al. assessed the value of topical capsaicin in alleviating the symptoms associated with PHN.[51] In a double-blind trial of 30 patients over the age of 60 years, patients were randomly allocated to receive either 0.025% capsaicin cream or placebo applied five times per day for 1 week and four times a day for 3 weeks. Drake et al. concluded that 0.025% topical capsaicin was not effective in treating PHN.

Other Therapies. Transcutaneous electrical nerve stimulation is not usually used for acute herpes zoster. Ice therapy is a counterirritation technique based on the gate control theory. It is sometimes used alone in the acute stage to cool the area. Acupuncture and hypnosis are not usually used in acute herpes zoster. Surgery and neurosurgery are not indicated. The acute stage is self-limiting and does not require such drastic measures.

Recommended Therapeutic Strategy for Acute Herpes Zoster

It is useful to categorize herpes zoster patients according to their immune status and age. This allows the clinicians to direct their efforts toward either antiviral, anti-inflammatory, or antinociceptive effects based on the probability of success and risk factors involved. Patients can be categorized into (1) immunocompetent young, (2) immunocompetent old, (3) immunosuppressed young, and (4) immunosuppressed old patients.

Immunocompetent Young Patients

Patients in this group suffer no defined underlying illness, are less than 50 years old, and possess normal immunologic responsiveness. Although they develop acute herpes zoster, their reaction to the infection is brisk, enabling them to confine the rash within the initial unit. Likewise, PHN is not an issue. Acute morbidity is low and healing is rapid. The rationale for treatment for such groups of patients is to relieve their intolerable pain and to prevent inflammatory damage of the tissues. Antiviral agents used in the first 72 hours may help stop the replication of the virus and the spread of the infection to the peripheral nerves. Anti-inflammatory agents (steroids administered locally or systemically) are very useful in decreasing tissue damage and keeping the inflammatory reaction of the host to a minimum. The obligatory treatment is to decrease the severe pain of neuralgia. This is best accomplished with sympathetic or epidural blocks in the first 3–4 weeks of onset of infection. Antidepressive agents are also helpful as adjuvant agents.

Immunocompetent Older Patients

The major objective of therapy in this group is to prevent PHN. Although suffering no underlying disease, response to VZV in this group may be less vigorous than in young individuals, leading to slower viral clearance and perhaps a higher incidence of spread beyond the initial unit of infection. Nonetheless, nervous system and visceral complications are still of lower incidence and, by themselves, probably do not warrant the use of potentially toxic therapy at this time. However, antiviral and anti-inflammatory therapies may help prevent PHN. Of these, only the latter has been prospectively shown to be effective in this group of patients. In two controlled studies, a course of corticosteroids administered in the acute phase of infection was reported to prevent the development of PHN pain in a significant percentage of patients.[12, 47] Although this finding deserves further investigative attention, it is reasonable, on the basis of the previously mentioned evidence, to treat patients suffering from acute herpes zoster who are immunologically normal (i.e., those who suffer from no underlying immunosuppressing condition) with a limited course of corticosteroids (e.g., 60 mg of prednisone or the equivalent daily for 5 days, then taper the dose over the following 2 weeks).

Pain relief needs to be addressed in these patients. Conventional narcotics should be avoided because the patients in this group are usually older and frail. In addition there is a high incidence of PHN. Nonnarcotic analgesics in association with nerve blocks (epidural and sympathetic blocks or local intracutaneous infiltration with bupivacaine and corticosteroids) are recommended.

Immunosuppressed Young Patients

The principal concern with immunodeficient younger patients is the spread of virus within and outside the primary ganglion nerve–dermatome unit. PHN is not a major issue for these patients. Therefore, therapy is directed at confining viral infection. At present, acyclovir is available, is of proven efficacy, and can be recommended for many patients. At this point, hospitalization should be recommended for patients in this group who are at greatest risk of developing complications, particularly those with lymphoproliferative disease or early dissemination. It must also be emphasized that, if the therapy is to be given, every effort should be made to start treatment early. As newer agents become available, they will require similar consideration, with convenience, cost, and toxicity weighed against the magnitude of potential benefit. It can be predicted, however, that as oral drugs are introduced, their efficacy proven, and toxicity demonstrated to be low, the indications for treatment will expand. Indeed, as the antiviral drugs live up to their promise, the clinical decision to give these drugs to this group of patients is an easy one, with virtually all patients within this group routinely receiving such treatment. Pain relief in such patients should be obtained by techniques that are common for acute pain management.[37, 38]

Immunosuppressed Older Patients

In this group of patients, therapeutic objectives include prevention of viral spread and PHN pain. As discussed previously, antiviral therapy may be helpful for both objectives. Acyclovir has proved to be effective in reducing infection and, possibly, in reducing PHN pain. The latter requires additional confirmation. More important, because of the risk of viral dissemination, patients in this group require antiviral treatment. On the other hand, the use of corticosteroids to prevent PHN warrants separate comment. Whereas in the older immunocompetent patient corticosteroids appear to present no special risk and to be therapeutically beneficial,[12, 46] in the immunosuppressed individual greater caution is required. These patients are more susceptible to viral spread and attendant central nervous system and visceral complications. Steroids may impair their remaining defenses beyond a critical level, thus increasing the risk of these complications. Data from the NIAID Collaborative Study suggest that steroids did not protect against PHN pain in this group. This issue certainly warrants separate investigation, particularly the effects of combined antiviral and steroid therapy. Under potent antiviral coverage, corticosteroids may prove safe. Pain relief is best provided by nerve blocks.

Prognosis

There is a close relationship between the duration of neuralgia and therapeutic efficacy. Prompt treatment shortens the progressive course of the disease and decreases its severity. There also appears to be a correlation between the age of the patient and the response to therapy. Patients under 60 years of age generally respond better to therapy and, even untreated, have a lower incidence of PHN than patients over 60 years of age. In addition, older patients do not respond as well as young patients to therapy and specifically to sympathetic nerve blocks.

Postherpetic Neuralgia

PHN is a sequela of acute herpes zoster. Although spontaneous resolution of herpes zoster may be expected in most patients, many older patients experience intractable pain. PHN has been variably defined arbitrarily as pain that persists after the crusting of lesions or that persists for more than either 4 weeks, 6 weeks, 2 months, or 6 months. PHN occurs in about 10% of patients over 40 years of

age and 20–50% of patients over 60 years of age. Some young patients may experience PHN for 1–2 weeks after the herpes zoster lesions heal, although hypoesthesia or hyperesthesia may persist.

PHN is one of the most difficult problems encountered by physicians. Few other conditions create such agonizing pain and suffering for patients. Many of these patients consider suicide as a means of relief from the debilitating pain.

Clinical Manifestation

Patients with PHN complain of unrelenting pain typically associated with depressed affect and vegetative signs, such as sleep disturbances, anorexia, lassitude, constipation, and diminished libido. The pain is often qualitatively similar to that of herpes zoster neuralgia, with some combination of burning, aching, or itching, accompanied by severe paroxysms of stabbing or burning pain. Many patients describe allodynia superimposed on the continuous component of the pain.

Marmikko and Bowsher assessed somatic sensory perception thresholds (warm, cold, hot pain, touch, pinprick, vibration, two-point discrimination), allodynia, and skin temperature in the affected area of 42 patients with unilateral PHN, and 20 patients who have had unilateral shingles not followed by PHN. They compared data obtained from these assessments between the two groups.[55] There was no difference between the two groups for age or length of time after the acute herpes zoster infection. The PHN group showed significant changes in all sensory threshold measurements when the affected area was compared with the mirror image area on the unaffected side, whereas the group without PHN exhibited no threshold changes. The mechanical allodynia was present in 87% of the PHN group. No differences in skin temperature were recorded. Their findings show a deficit of sensory functions mediated by both large and small primary afferent fibers and also suggest major central involvement in the pathophysiology of the condition.

Diagnosis

PHN can be confused with other chronic painful conditions, but the patient usually has a history of a previous unilateral skin eruption and there may be a residual scarring of the skin. Hyperesthesia, dysesthesia, and anesthesia may be present in the affected area. Skin eruption may be minimal in some herpes zoster cases so that the diagnosis becomes difficult. Laboratory diagnosis may help isolate antibodies specific to herpes zoster.

Pathogenesis

Many theories have been put forward to explain the intractable nature of PHN. Noxious impulses may become established in centrally located, closed, self-perpetuating loops, and progressive facilitation develops in these synapses. Eventually, pain that is entirely unaffected by surgical section of peripheral pathways occurs spontaneously. The possibility also exists that the infection involves higher pathways in the cord and brain than was formerly believed. If that is the case, the infection is outside the reach of extradural and intrathecal medication, and possibly beyond cordotomy.

The gate control theory might explain some of the features involved in the production and persistence of PHN. Pain is thought to be carried by small unmyelinated and small myelinated nerve fibers to the central nervous system, where the input is modified via pathways in larger myelinated nerve fibers. Nerve impulses are transmitted faster in large myelinated nerve fibers than in small unmyelinated nerve fibers. In acute herpes zoster, there is a tendency for more of the large fibers to be damaged and destroyed than the small fibers. They regenerate slower than small fibers, and their diameter after regeneration is usually smaller than originally. Hence, there is an increase in the percentage of smaller fibers over larger fibers.

The gate control theory purports that minimal small fiber stimulation might produce the sensation of pain because the normal modulation of large nerve fiber stimulation is no longer present. Older patients have fewer large fibers to begin with and thus lose more due to the infection. Therefore, older patients are more likely to feel a greater degree of pain than the younger patient and to be more susceptible to the intractable PHN pain.

Noordenbos, in his spectrographic study of intercostal fibers in four patients, describes a loss of myelinated fibers and a proportional increase in nonmyelinated fibers.[56] This has been confirmed by Watson et al.[57] Noordenbos proposed that the dysthesia present in the PHN could be due to excessive pro-

cessing of nociceptive pathway by the small fibers without the concurrent inhibitory action available from the large myelinated fibers. Watson et al. reported on an exhaustive cadaveric histopathologic study in a 67-year-old man who suffered severe pain due to herpes zoster for 5 years.[57] The eighth thoracic ganglion showed fibrosis and cellular loss, localized to one segment with a loss of large myelinated fibers. The posterior horn was atrophied from thoracic spinal levels 4–8, and affected both the axons and the myelin sheath. Biochemical markers for substance P, opiate receptors, dopamine, and serotonin showed no difference between the affected or the unaffected side of the spinal cord. Watson et al. believed that PHN pain was due to deafferentation and hypersensitivity in the posterior horn of the spinal cord.[57]

Treatment

Pharmacologic

A threefold purpose governs the role of drug therapy in the patient with PHN: (1) To provide analgesia for pain, (2) to reduce depression and anxiety, and (3) to decrease insomnia. Because a considerable degree of depression, anxiety, and insomnia accompany all chronic pain syndromes, hypnotics, tranquilizers, antidepressants, and anticonvulsants have frequently been used as analgesic adjuvants in the management of PHN. These adjuvants include barbiturates, flurazepam hydrochloride, *Rauwolfia* alkaloids, phenothiazine derivatives, benzodiazepines, amphetamines, tricyclic antidepressants, diphenylhydantoin, and carbamazepine.

However, it is equally important for the physician to adopt a positive approach regarding the medication. On average, 35% of patients benefit significantly from the placebo effect.[58] This can be used to advantage by enthusiastically describing the sought-after effects of each drug that, with time, may be obtained in some individuals. Patients are also less likely to stop taking their medication before it has had time to give the desired effect.

Antiviral Agents. As a rule, antiviral agents are inappropriate for PHN.[2] An exception may include their use to prevent the possible recurrence of herpes zoster infection in the susceptible patient. For example, patients with Hodgkin's disease are predisposed to recurrent herpes zoster; antiviral agents may be given prior to treatment of the primary disease (e.g., chemotherapy and radiation therapy) when the reactivation of the virus is most likely.

Analgesics. Analgesics may be required to control the severe intractable pain of PHN. Narcotics should be used with extreme caution, if at all, because: (1) They are addictive; (2) the problem is chronic; (3) patients are not usually terminally ill; (4) side effects such as nausea, loss of appetite, and constipation usually make these patients miserable; (5) there may be adverse drug interactions with antidepressants and other drugs; and, most importantly, (6) adequate pain relief may be obtained with other drugs. The temporary, initial use of narcotics to relieve extreme pain may be necessary, however, until the patient begins to respond to other therapies.

Antidepressants and Tranquilizers. Antidepressants and tranquilizers are frequently used in conjunction with analgesics.[59] Some patients become depressed as a reaction to their pain. The signs of depression may be so subtle that they are easily missed. Lindsay found that as many as 90% of the patients whom he had seen were depressed; about 85% of these patients responded to antidepressant drugs.

Tricyclic antidepressants are the most commonly used drugs for PHN. Antidepressants may act at a higher level than the neurotransmitter, perhaps on the hypothalamus or pituitary. This could explain why only some depressed patients fit the catecholamine hypothesis, which advocates that a deficit of serotonin or norepinephrine is the cause of the problem. It could also be that both chronic pain and depression represent neurotransmitter deficiencies and that the antidepressants restore these levels. The drugs should be given in appropriate dose levels and several different drugs should be tried before concluding that there is no response.

In one study, Nathan obtained excellent pain relief with chlorprothixene in one-third of patients who had not responded to other therapy.[60] A high-dose of chlorprothixene, 50 mg every 6 hours for 5 days, was used. The prominent side effects of this high dose necessitated hospitalization during the course of therapy, and many patients stopped taking the medication because they were unable to tolerate the side effects. This treatment is recommended only if all other methods fail and if pain is severe.[60]

Anticonvulsants. Raftery reported success with sodium valproate (Depakene), 200 mg two times a day, and amitriptyline, 10–15 mg two times a day. He characterized pain as stabbing, lancinating, burning, dull ache, and hyperesthesic. If the stabbing component of pain continued, he increased the dosage of sodium valproate to 200 mg three times a day. If the burning and hyperesthesia remained, the dosage of amitriptyline was increased. He found the dull ache component of pain to be most resistant to therapy. If it persisted, he infiltrated the scar with local anesthetic and steroids or started transcutaneous electrical nerve stimulation.[61]

The side effects of anticonvulsants tend to limit their use. These effects include bone marrow depression, ataxia, diplopia, nystagmus, abnormal liver function tests, nausea, lymphadenopathy, confusion, and vertigo.[59]

Nerve Blocks

The pathogenesis of PHN pain is unknown. However, autopsy studies have shown that the entire sensory pathway, including the brain and sympathetic ganglia, may be involved. There appear to be multiple areas along this pathway that are capable of initiating pain. This provides a rationale for the various methods of treatment and an explanation of treatment failures.

Analgesic blocks can be used as prognostic, therapeutic, and prophylactic tools in managing pain. As prognostic tools, blocks help predict the effects of prolonged interruption of nerve pathways achieved through injection of neurolytic agents or surgery. By interrupting pain pathways, therapeutic blocks influence the autonomic response to noxious stimulation. They break the vicious cycle of the disease. Patients with severe intractable pain who are not suited to other treatment regimens may be relieved by blocks with neurolytic agents.

Local Infiltration. Epstein used subcutaneous infiltration of steroids and obtained relief in about 64% of his patients. He injected a 0.2% solution of triamcinolone in normal saline daily under all areas of pain, burning, or itching until the desired effect was obtained. Maximum benefit was achieved within the first 12 treatments.[40] In a comparative study, Tio et al. used subcutaneous infiltration of 0.25% bupivacaine and 0.2% triamcinolone alone or in conjunction with medication and sympathetic blockade. Overall results showed moderate to significant improvement in 70% of patients. They noted a difference in response to treatment in relation to the duration of symptoms: Patients with symptoms less than 1 year responded better (85% success) than patients with symptoms for greater than 1 year (55% success).[62]

Somatic Nerve Block. Nerve root involvement being an obvious characteristic of PHN, sensory nerve blocks are used in early attempts to relieve its pain. Results are limited, depending primarily on the duration of the blocks, although there are some reports of success in managing pain in the early stages of the disease. Coincidental spontaneous resolution may be responsible. Nerve blocks are primarily used in PHN for diagnosis and prognosis, especially as a prognostic block prior to neurolytic block. Steroids injected around the dorsal nerve have had unpredictable and limited success.

Sympathetic Nerve Block. Bonica reported good, although temporary, results with a series of paravertebral somatic sympathetic blocks using 0.2% procaine at 4-day intervals. The best results were obtained in PHN of less than 2 months' duration.[63] In another study, 34 patients with PHN for 2 years were treated with sympathetic blocks. Each patient received an average of three or four blocks. The treatment seemed to be without any effect.[44]

Epidural Block. Because epidural steroids have been successful in treating a variety of lumbosacral conditions, Forrest experimented with this technique on PHN.[64] In a well-controlled study, he obtained a progressive decrease in pain. Patients began to have relief after the first steroid injection. Fifty-seven percent were pain free 1 month after the third steroid injection. At 6 months, 86% were pain free. Nine patients were followed for 1 year and, of these, eight were completely pain free. Forrest first identified the affected dorsal roots with segmental epidural injections of 0.5% bupivacaine, 2 ml in the lumbar and thoracic regions and 1 ml in the cervical area. This provided *complete* temporary relief. A series of three epidural steroid injections were then given 1 week apart. Methylprednisone, 80 mg, was used for a single-root involvement, 60 mg per root for a two-root involvement, and 40 mg per root for a three-root involvement—the total dose for any one visit not exceeding 120 mg. The patients were kept in a lateral position for 30 minutes and discharged 6 hours later. Complications included minor weight gain and a slight increase in resting blood pressure.[64] Other investigators using a significantly different technique have not had much success with epidural injections.

Neurolytic Block. Neurolytic blocks may be considered when other blocks have not significantly relieved the patient's pain. They should only be performed after a prognostic block has demonstrated that an effective block of the appropriate area can be achieved. Neurolytic agents such as ethyl alcohol or phenol are used for prolonged destruction of nerves. Fifty to 90% ethyl alcohol in aqueous solution or 6–10% phenol has been used. Ethyl alcohol causes a higher incidence of neuritis than phenol. This is primarily due to incomplete peripheral nerve block resulting from inaccurate needle placement or to spillage of the agent on somatic nerve fibers. The duration of effects may vary from days to years, but usually ranges from 2–6 months.

Ammonium compounds can also be used for peripheral nerve block. Pain relief is due to selective destruction of unmyelinated C fibers by the ammonium ion. A solution of 10% ammonium sulfate in 1% lidocaine or 15% ammonium chloride is used. The duration of action ranges from 4–24 weeks. Neuritis does not occur with either ammonium sulfate or chloride. The most annoying side effect is numbness, which can be as bad as the pain for some patients.[37]

Miscellaneous Therapies

Because many patients continue to have some residual pain of varying degrees that can be aggravating, they may require management with other techniques. The following techniques are used when all other modalities have failed.

Transcutaneous Electrical Neural Stimulation

Transcutaneous electrical neural stimulation has been used in an attempt to relieve the intractable PHN pain. Winnie reported a success rate of only 20%, but relief was sufficient to permit a return to normal activity without analgesic therapy.[65]

Ice and Other Cold Therapies

Ice is applied to the skin for 2–3 minutes several times a day, starting with the least sensitive area and approaching the most sensitive area. A vibrator is then used in the same manner in conjunction with psychotropic drugs. Ethyl chloride, or other cold sprays, may be used for treatment. Fluid is sprayed over the whole painful area, beginning at the upper area and working down. Evaporation cools the area. The procedure is repeated twice at 1-minute intervals until the skin is thoroughly cooled. When of value, treatments will relieve the pain for varying lengths of time. When pain returns to near its former intensity, the treatment can be repeated. If the patient responds satisfactorily, pain is relieved by two or three sets of sprays per day.[66, 67] Good to excellent pain relief was maintained in about 66% of patients with refractory PHN pain using cryocautery with a stick of solid carbon dioxide (dry ice) applied directly to the hyperesthetic skin areas of the cutaneous scars.[68]

Acupuncture

A preliminary report shows significant pain relief was obtained in 40% of PHN patients with acupuncture. Many of these patients had already had invasive or destructive procedures prior to acupuncture (Figure 27-5).[69]

Hypnosis

Hypnosis acts at the level of the cerebral cortex. Impulses are sent down from higher centers to close the neurophysiologic gate that controls pain. Pain relief through hypnosis is sometimes complete but usually is not. Hypnotism breaks up patterns of suffering to help patients with chronic unbearable pain change the pain to bearable discomfort.

Surgery and Neurosurgery

Surgery is the last resort for severe, intractable PHN pain. It is not always successful, however. More effective management techniques learned recently have further limited this option.

Surgery usually is done on the sites of the pain pathway in stages progressively higher. Because it was suspected that the origin of the pain lay in the scar and peripheral receptors, wide excision and skin grafting was tried but was found to be ineffective and is rarely tried today.

Prognosis

There is a close relationship between the duration of the PHN and therapeutic efficacy. Prompt treatment shortens the progressive course of the disease and also decreases its severity. There also appears to be a correlation between the age of the patient and his or her response to therapy. Patients under 60 years of age generally respond better to therapy and, even untreated, have a lower incidence of PHN than patients over 60. In addition, older patients do not respond as well as young patients to therapy and specifically to sympathetic nerve blocks. For unknown reasons, PHN lesions in the ophthalmic division of the trigeminal nerve are difficult lesions to treat successfully. The psychological make-up of the individual patient is also important. Lastly, one-fifth of patients with neoplasms who have had herpes zoster will get it at least once again.

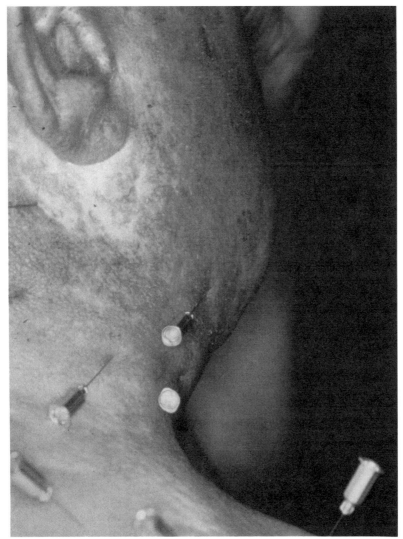

Figure 27-5. Acupuncture performed in a patient with postherpetic neuralgia affecting the cervical plexus.

References

1. Hope-Simpson RE. The nature of herpes zoster: A long-term study and a new hypothesis. Proc R Soc Med 1965;58:9.

2. Bokai J. Das Auftreten der Schafblattern unter be sonderen Umstanden. Ungar Arch Med 1892;1:159.

3. Head H, Campbell AW. The pathology of herpes zoster and its bearing on sensory localisation. Brain 1990;23:353.

4. Tyzzer EE. The histology of the skin lesions in varicella. Philippine J Sci 1906;1:349.

5. Bruusgaard E. The mutual relation between zoster and varicella. Br J Dermatol 1932;44:1.

6. Weller TH. Serial propagation in vitro of agents producing inclusion bodies derived from varicella and herpes zoster. Proc Soc Exp Biol Med 1953;83:340.

7. Hyman RW. Structure and Function of the Varicella-Zoster Virus Genome. In AJ Nahmias, WR Dowdle, RF Schinazi (eds), The Human Herpesviruses: An Interdisciplinary Perspective. New York: Elsevier, 1981;63.

8. Loeser JD. Review article: Herpes zoster and postherpetic neuralgia. Pain 1986;25:149.

9. Berger R, Florent G, Just M. Decrease of the lymphoproliferative response to varicella-zoster virus antigen in the aged. Infect Immunol 1981;32:24.

10. Burgoon CF, Burgoon JS, Baldridge GD. The natural history of herpes zoster. JAMA 1957;164:265.

11. DeMorages JM, Kierland RR. The outcome of patients with herpes zoster. Arch Dermatol Syphilis 1957;75:193.

12. Eaglstein WH, Katz R, Brown JA. The effect of early

corticosteroid therapy on skin eruption and pain of herpes zoster. JAMA 1970;211:1681.

13. Keczkes K, Basheer AM. Do corticosteroids prevent post-herpetic neuralgia? Br J Dermatol 1980;102:551.

14. Walsh FB, Hoyt WF. Clinical Neuro-Ophthalmology (3rd ed) Vol. 2. Baltimore: Williams & Wilkins, 1969;1351.

15. Arvin AM, Pollard RB, Rasmussen LE, et al. Cellular and humoral immunity in the pathogenesis of recurrent herpes viral infections in patients with lymphoma. J Clin Invest 1980;65:869.

16. Gershon AA, Steinberg SP. Cellular and humoral immune responses to varicella-zoster virus in immunocompromised patients during and after varicella-zoster infections. Infect Immunol 1979;25:170.

17. Gershon AA, Steinberg SP. Antibody responses to varicella-zoster virus and the role of antibody in host defenses. Am J Med Sci 1981;282:12.

18. Atkinson K, Meyers JD, Storb R, et al. Varicella-zoster virus infection after marrow transplantation for aplastic anemia or leukemia. Transplantation 1980;29:47.

19. Price RW. Herpes zoster: An approach to systemic therapy. Med Clin North Am 1982;66:1105.

20. Pernak JM, Blemans JCH. The Treatment of Acute Herpes Zoster in Trigeminal Nerve for the Prevention of Post-Herpetic Neuralgia. In W Erdmanov, T Oyama, JM Pernak (eds), The Pain Clinic (Vol. 1). Utrecht, The Netherlands: VNU Science Press, 1985.

21. Gershon A. Varicella-zoster virus. Prospects for active immunization. Am J Clin Pathol 1978;70:170.

22. Biron K, Elion GB. In vitro susceptibility of varicella-zoster virus to acyclovir. Antimicrob Agents Chemother 1980;18:443.

23. Hirsch MS, Swartz MN. Antiviral agents. N Engl J Med 1980;302:903,949.

24. Coen DM, Furman PA, Gelep PT, et al. Mutations in the herpes simplex DNA polymerase gene can confer resistance to 9-b-D-arabinofuranosyladenine. J Virol 1982;41:909.

25. Whitley RJ, Soong SJ, Dolin R, et al. Early vidarabine therapy to control the complications of herpes zoster in immunosuppressed patients. N Engl J Med 1982;307:971.

26. Peterslund NA, Seyer-Hansen K, Ipsen J, et al. Acyclovir in herpes zoster. Lancet 1981;2:827.

27. Bean B, Braun C, Balfour HH. Acyclovir therapy for acute herpes zoster. Lancet 1982;2:118.

28. Balfour H. Acyclovir therapy for herpes zoster: Advantages and adverse effects. JAMA 1986;255:387.

29. Shepp DH, Dandliker PS, Meyers JD. Treatment of varicella zoster virus infection in severely immunocompromised patients: A randomized comparison of acyclovir and vidarabine. N Engl J Med 1986;314:208.

30. Leyland-Jones B, Donnelly H, Groshen S, et al. 2'-Fluoro-5-iodoarabinosyl-cytosine, a new potent antiviral agent: Efficacy in immunosuppressed individuals with herpes zoster. J Infect Dis 1986;154:430.

31. Lopez C, Watanabe KA, Fox JJ. 2'-Fluoro-5-iodo-ana-cytosine: A potent and selective antiherpesvirus agent. Antimicrob Agents Chemother 1980;17:803.

32. Neumann M, Chung D. Intravenous acyclovir for the reduction of postherpetic neuralgia. Pain Suppl 1990;5:S57.

33. Gelfand ML. Treatment of herpes zoster with cortisone. JAMA 1954;154:911.

34. Appleman DH. Treatment of herpes zoster with ACTH. N Engl J Med 1955;253:693.

35. Elliot FA. Treatment of herpes zoster with high doses of prednisone. Lancet 1964;2:610.

36. Lycka BA. Postherpetic neuralgia and systemic corticosteroid therapy: Efficacy and safety. Int J Dermatol 1990;29:523.

37. Tio R, Moya F, Usubiaga L. Management of Intractable Pain. In M Lichtiger, F Moya (eds), Introduction to the Practice of Anesthesia. Hagerstown, MD: Harper & Row, 1978;485.

38. Basbaum AL, Fields HL. Endogenous pain control mechanisms: Review and hypothesis. Ann Neurol 1978;4:451.

39. Rosenak S. Procaine injection treatment of herpes zoster. Lancet 1938;2:1056.

40. Epstein E. Treatment of herpes zoster and postzoster neuralgia by subcutaneous injection of triamcinolone. Int J Dermatol 1981;20:65.

41. Epstein E. Intralesional triamcinolone therapy in herpes zoster and post zoster neuralgia. Eye Ear Nose Throat 1973;52:416.

42. Lipton JR, Marding SP, Wells JCD. The effect of early stellate ganglion block on post-herpetic neuralgia in herpes zoster ophthalmicus. Pain Clin 1987;1:247.

43. Colding A. The effect of regional sympathetic blocks in the treatment of herpes zoster. Acta Anaesth Scand 1969;13:133.

44. Riopelle JM, Maraghi M, Gursch KP. Chronic neuralgia incidence following local anesthetic therapy for herpes zoster. Arch Dermatol 1984;120:747.

45. Colding A. Treatment of pain: Organization of a pain clinic, treatment of herpes zoster. Proc R Soc Med 973;66:541.

46. Bauman J. Treatment of acute herpes zoster neuralgia by epidural injection or stellate ganglion block. Anesthesiology 1979;50(Suppl):223.

47. Toyama N. Sympathetic ganglion block therapy for herpes zoster [Japanese]. J Dermatol 1982;9:59.

48. Masud KZ, Forster KR. Sympathetic block in herpes zoster. Am Fam Pract 1975;12:142.

49. Perkins HM, Hanlon PR. Epidural injection of local anesthetic and steroids for relief of pain secondary to herpes zoster. Arch Surg 1978;113:253.

50. Berger JJ, Perkins HM. Comparison of epidural methylprednisolone alone or combined with lidocaine for relieving postherpetic neuralgia. Pain Suppl 1990;5:S1-S528.

51. Drake HF, Harries AJ, Gamester RE, et al. Randomised double-blind study of topical capsaicin for treatment of postherpetic neuralgia. Pain Suppl 1990;5:S1-S528.

52. Bernstein JE, Korman N-J, Bickers DR. Topical capsaicin treatment of chronic post-herpetic neuralgia. J Am Acad Dermatol 1989;21:263.

53. Morimoto M, Inamori K, Hyodo M. The effect of indomethacin stupe for post-herpetic neuralgia—particularly in comparison with chloroform-aspirin solution. Pain Suppl 1990;5:S1-S528.

54. DeBeneditio G, Lorenzetti A, Besana F. A new topical treatment for acute herpetic neuralgia and postherpetic neuralgia. Pain Suppl 1990;5:S1-S528.

55. Marmikko T, Bowsher D. Somatosensory findings in post-herpetic neuralgia. J Neurol Neurosurg Psychiatry 1990;53:135.

56. Noordenbos W. Problems pertaining to the transmission of nerve impulses which give rise to pain. Pain 1959;1:68.

57. Watson CPN, Deck JH, Morshead C, et al. Postherpetic neuralgia: Further post mortem studies of cases with and without pain. Pain 1991;44:105.

58. Moore ME. Use of drugs in the management of chronic pain. Anesthesiol Rev 1975;8:14.

59. Taub A. Relief of postherpetic neuralgia with psychotropic drugs. J Neurosurg 1973;39:235.

60. Nathan PW. Chlorprothixene (Taractan) in postherpetic neuralgia and other severe chronic pains. Pain 1978;5:367.

61. Raftery H. The management of postherpetic pain using sodium valproate and amitriptyline. Ir Med J 1979;72:399.

62. Tio R, Moya F, Vorasaran S. Treatments of postherpetic neuralgia. Anesth Sinica 1978;16:151.

63. Bonica JJ. Thoracic Segmental and Intercostal Neuralgia. In The Management of Pain. Philadelphia: Lea & Febiger, 1953;861.

64. Forrest JB. Management of chronic dorsal root pain with epidural steroid. Can Anaesth Soc J 1978;25:218.

65. Winnie AP. The Patient with Herpetic Neuralgia. In F Moya, H Gion (eds), Postgraduate Seminar in Anesthesiology, Program Syllabus. Miami Beach, Florida, 1983;165.

66. Crue BL Jr, Todd EM, Maline DB. Postherpetic Neuralgia: Conservative Treatment Regimen. In BL Crue (ed), Pain Research and Treatment. New York: Academic, 1975;289.

67. Lipton S. Postherpetic Neuralgia. In Relief of Pain in Clinical Practice. Oxford: Scientific Publications, 1979;231.

68. Suzuki H, Ogawa S, Nakagawa H, et al. Cryocautery of sensitized skin areas for the relief of pain due to postherpetic neuralgia. Pain 1980;9:355.

69. Lewith GT, Field J. Acupuncture and postherpetic neuralgia [letter]. Br Med J 1980;(August 30):622.

70. Hatangdi VS, Boas RA, Richards EG. Postherpetic Neuralgia: Management with Antiepileptic and Tricyclic drugs. In JJ Bonica, D Albe-Fessard (eds), Advances in Pain Research and Therapy (Vol. 1). New York: Raven, 1976;583.

71. Kishore-Kumar R, Max MB, Schafer SC, et al. Desipramine relieves postherpetic neuralgia. Clin Pharmacol Ther 1990;47:305.

72. Baker KA, Taylor JW, Lilly GE. Treatment of trigeminal neuralgia: Use of baclofen in combination with carbamazepine. Clin Pharm 1985;4:93.

73. Sklar SH, Wigand JS. Herpes zoster. Br J Dermatol 1981;104:351.

74. Galbraith AW. Prevention of post-herpetic neuralgia by amantadine hydrochloride (Symmetrel). Br J Clin Pract 1983;37:304.

75. Castelli M, Zanca A, Giubertoni G, et al. Griseofulvin-methisoprinol combination in the treatment of herpes zoster. Pharmacol Res 1986;18:991.

76. Farber GA, Burks JW. Chlorprothixene therapy for herpes zoster neuralgia. South Med J 1974;67:808.

Chapter 28

Biochemical Considerations of Nutrition

Michele Holevar

Malignant disease is commonly associated with anorexia and weight loss. Cachexia is present in more than two-thirds of patients with advanced, terminal disease,[1] 50% of patients have signs and symptoms of cachexia on initial presentation,[2] and cancer patients have the highest incidence of malnutrition of any hospitalized group. Fifty percent of cancer patients undergoing major surgical procedures will have evidence of significant malnutrition.[3] The development of cachexia has not been consistently related to the type or stage of cancer, the duration of disease, or the site and number of metastases.[4]

Malnutrition has several adverse effects and has been found to be an independent prognosticator of mortality.[5] In an autopsy study of 500 cancer patients, anorexia and cachexia, rather than the cancer itself, were found to be the cause of death in 22%. It was the second most common cause of death in patients with solid tumors, surpassed only by pulmonary complications.[6] Weight loss is a better predictor of death than performance index, tumor histology, or type of chemotherapy in patients with lung cancer.[7] Even a loss of only 5–10% of normal body weight can worsen the prognosis.[5]

The mechanism by which malnutrition adversely affects survival has not been completely delineated. The relative contributions of decreased immune function, increased susceptibility to infection, and delayed wound healing are uncertain. In addition, the therapeutic margin of safety of many chemotherapeutic and radiation therapy regimens may be narrowed in the cachectic cancer patient.

Finally, severe cachexia and anorexia result in discomfort, weakness, depression, and fatigue,

which interfere with the patient's quality of life. The steady loss of weight may serve as a painful reminder to both patient and family of the human frailty and life expectancy, thus reinforcing the perception of hopelessness.

Causes of Malnutrition in Cancer

Weight loss develops as a result of the negative balance between nutrient intake and energy expenditure such as when intake is decreased with normal caloric expenditure, when intake remains stable in the face of increased caloric expenditure, or as a combination of both mechanisms. In cancer patients, this imbalance can result from decreased oral intake as a result of anorexia, taste changes, food aversions, protracted emesis, psychological reluctance to eat, mechanical interference with nutrient consumption, or obstruction; malabsorption of nutrients; increased energy expenditure; and abnormal metabolism of protein, carbohydrates, and fat.

Tumor Effects

Decreased Intake

Although most of the weight loss has been attributed to metabolic effects such as increased basal metabolic rate and inefficient metabolism of nutrients, one could theoretically argue that the organism should compensate for increased energy requirements by increasing the intake of nutrients. Therefore, the ultimate cause of weight loss may be the inadequate intake of nutrition. There are many reasons for this failure. The cause of decreased oral intake may be obvious (such as an obstructing lesion of the esophagus) or more subtle (such as the anorexia that may accompany even small, undiagnosed neoplasms). In addition, most chemotherapeutic agents produce significant nausea and vomiting, with subsequent weight loss and cachexia.

Anorexia

Anorexia exists in 25% of patients at the time of presentation and is usually always present during the terminal stage of the disease. Anorexia may be caused by physical, metabolic, and psychological factors.

Increased Satiety

The hypothalamus controls oral intake. Occasionally, anorexia may be the result of brain metastasis or increased intracranial pressure. The hypothalamic control of appetite is influenced by changes in blood glucose and amino acid levels, both of which may be deranged in certain types of cancer.[8] Lactate produced by tumor cells may also cause anorexia and nausea. It is unlikely, however, that altered hypothalamic function is the only cause of cancer cachexia because ablation of the hypothalamus in rats does not prevent the anorexia associated with advanced carcinoma.[9]

Hormones, such as insulin, glucagon, epinephrine, enterogastrone, and cholecystokinin are also thought to affect nutrient intake.[10] The glucose intolerance present in many cancer patients results in a prolonged elevation of blood glucose after a meal.[11] Because hunger corresponds with return of blood glucose to normal, hunger in cancer patients may be delayed after a meal. A few tumors secrete mediators such as bombesin and serotonin that can lead to paraneoplastic syndromes and anorexia.[12] Anorexia can also be caused by the release of cytokines such as interferon, cachectin and tumor necrosis factor (TNF), and interleukin 1 (IL-1), by lymphocytes and monocytes in response to the tumor.[2] The contribution of these circulating factors is evidenced by the fact that an improvement in anorexia may precede objective measures of tumor shrinkage following successful oncologic treatment.[13]

Increased fullness and early satiety may contribute to gastrointestinal changes. Likewise, taste aberrations may result in decreased digestive secretions, thus delaying digestion. Atrophic changes in the small intestine due to malnutrition may also slow digestion. The loss of stomach wall muscle in response to starvation parallels the loss of skeletal muscle mass, producing delayed gastric emptying. All of these factors help explain the clinical observation of an inability for cancer patients to eat later in the day.[8]

Taste Changes (Dysgeusia)

De Wys and others have delineated changes in taste and olfactory sensation in cancer patients that inversely correlate with food intake.[8] The most frequent taste aberration is an elevation of the threshold for sweet sensation, which occurs in approximately one-third of patients. A lowering of the threshold for bitter tastes is noted in one-sixth of patients, and this observation has been correlated with an aversion for meat.[8] Abnormalities in smell may result in less pleasant associations and even distortions of food odors. Some investigators have found that taste alterations equated with the spread of the tumor and paralleled the change in disease status in response to therapy.[14] Unfortunately, weight loss itself may alter taste sensation; increasing nutrient intake has been shown to reduce taste aberrations.[15]

Psychological Effects

Depression

Psychologic factors play an important role in the development of anorexia. Feelings of worthlessness, hopelessness, guilt, loss of self-esteem, and suicidal ideation are common in cancer patients. In one study, cachectic cancer patients had a higher incidence of depression than noncachectic patients.[16] The incidence of taste changes and vomiting was similar in both groups of patients. Transient anorexia often occurs at the time of diagnosis. Renewed optimism occurs once the diagnosis has been made and a treatment plan instituted. If, however, patients are uninformed as to the physical changes associated with cancer treatment, they may become depressed by their deteriorating physical condition and appearance. If recurrent disease is diagnosed, anxiety and depression may recur.

Learned Food Aversions

Learned food aversions are dislikes for specific foods that develop as a result of the association of those foods with unpleasant symptoms, such as nausea and vomiting. They are a form of classic conditioning where the unconditioned stimulus is the illness or malaise felt during tumor growth or chemotherapy; and the conditioned stimulus is the taste associated with the food ingested while the malaise is experienced. The learning or conditioned response is the rejection of food associated with the unpleasant symptoms. This learning occurs rapidly, and there may be a delay of many hours between the conditioned stimulus (the taste) and the unconditioned stimulus (the illness). However, the food aversion still develops.[17] Although food aversions are more likely to develop with new foods, they may develop to familiar or preferred foods. Perhaps the most disturbing aspect of learned food aversions is that they may persist long after gastrointestinal symptoms have resolved.

Patients may also induce nutritional imbalances by avoiding foods they believe were responsible for the development of their tumor. Alternatively, they may start questionable "nutritional" therapies that they perceive have therapeutic value as far as their cancer is concerned, but which, in fact, are nutritionally inadequate.

Abnormal Gastrointestinal Function

Neoplastic invasion of the gastrointestinal tract may result in mechanical interference with food intake. Obstructing or fungating lesions of the head and neck or esophagus may result in pain and inability to swallow. Intrinsic gastric neoplasms or extrinsic compression of the stomach by metastasis or ascites decrease the gastric reservoir. Mechanical obstruction of the small intestine may be caused by a primary neoplasm or diffuse carcinomatosis associated with malignancies of the colon, pancreas, ovaries, and breast.

The obstruction of small bowel mesenteric lymph nodes may result in an intestinal malabsorption syndrome of steatorrhea and protein-wasting enteropathy.[18] Partial bowel obstruction may produce bacterial overgrowth with steatorrhea and vitamin B_{12} deficiency. Malnutrition alone causes intestinal mucosal atrophy ("cancer enteropathy"), resulting in a continuous cycle of malabsorption and worsening cachexia.

Increased Energy Expenditure

Although decreased intake is the predominant cause of cachexia in cancer patients, weight loss may occur in the absence of nutrient restriction. In addition, the degree of weight loss may be disproportional to the degree of decreased intake, with a loss of weight of more than the 2–4 pounds per week seen in normal starvation.[19] This may be the result of an increased metabolic rate or alterations in host metabolism with inefficient use of nutrients.

Increased Metabolic Rate

One interesting characteristic of cancer cachexia is the frequent elevation of basal metabolic rate. Knox measured the resting energy expenditure (REE) in 200 malnourished cancer patients via indirect calorimetry. Forty-one percent of patients demonstrated normal REE, 26% had an increased REE, whereas only 10% had a decrease.[20] The alteration in metabolic rate varies with the type of tumor.[21] Although nutritional support has not been shown to decrease the elevation in metabolic rate, the increase in metabolic rate is reversed in some patients by complete response to chemotherapy[22] and tumor resection.[23]

More interesting than the variation in metabolic rates among different tumors, however, is the failure of malnourished cancer patients to adapt to simple starvation by decreasing their metabolic rate. Possible mechanisms of this phenomenon include inefficient utilization of nutrients with tumor-induced futile substrate cycling or tumor-induced cytokines, such as cachectin and TNF.

TNF is a soluble protein secreted by macrophages in response to cancer. It has been found to increase catabolism (particularly muscle catabolism). Its role in cancer cachexia is not fully established because serum levels have only shown conflicting results. In some patients levels are increased but in others they are undetectable.

Abnormal Metabolism (Impaired Adaptation to Starvation)

Protein

During simple starvation, skeletal muscle is initially catabolized to provide amino acids for gluconeogenesis. With chronic starvation, however, the body decreases muscle breakdown and conserves nitrogen to maintain lean body mass. This ability to preserve body mass is impaired in cancer patients. Despite the variability in REE, all cancer patients have an increase of more than 50% in total body protein turnover.[24] Unlike simple starvation, no correlation exists between hypermetabolism and hypercatabolism.

The net loss of protein is most likely due to decreased synthesis of protein in nonmalignant tissues and to increased skeletal muscle catabolism.[25] The tumor appears to grow according to its genetic predisposition, oblivious to the state of the host. Clinically, the net loss of protein manifests as wasting of skeletal muscle, visceral atrophy, hypoalbuminemia, and impaired immunity.

In addition, an imbalance occurs in the levels of free amino acids. In simple starvation, levels of branched-chain amino acids (leucine, isoleucine, and valine) are decreased. In contrast, starving cancer patients maintain normal or increased levels of branched-chain amino acids.[26] It is likely that these branched-chain amino acids are used for tumor metabolism and gluconeogenesis. Alanine liberated by muscle catabolism is the major substrate for gluconeogenesis.[27] In experiments in animals, the administration of TNF and IL-1 has been found to induce similar imbalances in free amino acids. A definitive answer to the issue is difficult because of the fact that circulating levels of TNF and IL-1 are difficult to detect in cancer patients.

Carbohydrate

Although tumor cells are derived from the host's cells, they lack some of the metabolic capabilities of normal cells but retain some of those present in fetal tissue. One capability lacking in tumor cells is the efficient metabolism of glucose, which results in increased reliance on elevated glycolysis. Neoplasms, particularly sarcomas, metabolize glucose through anaerobic pathways, thus generating lactate. Lactate is converted by the liver to glucose via the Cori cycle. This process consumes much of the patient's energy. Therefore, the tumor gains energy at the expense of the host. In addition, gluconeogenesis is enhanced in the cancer patient's liver, and this process requires energy. Thus, the combination of inappropriate stimulation of gluconeogenesis combined with inefficient use of the glucose produced results in "futile cycling" and a significant energy drain on the patient.[28] This accelerated glucose turnover is particularly prominent in cancer patients with weight loss.

As mentioned, glucose intolerance secondary to insulin resistance is common in cancer patients. It may occur prior to detection of cachexia and is related to the degree of tumor burden.[29]

Fat

Cachectic cancer patients experience a depletion in body fat stores that are disproportionate to the loss of protein. These alterations in lipid metabolism are associated with both decreased immune response and reduced survival in cancer patients.[30]

It is not known if TNF, interferon, or some other circulating tumor-produced lipolytic factor is responsible for these alterations. TNF suppresses lipoprotein lipase, which is responsible for conversion of circulating free fatty acids to fat. Insulin resistance may also contribute by preventing the stimulation of lipoprotein lipase and the inhibition of hormone-sensitive lipase, thus further exacerbating mobilization of fat stores. This might explain the failure of glucose infusion to suppress fatty acid mobilization to the extent that it does in normally functioning patients.

In cancer patients, the increase of serum free fatty acids is due to an increase in mobilization and in clearance of fat.[31] Patients with localized neoplasms have a 20% increase in fat oxidation compared with a 40% increase seen in patients with metastatic disease.[32] It is likely that the neoplasm uses fatty acids to synthesize tumor lipids at the expense of the host.

Treatment Effects

In addition to the problems caused by the tumor, treatment modalities for cancer such as radical surgery, chemotherapy, and radiation therapy may carry their own severe nutritional consequences. Some are obvious such as with the nausea and vomiting resulting from chemotherapy; others are more subtle such as with the fat malabsorption that may occur after gastric, pancreatic, or intestinal resections.

Surgery

Notwithstanding the stress and increased nutritional requirements, surgery may also create other difficulties in maintaining adequate nutrition, depending on the location of the tumor and the extent of resection. Resection of tumors involving the tongue, mandible, or oropharynx interfere with mastication and swallowing. Stenosis of the esophagus following surgical procedures may produce a mechanical obstruction to swallowing. Both esophagectomy and gastrectomy have been associated with fat malabsorption and a form of the dumping syndrome, probably due to the vagotomy.

Gastric resection also results in the loss of the gastric reservoir, which limits the amount of food that can be comfortably eaten at one sitting. Other nutritional deficiencies include decreased absorption of iron and vitamin B_{12}.

Small bowel resection does not result in malabsorption until more than 75% of the bowel is resected. This is usually followed by progressive adaptation of the small bowel, which serves to limit the malabsorption. Deficits also depend on the area of resection. Fat malabsorption occurs when more than 100 cm of ileum are removed. In addition, the distal ileum is where bile salts and vitamin B_{12} are absorbed, thus imposing further deficits. Some patients have a syndrome of gastric hypersecretion in response to small bowel resection which exacerbates their diarrhea.[33] Furthermore, the increase in intraluminal acid can inhibit the enzymatic digestion of nutrients. Finally, pan-

creatic resection results in exocrine insufficiency and diabetes mellitus.

Chemotherapy

Almost all chemotherapeutic agents produce anorexia as well as some degree of nausea and vomiting. Some agents also produce a metallic taste in the mouth. Chemotherapeutic agents have also been associated with the development of the conditioned behaviors of learned food aversions and anticipatory nausea and vomiting. Because these drugs are effective against the most rapidly proliferating cells, it is not surprising that they affect the mucosal cells of the gastrointestinal tract to produce mucositis, which presents as painful oral lesions or bloody diarrhea. Indirect effects of chemotherapy include candidiasis of the oropharynx or esophagus. The symptoms of mouth pain and odynophagia may limit the amount of oral nutrition tolerated by the patient.

The *Vinca* alkaloids may produce abdominal pain, constipation, ileus, or diarrhea. This may be more severe in the elderly,[34] and typically lasts up to 2 weeks.

Radiation Therapy

Anorexia and fatigue are general effects from radiation that usually occur regardless of the site, extent, and duration of therapy. Other side effects are related to the site undergoing therapy and can be divided into those that occur early and those that occur late.

Radiation to the head and neck may produce a decrease in the amount of saliva and an increase in the viscosity, thus resulting in a dry, painful mouth and difficulty swallowing. Mucositis may be severe, with oral ulcerations limiting oral intake. The decrease in saliva and direct radiation damage of the teeth results in loosening of the teeth and accelerated dental caries. Changes in the underlying bone structure as well as weight loss may affect the fit of dentures, thus lacerating the already damaged, vulnerable buccal mucosa. Delayed effects include an inability to taste food ("mouth blindness") and mandibular necrosis.

Radiation to the thorax may cause dysphagia secondary to esophageal irritation that can persist for several weeks after completing the treatment. Late radiation sequelae include esophageal stenosis. Nausea, vomiting, diarrhea, and malabsorption occur acutely following radiation to the abdomen. Symptoms of chronic radiation enteritis include chronic diarrhea with weight loss, intermittent bowel obstruction, ulceration, perforation, fibrosis, or fistula.

Other Drugs (Protected Environment and Intestinal Sterilization)

Patients undergoing intensive chemotherapy may receive intestinal sterilization with nonabsorbable antibiotics in an attempt to reduce infections. Commonly used drugs include neomycin, polymyxin B, vancomycin, gentamycin, and nystatin. Neomycin inhibits pancreatic lipase, precipitates bile salts, and damages mucosa. In one study of patients receiving methotrexate, those patients who also received gastrointestinal sterilization lost more weight than those not on antibiotics.[35]

Rationale for Nutritional Therapy

Advantages and Disadvantages of Nutritional Repletion

The pertinent question in the nutritional management of cancer patients is whether the benefits of nutritional therapy, such as improved morbidity and mortality, outweigh the disadvantages of this therapy, such as the potentially enhanced tumor growth and the complications of nutritional therapy.

Impact on Malignancy

There are several different situations in which nutritional support may benefit the cancer patient. Nutritional support may be lifesaving for patients who have been cured of their tumor but are left with short bowel syndrome or chronic radiation enteritis. Few would disagree that such patients should be supported nutritionally. Patients with a potentially curable tumor who are so depleted that they may not tolerate the treatment may be considered for alimentation. Finally, patients who

have failed to respond to antineoplastic therapy but who wish to remain alive to accomplish personal goals, e.g., to see their children get married or graduate, might choose to undergo nutritional support, despite the fact that it would be palliative and not curative.

As previously stated, malnutrition is associated with decreased survival. Intensive nutritional support can reverse many of the nutritional deficits found in cancer patients. Weight gain, nitrogen retention, and improved immunity have been accomplished with nutritional repletion. If malnutrition is the cause of decreased survival, a reversal of these deficits might decrease the morbidity and mortality associated with cachexia. If, however, cachexia is merely a predictor of patients who will not survive, then reversing the cachexia should not affect morbidity and mortality.

Possible Tumor Stimulation

A theoretic concern of providing nutritional support has been the potential for stimulating the tumor growth. This theory has been supported by numerous animal studies evaluating enteral and parenteral supplementation in which starvation resulted in decreased tumor growth.[36] Although anecdotal reports appear in the literature, clinical series have not demonstrated stimulation of cancer in humans. Similarly, parenteral hyperalimentation has been shown to both induce[37] and have no effect[38] on the mitotic activity and protein synthesis rate of tumor tissue cells compared with host cells.

Some tumors appear to prefer glutamine and alanine. Studies are being conducted on specialized diets enriched with these amino acids to see if they can increase the number of tumor cells in a phase of mitosis that makes them more susceptible to cell cycle–specific chemotherapy.

Survival and Tolerance for Therapy

Numerous retrospective studies have supported the conclusion that nutritional support is efficacious for treating cancer. They have found increased response rates and tolerance for various forms of therapy. These studies, however, often have used historic controls, and thus must be considered skeptically.

Unfortunately, the results of prospective, randomized clinical studies evaluating the effect of nutritional support on the morbidity and mortality of patients undergoing surgery, chemotherapy, or radiation therapy have been conflicting. Therefore, this remains a controversial topic. Most of these studies are deficient because they include an inadequate number of patients, do not restrict the study to malnourished patients, and do not provide optimal nutritional support. This was precisely the case in the studies used for a meta-analysis of the benefit of parenteral hyperalimentation in patients receiving chemotherapy.[39] This study found that there was no statistically significant improvement in mortality, therapy toxicity or tolerance, or tumor response in patients receiving parenteral hyperalimentation. A fourfold increase was found in the risk of infection with hyperalimentation. This meta-analysis has been criticized on the basis of the quality of the papers chosen to review. Because many of the papers reviewed excluded severely malnourished patients, conclusions cannot be drawn on the potential benefit to this patient group or patients unable to maintain adequate nutritional intake.

There is some consensus, however, that preoperative nutritional support is beneficial and reduces morbidity in the severely malnourished patient. In the meta-analysis previously mentioned,[39] an evaluation of the value of total parenteral nutrition (TPN) in cancer patients documented that it significantly reduced major surgical operations and operative mortality in patients with gastrointestinal tumors. There remains controversy, however, as to the best duration of nutritional support. Notwithstanding the inadequate literature, the American Society of Parenteral and Enteral Nutrition has recommended nutritional support for patients who are severely malnourished preoperatively or who can be anticipated to have inadequate caloric intake for 10–14 days postoperatively.[40] The commonly accepted duration of preoperative nutritional support has been 7–10 days.

Impact on Quality of Life

Few studies exist regarding the impact of nutrition on the cancer patient's quality of life. This aspect is especially important because, in many cases, the available antitumor therapy can only prolong the patient's life and perhaps limit physical discomfort. For these patients particularly, the risks and inconveniences of nutritional support must be weighed against the possible benefits.

The elements of quality of life include psychological and physical well-being and symptom control. In one study of cancer patients receiving chemotherapy or radiotherapy, the quality of appetite and ability to eat were the most important aspects determining physical well-being. Control of nausea and vomiting were reported to be more important than pain control.[41] Another report followed patients with advanced, symptomatic malignancies who received chemotherapy with adjuvant parenteral hyperalimentation. These patients demonstrated improved performance status measured by activity and mental alertness, increased appetite and oral intake, and decreased analgesic requirements.[42]

The progressive inanition that may accompany terminal cancer leads to a deterioration of mental and physical functioning, which obviously affects the quality of the patient's remaining life. Some patients find consolation in enteral nutrition because it relieves them of the responsibility of eating. It also gives family members a sense that "something is being done," that the patient is not being abandoned, and also relieves them of the responsibility of constantly encouraging the patient to eat.

Assessment of Nutritional Status

Nutritional assessment is performed to identify those patients who are malnourished as well as to identify those patients who are at risk for becoming malnourished. The prevention of nutritional deficits is a more realistic than treating malnutrition after it is severe. Therefore, *all* patients should be screened at the time of diagnosis. This process will not only identify patients in need of nutritional management, but also help establish realistic goals in terms of weight gain or weight maintenance. The nutritional status should then be reevaluated periodically to ensure that those goals are being met.

Methods of Primary Assessment

The initial assessment should include a dietary history, a 3-day food diary, and a series of objective anthropometric measurements, biochemical tests, and recall skin antigen testing. Anthropometric measurements include the triceps skinfold measurement to assess body fat mass and the creatinine-height index to estimate lean body mass. Biochemical tests include the transferrin level, which indicates visceral protein depletion when less than 170 g per dl. Recall skin antigen testing commonly includes *Candida*, mumps, and dermatophyten or tetanus toxoid skin tests. Lack of response to these antigens indicates immunodeficiency, which supports a diagnosis of clinically significant protein-calorie malnutrition. Nutritional support may be applied before therapy such as for severely malnourished patients who are to undergo surgery. The second situation would be to provide nutritional support during therapy such as for patients receiving radiotherapy for an esophageal lesion that temporarily obstructs. The third group consists of patients who experience a complication of therapy, such as a fistula following abdominal surgery. The final group includes patients with advanced disease in whom nutritional support is palliative.

Dietary History

In addition to the location of tumor and presence of absence of metastasis, the patient's pre-illness weight, current weight, and timeframe of weight loss are recorded. Patients may underestimate their customary weight in an attempt to minimize degree of weight loss.[43] They should be questioned as to changes in appetite, taste, or smell, difficulties with chewing, swallowing, or digesting food, presence of nausea or vomiting, oral ulcerations, altered bowel habits, food allergies, preferences, and aversions, the time of day when appetite is greatest, religious or ethnic food restrictions, grocery budget, and cooking facilities. Other factors that may increase the risk of malnutrition include the inability of patients to feed themselves, due to weakness or pain, postoperative considerations, chemotherapy, or radiation therapy within the past 6 months, and the presence of chronic pain.

Physical Examination

The physical examination should focus on signs of protein-calorie malnutrition (Tables 28-1 and 28-2).

Table 28-1. Physical Signs of Protein-Calorie Malnutrition

Mentation
    Irritability
    Apathy
    Confusion
    Decreased concentration
Musculature
    Generalized wasting
    Weakness
Eyes
    Dull, dry conjunctivae
    Dark areas under the eyes
Nails
    Thin and brittle
    Ridged
Skin
    Dry, flaky, itchy
    Decreased turgor
    Easily bruised
    Delayed wound healing
Hair
    Sparse
    Dry, dull, brittle
    Areas of color change
    Easily pluckable
Lips
    Red, swollen
    Dry
    Cheilosis and angular fissure
Gums
    Tender and bleeding
    Ulcerations
Other
    Diarrhea or constipation
    Anorexia
    Nausea and vomiting
    Cold intolerance
    Decreased physical activity
    Enlarged parotid glands, liver, spleen

Source: Reprinted with permission from CL Buss. Nutritional support of cancer patients. Primary Care 1987;14:325.

Three-Day Food Records

A 3-day calorie count identifies trends in the patient's nutritional intake. These data can be compared with standard values to decide if the patient's caloric and protein intake is adequate.

Laboratory Analysis

Composite indices, such as the Prognostic Nutritional Index, seem to be more accurate than individual measurements. Although some authors consider serum albumin to be as accurate as composite indices,[44] others have questioned its value due to the 20-day biological half-life of albumin,[45] considering that this value falls only in severe malnutrition. Other authors have stated that physical examination is equal or superior to any single objective measurement in the prediction of nutritionally related complications.[46]

One simple technique for nutritional assessment is described by Dudrick, who uses weight loss, albumin level, and skin reactivity.[47] Nutritional depletion is defined as a weight loss of 10% or more of body weight, a serum albumin of less than 3.4 g per dl, and a negative reaction to a series of recall skin test antigens.

Reassessment

To monitor weight accurately, the patient should be weighed twice a week on the same scale at the same time of day, while wearing similar clothing. Weight changes are most valuable when edema and ascites are absent. Nitrogen balance and albumin levels are determined weekly, and the anergy battery of recall skin antigen testing repeated monthly. Outpatients should be reevaluated every 2 weeks.

Patients who are determined not to require nutritional supplementation at the time of initial evaluation, but who are still deemed to be at risk for nutritional deficits, should be evaluated periodically to ensure satisfactory nutritional status.

Determination of Nutritional Needs

Caloric Requirements

Daily caloric requirements can be estimated by determining the patient's basal energy expenditure (BEE) by direct measurement with an indirect calorimeter or using the Harris and Benedict equation[48]:

$$\text{Men: } 66 + (6.2 \times wt^{lb}) + (12.7 \times ht^{in}) - (6.8 \times age^{yrs})$$

$$\text{Women: } 644 + (4.4 \times wt^{lb}) + (4.3 \times ht^{in}) - (4.7 \times age^{yrs})$$

Table 28-2. Clinical Signs of Nutrient Deficiencies

Vitamin A
  Dry, scaly skin
  Night blindness
  Eye irritation
  Follicular hyperkeratosis
Vitamin C
  Petechiae, purpura
  Easy bruising
  Delayed wound healing
  Bleeding gums
  Edema
Folate
  Anorexia
  Glossitis
  Diarrhea, malabsorption
  Fatigue and irritability
  Leukopenia
  Megaloblastic anemia
B_{12}
  Paresthesias of hands and feet
  Agitation, moodiness
  Sore tongue
  Incoordination, ataxia
  Anorexia, nausea
Thiamine
  Burning feet
  Peripheral neuropathies
  Wrist or foot drop
  Decreased reflexes
  Calf muscle tenderness
Pyridoxine
  Seborrhea of face and neck
  Tingling paresthesia
  Disequilibrium
  Depression
Zinc
  Loss of taste acuity
  Decreased olfactory sensations
  White spotting of nails
  Facial hyperpigmentation
Magnesium
  Numbness and tingling
  Muscle twitching and tremor
  Muscle cramps
  Cardiac arrhythmias
  Chvostek's sign
Essential fatty acids
  Dry, flaky skin
  Hair loss
  Skin thickening
  Delayed wound healing

Source: Adapted from CL Buss. Nutritional support of cancer patients. Primary Care 1987;14:2.

The BEE is then multiplied by various activity and stress factors:

calories for weight maintenance = BEE × activity factor × stress injury factor

Activity factor:
1.2 = Bed rest
1.3 = Ambulating ad lib

Stress/injury factors:
1.13 per degree, Centigrade fever
1.0–1.2, Elective surgery
1.3–1.5, Cancer cachexia[48]

If the patient continues to lose more than 2.2 pounds per week, the caloric intake should be increased by 2 calories per pound until the weight stabilizes or increases. Patients receiving chemotherapy or radiation therapy should also have caloric intake increased by 2 calories per pound to avoid significant weight loss.[49]

Protein Requirements

To allow for anabolism, 1.2–1.5 g of protein per kg of actual body weight are required.[50] Specific disease states may require adjustment of protein requirements. For example, patients with graft-versus-host reaction should receive 2 g of protein per kg of body weight.[51]

Methods of Nutritional Support

Oral Method

Advantages Versus Disadvantages

Voluntary oral feeding is the preferred method of nutritional support for as long as the patient can receive nutrients this way. With preventative nutritional counseling, weight loss may be minimized or avoided. Although this is ideally accomplished using normal foods, if the patient continues to lose weight, nutritional supplements may be necessary. It is only when patients are unable to provide their nutritional needs orally that other techniques, such as enteral or parenteral feeding, should be used.

A variety of oral supplements are available, and the patient with taste changes should be allowed to "taste-test" a number of them in hopes of finding the supplements that are most palatable. Although most supplements are sufficiently sweetened for most cancer patients, spices, seasoning, or food color may be added to increase palatability. Generally, the supplements provide 240–480 calories and 7–20 g of protein per 240 ml serving. If a supplement is prescribed, it should be prescribed as a medication with a certain amount to be taken every day. The patient should then record the amount actually taken.

Techniques and Formulas

Anorexia. Patients with anorexia and early satiety should be encouraged to eat small, highly nutritious meals frequently. Because anorexia seems to be worse later in the day, meals should be planned so that breakfast contains more than one-third of the day's requirement for protein and calories. Nutritious snacks and leftovers should be readily available for between-meal snacking. If the patient is in the hospital and nothing per mouth is allowed during the day for tests, nighttime food service should be available so the patient can "catch up" with food intake missed during the day.

The protein content of foods may be increased by adding skim milk powder to make double-strength milk to recipes containing milk and to ground meats, and by using half-and-half cream instead of water. Butter, margarine, sour cream, mayonnaise, whipped cream, peanut butter, and commercially available carbohydrate supplements can be added to various foods. Food colors and textures should be varied. Calorically dense "fast foods" might also be offered.

If possible, the patient should be involved in meal planning. This input not only gives patients a sense of control over their lives, but intake seems to improve if patients can select food items shortly before the meal is served.

Patients should be encouraged to think of food as a form of medication, and this may increase intake. However, family and staff should avoid nagging patients to "take one more bite." This only frustrates patients, who are being asked to eat past the point of satiety.

Mealtimes should be made as pleasurable as possible, with visually appealing meals, good conversation, music, and pleasant table settings. A glass of beer or wine and light exercise, such as a walk before mealtimes, may stimulate the appetite. Taste impairment may be improved by supplemental oral zinc sulfate, 30–40 mg daily.[52]

Taste Changes

FOOD LACKS TASTE. For patients with decreased taste, food with strong flavors and smells are often preferable, such as Italian, Mexican, and foods that contain curry. Tart flavors, such as lemon juice, may stimulate taste unless they result in burning or a metallic taste. Herbs, spices, mint, additional salt and sugar, and marinades, such as soy, wine, or barbecue sauce, may be helpful. In addition, warm foods generally have more taste than cold foods.

FOOD TASTES BITTER. Patients should be asked to identify the changes in their taste and smell. If meat is unpalatable, milder-flavored sources of protein may be used, such as eggs, soy products (tofu), poultry, fish, milk, cheese, legumes, and peanut butter. Meats may be better tolerated if marinated in fruit juices or served with fruit sauces. Smells from cooking foods should be minimized. Metal serving utensils and pans should be avoided.

Dry Mouth and Thick Saliva. Foods moistened with gravies, sauces, melted butter, or mayonnaise may be easier to swallow. Patients should sip water and juice or suck on ice throughout the day. If patients do not have open mouth lesions, lemon juice or tart candy may stimulate saliva. A room humidifier may lessen the symptoms of dry lips and mouth. The patient's lips should be lubricated with a water-soluble gel. Commercial mouthwashes should be avoided, using one-half hydrogen peroxide and one-half water to rinse the mouth before and after meals. Artificial saliva may be useful, although some patients dislike the taste.

Stomatitis, Painful Chewing, and Dental Extractions. Soft or pureed foods, such as applesauce, cooked cereal, cream soups, casseroles, mashed potatoes, cheesecake, custard, ice cream, milk shakes, and puddings, are better tolerated than hard, crusty foods, such as dry toast, coarse cereals, or raw fruits and vegetables. Extreme temperatures may be irritating, as are spicy, hot foods, and acidic fruits and fruit juices.

Commercial mouthwashes containing alcohol should be avoided; instead, use normal saline or baking soda and water (1 teaspoon per half L). The

patient's dentures should be checked for proper fit because ill-fitting dental prosthetics may result in oral ulcerations. A local anesthetic such as viscous lidocaine may be applied to mouth lesions prior to eating, although patients should be discouraged from consuming hot foods and beverages that may burn their mouths. Patients may rinse with half liquid diphenhydramine and half kaolin and pectin suspension for 15 minutes prior to meals.[53] Ulcerated areas may be painted with an antacid or kaolin and pectin suspension.

Nausea and Vomiting. Eliminate any factors that cause nausea including drug reactions (especially meperidine and codeine) and electrolyte abnormalities. Medications such as digitalis and anticholinergics may exacerbate anorexia.

Dry toast, crackers, or ginger ale taken on rising or prior to mealtimes may increase food tolerance. Patients should avoid foods that seem to trigger nausea, such as spicy foods, foods with strong odors, and greasy foods such as fried foods, cream soups, gravies, cold cuts, and whole milk. Cold foods may be better tolerated. Several small meals should be eaten slowly throughout the day.

Patients should wear loose clothing and avoid lying flat after eating. They should also avoid forced eating past the point of tolerance. Relaxation techniques (sitting quietly, deep breathing, and progressively relaxing body muscles) have been found to increase food intake.[54]

If patients require antiemetics, the administration should be timed to provide peak effect at mealtimes. Antiemetics should be given prophylactically, not after symptoms are present. Patients should also have access to antiemetic rectal suppositories for vomiting episodes.

Constipation. The patient should be encouraged to drink 8–10 glasses of fluid per day. Fiber can be added to the diet by eating raw fruits and vegetables, nuts, whole-grain breads, and bran. Prune juice may be helpful, but medications may become necessary.

Diarrhea, Lactose Intolerance, and Dumping Syndrome

Small, frequent meals and boiled rice, bananas, and potatoes may help control diarrhea. Consider enzyme supplements if the patient has evidence of steatorrhea.

If lactose intolerance seems to be a problem, lactose-free milk substitutes, such as soy milk, may be substituted for milk. If milk products are eliminated from the diet, calcium supplements should be prescribed. If milk products are to be consumed, lactase enzyme (Lact-Aid) may be added. Yogurt and some cheeses may be tolerated.

The patient with dumping syndrome should eat a high-protein, low-carbohydrate diet, avoiding concentrated sweets. Solid foods should be eaten alone, with liquids consumed 30 minutes later. Meals should be small and frequent, and the supine position should be avoided for 30 minutes after eating.

Exacerbating Symptoms

FATIGUE. Any unnecessary activity should be avoided around mealtimes. Breakfast should be emphasized, because the patient may have more strength earlier in the day. Soft foods may decrease the energy required for chewing.

DYSPNEA AND COUGH. Cough medications should be administered prior to meals. The patient should eat in a sitting position, and supplemental oxygen may be provided via nasal prongs.

ODOR. Unpleasant odors may contribute to anorexia and nausea. Therefore, dressing changes should be timed separately from mealtime. Dressings should be disposed in an area other than where the patient eats, and waste baskets should be kept clean and odor-free.

ASCITES. Small, frequent meals should be taken in a sitting position.

PAIN. Pain may significantly interfere with eating, and pain medications should be scheduled so that the maximal effect is experienced during mealtimes.

HICCUPS. Medications should be timed to provide hiccup-free periods for eating.

ERUCTATION AND FLATUS. Gas-producing foods such as cabbage, broccoli, beans, onions, and carbonated beverages should be avoided. Meals should be consumed slowly, and air swallowing may be decreased by minimizing conversation while swallowing.

Artificial Feeding Methods

Enteral Method

Advantages Versus Disadvantages. Patients who have inadequate oral intake but a functioning gas-trointestinal tract are candidates for enteral alimentation. Advantages of using the enteral rather than the parenteral route include ease of administration, lower cost,[55] comparable efficacy in maintaining or improving nutritional status,[56] both in terms of suppressing gluconeogenesis and preserving lean body mass,[57] and decreased severity of complications.[58] The intestinal mucosal mass is stimulated by enteral feeding, decreasing septic complications in postoperative patients,[59] and exogenous insulin is usually not required.

Delivery Approaches. The gastrointestinal tract can be accessed through the use of transnasal tubes or enterostomy tubes. The choice depends on the proficiency of the gastrointestinal tract in absorbing and digesting nutrients, the expected duration of nutritional support, and patient tolerance and preference.

NASOGASTRIC AND NASODUODENAL TUBES. A soft, small-bore silicone tube with a weighted tip is passed transnasally or transorally into the stomach, duodenum, or proximal jejunum. These tubes are generally well tolerated, and the patient may continue to eat and drink with the tube in place. Owing to the small diameter, these tubes have the following characteristics: (1) they can only be used with formulas of low viscosity, (2) they require periodic flushing to maintain patency, and (3) they may require the use of a pump.

GASTROSTOMY. If the anticipated length of feeding is longer than 6 weeks, a gastrostomy or jejunostomy is performed, and the appropriate tube inserted. Some patients will not tolerate a transnasal tube, or will feel embarrassed to go out in public. These patients may prefer a gastrostomy or jejunostomy tube. Some patients find gastrostomy tubes more convenient because bolus feedings are well tolerated and because they do not spend hours attached to a pump.

A gastrostomy tube may be placed surgically at the time of other intra-abdominal procedures or as a separate laparotomy performed under local or general anesthesia. Another alternative is a percutaneous endoscopic gastrostomy tube placed under local anesthesia. The size of the tube placed should be at least 28 French to allow the use of thick blenderized diets.

JEJUNOSTOMY. If the patient is at a high risk for pulmonary aspiration, a jejunostomy tube is preferred over a gastrostomy tube, which may be associated with aspiration pneumonitis. The jejunostomy tube can be placed surgically or endoscopically.

Formulas. There are four categories of enteral feeding formulas: (1) complete, (2) chemically defined, (3) modular, and (4) disease specific. Complete formulas can be blenderized table food or commercially available lactose-containing or lactose-free nutritional supplements. The commercial formulas consist of whole proteins, complex sugars, and long and medium chain triglycerides. These formulas are generally the least expensive of all and can be used with nasogastric tubes or gastrostomies.

Chemically defined, or "elemental" formulas contain amino acids, simple carbohydrates, and small quantities of essential fat, minerals, and vitamins. They require little or no enzymatic activity for absorption and are indicated for patients with malabsorption syndromes, pancreatitis, or jejunal feeding. Many of the solutions are hyperosmolar and may require dilution or continuous pump infusion.

Modular components contain one nutrient, such as protein, carbohydrate, or fat. They may be combined to produce a nutritionally complete formula, but are more often used individually to customize a commercially available product.

Disease-specific compounds are designed for the nutritional needs of patients with disease states such as renal, hepatic, or pulmonary failure. They vary substantially in the amount of protein, carbohydrate, and fat contained in each formula.

Methods of Administration. Enteral feedings may be administered by bolus, intermittent, or continuous methods. Bolus methods entail administering 200–400 ml over 5–10 minutes. However, they may cause cramping, bloating, and nausea, and can only be used with gastric feedings, due to the reservoir capacity of the stomach. Intermittent feeding involves giving 200–400 ml by gravity drip over 20–30 minutes, up to eight times per day. This method is also limited to gastric feedings and is usually better tolerated than bolus feeds. With either bolus or intermittent methods, the tube should be irrigated after infusion of the solution to ensure patency.

Continuous feedings are given over 12–24 hours by gravity or by an infusion pump. They are administered with 50-ml half-strength formula per hour; volume is increased by 25 ml per hour every 8 hours

until the desired rate is reached. The concentration is gradually increased according to patient tolerance.

Complications. Pulmonary aspiration is the most serious complication of enteral alimentation. Patients particularly at risk for this complication are those with functional or mechanical bowel obstruction, gastric atony, and decreased mentation. The incidence of aspiration can be decreased by feeding the patient in a semireclining position and aspirating residuals periodically.

The most common complication is the development of bloating and an osmotic diarrhea due to the hypertonic composition of many enteral formulas. Generally, the lower the osmolality of the feeding, the fewer problems with diarrhea. This complication can be treated by slowing the rate of infusion or diluting the solution to an isotonic concentration. Alternatively, gradually increasing the strength of the feeding lessens the reaction. If the serum albumin is low, absorption is often inefficient, and the administration of exogenous albumin may correct the diarrhea.[60] If malabsorption continues, antidiarrheals or changing the patient to an elemental diet may successfully control the diarrhea.

Parenteral Method

Advantages Versus Disadvantages. Parenteral nutrition is indicated when contraindications to enteral nutrition exist. Common applications for this approach include patients with fistulas, malabsorption, persistent vomiting, and bowel obstruction. Parenteral nutrition is often initiated in the severely malnourished patients, thus allowing a slower transition to enteral feedings as the gut regains its absorptive ability.

Disadvantages of parenteral nutrition include difficulty of administration, cost, and increased severity of complications compared with enteral nutrition. Patients who require long-term parenteral nutrition, such as those with chronic radiation enteritis, short bowel syndrome, or fistulae, may benefit from home hyperalimentation. Not only does it allow the patient to go home and live a productive life, but it also costs approximately one-third the cost of in-hospital hyperalimentation. Selected patients with terminal cancer or malignant, unresectable bowel obstruction may live a more normal lifestyle at home, rather than being confined to the hospital for their last remaining days. The use of home hyperalimentation requires a significant commitment by the patient and the family to learn the appropriate techniques of administration.

Delivery Techniques. TPN is usually delivered through a catheter placed percutaneously into the subclavian vein, although the internal jugular vein has been frequently used. However, the subclavian vein offers the advantage of ease in maintaining a stable sterile dressing. A prior radical mastectomy may alter the location of the vein, and maintenance of a sterile dressing will be difficult due to the absence of the pectoralis major muscle.[61] The internal jugular vein may not be available in patients with head and neck cancer, in whom a radical neck dissection has been performed or is planned, and in patients with a tracheostomy. Double- and triple-lumen catheters provide additional ports for blood drawing, administering antibiotics, and chemotherapy.

When the anticipated duration of hyperalimentation is longer than 6 weeks, surgical placement of a silicone catheter with Dacron cuff is indicated. These catheters are tunneled subcutaneously to the lower chest wall, where they exit from the skin.

A subcutaneous implantable injection port may be used for parenteral alimentation as well as for chemotherapy. The reservoir is accessed percutaneously with a noncoring needle. This device is particularly indicated for active patients, such as those who swim regularly. Patients who abhor needlesticks, however, would be less inclined to prefer this system.

Composition of Solutions. The solutions used for TPN include a mixture of carbohydrates, protein, fat, vitamins, and minerals. The source of carbohydrate is dextrose, and the concentration is determined by the total calorie to nitrogen ratio and the patient's glucose tolerance. The calorie to nitrogen ratio is determined by the following formula:

$$\text{Calories: Nitrogen} = \frac{\text{total calories} (\text{g of dextrose} \times 2.3) + (\text{g of nitrogen} \times 6.25 \times 4)}{(\text{g of nitrogen}) \ (\text{g of amino acid} \times 1/6)}$$

Commonly used ratios range between 135 to 1 and 150 to 1 to provide optimal retention of nitrogen (while minimizing the glucose transformation to fat), resulting in hepatic fat infiltration.

Amino acid solutions are available in concentrations from 3.5–10.0%. The most commonly used solution, 8.5%, is usually mixed with an equal amount of 50% dextrose to yield a solution of 4.25% amino acids with 25% dextrose. This provides a calorie to nitrogen ratio of 150 to 1, and consists of approximately 3,000 calories and 128 g of protein. The more concentrated solutions are used in patients who require fluid restriction or additional protein.

Several lipid preparations are available as 10% or 20% solutions. These fat emulsions may be administered once a week, 1,000 ml of a 10% solution, to prevent essential fatty acid deficiency or to be used as a source of calories. Provision of up to 50% of the nonprotein calories as fat may prevent some of the complications seen with excessive carbohydrate administration, such as fatty liver and excessive production of carbon dioxide, which exacerbates respiratory failure.[62]

Electrolytes, vitamins, and minerals must be added to these solutions in amounts compatible with daily requirements. One ampule of Multiple Vitamin Infusion should be added to the hyperalimentation solution daily. The customary electrolyte additives include approximately 120 mEq of sodium, 100 mEq of potassium, 30 mEq of magnesium, 20 mEq of calcium, and 300–400 mg of phosphorus daily. Because the amino acids are commercially available as acetate, chloride, or hydrochloride salts, they are acidic, and additional sodium chloride and potassium chloride may cause hyperchloremic metabolic acidosis. Therefore, electrolytes should be added as the acetate, bicarbonate, lactate, chloride, or acid phosphate salt, depending on the patient's acid–base status.

When large amounts of dextrose are given, 400–800 mg of phosphorus may be required when TPN is initiated. Phosphorus enters the cells with glucose, and debilitated patients have an inadequate phosphorous reserve. As the serum level of phosphate increases and reaches 3.0 mg per dl, the exogenous phosphorus can be decreased.

Trace minerals are added daily per the recommendations of the American Medical Association (Table 28-3).[63] Additional amounts of zinc are given to patients who are acutely catabolic or who have intestinal losses.

To avoid hyperglycemia and osmotic diuresis, the infusion is commenced at 50 ml per hour and gradually advanced over the next 48 hours. When

Table 28-3. Trace Minerals Administered to Cancer Patients

Mineral	Stable Adult	Adult Acutely Catabolic	Intestinal Losses
Zinc	2.5–4.0 mg	Additional 2.0 mg	12.2 mg/L bowel fluid lost; 17.2 mg/kg stool/ileostomy output
Copper	0.5–1.5 mg	—	—
Chromium	10–15 μg	—	20 μg
Manganese	0.15–0.8 mg	—	—

TPN is discontinued, it should also be done gradually over 12–24 hours, so as to decrease the incidence of biochemical complications including reactive hypoglycemia

Complications. One of the most worrisome complications of parenteral hyperalimentation is the risk of catheter sepsis. Catheter infections occur in 3–5% of patients and may be more frequent in patients with tracheostomies, in whom it is difficult to maintain a dry, sterile dressing. The usual organisms are gram-positive cocci or fungi. Catheter sepsis may be minimized by attention to rigid sterile techniques and by avoiding use of the catheter for antibiotics, blood products, and chemotherapy.

Mechanical complications associated with the insertion of the catheter include pneumothorax, hemothorax, catheter embolus, and injury to the heart or thoracic duct. Hyperglycemia can be controlled with the addition of regular insulin to the hyperalimentation bag after determining the patient's needs; hypoglycemia can be prevented by gradually tapering the hyperalimentation when it is no longer necessary.

Pharmacologic Interventions to Stimulate Appetite

A variety of agents have been used in an attempt to stimulate appetite, including steroids, growth hormones, cyproheptadine, hydrazine sulfate, cannabinoids, and megestrol acetate.

Glucocorticoids

Prednisolone has been evaluated in several studies.[64, 65] Although it has been associated with short-term subjective improvement in appetite, it has not affected objective measures of caloric intake or body weight.

Growth Hormone

The recent availability of recombinant human growth hormone has led to studies that indicate that it promotes lean body nitrogen retention in stable patients.[66] Its effect on stressed, cachectic patients is unknown. A theoretical objection to its use in cancer patients is the potential mitogenic effect of growth hormone.

Cyproheptadine

Cyproheptadine, a serotonin antagonist, has shown minimal effects on appetite and weight loss in randomized trials.[67]

Hydrazine Sulfate

Hydrazine sulfate inhibits the enzyme phosphoenolpyruvate carboxykinase and decreases gluconeogenesis in animals. Prospective, randomized trials are inconclusive as to its efficacy in improving appetite and weight gain.[68, 69] This agent continues to be evaluated, and recommendations await further clinical trials.

Cannabinoids

Dronabinol has been used to control chemotherapy-induced vomiting and has anecdotally stimulated appetite in patients with malignancies.[70] In an open pilot study, dronabinol (Marinol) improved appetite but had no effect on weight in a small number of cancer patients.[71]

Megestrol Acetate

The progestational agent megestrol acetate was noted to cause weight increase in postmenopausal women with breast cancer.[72] A randomized, double-blind, placebo-controlled trial demonstrated statistically significant increases in appetite and food intake, with a trend toward increased weight gain in the megestrol group.[73] Maximal effect has been reported with doses of 480–800 mg per day.[74] Side effects include impotence in men and vaginal bleeding in women. Thromboembolism is a theoretical risk, although it has not been reported in these studies.

Psychosocial Aspects of Artificial Feeding

Artificial feeding has been associated with unique psychological problems in cancer patients. This response has been found to depend on the diagnosis and prognosis of the patient's cancer, and the personality characteristics of the patient and the patient's family.[75] Disheartened patients tend to feel passive and helpless, whereas independent patients fight for a sense of control. Patients and families who are predominantly anxious tend to be extremely concerned with eating and maintaining weight.

Patients receiving parenteral nutrition initially tend to develop moderate-to-severe depression, which resolves with increased comfort in handling the nutritional devices.[76] In the first 3 months, patients fear equipment problems and complications associated with parenteral nutrition.[77] Patients receiving enteral support complain of irritation from the tube and limited mobility, but generally seem to tolerate enteral nutrition better than patients receiving parenteral nutrition.[78]

Because these reactions may influence the compliance with nutritional regimens, they need to be addressed for optimal management of the patient.[79] Patients who are independent should be involved with the feeding regimen, so that they may obtain a sense of control. The nutritional team should work in conjunction with the patient and family to increase the comfort level associated with the nutritional apparatus. Finally, if possible, enteral nutrition should be chosen over parenteral nutrition if feasible, because it is not only physiologically equivalent, but is also associated with less patient distress.

Acknowledgment

I acknowledge Dorothy Holevar for her editorial assistance and thank Joyce Federczko, MALS, and the library staff of Advocate Health Sciences Library Network for their valuable research assistance.

References

1. Bruera E, MacDonald RN. Nutrition in cancer patients: An update and review of our experience. J Pain Symptom Manage 1988;3:134.
2. Langstein HN, Norton JA. Mechanisms of cancer cachexia. Hematol Oncol Clin North Am 1991;4:103.
3. Daly JM, Redmond HP, Lieverman MD, et al. Nutritional support of patients with cancer of the gastrointestinal tract. Surg Clin North Am 1991;71:523.
4. Costa G, Donaldson SS. Effects of cancer and cancer treatment on the nutrition of the host. N Engl J Med 1979;300:1471.
5. Wys WD, Begg D, Lavin PT, et al. Prognostic effect of weight loss prior to chemotherapy in cancer patients. Am J Med 1980;69:491.
6. Warren S. The immediate causes of death in cancer. Am J Med Sci 1932;184:610.
7. Costa G, Donaldson S. The nutritional effects of cancer and its therapy. Nutr Cancer 1980;2:22.
8. DeWys WD. Anorexia as a general effect of cancer. Cancer 1979;43:2013.
9. Baillie P, Millar FK, Pratt AW. Food and water intakes and Walker tumor growth in rats with hypothalamic lesions. Am J Physiol 1965;209:293.
10. Novin D, Wyricko W, Bray G (eds). Hunger: Basic Mechanisms and Clinical Implications. New York: Raven, 1976.
11. Kern KA, Norton JA. Cancer cachexia. J Parenter Enter Nutr 1988;12:286.
12. McNamara M, Alexander R, Norton J. Cytokines and their role in the pathophysiology of cancer cachexia. J Parenter Enter Nutr 1992;16:50S.
13. Theologides A. Pathogenesis of cachexia in cancer: A review and a hypothesis. Cancer 1972;29:484.
14. DeWys WD, Walters K. Abnormalities of taste sensation in cancer patients. Cancer 1975;36:1888.
15. DeWys WD. Changes in Taste Sensation in Cancer Patient. In MR Kare, O Maller (eds), The Chemical Senses and Nutrition. London: Academic Press, 1977;281.

16. Bruera E, Carraro S, Roca E, et al. Association between malnutrition and caloric intake, emesis, psychological depression, glucose taste, and tumor mass. Cancer Treat Rep 1984;68:873.
17. Garcia J, Ervin FR, Koelling RA. Learning with prolonged delay of reinforcement. Psychon Sci 1966;4:121.
18. Waldmann TA, Broder S, Stroeber W. Protein-losing enteropathies in malignancy. Ann NY Acad Sci 1974;230:306.
19. Douglas HO. Hyperalimentation in gastrointestinal cancer. Contemp Surg 1978;13:35.
20. Knox LS, Crosby LO, Feurer ID, et al. Energy expenditure in malnourished cancer patients. Ann Surg 1983;197:152.
21. Shaw JM, Humberstone DM, Wolfe RR. Energy and protein metabolism in sarcoma patients. Ann Surg 1988;207:283.
22. Russell DM, Shike M, Marliss EB, et al. Effects of total parenteral nutrition and chemotherapy on the metabolic derangements in small cell lung cancer. Cancer Res 1984;44:1706.
23. Arbeit JM, Lees DE, Corsey R, et al. Resting energy expenditure in controls and cancer patients with localized and diffuse disease. Ann Surg 1984;200:292.
24. Fearon KCH, Hansell DT, Preston T, et al. Energy expenditure in malnourished cancer patients. Ann Surg 1983;197:152.
25. Lundholm K, Bennegard K, Eden E, et al. Efflux of 3-methylhistidine from the leg in cancer patients who experience weight loss. Cancer Res 1982;42:4807.
26. Norton JA, Gorschboth CM, Wesley RA, et al. Fasting plasma amino acid levels in cancer patients. Cancer 1985;56:1181
27. Felig P, Pozefsky T, Marliss E, Cahill Jr GR. Alanine: Key role in gluconeogenesis. Science 1989;83:1614.
28. Marks PA, Bishop J. Glucose metabolism in subjects with neoplastic disease: Response to insulin and glucose tolerance: Follow-up studies. Proc Am Assoc Cancer Res 1957;2:228.
29. Holroyade CP, Gabuzda TG, Putnam RC, et al. Altered glucose metabolism in metastatic carcinoma. Cancer Res 1975;35:3710.
30. Olgilvie GK, Vail DM. Nutrition and cancer: Recent developments. Vet Clin North Am 1990;20:969.
31. Waterhouse C, Nye WHR. Metabolic effects of infused triglyceride. Metabolism 1961;10:403.
32. Arbeit JM, Lees DE, Corsey R, et al. Determination of resting energy expenditure in patients with and without extremity sarcomas. Proc Am Assoc Cancer Res Am Soc Clin Oncol 1981;22:194A.
33. Buxton B. Small bowel resection and gastric hypersecretion. Gut 1974;14:229.
34. Holland JF, Scharlau C, Gailani S, et al. Vincristine treatment of advanced cancer: A cooperative study of 392 cases. Cancer Res 1973;33:1258.
35. Cohen M. Effects of oral prophylactic broad spectrum non-absorbable antibiotics on GI absorption of nutrients and methotrexate in small cell bronchogenic carcinoma patients. Cancer 1976;38:1856.
36. Torosian M, Daly J. Nutritional support in the cancer-bearing host. Cancer 1986;58:1914.
37. Baron PL, Lawrence WH, Chan WM, et al. Effects of parenteral nutrition on cell cycle kinetics of head and neck cancers. Arch Surg 1986;121:1282.
38. Mullen JL, Buzby GP, Gertner MH, et al. Protein synthesis dynamics in human gastrointestinal malignancies. Surgery 1980;87:331.
39. Klein S, Simes J, Blackburn G. Total parenteral nutrition and cancer clinical trials. Cancer 1986;58:1378.
40. American Society of Parenteral and Enteral Nutrition Board of Directors. Guidelines for use of total parenteral nutrition in the hospitalized adult patient. J Parenter Enteral Nutr 1986;10:441.
41. Padilla GV, Presant C, Grant MM, et al. Quality of life index for patients with cancer. Res Nurs Health 1983;6:117.
42. Schwartz G. Combined parenteral hyperalimentation as an adjunct to cancer chemotherapy. Am J Surg 1971;121:167.
43. Morgan DB, Hill GL, Burkinshaw L. The assessment of weight loss from a single measurement of body weight: The problems and limitations. Am J Nutr 1980;33:2101.
44. Leite JF, Antunes CF, Monteiro JC, et al. Value of nutritional parameters in the prediction of postoperative complications in elective gastrointestinal surgery. Br J Surg 1987;74:426.
45. Dempsey DT, Mullen JL, Buzby GP. The link between nutritional status and clinical outcome: Can nutritional intervention modify it? Am J Clin Nutr 1988;47:352.
46. Daly JM, Redmond HP, Lieberman MD, et al. Nutritional support of patients with cancer of the gastrointestinal tract. Surg Clin North Am 1991;71:523.
47. Copeland EM, Daly JM, Dudrick SJ. Nutrition as an adjunct to cancer treatment in the adult. Cancer Res 1977;37:2451.
48. Harris JA, Benedict FG. Biometric studies of basal metabolism in man. Carnegie Institute of Washington, Publication No. 279, 1919.
49. Nunnally C, Donoghue M, Yasko JM. Nutritional needs of cancer patients. Nurs Clin North Am 1982;17:557.
50. Blackburn GL, Bistrian BR, Maini BS, et al. Nutritional and metabolic assessment of the hospitalized patient. J Parenter Enter Nutr 1977;1:11.
51. Gauvreau JM, Lenssen P, Cheney CL, et al. Nutritional management of patients with intestinal graft vs host disease. J Am Diet Assoc 1981;79:673.
52. Yardumian H. Oral nutrition of cancer patients. J Am Osteopath Assoc 1983;82:393.
53. D'Agostino NS. Managing nutrition problems in advanced cancer. Am J Nurs 1989;1:50.
54. Dixon J. Effect of nursing interventions on nutritional and performance status in cancer patients. Nurs Res 1984;33:330.

55. Roberts DR, Thelen D, Weinstein S. Parenteral and enteral nutrition: A cost-benefit audit. Minn Med 1982;65:707.

56. Burt ME, Gorschboth BS, Brennan MF. A controlled, prospective, randomized trial evaluating the metabolic effects of enteral and parenteral nutrition in the cancer patient. Cancer 1982;49:1092.

57. Jensen S. Clinical effects of enteral and parenteral nutrition preceding cancer surgery. Med Oncol Tumor Pharmacother 1985;2:225.

58. Heymsfield SB, Bethel RA, Ausley JD, et al. Enteral hyperalimentation: An alternative to central venous hyperalimentation. Ann Intern Med 1979;90:63.

59. Moore EE, Jones TN. Benefits of immediate jejunostomy feedings after major abdominal trauma: A prospective randomized study. J Trauma 1986;26:874.

60. Brinson R, Guild R, Kolts B. Diarrhea and hypoalbuminemia in a medical intensive care unit. Gastroenterology 1986;88:1336.

61. Ota DM, Kleman G, Diamond K. Practical considerations in the nutritional management of the cancer patient. Curr Probl Cancer 1986;10:345.

62. Askanazi J. Nutrition and the respiratory system. Crit Care Med 1982;10:163.

63. Guidelines for essential trace element: Preparations for parenteral use. JAMA 1979;241:2051.

64. Bruera E, Roca E, Cedaro L, et al. Methylprednisolone use in patients with cancer. Cancer Treat Rep 1985;69:751.

65. Willox JC, Cou J, Shaw J, et al. Prednisolone as an appetite stimulant in patients with cancer. Br Med J 1984;288:27.

66. Pontin GA, Halliday D, Teale JD, et al. Postoperative positive nitrogen balance with intravenous hyponutrition and growth hormone. Lancet 1988;1:438.

67. Kardinal CG, Loprinzi C, Schaid DJ, et al. A controlled trial of cyproheptadine in cancer patients with anorexia and/or cachexia. Cancer 1990;65:2657.

68. Chlebowski RT, Bulcavage L, Grosvenor M, et al. Hydrazine sulfate influence on nutritional status and survival in non-small-cell lung cancer. J Clin Oncol 8:9.

69. Chlebowski RT, Herber D, Richardson B, et al. Influence of hydrazine sulfate on abnormal carbohydrate metabolism in cancer patients with weight loss. Cancer Res 1984;44:857.

70. Regelson W. THC in Patients with Cancer. In MC Braude, S Szara (eds), The Pharmacology of Marijuana. New York: Raven, 1976;763.

71. Plasse TF, Gorter RW, Ksnow SH, et al. Recent clinical experience with Dronabinol. Pharm Biochem Behav 1991;40:695.

72. Tchekmedyian NS, Tait N, Moody M, et al. High-dose megestrol acetate. A possible treatment for cachexia. JAMA 1987;257:1195.

73. Tchekmedyian NS, Hickman M, Stau J, et al. Megestrol acetate in cancer anorexia and weight loss. Cancer 1992;69:1268.

74. Loprinzi CI, Mailliard J, Schaid D. Dose/response evaluation of megestrol acetate (MA) for the treatment of cancer anorexia/cachexia. Proc ASCO 1992;11:378.

75. Peteet JR, Medeiros C, Slavin L, et al. Psychological aspects of artificial feeding in cancer patients. J Parenter Enter Nutr 1981;5:138.

76. Price BS, Levine EL. Permanent total parenteral nutrition: Psychological and social responses of the early stages. J Parenter Enter Nutr 1979;3:48.

77. Perl M, Hall RCW, Dudrick SJ. Psychological aspects of long-term home hyperalimentation. J Parenter Enter Nutr 1980;4:544.

78. Padilla GV, Grant MM. Psychosocial aspects of artificial feeding. Cancer 1985;55:301.

79. Hughes BA, Fleming R, Berkner S. Patient compliance with a home parenteral nutrition program. J Parenter Enter Nutr 1980;4:12.

Chapter 29

Nutrition Management for Selected Types of Cancer

Joan M. Payne

Practical Considerations

Nutrition intervention and diet management are important parts of the cancer patient's treatment plan. Malnutrition and cachexia may develop prior to the actual cancer diagnosis, during treatment, and in the end-stage disease state. Weight loss is usually the most obvious sign of decreased nutritional status, which also includes wasting of body fat and lean body mass. In comparing a similar amount of weight loss between a healthy person and the patient diagnosed with cancer, the cancer patient loses much more muscle mass. This lean mass includes both skeletal and cardiac muscle.[1] The overall weight loss may be a result of negative energy balance. The cancer patient may experience a decreased caloric intake, increased caloric expenditure, or a combination of both.[1, 2] As a biochemical response of the pain process, decreased caloric intake is exacerbated in the cancer patient with chronic pain. A negative energy balance may also result from competition of the neoplastic tissue for nutrients, increased energy requirements to maintain sodium and potassium gradients, and increased energy need for protein synthesis.[3, 4] Increased nutritional uptake results in an increased resting metabolic rate.[4]

Metabolic rates in patients with cancer have been reported to be increased by as much as 35–74% of resting metabolic rates.[4] In many patients, the tumor burden is not great enough to produce an observed amount of wasting[4] and resting metabolism is not consistently elevated in cancer patients.[5] In patients with small cell lung carci-

noma, leukemia, and lymphoma, there may be an increased resting metabolic rate.[5]

The metabolism of carbohydrate, protein, and lipid may be altered but this has not proved to be the sole reason for the degree of malnutrition.[3] Besides tumor burden, the use of multimodal antineoplastic therapy may contribute to the deterioration of nutritional status and malnutrition.[6] Surgery, chemotherapy, and radiation can cause nutritional disabilities such as decreased oral intake and malabsorption of nutrients, which may lead to nutritional deficiencies.[6] If the patient's nutritional status has already started to decline, antitumor modalities can enhance morbidity and, for some patients, it may lead to mortality.[6] Morbidity and mortality can be increased due to organ function impairment from malnutrition.[7]

Nutritional management and the type of nutritional support are based on factors such as nutritional deficit, feasibility, convenience, and cost.[1] Not all cancer patients need aggressive nutrition support such as tube feeding or parenteral nutrition. Special attention regarding nutrition should be given to the cancer pain patient. The patient may be able to maintain adequate nutritional status through oral intake with appropriate diet counseling. The registered dietitian plays an important role in the oncology team. The dietitian can assess and monitor the cancer patient's nutritional status, both in the acute care and outpatient setting. After an initial assessment, the dietitian can recommend and implement interventions to improve or maintain the nutritional status of the patient. The nutrition care plan for the cancer patient should consist of short-

and long-term goals. Short-term goals include the following:

1. Provide optimal nutrition support by treating symptoms
2. Maintain desirable body weight
3. Correct vitamin and mineral abnormalities[8]

Long-term goals are based on long-term medical goals:

1. Supportive nutrition care should be given to those patients receiving palliative treatment or no treatment due to a poor prognosis. An emphasis on provision of comfort for the patient and family is recommended. Parenteral nutrition should not be initiated unless it is of emotional benefit to the patient and family.
2. Aggressive nutrition support to maintain desirable body weight and minimize overall weight loss
3. Provide adequate calories, protein, vitamins, and minerals
4. Oral nutritional supplementation or enteral nutrition support via tube feeding
5. Total parenteral nutrition (TPN) support only if enteral support is not medically feasible
6. A combination of enteral and parenteral nutrition support[8]

When considering nutrition support, Guidelines for the Use of Parenteral and Enteral Nutrition in Adult and Pediatric Populations, established by the American Society for Parenteral and Enteral Nutrition, may be used and are as follows:

1. Enteral tube feeding and parenteral support may benefit some severely malnourished cancer patients or those in whom gastrointestinal or other toxicities are anticipated to preclude adequate oral nutrition intake for more than 1 week. Patients who are candidates for nutrition intervention under these circumstances should receive nutrition support, if possible, in conjunction with the initiation of oncologic therapy.

2. Specialized nutrition support is not routinely indicated for well-nourished or mildly nourished patients undergoing surgery, chemotherapy, or radiation treatment in whom adequate oral intake is anticipated.

3. TPN is unlikely to benefit patients with advanced cancer whose malignancy is documented as unresponsive to chemotherapy or radiation therapy.[9]

Pain from the cancer itself (especially in a metastatic process), postsurgical pain, pain from chemotherapy, and radiation side effects can impose negative nutritional consequences. Many cancer pain patients lack or do not have the desire to eat or drink, which can lead to a decreased solid food and fluid intake. If the patient does not receive adequate nutrients and water, dehydration can result. Dehydration has nutritional implications related to fluid and electrolyte imbalance that have their own clinical manifestations.

Effective pain control management for cancer patients involves the use of pain medications. The use of narcotics (and nonnarcotic analgesics) can produce significant food–drug interactions. Continuous narcotic use may require necessary nutritional interventions in the hospital or home environment. Table 29-1 shows a listing of analgesics and narcotics and food–drug interactions.[10]

Basic Nutrition Guidelines for the Cancer Patient

As cancer patients undergo antineoplastic therapies, it is important that they maintain adequate nutrient intake to combat the metabolic stress of the disease process itself and the side effects of treatment modalities. A balance of foods is necessary to meet the needs for tissue repair and to maintain lean body mass. The diet must include both macronutrients and micronutrients. For the healthy person, the Recommended Dietary Allowances have been developed as a guide for maintaining optimal nutrition status. The food groups shown below are classified in the Food Guide Pyramid (Figure 29-1):

1. Milk and dairy products
2. Meats or meat substitutes
3. Fruits and vegetables
4. Breads, cereals, and starches
5. Fats, alcohol, and sweets

The cancer patient may require specialized diet plans during treatment and recovery. Modifications in the diet plan are based on oral intake, food tolerances, type of cancer, stage of disease, and side effects from treatment modalities used.

Table 29-1. Food–Drug Interactions of Medications Commonly Prescribed for Oncology Patients

Medication	Classification	Precautions and Side Effects
Acetaminophen Datril	Analgesic, antipyretic	Take with food to ⇓ GI distress. Avoid alcohol
Acetysalicylic acid Aspirin Ecotrin Empirin	Analgesic, nonsteroidal anti-inflammatory drug, antipyretic	Take with 8 oz water after meals or with food to ⇓ GI upset. Food ⇓ rate of absorption. Ensure adequate fluid intake. Need foods ⇑ in vitaminC and folic acid. Not for patient prone to vitamin K deficiency. Caution with diabetic. Avoid alcohol
Diflunisal Dolobid	Analgesic, anti-inflammatory, antipyretic	Take with food to ⇓ GI irritation, nausea, vomiting, GI pain, diarrhea, constipation, flatulence. Avoid alcohol
Fioricet	Analgesic, sedative	Take with food. Avoid alcohol. Can cause nausea, vomiting, heartburn, flatulence
Fiorinal	Analgesic, sedative	Take with food. Avoid alcohol. Can cause nausea, vomiting, flatulence, heartburn
Hydromorphone HCl Dilaudid	Analgesic, narcotic	Take with 8 oz water. Avoid alcohol. Can cause constipation, nausea, vomiting, GI distress, edema, anorexia, dry mouth. Delays digestion of food
Meperidine HCl Demerol	Analgesic, narcotic	Dilute in 4 oz water. Can cause nausea, vomiting, anorexia, dry mouth. Avoid alcohol
Methadone HCl Dolophine	Analgesic, narcotic	Dissolve tabs in juice or water. Can cause constipation, nausea, vomiting, anorexia, dry mouth. Avoid alcohol
Morphine sulfate	Analgesic, narcotic	Nausea, vomiting, constipation, dry mouth, anorexia. Digestion of food delayed in small intestines
Oxymorphone HCl Numorphan	Analgesic, narcotic	Constipation, nausea, vomiting, anorexia, dry mouth. Avoid alcohol
Pentazocine HCl plus naloxone HCl Talwin NX	Analgesic, narcotic	Nausea, vomiting, constipation. Avoid alcohol. Anorexia, dry mouth, altered taste
Oxycodone HCl plus acetaminophen Percocet-5	Analgesic, narcotic	Nausea, vomiting, ⇓ appetite, dry mouth. Avoid alcohol
Oxycodone plus aspirin Percodan	Analgesic, narcotic	Take with food or 8 oz water to ⇓ GI distress. Nausea, vomiting, constipation, dry mouth. Avoid alcohol
Propoxyphene HCl Darvon	Analgesic, narcotic	Take with 8 oz water on empty stomach. May take with food to prevent irritation. Nausea, vomiting, constipation, abdominal pain, dry mouth. Avoid alcohol
Hydrocodone plus bitartrate plus acetaminophen Vicodin	Analgesic, narcotic, antitussive	Nausea, vomiting, constipation, dry mouth. Avoid alcohol

GI = gastrointestinal; ⇓ = decreased; ⇑ = increased.

Looking at the Pieces of the Pyramid

The Food Guide Pyramid emphasizes foods from the five major food groups shown in the three lower sections of the Pyramid. Each of these food groups provides some, but not all, of the nutrients you need. Foods in one group can't replace those in another. No one food group is more important than another – for good health, you need them all.

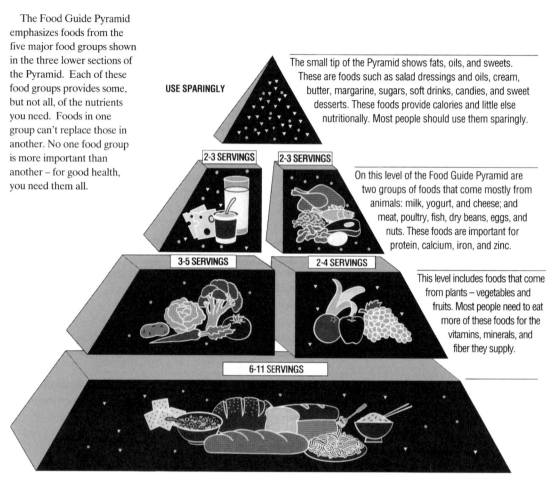

USE SPARINGLY

The small tip of the Pyramid shows fats, oils, and sweets. These are foods such as salad dressings and oils, cream, butter, margarine, sugars, soft drinks, candies, and sweet desserts. These foods provide calories and little else nutritionally. Most people should use them sparingly.

2-3 SERVINGS   **2-3 SERVINGS**

On this level of the Food Guide Pyramid are two groups of foods that come mostly from animals: milk, yogurt, and cheese; and meat, poultry, fish, dry beans, eggs, and nuts. These foods are important for protein, calcium, iron, and zinc.

3-5 SERVINGS   **2-4 SERVINGS**

This level includes foods that come from plants – vegetables and fruits. Most people need to eat more of these foods for the vitamins, minerals, and fiber they supply.

6-11 SERVINGS

At the base of the Food Guide Pyramid are breads, cereals, rice, and pasta — all foods from grains. You need the most servings of these foods each day.

Figure 29-1. Food Guide Pyramid. (Reprinted from The Food Guide Pyramid. U.S. Department of Agriculture, 1992.)

The milk and dairy product group provides carbohydrate, protein, fat (unless fat-free or skim milk products are used) as well as vitamin A, vitamin D, riboflavin (B_2) and vitamins B_1, B_6, B_{12}, niacin, calcium, and magnesium. Milk and milk products are good sources of high biological protein that is more readily available to the body.

During various chemotherapy or radiation protocols, the patient may become lactose intolerant. There are several over-the-counter products that contain the enzyme lactase, e.g., Lactaid or Dairy Ease, which can be combined with milk products to aid in lactose digestion.

The meat and meat substitute group provides protein. Red meats, especially organ meats, are good sources of iron. Poultry and fish provide less iron. Meat also provides zinc, phosphorus, vitamins B_1, B_2, B_6, B_{12}, and niacin. Meat substitutes such as dried beans, dried peas, peanut butter, and tofu are good sources of iron but have a lower biological value. Eggs are also classified in this group. Although eggs are high in fat and cholesterol, they are a complete protein source.

Foods from the fruit and vegetable group provide vitamins A and C, folic acid, magnesium, and iron. Fruits and vegetables, especially fresh fruits provide fiber. Increasing the intake of high-fiber fruits and vegetables may be recommended for patients experiencing constipation, a common side effect when narcotics are used to control pain.

The bread-cereal-starch group is important as a main source of carbohydrates as well as small amounts of protein, fiber, niacin, B_1, and B_2. Whole wheat or whole grain products contribute a significant amount of fiber.

The other food group contains foods that provide calories from fat and carbohydrate, mainly from simple sugars. Vitamin E may be obtained from vegetable oils and vitamin A from fortified margarine. Foods from this food group may be beneficial as concentrated caloric sources when the patient is unable to consume adequate amounts of food or liquids. This group must not be relied on as a sole source of calories for the patient.

Vitamins and Minerals

The micronutrients are nonyielding energy sources but necessary for various metabolic functions and prevention of nutrient-deficient diseases. The requirements for the cancer patient may vary from those for the healthy individual. The variants required may be due to effects of the tumor, chemotherapy, or treatment modalities.

Vitamins are divided into two groups: fat soluble and water soluble. The fat-soluble vitamins are A, D, E, and K. Fat-soluble vitamins are soluble in fat solvents. Bile and pancreatic lipase are required for absorption. Excessive intakes of the vitamins are stored in the liver and in other organs. Two of the fat-soluble vitamins, A and D, are toxic when megadoses are ingested. The second group of vitamins are water soluble. These vitamins are soluble in water and are readily absorbed. Excessive intakes are excreted in the urine; thus body reserves are limited.

Researchers continue to study the use of vitamins as adjunctive therapy in the treatment of cancer and the role of vitamins in cancer prevention. In the treatment of cancer, administration of vitamins alone has not gained acceptance. Studies have proved that the cancer patient, especially those undergoing chemotherapy and radiation therapy have increased vitamin requirements.[11] Fluorouracil (Adrucil) and floxuridane (FUDR) can deplete niacin and thiamine.[12] Attention should also be given to increased intakes of fat-soluble vitamins, vitamins B_{12} and C, and folic acid. These vitamins need to be replenished due to increased cell growth and turnover.[13] Patients with cancer cachexia need increased vitamins to improve nutritional status (see Appendix I).

Minerals, like vitamins, are active in many metabolic processes. Minerals are divided into three groups: (1) major minerals, (2) essential trace elements, and (3) probably essential ultratrace elements. The major minerals contribute 60–80% of all the inorganic material in the human body.[14] Trace elements make up the remaining percentage.

A depletion of minerals occurs from decreased intake, medications, and chemotherapy. Corticosteroids can cause hypocalcemia and electrolyte imbalance. Cisplatin (Platinol) can deplete magnesium, calcium, potassium, phosphorus, and electrolytes. Daunorubicin (Cerubidine) can decrease iron stores. Etopside (VePesid) can result in loss of fluids and electrolytes.[12]

Small bowel or colon cancer may result in malabsorption of magnesium, calcium, and zinc. Calcium supplementation is important for patients who become lactose intolerant or who may have their intake of milk and milk products reduced or eliminated.[15]

Intakes of vitamins and minerals should be emphasized during the cancer treatment and especially during the recovery phase. Electrolyte and zinc levels should be monitored to assess the need for repletion. The amount prescribed should be individualized depending on adequacy of oral intake, serum levels, gastrointestinal losses, and clinical deficiency symptoms[15] (see Appendix I).

Diets for Specific Cancers

Head and Neck Cancer

Head and neck cancer patients can present initially with preestablished malnutrition. In many cases, patients avoid medical attention until weight loss is quite pronounced. Severe weight loss is defined as

1–2% of total body weight in 1 week, more than 5% in 1 month, more than 7.5% in 3 months, and more than 10% in no more than 6 months.[16] These patients need nutritional intervention early in the treatment phase.

Several factors contribute to malnutrition of the head and neck cancer patient. The tumor itself can interfere with swallowing. Treatment modalities (surgery, chemotherapy, radiation therapy) can result in nutritional deficiencies. The diet often has to be modified for consistency when patients experience pain, swallowing, or chewing difficulties. Foods high in calories and protein must be incorporated into the diet with frequent feeding times (five to six times per day) as these patients can tolerate only small amounts of liquids or solid foods at one time. Liquid diets include clear liquid (broth, gelatin, clear soda or fruit-flavored drinks, tea, coffee) and full liquid (cream soups, milk-based products such as puddings, ice cream, gruel, fruit juice). Consistency modifications are prescribed according to a patient's tolerance. Modifications include Pureed, Dysphagia I and II, and Mechanical Soft and Soft Diets (see Appendixes II–V for diet guidelines).

Aggressive nutrition support is needed if the patient is severely depleted prior to treatment, if frequent cycles of chemotherapy are planned, and if the patient cannot meet 60% of assessed nutritional needs for 7 days.[16] Oral liquid supplementation is necessary for patients on a clear, full, or pureed diet as they do not meet 100% of macronutrient and micronutrient needs.[16] Enteral nutritional support can be delivered by various routes using a nasogastric tube, percutaneous endoscopic gastrostomy (PEG), gastrostomy, and jejunostomy. The route and method of delivery depends on the cancer type and accessibility for tube placement. The placement of a PEG tube is a simpler procedure that does not usually require general anesthesia. PEG tube placement may result in a shorter hospitalization, lower risks, and reduced costs compared with placement of the gastrostomy tube. Another advantage of the PEG tube is greater psychological acceptance of this type of tube over the Dobb-Hoff or other nasogastric tube.[16] The tube feeding formula chosen should provide high protein and high calories. Depending on the gut function and ability of absorption, formula choice may also need to consider osmolarity, protein base and lactose content (see Appendix VI for suggested Oral Supplement and Tube Feeding Products).

TPN support is infrequently used for this type of patient because most head and neck cancer patients have a functioning gut. TPN may be required if there is a complete upper bowel obstruction, history of paralytic ileus, chyle fistula that does not resolve with a fat restricted diet or formula, or if there is a high risk for aspiration.[16] There are also protocols for certain types of head and neck cancers that require a lengthy radiation treatment.

Side effects from such treatment include mucositis, esophagitis, dysphagia, anorexia, and nausea and vomiting, which can prevent the use of enteral nutrition support whereby hyperalimentation is the appropriate choice to provide adequate nutritional intake.

Esophageal Cancer

The occurrence of esophageal cancer makes up about 1.5% of all cancers and about 5% of the gastrointestinal cancers in the United States.[17] Esophageal cancer is usually associated with the above average consumption of alcohol and tobacco use, particularly when used in combination. In the past 10 years, the role of nutrition and diet in the etiology of the disease has received an increasing amount of attention.[18] Dysphagia (i.e., difficulty swallowing progressing from bulky foods to liquids) is usually a first symptom of esophageal cancer. Other symptoms include weight loss, regurgitation, and aspiration pneumonia.[19]

The esophageal cancer patient's dietary habits must be evaluated for dysphagia (difficulty in swallowing) and odynophagia (pain on swallowing). The severity of these two conditions must be determined by ascertaining information such as adequacy of diet to meet daily nutritional requirements, swallowing ability of the patient, and amount of fluids that the patient can consume per day. Often, as treatment modalities progress (chemotherapy and radiation therapy) and the tumor size decreases, dysphagia may improve. If dysphagia is severe or progressive, such as in an advanced disease state, esophageal dilatation and laser therapy may increase the patency of the esophagus and swallowing foods and liquids may become easier for the patient.[20]

Reflux is often encountered while eating or shortly after eating. Two mechanisms can possibly account for this: (1) weakened antireflux barrier by a direct reduction in pressure of the lower esophageal sphincter (LES) and (2) inflammatory lesions of the esophagus caused by irritative foods. There have been tests on certain foods such as chocolate, fats, alcohol, coffee, and carminatives that lower the LES tone, thus causing heartburn, gas, and regurgitation. Other foods that do not affect the LES pressure and are associated with high acidity and esophagitis that may cause discomfort for the patient include coffee, orange juice, tomato juice, lemon juice, pineapple juice, and grapefruit juice. The main problem with these juices is not necessarily the acid content, but the high osmolality. Proteins increase the LES pressure and carbohydrates have a neutral effect on LES pressure.[19] Dietary recommendations include food choices from the Food Guide Pyramid. Emphasis should be placed on inclusion of lean meats, low-fat dairy products, whole grain breads, cereals, rice, and pasta. Fats, oils, and sweets should be used sparingly.

The patient who has a severe degree of dysphagia and who is prone to develop aspiration pneumonia should be advised to follow a Dysphagia I or II diet (see Appendix III for diet guidelines). These diets progress in consistency of liquids and foods with varied thickness. Many times esophageal cancer patients can tolerate pureed foods, mechanically altered soft foods, and soft or regular diets. High-calorie, high-protein diets with small frequent meals throughout the day are recommended. Usually, five to six small meals are needed to meet the nutrient requirements. Oral supplementation with liquid products made at home or commercial products can be used for snacks or between meal feedings to help meet the nutrient needs (see Appendix VI for Oral Nutritional Supplements). Patients with esophagastrectomies need to be monitored for vitamin B_{12} and iron deficiency.[19]

If the patient's nutritional status continues to decline, nutrition support should be initiated. As for enteral nutritional support, the selection of the type of tube depends on the type and location of the tumor. A tumor may not allow a nasogastric tube to pass through the esophagus to the stomach. If the treatment plan calls for an esophageal resection, a gastrostomy or PEG tube is usually not placed due to the ostomy that would be formed in the stomach, which can compromise the gastric pull-up procedure. TPN support should be instituted if the patient's dysphagia hampers overall oral nutrition intake and if a tube cannot be used.

In the course of treatment, radiation is routinely used for protocols for esophageal cancer or palliative therapy for dysphagia. The side effects of radiation include esophagitis, stomatitis, xerostomia, early satiety, and reflux, which potentially decreases oral intake and negatively affects nutritional status. A nutrition plan should include avoiding irritants that cause pain on swallowing and foods difficult to chew or swallow. Diet recommendations include altering consistency of foods as appropriate, supplementation, and the inclusion of five to six high-protein, high-calorie meals per day.

Chemotherapy treatments produce side effects such as nausea, vomiting, xerostomia, esophagitis, diarrhea, early satiety, steatorrhea, and malabsorption syndrome. Vitamin B_{12} and iron deficiency can occur in this group. The patient who experiences these side effects will need to select a diet as tolerated, such as clear liquids (maximum of 1–3 days for intractable vomiting), full liquid, or high-protein, high-calorie soft diet. Oral supplements may be used to meet needed nutrient requirements.

Gastric Cancer

The United States has a relatively low incidence of gastric cancer compared with Japan, Chile, Columbia, Iceland, and Scandinavia.[19] Many contributing factors are possibly linked to gastric cancer including diet and other environmental factors. Gastric cancer can affect nutritional status by way of absorption, food passage, and proper mixing of digestive juices.[19]

Patients with cancer of the upper gastrointestinal tract such as in the stomach become malnourished as a result of the disease processes. This can affect antineoplastic therapy including surgical treatment.[21] The maintenance or improvement of nutritional status is thought to be important in the preoperative gastric cancer patient. A preoperative nutritional assessment should be performed by a registered dietitian. The patient is considered to be at nutritional risk if there has been a 15% body weight loss within 6 months or a 10% weight loss within 3 months. The patient is also considered to be at nutritional risk if body weight is 15% or less of the desirable weight.[19]

Many studies have been conducted on perioperative nutritional support in the gastric cancer patient. One study showed that perioperative nutritional support with TPN could improve the immunocompetence of gastric patients to some extent and help promote the recovery of immune depression as a result of surgery. The immune depressing factors from the tumor could not be eliminated. Intralipid used for nutrition support does not exhibit any immunodepressant effects.[22] Another study by Nishi and Yamamoto also found that TPN inhibited the depression of cell-mediated immunity, increased tolerance to antineoplastic therapies adjunct to surgery, and prolonged intervals of no disease in patients undergoing absolute noncurative gastrectomy for advanced stage cancer. The effects of chemotherapy were better in patients with upper gastrointestinal cancer whose nutritional parameters were within a normal range or improved after 2 weeks of TPN.[21]

For the gastric cancer patient who has had a surgical procedure, the nutrition plan must be individualized according to whether a partial or total gastrectomy was performed. After a partial gastrectomy, reflux may be a problem if both sphincters have been removed. Also, rapid transit of foods can cause some difficulty with certain types of foods. Rapid transit can produce "dumping syndrome," abdominal cramping, distention, and diarrhea. Foods with high osmotic load such as concentrated sweets and sweetened fluids can increase dumping. Recommendations for dietary modification to reduce dumping include eating slowly, consuming small, frequent meals low in sugar content and sipping liquids. A partial gastrectomy in which the upper part of the stomach has been removed reduces the volume of food and fluid the patient can tolerate per meal. For these patients, a high-protein and high-calorie diet with five to six small feedings per day is recommended. If an adequate intake of vitamins and minerals is not achieved through oral intake, a vitamin and mineral daily supplement may be needed. If the vagus nerve was severed during surgery, fat intolerance may become a problem. Poor tolerance to food substances such as fat and milk can result in decreased protein and calorie consumption. A low-fat diet is recommended until the patient can tolerate larger amounts of fat at one time. Decreasing fat intake in the diet will eliminate calories. Therefore, emphasis needs to be given to increasing the intake of complex carbohydrates such as whole grains and starches.[19] Protein intake can be maintained using low-fat meats such as baked chicken, turkey, fish, or lean red meat and fat-free or skim milk products. Milk intolerance may be prevalent due to poor digestion of lactose. Amounts tolerated by the patient are individualized. Over-the-counter products such as Lactaid or Dairy Ease may be helpful in maintaining an adequate amount of milk products in the diet. If necessary, the diet should be restricted to low lactose (limiting milk to one cup per day used in cooking or for drinking) or lactose free (eliminates all milk and milk products including that used in prepared foods).

As previously mentioned, the patient with gastric cancer may benefit from the use of TPN. Tube feedings may also aid in providing adequate nutrition. The nasoenteric or jejunostomy tubes can be used successfully. The selection depends on the tumor status and type of surgical procedure performed. If the patient is a candidate for tube feeding as defined by an acceptable tube placement and the anticipated need for long-term nutrition support, enteral feeding is an appropriate choice to maintain the gastric patient's nutritional status (see Appendix VI for Enteral Feeding Products).

Small Bowel and Colon Cancer

Carcinomas of the large bowel are fairly common, whereas adenocarcinomas of the small bowel are rare. Small bowel cancer is most common in the duodenum, less common in the jejunum and least common in the ileum.[17] Many nutrition problems result from the treatment modalities, including chemotherapy, surgery, and radiation.

Bowel surgery can affect nutrient digestion and absorption. The effects depend on the extent and site of resection, integrity of the ileum, and function of the residual gastrointestinal tract.[15]

For the patient with colon cancer, a partial or total colectomy may be part of the treatment protocol. Colectomies can induce significant losses of fluid and electrolytes. Potassium is usually depleted, depending on the length of the colon removed.[15]

Resection of the ileum can be detrimental to the nutritional status of the patient. Resection of the ileus can be divided into two categories: minor loss and major loss. The ileum plays an important role in the transportation and reabsorption of conjugated bile salts, absorption of intrinsic factor, vitamin B_{12} complex, and, possibly, reabsorption of vitamin D metabolites that are excreted into the bile. Increased infusion of bile salts and vitamin B_{12} across the jejunal mucosa can partially compensate for the lost ileal function.[23, 24]

A minor loss of the ileum is a resection of approximately 100 cm and this can result in diarrhea and steatorrhea.[24] A major loss of the ileum can result in steatorrhea as a result of depleted enterohepatic pool of bile salts. With the decrease of bile salt secondary to poor reabsorption, bile salt micelle formation (responsible for fat absorption) decreases. Furthermore, a reduction in absorption of water soluble 2-monoglycerides, 1-lysophospholipids, fatty acids, and fat-soluble vitamins occurs.[23] Unabsorbed fats and bile salts enter the colon and are acted on by bacteria to produce substances that hamper water and electrolyte absorption. This contributes to the increase of diarrhea and steatorrhea from the major loss of the ileum.[23] Significant losses of fat-soluble vitamins have nutritional implications (see Appendix I).

After a small bowel resection, gastric hypersecretion and hypergastrinemia occurs. Hypersecretion inactivates pancreatic lipase, which contributes to steatorrhea production. Osmolality in the gut increases, causing diarrhea production. Minerals (iron, calcium, and magnesium) are mainly absorbed along the entire length of the small bowel. Thus, after major loss of the small bowel, deficiencies may occur. With the decreased absorption of vitamin D metabolites, calcium deficiency may occur. Others have noted a decrease in zinc and some trace metals in the patient with a shortened bowel.[23] Water-soluble vitamins are not usually depleted. Apparently, the ileum can adequately absorb these vitamins without the jejunum.[23]

Manipulation of macronutrients has also been researched. Carbohydrates may need to be restricted if the patient experiences osmotic type diarrhea. Lactose may need to be eliminated from the patient's diet depending on individual tolerances. Lactose enzyme products such as Lactaid or Dairy Ease can be used because they may increase tolerance to milk and milk products. The villi regenerate and digestion of lactose may improve, but will probably not return to normal.[15]

Osmotic load may increase diarrhea. A diet low in simple carbohydrates may decrease intestinal transit time. A recommended diet is one without concentrated sugar, depending on the patient's tolerance to simple carbohydrates. Restriction of fiber is also recommended as fiber can increase malabsorption. Foods to be eliminated include whole grain products, fresh fruits, fibrous vegetables, and legumes.[15] Guidelines for short bowel syndrome address three phases of feeding. Phase I is the immediate postoperative phase. Parenteral nutrition is recommended in this stage, especially if less than 60–80 cm of small bowel remain. Phase II discusses transition to enteral feeding. Patients may be advanced to oral electrolyte solutions, tube feeding, or oral diet. In patients who have more than 60–80 cm of remaining bowel, the goal should be to progress to a normal or modified oral diet. Oral electrolyte solutions may be used to treat high output diarrhea. If glucose absorption is not impaired, sodium and water are absorbed along with glucose, thus reversing net water secretion. Controversy exists whether an elemental formula is better tolerated than a polymeric formula. At this time, it is thought that, due to increased gastric motility and decreased surface area associated with short bowel syndrome, a defined formula may be better absorbed and tolerated. Whatever formula is selected, it should be low fat, low residue, and lactose free. The patient should start with full strength formula at 20–25 ml per hour. Hypotonic formulas are not recommended because they promote salt and water losses from the jejunum. When oral feedings are begun, guidelines include small, frequent feedings, low-lactose, low-fiber, low-fat diet (< 50 g per day) no caffeine, no alcohol, isotonic liquids taken between meals, supplementation of fat-soluble vitamins, B_{12}, folate, magnesium, calcium, zinc and iron; and limitation of simple carbohydrates. Phase III is the diet following adaption. This phase includes the advantages and disadvantages of a high fat diet and other suggestions to aid the patient's dietary adaptation.[25]

A bowel cancer patient receiving radiation treatment may suffer from radiation enteritis and other induced acute and chronic bowel changes such as shortening of the villi, mucosal ulcerations, and a reduced absorptive surface.[15] A low-fat, low-fiber, low-lactose diet is recommended. The following are specific guidelines:

Dietary fat: less than 40 g per day
Fruits and vegetables: less than 2 g of fiber per serving
Breads, grains, and cereals: less than 1.5 g of fiber per serving
Lactase enzyme products may be used to improve lactose tolerance[15]

Other complications that may arise from radiation of the bowel may require a low-residue diet. The patient with bowel cancer who has been previously treated with radiation may develop bowel obstructions. This requires bowel rest (longer than 3 days will require initiation of TPN). With the resolution of the obstruction, the initial diet is clear liquids and advanced as tolerated. Diet education is important as the patient may remain at risk for further obstruction with the addition of fibrous foods.[15]

Bowel surgery may not always result in a resection, but an ostomy may be necessary. The ileostomy and jejunostomy can have significant influence on gastrointestinal fluid losses because the colon is bypassed. Colostomies have little effect on bowel movements, particularly if a large portion of the bowel is functional. An ostomy diet alleviates some of the difficulties encountered with an ostomy. Guidelines for short bowel syndrome may need to be considered for the ostomy patient as well (see Appendix VII for Ostomy Diet Guidelines).

The patient with bowel cancer may require nutritional support. Nutrition support may be necessary prior to treatment or elective surgery. The decision is made after completion of a nutrition assessment by a registered dietitian. Nutritional support of the malnourished patient with gastrointestinal cancer, prior to the surgery may be of great benefit. Brennan showed a decrease in perioperative morbidity and mortality in that patient group.[26]

Pancreatic Cancer

Pancreatic cancer is the fourth most common cancer in the United States today and, by the time most patients are diagnosed, the lesions are unresectable.[27, 28] Surgery is the treatment of choice in conjunction with chemotherapy and radiation therapy. In most cases, symptom management or palliative care is the goal to maintain quality of the remaining life for the pancreatic cancer patient. These symptoms include severe abdominal pain, weight loss, anorexia, jaundice secondary to biliary compression, and sometimes digestive consequences from surgery.[29]

If the patient is a candidate for resection, preoperative and postoperative nutrition must be considered. Many pancreatic cancer patients are already severely malnourished at the time of diagnosis.[30] The patient may experience diarrhea, constipation, nausea, vomiting, early satiety, anorexia, and weight loss that compromises the patient's nutritional status. For the patient who is unable to eat, small frequent feedings (five to eight times per day) that include high-

calorie, high-protein foods are recommended. The patient may be able to drink supplements to achieve adequate caloric, protein, and fluid intake. A vitamin and mineral supplement should be considered, especially if malabsorption is present. For patients who cannot tolerate fat, a low-fat diet is best tolerated and possibly a pancreatic enzyme replacement is needed depending on the extent of the disease. Vitamin K may be used in the obstructive jaundice patient as bile salts are decreased and are needed in gastrointestinal absorption of the vitamin.[28]

If the patient with pancreatic cancer cannot tolerate oral feedings, the patient could be maintained on a tube feeding. A nasoenteric tube should be placed in the small bowel to avoid pancreatic enzyme secretion.[28] If the patient cannot tolerate enteral feedings, parenteral nutrition support should be the next choice to optimize nutrition status. A surgical procedure called the Whipple may require the patient to take a pancreatic enzyme replacement to aid in digestion and prevent malabsorption. In this procedure, the common bile duct is reattached to the jejunum, thereby minimizing fat malabsorption. Fluids are limited to 4 oz every 1–2 hours after a small meal. A restriction of simple carbohydrates should be emphasized to minimize diarrhea.

The pancreatic cancer patient usually develops early satiety. High-calorie foods should be incorporated into small feedings and a medium-chain triglyceride oil can be used to supplement calories. Medium-chain triglycerides are also useful for patients who are experiencing steatorrhea.

In patients having a total pancreatectomy, the entire pancreas is removed and the patient must take insulin and pancreatic enzyme replacement. Diet therapy consists of a no added sugar food plan (low simple carbohydrates) and small, frequent feedings to regulate blood glucose levels. If steatorrhea occurs even with the use of a pancreatic enzyme, low-fat diet guidelines and H_2-blockers should be added to the diet regimen.[28] Supplemental use of medium-chain triglycerides can be a significant caloric source.

Liver Cancer

Primary liver cancer represents only 1–2% of all carcinomas. There is a greater chance to develop liver metastases (about 20 times greater) with nearly all types of neoplasms, except for brain tumors.[28]

Carbohydrate metabolism changes may occur in the primary or secondary liver cancer patient. One carbohydrate glucose regulation problem is hypoglycemia. Dietary manipulation includes a low concentrated sweets diet with small, frequent meals. Fluids can be taken with meals, but not in large volume if the patient experiences early satiety. This type of patient can experience early satiety, especially in the presence of ascites.

Steatorrhea is common in the patient with liver cancer who also has underlying cirrhosis. Without cirrhosis, the patient can experience steatorrhea from tumor obstruction of the biliary drainage system, which prohibits the secretion of bile salt into the gut. Recommended dietary management is a low-fat diet and possible use of medium-chain triglyceride oil as a caloric source. The use of medium-chain triglyceride oil depends on the severity of the liver disease as metabolism may be altered.[28] With the presence of steatorrhea, the patient may develop fat-soluble vitamin deficiencies. Patients with poor oral intake are likely not meeting other vitamin and mineral needs. A multivitamin and mineral supplement may be beneficial but should not be administered in megadoses.

In some cases, a tube feeding with a nasoenteric tube can provide nutrient requirements. However, if the patient is experiencing frequent vomiting, tube feeding is contraindicated as the patient would be at risk for developing aspiration pneumonia. In some cases, TPN support is used. The initiation of enteral or parenteral support depends on the prognosis.

Breast Cancer

The incidence of breast cancer increases annually in women. Some studies have suggested that obesity is a factor in the development of breast cancer and is even noted as a possible risk for relapse of breast cancer.[31] During chemotherapy, weight gain has been observed to occur in patients. A recent study, the Nutrition Adjuvant Study, consisted of a randomized population of women aged 50–75 with stage II breast cancer. The study demonstrated that a significant dietary fat reduction as a secondary prevention can play a role in adjuvant breast cancer therapy.[32] Several other studies have shown weight gain during the time of breast cancer therapy. Knobf found that 43.6% of 89 cases reviewed gained

greater than 10 pounds (4.5 kg) and 28.7% gained more than 10% of their weight over the course of treatments.[33] Heasman et al. reviewed 237 patients and found 96% gained an average of 4.3 kg and none of the subjects lost weight.[33] This weight gain is thought to be multifactorial. Psychological factors, such as depression and anxiety can change eating habits. Daily activities in both social and employment environments may decrease thus energy requirements decrease. Oral intake may be increased because of thoughts related to improving the prognosis or to alleviate chemotherapy side effects such as nausea and a bad taste in the mouth.[31]

Control of weight gain in the breast cancer patient may be beneficial. After the initial assessment, education should include necessary dietary modifications, exercise, social activities, behavior modification, and management of therapy side effects.

There is no substantial evidence that reduced dietary fat intake can influence breast cancer patients but it may help them avoid weight gain. A low-fat diet of less than 30% of calories from fat can be incorporated into the patient's daily meal plan. Other sources of calories and nutrition are provided from protein and carbohydrates that the patient is able to tolerate.

Other diet modifications include those that help manage the side effects of chemotherapy and radiation therapy. These diets include liquid and soft diets. The patient who experiences early satiety will need five to six small, frequent meals with nutritious foods that meet all requirements for calories, protein, vitamins, and minerals.

Women diagnosed with breast cancer may have an interest in nutrition as a part of their treatment plans, and to prevent further disease and relapse. One study to assess the needs of the breast cancer patient included 143 Reach to Recovery (a cancer rehabilitation program of the American Cancer Society) participants with a response rate of 72%. The major concerns participants wanted to discuss with the dietitian were:

1. Recommendations for cancer prevention (45.6%)
2. How to lose weight (38.8%)
3. Low-fat diet information (35.9%)
4. Use of vitamin supplements (26.2%)
5. Use of mineral supplements (23.3%)
6. Low-caffeine diets (22.3%)
7. Macrobiotic diets (10.7%)

8. Use of health food products (8.7%)
9. Guidelines for weight gain (2.9%)[33]

Another study from Stockholm, Sweden, by Nordevong et al. suggested that dietary habits and intake of nutrients can be altered through dietary counseling with breast cancer patients and that these changes can be long lasting.[34]

Clinicians in the acute care or outpatient setting can use studies and questionnaires to gather information to develop or expand educational programs to meet the needs of the breast cancer patient. Education materials and the extent of nutritional counseling necessary can be developed to meet the patient's needs and satisfaction level and improve his or her quality of life.

Summary

Nutrition management of the cancer patient is an integral component of the treatment plan. It helps increase and maintain the well-being of the patient. Several factors have been identified that contribute to the death of many cancer patients and these include cancer cachexia, malnutrition, and inadequate oral intake. Malnutrition varies with the type of tumor, stage of disease, response to antineoplastic therapy, and standards used to measure malnutrition.[9] There is evidence that effective nutritional repletion can reduce postoperative complications and mortality after surgery in severely malnourished cancer patients. Weight gain and maintenance of nutritional status may improve the functioning immune system.[35]

Pain can be a contributing factor to malnutrition. The cancer patient may experience pain to such a degree that oral nutrition is decreased or diminished. Management of cancer pain allows the patient to focus on improving or maintaining adequate intake.

Even though everything is not understood about the cancer patient's metabolic alterations and effects of tumor progression with nutrition intervention, attention should be given to the nutritional status of the patient and comprehensive nutrition assessment and monitoring should be included in every cancer patient's care plan.

Many questions arise when nutrition intervention becomes an ethical issue: feeding a patient with cancer and meeting nutrient needs that sustain metabolic functions necessary for life versus providing nutrients that may alter or reverse the effects of the disease process.[9]

Goals for nutrition repletion and maintenance are to improve response to therapy and to aid in recovery from adverse effects of antineoplastic treatments and improve quality of life. For a patient receiving palliative care, quality of life is of primary importance.

References

1. DeWys W. Management of cancer cachexia. Semin Oncol 1985;12:452.
2. Hulroyde CP, Reichard GA. General metabolic abnormalities in cancer patients: Anorexia and cachexia. Surg Clin North Am 1986;66:947.
3. Thom AK, Daly JM. Nutritional Support of the Cancer Patient. In RE Wittes (ed), Manual of Oncologic Therapeutics 1991/1992. Philadelphia: Lippincott, 1991;356.
4. Zeman FJ. Clinical Nutrition and Dietetics (2nd ed). New York: Macmillan, 1991.
5. Gottschlich MM, Matarese LE, Shronts EP. Nutrition Support Dietetics Core Curriculum. Silver Spring, MD: Aspen, 1993.
6. McAnena OJ, Daly JM. Impact of antitumor on nutrition (Review). Surg Clin North Am 1986;66:1213.
7. Thiel HS, Fietkau R, Sauer R. Malnutrition and the role of nutritional support for radiation therapy patients. Recent Results Cancer Res 1988;108:205.
8. Twin Cities District Dietetic Association. Manual of Clinical Nutrition (3rd ed). St. Paul, MN: DCI Publishing, 1988.
9. Block AS. Feeding the cancer patient: Where have we come from, where are we going? Nutr Clin Pract 1994;9:87.
10. Allen AM. Food Medication Interactions. Tempe, AZ: Ann Moore Allen Publishers, 1991.
11. Berger MR, Berger I, Schmahl D. Vitamins and Cancer. In IR Rowland (ed), Nutrition, Toxicity, and Cancer. Boca Raton, FL: CRC Press, 1991;517.
12. Ignoffo RJ, Ramstack JL, Rosenbaum EH. Description of Chemotherapeutic Drugs. In JL Ramstack, EH Rosenbaum (ed). Nutrition for the Chemotherapy Patient. Palo Alto, CA: Bull Publishing Company, 1990;205.
13. Schreurs WHP, Odnik J, Egger RJ, et al. The influence of radiotherapy and chemotherapy on the vitamin status of cancer patients. Int J Vit Nutr Res 1985;55:425.
14. Williams SR. Minerals. In SR Williams (ed). Nutrition and Diet Therapy (7th ed). St. Louis: Mosby, 1993;220.
15. Hermann-Zaidins M. The Gastrointestinal Tract: Small Bowel and Colon. In AS Block (ed), Nutrition Management of the Cancer Patient. Rockville, MD: Aspen, 1990;53.

16. Kyle UG. The Patient with Head and Neck Cancer. In AS Block (ed), Nutrition Management of the Cancer Patient. Rockville, MD: Aspen, 1990;53.

17. Macdonald JS. Gastrointestinal Cancers. In RE Wittes (ed), Manual of Oncologic Therapeutics. Philadelphia: Lippincott, 1991;161.

18. Ghadirian P, Ekoe JM, Thouez JP. Food habits and esophageal cancer: An overview [abstract]. Cancer Detect Prevent 1992;16:163.

19. Block AS. Nutritional Implications in Esophageal and Gastric Cancer. In AS Block (ed), Nutrition Management of the Cancer Patient. Rockville, MD: Aspen, 1990;73.

20. Boyce GA. Palliation of malignant esophageal obstruction [abstract]. Dysphagia 1990;5:20.

21. Nish, M. Yamamoto M. Nutritional support as an adjunct to the treatment of upper gastrointestinal cancer patients: Esophageal and gastric cancer [abstract]. Gan To Kagaku Ryoho 1988;15:854.

22. Yan M. Effects of perioperative parenteral nutrition on immunocompetence in patients with gastric cancer. Chung Hua Wai Ko Tsa Chih 1990;28:739, 741, 782.

23. Weser E. Nutritional aspects of malabsorption: Short gut adaptation. Clin Gastroenterol 1983;12:443.

24. Tilson MD. Pathophysiology and treatment of short bowel syndrome. Surg Clin North Am 1980;60:1273.

25. Nashville District Dietetic Association, Inc. Manual of Nutrition and Dietetics (4th ed). Nashville, TN: Tennessee Hospital Association, 1991.

26. Brennan MF. Malnutrition in patients with gastrointestinal malignancy. Significance and management. Dig Dis Sci 1986;31(Suppl. 9):775.

27. Friedman MA. Cancers of the Pancreas and Hepatobiliary System. In RE Wittes (ed), Manual of Oncologic Therapeutics. Philadelphia: Lippincott, 1991;175.

28. Bowers DF. Nutrition Problems Caused by Pancreatic, Liver or Renal Cancer. In AS Block (ed), Nutrition Management of the Cancer Patient. Rockville, MD: Aspen, 1990;85.

29. Bernades P. Conclusions concerning the symptomatic treatment of cancer in the pancreas. Bulletin du Cancer 1990;77:295.

30. Higashiguchi T, Noguschi KT, Kawarada Y, Mizumoto R. Importance of nutritional management for the treatment of carcinoma of the pancreas [abstract]. Gan To Kagaku Ryoho 1988;15:847.

31. See J. Nutrition Management of the Patient with Breast Cancer. In AS Block (ed), Nutrition Management of the Cancer Patient. Rockville, MD: Aspen, 1990;149.

32. Clifford C, Kramer B. Diet as risk and therapy for cancer. Med Clin North Am 1993;77:725

33. Monnin S, Schiller MR. Nutrition counseling for breast cancer patients. J Am Diet Assoc 1993;93:72.

34. Nordevang E, Ikkala E, Callmer E, et al. Dietary intervention in breast cancer patients: Effects of dietary habits and nutrient intake. Eur J Clin Nutr 1990;44:681.

35. Daly JM, Hoffman K, Lieberman M, et al. Nutritional support in the cancer patient. J Parenter Enter Nutr 1990;14(Suppl. 5):245S.

Appendix I
Vitamins, Minerals, and Trace Elements

Table AI-1. Known Essential Vitamins, Minerals, and Trace Elements

Nutrient	Functions	Deficiency Signs	Toxicity Potential	Biochemical Measures of Status	Common Food Sources	Adult RDA
Fat-soluble vitamins						
Vitamin A (Retinol)	Involved in maintenance of mucous membranes; constituent of visual pigments	Impaired dark adaptation; rough, dry skin; damaged ocular tissues; night blindness, Bitot's spots	Toxic; greater than 7,500 RE/day not prudent; headache, nausea, vomiting, pseudotumor cerebri	Plasma retinol	Dark green and dark yellow vegetables; fruits; tomatoes; egg yolk; butter; fortified margarine; liver	Women, 800 RE; men, 1,000 RE
Vitamin D (ergocalciferol and cholecalciferol)	Regulates calcium and phosphorous metabolism; intestinal absorption of calcium or phosphorus; mineralization of bone matrix	Rickets, osteomalacia, poor teeth, soft bones	Toxic; intakes should closely approximate RDAs; renal failure; hypercalcemia	Serum alkaline phosphatase	Fatty fish, fish liver oils; egg yolk; liver; fortified milk; action of sunlight (ultraviolet irradiation)	7.5 µg
Vitamin E	Antioxidant protects cell structure	Fragility of blood cells; muscle loss; deposition of ceroid pigment in musculature of small intestine	Undocumented in humans and animals; deposition of cholesterol in aorta; decreased hepatic tolerance to alcohol	Plasma tocopherols	Vegetable oils; wheat germ; cereal and other whole grain products; egg yolk; greens; nuts; dried peas and beans; margarine	Women, 8 mg; men, 10 mg
Vitamin K (phylloquinone, menaquinones)	Catalysts in synthesis prothrombin and other blood-clotting factors (catalyst)	Defective blood coagulation; hemorrhagic disease in newborn	Toxic, therapeutic preparation, menadione, may be toxic because of its configurations	Prothrombin	Green leafy vegetables; fruits; cereals; dairy products; meat; liver	70–140 µg*
Water-soluble vitamins						
Vitamin C (ascorbic acid and dehydroascorbic acid)	Enhances iron absorption; possible role in hydroxylation of proline in collagen formation	Scurvy; decreased wound healing; sore mouth; bleeding gums; weak-walled capillaries	2,000–4,000 mg; reproductive failure; interferes with tests for glycosuria; inactivates vitamin B_{12}	Ascorbate in plasma, leukocyte, whole blood, red blood cells, urine	Citrus fruits; tomatoes; potatoes; leafy vegetables; cantaloupe; berries; fortified drinks; liver; green pepper	60 mg

Table AI-1. Continued

Nutrient	Functions	Deficiency Signs	Toxicity Potential	Biochemical Measures of Status	Common Food Sources	Adult RDA
Thiamin	Coenzyme in metabolism of alphaketo acids and 2-keto sugars; cofactor in carbohydrate metabolism	Beriberi; mental confusion; anorexia; muscle weakness and wasting; ataxia; peripheral paralysis; edema; tachycardia; enlarged heart; cardiac failure	Undocumented	Erythrocyte transketolase activity; urinary excretion of thiamin or its metabolites	Meat, especially pork; poultry; organ meats; oysters; whole grain and enriched cereal products; potatoes; melons; wheat germ; soybeans; brewer's yeast	Women, 1.1 mg; men, 1.5 mg
Riboflavin	Cofactor in biological oxidations	Cheilosis; angular stomatitis; scrotal skin changes; seborrheic dermatitis; eye sensitivity	Undocumented	Urinary excretion of riboflavin; erythrocyte glutathione reductase	Milk and dairy products; organ meats; meats; poultry; eggs; oysters; enriched bread	Women, 1.2 mg; men, 1.7 mg
Niacin (nicotinic acid and nicotinamide)	Component of coenzymes NAD: NADP necessary for glycolysis, fat synthesis, tissue respiration	Diarrhea; pellagra; dermatitis; inflammation of mucous membrane; dementia; death	100–2,000 mg may produce vascular dilation or "flushing"; carbohydrate intolerance; gastritis	Urinary metabolites of niacin	Organ meats; meats; poultry; fish; peanut butter; whole grain and enriched cereal products; mushrooms; peas	Women, 14 mg; men, 19 mg
Vitamin B_6 (pyridoxine, pyridoxal pyridoxamine)	Coenzymes in amino acid metabolism	Convulsions; loss of weight; abdominal distress; vomiting; hyperirritability; depression, confusion	Abnormal hepatic enzymes	Urinary excretion of B_6 or its metabolite, 4-pyridoxic acid	Meat, especially pork; organ meats; fish; milk; whole grain products; dried peas and beans	Women, 2.0 mg; men, 2.2 mg
Folacin	Coenzyme in synthesis of nucleic acid and metabolism of some amino acids; blood formation; growth	Megaloblastic anemia; glossitis; diarrhea	Undocumented	Serum folacin	Liver; kidney; leafy green vegetables; nuts; legumes; whole grain breads; meat; fish; orange juice; bananas	400 µg

Nutrient	Function	Deficiency	Toxicity	Assessment	Food sources	Amount
Vitamin B$_{12}$ (cobalamin)	Blood formation; choline synthesis; amino acid metabolism; maintenance of nervous system	Megaloblastic anemia; pernicious anemia	Undocumented	Urinary methylmalonate; serum B$_{12}$	Liver; kidney; meat; seafood; eggs; dairy products	3 µg
Biotin	Component of carboxylating enzymes in metabolism of fat and carbohydrate	Anorexia; vomiting; nausea; glossitis; pallor; mental depression; dry, scaly dermatitis	Nontoxic	Serum and urinary levels of biotin	Liver; kidney; mushrooms; peas; nuts	100–200 µg*
Pantothenic acid	Component of coenzyme A (cofactor for acyl group activation); important for release of energy from carbohydrate in gluconeogenesis, in synthesis and degradation of fatty acids, in synthesis of sterols and steroid hormones	Tissue failure, including infertility, abortion, abnormalities of skin and hair; abdominal soreness; leg cramps; insomnia	Nontoxic	Urinary pantothenic acid	Organ meats; meat; milk; eggs; whole grain products; peanuts, legumes; poultry; potatoes; tomatoes	407 µg*
Minerals						
Calcium	Skeleton and tooth formation; involved in excitability of peripheral nerves and muscle; blood coagulation; myocardial function	Poor skeletal growth and bone density; may be associated with development of osteoporosis	Undocumented	Plasma and urinary calcium	Milk, milk products; green vegetables	800 mg
Phosphorus	Component of supportive structures of body including bones and teeth; important in many chemical reactions within body; lipid protein, carbohydrate, energy-transfer enzymes: part of DNA and RNA; many B complex vitamins only effective when combined with phosphate	Weakness; anorexia; malaise, pain in bones	Undocumented	Serum phosphate	Organ meats; meat; poultry; fish; milk; most foods	800 mg

Table AI-1. Continued

Nutrient	Functions	Deficiency Signs	Toxicity Potential	Biochemical Measures of Status	Common Food Sources	Adult RDA
Magnesium	Predominant cation in living cells; component of many enzyme systems and bone; important in maintaining electrical potential in nerves and muscle membranes	Neuromuscular dysfunction (tremor convulsions)	Undocumented	Serum magnesium	Most foods, especially vegetables, nuts, legumes, milk, meat	Women, 300 mg; men, 350 mg
Trace elements						
Iron	Constituent of hemoglobin, myoglobin, number of enzymes	Iron deficiency anemia	Hemosiderosis	Hemoglobin; free erythrocyte protoporphyrin; serum iron-binding capacity; transferrin saturation; serum iron	Organ meats; meat; poultry; fish; oysters; egg yolk; peas; tomatoes; dried fruits	Women, 18 mg; men, 10 mg
Zinc	Constituent of enzymes involved in most major metabolic pathways; sexual maturation; wound healing; taste acuity	Decreased cellular growth and repair; loss of appetite; failure to grow; skin changes; impaired regeneration of wound tissues; decreased taste acuity; hypogonadism; dwarfism	Toxic	Serum zinc; urinary zinc	Meat; egg; seafood; milk; liver	15 mg
Iodine	Integral part of thyroid hormones, thyroxin, and triiodothyronine	Thyroid enlargement	Toxic	Urinary iodine	Iodized salt; seafood	150 µg
Copper	Component of enzyme systems; use of iron in hemoglobin synthesis	Bone disease; anemia; neutropenia; many skeletal defects, demyelination; degeneration of nervous system and defects in	Nontoxic	Serum copper	Liver; meat; fish; poultry; oysters; mushrooms; coffee; nuts; dried peas and beans	2–3 mg*

Mineral	Function	Deficiency	Toxicity	Assessment	Food Sources	Amount
Manganese	Essential in several enzyme systems in protein and energy metabolism; formation of mucopolysaccharides	pigmentation and structure of hair; Undocumented	Undocumented by ingestion; injected or inhaled adverse effects on central nervous system	Serum manganese	Nuts; unrefined grains; vegetables; fruits; tea	2.5–5.0 mg*
Fluoride (ine)	Increase caries resistant teeth; fluorosis	Mottling of teeth; bone fluorosis	Toxic; bone fluorosis	Serum fluoride	Fluoridated water; seafood	1.5–4.0 mg*
Chromium	May be cofactor of insulin and in maintenance of glucose metabolism	Disturbances of glucose metabolism	Undocumented	Urinary chromium	Brewer's yeast; meat; cheese; whole grains	0.05–0.2 mg*
Selenium	Enzyme of glutathione peroxidase (antioxidant)	General muscle soreness, especially cardiac and thigh	Selenosis in animals	Plasma selenium	Seafoods; kidney; liver; meat	0.05–0.2 mg*
Molybdenum	Essential to function of enzymes involved in production of uric acid and oxidation of aldehydes and sulfites	Undocumented	Toxic	Serum molybdenum	Meat; grains; legumes	0.15–0.5 mg*

*RDA not established; estimated safe and adequate daily dietary intake.

RE = retinol equivalent.

Source: Adapted from NJ Grills, MV Bosscher. Manual of Nutrition and Diet Therapy. New York: Macmillan, 1981:8.

Appendix II
Pureed Diet

Purpose

The pureed diet is designed for alert individuals who have difficulty chewing and swallowing and do not tolerate a mechanical diet such as in cases of stroke, poor dentition, oral surgery, oral or esophageal cancer, and esophageal stricture.

Description

The diet consists of regular foods that are blenderized or strained and liquids. It may be modified for other therapeutic regimens (i.e., fat controlled, diabetic, etc.) as appropriate.

Adequacy

The diet will meet the Recommended Dietary Allowances if a wide variety of foods are selected and adequate quantities are consumed. Oral supplements may be used to meet nutritional needs.

General Guidelines

1. It is important to evaluate each individual's swallowing ability and modify consistency of foods accordingly.
2. Additional liquids such as broth, milk, gravy, or sauces may be added to achieve appropriate consistency.
3. To increase calories, add margarine to cereals, starches and vegetables; add sweeteners (i.e., sugar, honey, etc.) to beverages, cereals, and fruits.
4. Serve food attractively to enhance acceptance.

Table AII-1. Pureed Diet Recommendations

Foods	Recommended	Not Recommended
Milk	Milk, plain yogurt, milkshakes, malts	None
Meat and protein foods	Strained or pureed meat, fish, and poultry; pureed cottage cheese, cheese sauce; soft poached, scrambled or boiled eggs, egg substitutes	Whole meats, fish, or poultry; hard cooked or fried eggs
Vegetables	Vegetable juices, pureed cooked vegetables without seeds	All others
Fruits	Fruit juices and nectars, fruit drinks, pureed fruits without seeds or large chunks	All others
Breads, cereals, and starches	Cooked cereals without fruit or nuts; mashed or creamed potatoes, pureed rice or noodles thinned with a sauce	Dry cereals, cooked cereals with fruit and nuts; all breads; sweet potatoes
Fats and oils	Margarine, oil, cream, cream substitutes, gravies, cream sauces, whipped topping	All others
Soups	Broth, bouillon, consommé, soups with pureed vegetables, strained cream soups	All others
Desserts	Gelatin, plain custard or pudding, ice cream, ice milk, sherbet, flavored fruit ices, popsicles, fruit whips, plain Bavarian creams	Any made with coconut, nuts, or whole fruit
Beverages	Coffee, decaffeinated coffee, tea, and carbonated beverages	Any not tolerated, alcohol
Miscellaneous condiments	Catsup, mustard, vinegar	Horseradish, chili sauce, olives, pickles, seeds
Seasonings	Salt, pepper, powdered herbs, and spices	None
Sweets	Sugar, syrup, honey, jelly, chocolate syrup	Jams, preserves, candy

Source: Reprinted with permission from Nashville District Dietetic Association, Inc. Manual of Nutrition and Dietetics (4th ed). Nashville, TN: Tennessee Hospital Association, 1991.

Table AII-2. Sample Menu

Breakfast	Lunch or Supper	Dinner
½ cup orange juice	1 cup strained cream of pea soup	1 cup strained cream of asparagus soup
½ cup oatmeal	3 oz pureed beef	3 oz pureed chicken
1 soft scrambled egg	½ cup mashed potatoes	½ cup pureed noodles in sauce
2 tsp margarine	½ cup pureed beets	½ cup pureed green beans
1 cup low-fat milk	½ cup pureed peaches	½ cup chocolate ice cream
3 tsp sugar	1 cup low-fat milk	2 tsp margarine
Coffee/tea	½ cup pear nectar	1 cup low-fat milk
	½ cup pineapple juice	2 tsp sugar
	2 tsp sugar	Coffee/tea
	Coffee/tea	

Source: Reprinted with permission from Nashville District Dietetic Association, Inc. Manual of Nutrition and Dietetics (4th ed). Nashville, TN: Tennessee Hospital Association, 1991.

Appendix III
Dysphagia Diet

Purpose

This diet is designed to maximize oral and pharyngeal management of foods by persons having conditions secondary to neurologic impairment (cerebrovascular accident, Parkinson's disease, tumor) or structural head and neck anomalies (partial glossectomy, partial or total laryngectomy, radical neck dissection, radiation). Further, it is designed to reduce the risks associated with choking, gagging, and aspiration, and to stimulate reestablishment of the swallow reflex.

Description

The dysphagia diet contains foods that stimulate the swallowing muscles because of extreme temperatures or seasoning and have a texture that will stimulate chewing. It avoids foods that cause excessive mucus and saliva production such as whole milk products, chocolate, and caffeine. Straws are avoided because of increased risk of aspiration.

The diet consists of two stages. The first stage contains thick liquids and other foods of a thick consistency that are easy to swallow, do not have to be well chewed, and will not be readily pocketed. The second stage contains foods that stimulate the swallowing muscles because of extreme temperatures and have a texture that will require chewing. All liquids should be thickened to nectar consistency in both dysphagia stages. Extra sauces or gravy should be included to provide appropriate consistency to meat items. Both diets may be individualized as necessary by the speech pathologist, occupational therapist, and dietitian. It is advisable for an occupational therapist, speech pathologist, or other specialist to evaluate the patient for swallowing ability before a diet is ordered.

Adequacy

This diet will meet the Recommended Dietary Allowances if carefully planned.

General Guidelines

1. Use foods and liquids with distinct tastes.
2. Eliminate pureed consistency foods as other textures are tolerated.
3. Avoid foods that tend to fall apart in the mouth.
4. Use hot or cold foods. Avoid foods that are tepid or at room temperature.

Table AIII-1. Dysphagia Diet Stage 1

Foods	Recommended	Not Recommended
Milk	Low-fat yogurt, frozen yogurt (without fruit pieces, nuts, coconut, chocolate, etc.) thickened liquid supplements	All other milk products except sherbet, cheese sauce and low-fat puddings; chocolate items
Meat and protein foods	Pureed meats, soft scrambled eggs	All others
Vegetables	Any pureed	Corn
Fruits	Any pureed fruit, fruit nectars; thickened juices	Raw fruit, dried fruit, thin juices (that are not thickened)
Breads, cereals, and starches	Baby cereals, oats; blended pasta with gravy, margarine, or sauce	All others including popcorn, corn chips, potato chips, pretzels, and toast
Fats and oils	Butter, margarine; smooth, nonspicy dressing, gravy, oils, cheese sauce	Bacon, nuts; nonsmooth, spicy salad dressings
Soups	Broth, thickened	All others
Desserts	Sherbet, low-fat, plain pudding; pureed fruit whip	Popsicles, ices, gelatin, all others
Beverages	Thickened: carbonated beverages, fruit drinks, coffee, and water	All others including ice chips, chocolate beverages
Miscellaneous condiments	Catsup, mustard, vinegar	Horseradish, pickles, chili sauce, dried herbs, garlic buds
Seasonings	Salt, pepper, powdered herbs and spices	
Sweets	Sugar, syrup, honey, jelly	Jams, preserves, candy

Source: Reprinted with permission from Nashville District Dietetic Association, Inc. Manual of Nutrition and Dietetics (4th ed). Nashville, TN: Tennessee Hospital Association, 1991.

Table AIII-2. Sample Menu

Breakfast	Lunch or Supper	Dinner
½ cup peach nectar	3 oz pureed hamburger with gravy	3 oz pureed chicken with gravy
¾ cup Cream of Wheat	½ cup mashed potato with 1 tablespoon gravy	½ cup mashed sweet potato
1 pureed egg	½ cup pureed carrots	½ cup applesauce
2 tsp margarine	½ cup pureed pears	½ cup pureed asparagus, 2 tsp margarine
1 cup liquid supplement, thickened	2 tsp margarine	2 tsp margarine
	1 cup liquid supplement, thickened	½ cup low-fat butterscotch pudding
		1 cup liquid supplement, thickened

Mid-Morning	Mid-Afternoon	Evening
1 cup low-fat vanilla yogurt	1 cup low-fat lemon custard	1 cup low-fat frozen strawberry yogurt
½ cup pureed peaches		

Source: Reprinted with permission from Nashville District Dietetic Association, Inc. Manual of Nutrition and Dietetics (4th ed). Nashville, TN: Tennessee Hospital Association, 1991.

Table AIII-3. Dysphagia Diet Stage II

Foods	Recommended	Not Recommended
Milk	Skim and low-fat milk, low-fat yogurt without nuts or chocolate; thickened liquid supplements	Chocolate items; all others except those recommended
Meat and protein foods	Moist, tender chopped meat, fish, and poultry including ground beef or meat loaf with gravy, chopped tetrazzini, lasagna; eggs (scrambled, poached, or deviled); cottage cheese	Any difficult-to-chew meat, fried meat, hard cheeses, hard cooked eggs, pizza
Vegetables	Any very tender or canned except those not recommended; thickened vegetable juice	Fried vegetables; beets, broccoli, cauliflower, hash browns, cabbage, corn, raw onions, sauerkraut, spinach, raw tomatoes, greens, brussels sprouts
Fruits	Any soft canned; ripe bananas, ripe peeled peaches, plums, fruit nectars; thickened juices	Other raw fruit; dried fruit
Breads, cereals, and starches	Whole wheat bread without seeds or nuts; pastas, macaroni and cheese, hot cereals, pancakes and french toast with syrup, crackers in soup, soft muffins, plain roll, waffles, bread dressing, soft graham crackers	White bread, cornbread, hard rolls, dry crackers, toast, fried bread with seeds or nuts; rice, popcorn, potato chips, corn chips and pretzels
Fats and oils	Butter, margarine; smooth, nonspicy dressings, gravy, oils, cheese sauce	Bacon; nuts; nonsmooth, spicy salad dressings
Soups	Strained cream soups made with recommended ingredients; thickened broth	All others
Desserts	Sherbet, plain low-fat pudding, plain bread pudding, moist cookies (without fruits or nuts); soft pies and cakes	Popsicles, ices; chocolate items; all others
Beverages	Thickened: carbonated beverages, fruit drinks, coffee, tea, and water	Chocolate beverages; all others including ice chips
Miscellaneous condiments	Catsup, mustard, vinegar	Horseradish, chili sauce
Seasonings	Salt, pepper, powdered herbs and spices	Dried herbs, garlic buds
Sweets	Sugar, syrup, honey, jelly	Jams, preserves, candy

Source: Reprinted with permission from Nashville District Dietetic Association, Inc. Manual of Nutrition and Dietetics (4th ed). Nashville, TN: Tennessee Hospital Association, 1991.

Table AIII-4. Sample Menu

Breakfast	Lunch or Supper	Dinner
½ cup pear nectar	1 cup spaghetti with 2 oz. meat sauce	3 oz ground turkey with 2 tbsp gravy
1 soft-boiled egg	½ cup buttered carrots	½ cup mashed potato with 1 tbsp gravy
1 slice whole wheat toast or bread	1 slice whole wheat bread	½ cup green bean casserole, white sauce
2 tsp margarine	2 tsp margarine	½ cup fruit cocktail
2 tsp jelly	½ cup sherbet	1 slice whole wheat bread
1 cup coffee	1 cup skim milk	2 tsp margarine
		1 cup skim milk
Mid-Morning	**Mid-Afternoon**	**Mid-Evening**
1 cup liquid supplement, thickened	½ cup peach nectar	1 cup skim milk
	1 cup low-fat fruit yogurt	½ cup apple cobbler

Source: Reprinted with permission from Nashville District Dietetic Association, Inc. Manual of Nutrition and Dietetics (4th ed). Nashville, TN: Tennessee Hospital Association, 1991.

Appendix IV
Mechanical Diet

Purpose

The mechanical diet is designed for individuals who have chewing and swallowing difficulties requiring modification in texture to minimize the amount of chewing necessary for ingestion of food.

Adequacy

The diet will meet all Recommended Dietary Allowances.

Description

The diet contains all foods from the regular diet as well as chopped or ground foods. It must be individualized according to tolerance and acceptance.

Table AIV-1. Sample Menu

Breakfast	Lunch or Supper	Dinner
½ cup orange juice	1 cup vegetable soup	½ cup fruit juice
½ cup oatmeal	3 oz lean ground beef with barbecue	3 oz ground chicken
1 scrambled egg	sauce	⅓ cup buttered rice
1 slice whole wheat toast	1 medium bun	½ cup chopped broccoli with lemon butter
2 tsp margarine	½ cup green beans	1 medium soft roll
1 tbsp grape jelly	2 halves canned peaches	2 tsp margarine
1 cup low-fat milk	1 cup low-fat milk	½ cup fruit-flavored gelatin
3 tsp sugar	2 tsp sugar	1 cup low-fat milk
Coffee/tea	1 tsp mustard	2 tsp sugar
	1 tbsp catsup	Coffee/tea
	Coffee/tea	

Source: Reprinted with permission from Nashville District Dietetic Association, Inc. Manual of Nutrition and Dietetics (4th ed). Nashville, TN: Tennessee Hospital Association, 1991.

Appendix V
Soft Diet

Purpose

This diet is used most commonly after surgery in the transition from a liquid to a regular diet to minimize gastrointestinal discomfort.

Adequacy

This diet will meet the Recommended Dietary Allowances.

Description

This diet usually includes three meals. Foods that arc difficult to digest or are excessively gas forming are eliminated.

Table AV-1. Soft Diet Recommendations

Foods	Recommended	Not Recommended
Milk	Milk, milkshakes, "instant breakfast" beverages, cocoa, eggnog, yogurt	None
Meat and protein foods	Lean beef, ham, lamb, liver, pork, veal, chicken, duck, turkey, fish (baked, broiled, roasted or stewed); mildly flavored cheeses, cottage cheese; eggs, egg substitutes; smooth peanut butter	Fried meats, poultry and fish; cold cuts, salami, sausages, other spiced meats, wieners; strongly flavored cheeses; fried eggs; chunky peanut butter; nuts; textured vegetable protein
Vegetables	Asparagus, beets, carrots, eggplant, green beans, mushrooms, okra, green peas, pumpkin, spinach, squash, tomatoes (all should be cooked until tender); tender lettuce; raw tomatoes; tomato juice, vegetable juice cocktail	All fried vegetables; broccoli, brussels sprouts, cabbage, cauliflower, corn, cucumber, dried beans and peas, green peppers, greens (except spinach), hominy; onions, pimiento, radishes, rutabagas, sauerkraut, sauerkraut juice, turnips
Fruits	Canned fruit according to individual tolerance, bananas, fruit juices	Coconut, other raw fruit

Table AV-1. Continued

Foods	Recommended	Not Recommended
Breads, cereals, and starches	Refined wheat bread, white bread, bagels, biscuits, cornbread, croissants, rolls; graham crackers, rusk, soda crackers, zwieback; cooked cereals; dry cereals (except those not recommended); macaroni, noodles, potatoes (sweet or white), rice, spaghetti	Whole grain breads and dry cereals containing fruits not tolerated, nuts and wheat bran, fried potatoes
Fats and oils	Bacon; butter, cooking oils, margarine; cream, cream cheese, nondairy creamer, sour cream; mildly seasoned salad dressings, mayonnaise, mayonnaise-type salad dressing, oil and vinegar; whipped topping	Fried foods, lard, meat drippings
Soups	Commercial or homemade broth-based or cream soups made with recommended ingredients	Soups containing ingredients not recommended
Desserts	Cake, cookies, custard, gelatin, ice cream, pudding sherbet; tolerated fruits, fruit whips	All desserts containing coconut, nuts, or other ingredients not tolerated
Beverages	Carbonated beverages, coffee, fruit drinks and juices, lemonade, milk beverages, tea	All alcoholic beverages
Miscellaneous condiments	Catsup, lemon juice, mild sauces and spreads, vinegar, gravy	Sauces and condiments containing chili powder or hot pepper such as taco sauce and barbecue sauce
Seasonings	Butter substitutes, butter-flavored salt, garlic powder, onion powder, paprika, salt, seasoned salt, spices in moderation as tolerated, vanilla and other flavor extracts	Chili powder, curry, ginger, hot pepper, all others that cause discomfort
Sweets	Any except those containing nuts or other ingredients not recommended	All containing ingredients not recommended

Source: Reprinted with permission from Nashville District Dietetic Association, Inc. Manual of Nutrition and Dietetics (4th ed). Nashville, TN: Tennessee Hospital Assocaition, 1991.

Table AV-2. Sample Menu

Breakfast	Lunch or Supper	Dinner
½ cup orange juice	1 cup vegetable soup (prepared with recommended ingredients)	3 oz broiled chicken
½ cup oatmeal		⅓ cup buttered rice
1 scrambled egg	3 oz lean hamburger	½ cup green peas
1 slice whole wheat toast	1 medium bun	1 cup lettuce salad
2 tsp margarine	Lettuce and tomato	2 tsp French dressing
1 tbsp grape jelly	½ cup green beans	1 medium roll
1 cup low-fat milk	2 halves canned peaches	2 tsp margarine
3 tsp sugar	1 cup low-fat milk	1 small peeled baked apple
Coffee/tea	2 tsp sugar	1 cup low-fat milk
	1 tsp mustard	2 tsp sugar
	1 tbsp catsup	Coffee/tea
	Coffee/tea	

Source: Reprinted with permission from Nashville District Dietetic Association, Inc. Manual of Nutrition and Dietetics (4th ed). Nashville, TN: Tennessee Hospital Assocaition, 1991.

Appendix VI

Enteral Feeding Products

Table AVI-1. Standard Formulas (Intact Macronutrients; Low Residue; Lactose-Free; 1.0–1.4 Calories/ml)

	Attain	Ensure	Isocal	Isosource	Newtrition[a]	Newtrition Isotonic[b]	Nutren 1.0
Calories (ml)	1	1.06	1.06	1.20	1.06	1.06	1.0
Carbohydrate source	Maltodextrin	Corn syrup sucrose	Maltodextrin	Hydrolyzed corn-starch	Maltodextrin, sugar	Maltodextrin	Maltodextrin, corn syrup solids
Protein source	Caseinate	Sodium and calcium caseinates, soy protein isolate	Sodium and calcium caseinates, soy protein isolate	Sodium and calcium caseinates, soy protein isolate	Sodium and calcium caseinates	Sodium and calcium caseinates	Casein
Fat source (MCT:LCT)	Corn oil, MCT (50:50)	Corn oil (NA)	Soy oil, MCT (20:80)	Canola oil, MCT (50:50)	Corn oil, MCT (19:81)	Corn oil, MCT (50:50)	Corn oil, MCT (NA)
Carbohydrate (g/liter)	135	145	133	170	143	144	127
(% Kcals)	54	54.5	50	56	54.1	54.3	51
Protein (g/liter)	40	37	34	43	38	40	40
(% Kcals)	16	14	13	14	14.4	15.1	16
Fat (g/liter)	35	37	44	41	37	36	38
(% Kcals)	30	31.5	37	30	31.5	30.6	33
% Free water	84	84.5	84	80	NA	NA	85
Volume (ml) for 100% RDA (adult)	1,250	1,887	1,887	1,500	1,585	1,250	1,500
mOsm/kg H$_2$O	300	470	300	360	450	300	300
Na (mEq/liter)	35.0	36.8	23.0	32.0	27.5	30.0	21.7
K (Meq/liter)	41.0	40.0	34.0	43.0	27.1	30.0	32.1
Cl (Meq/liter)	38.0	37.5	3.0	31.0	20.8	31.0	28.2
Manufacturer	Sherwood Medical	Ross Labs	Mead Johnson	Sandoz Nutrition	O'Brien/KMI[c]	O'Brien/KMI[c]	Clintec Nutrition
Available flavors/forms	Unflavored; ready to use liquid; available in closed system	Vanilla, chocolate, strawberry, black walnut, coffee eggnog; ready to use liquid, powder	Unflavored; ready to use liquid	Vanilla; ready to use liquid; available in closed system	Vanilla; ready to use liquid; available in closed system	Unflavored; ready to use liquid; available in closed system	Unflavored; ready to use liquid
Description/features		Fortified with selenium, chromium and molybdenum					

MCT = medium-chain triglyceride; LCT = long-chain trigyceride; NA = not available.

[a]Newtrition is now called Nitrolan.

[b]Newtrition Isotonic is now called Isolan.

[c]O'Brien/KMI is now called Elan.

Source: Reprinted with permission from Nashville District Dietetic Association, Inc. Manual of Nutrition and Dietetics (4th ed). Nashville, TN: Tennessee Hospital Association, 1991.

Table AVI-2. High-Nitrogen Standard Formulas (Intact Macronutrients; Low Residue; Lactose-Free)

	Ensure HN	Entrition HN	Isocal HN	Isosource NH	Newtrition HN[a]	Osmolite HN	Replete
Calories (ml)	1.06	1	1.06	1.2	1.24	1.06	1
Carbohydrate source	Corn syrup, sucrose	Maltodextrin	Maltodextrin	Hydrolyzed corn starch	Maltodextrin	Glucose polymers	Maltodextrin, sucrose
Protein source	Sodium and calcium caseinates, soy protein isolate	Casein, soy	Sodium and calcium caseinates, soy protein isolate	Sodium and calcium caseinates, soy protein isolate	Sodium and calcium caseinates	Sodium and calcium caseinates, soy protein isolate	Casein
Fat source	Corn oil	Corn oil	Soy oil, MCT	Canola oil, MCT	Corn oil, MCT	MCT,corn oil, soy oil	Corn oil
(MCT:LCT)	(NA)	(NA)	(40:60)	(50:50)	(50:50)	(50:50)	(NA)
Carboydrate (g/liter)	141.2	114.0	124.0	160	160.0	141.2	112.8
(% Kcals)	53.2	45.6	47	52	51.6	53.3	45.0
Protein (g/liter)	44.4	44.0	44.0	53	60.0	44.4	62.5
(% Kcals)	16.7	17.6	17	18	19.4	16.7	25.0
Fat (g/liter)	35.5	41.0	45.0	41	40.0	36.8	33.0
(% Kcals)	30.1	36.8	36	30	29.0	30.0	30.0
% Free water	84.1	84	84	80	NA	84.1	85
Volume (ml) for 100% RDA (adult)	1,321	1,300	1,200	1,500	1,250	1,321	1,500
mOsm/kg H2O	470	300	300	330 (373 flavored)	310	300	350
Na (mEq/liter)	40.4	40	40.4	32	30	40.4	21.7
K (Meq/liter)	40.4	40.5	40.7	43	30	40	39.5
Cl (Meq/liter)	40.5	43.4	41.1	31	31	40.5	28.2
Ca (mg/liter)	758	770	850	670	800	758	800
Phos (mg/liter)	758	770	850	670	800	758	720
Mg (mg/liter)	303	308	340	270	320	304	400
Manufacturer	Ross Labs	Clintec Nutrition	Mead Johnson	Sandoz Nutrition	O'Brien/KMI[b]	Ross Labs	Ross Labs
Available flavors/forms	Vanilla chocolate; ready to use liquid	Unflavored; ready to use liquid and closed delivery system	Unflavored; ready to use liquid	Vanilla; ready to use liquid; available in closed system	Unflavored; ready to use liquid; available in closed system	Unflavored; ready to use liquid and closed delivery system	Vanilla; ready to use liquid
Description/ features	Fortified with chromium, selenium and molybdenum					Fortified with taurine, carnitine, chromium, selenium, molybdenum	

MCT = medium-chain triglyceride; LCT = long-chain triglyceride; NA = not available.
[a]Newtrition HN is now called Nitrolan.
[b]O'Brien/KMI is now called Elan.
Source: Reprinted with permission from Nashville District Dietetic Association, Irc. Manual of Nutrition and Dietetics (4th ed). Nashville, TN: Tennessee Hospital Association, 1991.

Table AVI-3. Standard and Fiber-Containing Formulas

	Standard Formulas			Fiber-Containing Formulas			
	Osmolite	Resource	Sustacal	Compleat	Compleat Modified	Enrich	Fiber-Source
Calories (ml)	1.06	1.06	1.0	1.07	1.07	1.1	1.2
Carbohydrate source	Glucose polymers	Maltodextrin, sucrose	Sugar, corn syrup	Maltodextrin, green beans, peas, non-fat milk, peaches, orange juice	Maltodextrin, peas, green beans, peaches, orange juice	Hydrolyzed corn starch, sucrose, soy polysaccharide	Hydrolyzed corn starch, soy polysaccharide
Protein source	Sodium and calcium caseinates, soy protein isolate	Sodium and calcium caseinates, soy protein isolate	Sodium and calcium caseinates, soy protein isolate	Beef, non-fat milk	Beef, calcium caseinate	Sodium and calcium caseinates, soy protein	Sodium and calcium caseinates
Fat source (MCT:LCT)	MCT, corn oil, soy oil (50:50)	Corn oil (NA)	Partially hydrogenated soy oil (NA)	Corn oil, beef (NA)	Beef, corn oil (NA)	Corn oil (NA)	Canola oil, MCT (NA)
Carbohydrate (g/liter)	145	145	140	127.9	141.2	162	170
(% Kcals)	54.6	54.5	55	48.0	53.0	55.0	56
Protein (g/liter)	37.2	37.2	61	42.6	42.6	39.7	43
(% Kcals)	14.0	14.0	24	16.0	16.0	14.5	14
Fat (g/liter)	38.5	37.2	23	42.6	36.6	37.2	41
(% Kcals)	31.4	31.5	21	36.0	31.0	30.5	30
% Free water	84.1	82.0	84.0	78.0	78.0	82.9	NA
Volume (ml) for 100% RDA (Adult)	1,887	1,887	1,080	1,500	1,500	1,391	1,800
mOsm/kg H$_2$O	300	400	620 (choc. 700)	450	300	480	390
Na (mEq/liter)	27.6	36.7	41.0	55.0	43.4	36.8	38.0
K (mEq/liter)	25.9	41.1	54.0	35.8	35.8	40.0	46.0
Cl (mEq/liter)	23.8	39.9	42.0	32.3	32.3	40.5	31.0
Ca (mg/liter)	530	549	1,010	666	666	719	670
Phos (mg/liter)	530	549	930	1,199	932	719	670
Mg (mg/liter)	212	211	380	266	266	287	270
Manufacturer	Ross Labs	Sandoz Nutrition	Mead Johnson	Sandoz Nutrition	Sandoz Nutrition	Ross Labs	Sandoz Nutrition

Table AVI-3. Continued

| | Standard Formulas | | | Fiber-Containing Formulas | | |
	Osmolite	Resource	Sustacal	Compleat	Compleat Modified	Enrich	Fiber-Source
Available flavors/forms	Unflavored; ready-to-use liquid and closed delivery system	Vanilla, chocolate; ready-to-use liquid, instant crystals	Vanilla, chocolate, strawberry, eggnog; ready-to-use liquid, powder	Unflavored; ready-to-use liquid	Unflavored; ready-to-use liquid	Vanilla, chocolate; ready-to-use liquid	Vanilla; ready-to-use liquid
Description/features	Fortified with selenium, chromium, molybdenum, carnitine, and taurine		General dietary supplement	Formulated from blenderized foods, provides dietary fiber; contains lactose	Blenderized tube feeding formulated from foods; provides dietary fiber; lactose-free; isotonic	3.4 g dietary fiber per 8 fl. oz. fortified with selenium, chromium, and molybdenum	2.4 g dietary fiber per 8 fl. oz.

MCT = medium-chain triglyceride; LCT = long-chain triglyceride; NA = not available.

Source: Reprinted with permission from Nashville District Dietetic Association, Inc. Manual of Nutrition and Dietetics (4th ed). Nashville, TN: Tennessee Hospital Association, 1991.

Table AVI-4. Fiber-Containing Formulas

	Fibersource HN	Jevity	Newtrition Isofiber[a]	Nutren 1.0 with Fiber	Profiber	Sustacal with Fiber	Ultracal
Calories (ml)	1.2	1.06	1.2	1.0	1.0	1.06	1.06
Carbohydrate source	Hydrolyzed corn starch, soy polysaccharide	Hydrolyzed corn starch, soy polysaccharide	Maltodextrin, soy polysaccharide	Maltodextrin, corn syrup solids, soy polysaccharide	Hydrolyzed corn starch, soy polysaccharide	Maltodextrin, sugar, soy polysaccharide	Maltodextrin, soy polysaccharide, oat flour
Protein source	Sodium and calcium caseinates	Sodium and calcium caseinates	Sodium and calcium caseinates	Casein	Sodium and calcium caseinates	Sodium and calcium caseinates, soy protein isolate	Sodium and calcium caseinates
Fat source (MCT:LCT)	Canola oil, MCT	Corn oil, MCT, soy oil (50:50)	Corn oil, MCT	Corn oil, MCT	Corn oil	Corn oil	Soy oil, MCT
	(NA)	(NA)	(NA)	(NA)	(NA)	(NA)	(NA)
Carbohydrate (g/liter)	160	151.5	160	127	132	139.3	123
(% Kcals)	52	53.3	53.3	51	48	53.0	46
Protein (g/liter)	53	44.4	50	40	40	45.6	44
(% Kcals)	18	16.7	16.7	16	16	17.0	17
Fat (g/liter)	41	36.7	40	38	40	35.0	46
(% Kcals)	30	30	30	33	36	30.0	37
% Free water	(NA)	83.1	(NA)	(NA)	84.5	84.4	(NA)
Volume (ml) for 100% RDA	1,800	1,321	1,250	1,500	1,500	1,420	1,250
mOsm/kg H_2O	390	300	310	303 (373-flavored)	300	480	310
Na (mEq/liter)	38	40.4	40	21.7	32	31.2	31
K (mEq/liter)	46	40.3	40	32.1	32	35.6	36
Cl (mEq/liter)	31	36.9	39	28.2	34	39.8	39
Ca (mg/liter)	670	909	800	700	667	844	840
Phos (mg/liter)	670	758	800	700	667	705	700
Mg (mg/liter)	270	304	320	340	267	283	280
Manufacturer	Sandoz Nutrition	Ross Labs	O'Brien/KMI[b]	Clintec Nutrition	Sherwood Medical	Mead Johnson	Mead Johnson
Available flavors/forms	Vanilla; ready-to-use liquid	Unflavored; ready-to-use liquid and closed delivery system	Unflavored; ready-to-use liquid	Unflavored, vanilla, chocolate; ready-to-use liquid	Unflavored; ready-to-use liquid	Vanilla; ready-to-use liquid	Unflavored; ready-to-use liquid
Description/features	1.6 g dietary fiber per 8 fl. oz	3.4 g dietary fiber per 8 fl. oz; fortified with carnitine, taurine, chromium, selenium, molybdenum	3.4 g dietary fiber per 8 fl. oz	3.3 g dietary fiber per 8 fl. oz	2.8 g dietary fiber per 8 fl. oz	5.6 g dietary fiber per 8 fl. oz	3.4 g dietary fiber per 8 fl. oz

MCT = medium-chain triglyceride; LCT = long-chain triglyceride; NA = not available.
[a]Newtrition Isofiber is now called Fibrolan.
[b]O'Brien/KMI is now called Elan.
Source: Reprinted with permission from Nashville District Dietetic Association, Inc. Manual of Nutrition and Dietetics (4th ed). Nashville, TN: Tennessee Hospital Association, 1991.

Table AVI-4. Continued

	Vitaneed
Calories (ml)	1
Carbohydrate source	Maltodextrin, green beans, peaches, carrots; soy fiber
Protein source	Beef, sodium and calcium caseinates
Fat source	Corn oil
(MCT:LCT)	(NA)
Carbohydrate (g/liter)	128
(% Kcals)	48
Protein (g/liters)	40
(% Kcals)	16
Fat (g/liter)	40
(% Kcals)	36
% Free water	84.5
Volume (ml) for 100% RDA	1,500
mOsm/kg H_2O	300
Na (mEq/liter)	30
K (mEq/liter)	32
Cl (mEq/liter)	28
Ca (mg/liter)	667
Phos (mg/liter)	667
Mg (mg/liter)	267
Manufacturer	Sherwood Medical
Available flavors/forms	Unflavored; ready-to-use liquid; available in closed system
Description/features	Formulated from blenderized foods; 2 g dietary fiber per 8 fl. oz.; lactose free

MCT = medium-chain triglyceride; LCT = long-chain trigyceride; NA = not available.
Source: Reprinted with permission from Nashville District Dietetic Association, Inc. Manual of Nutrition and Dietetics (4th ed). Nashville, TN: Tennessee Hospital Association, 1991.

Table AVI-5. High-Caloric Density Formulas (1.5–2.0 Calories/ml)

	Comply	Ensure Plus	Ensure Plus HN	Isocal HCN	Magnacal	Newtrition One and a Half[a]	Nutren 1.5
Calories (ml)	1.5	1.5	1.5	2.0	2.0	1.5	1.5
Carbohydrate source	Hydrolyzed corn starch	Corn syrup, sucrose	Corn syrup, sucrose	Corn syrup	Maltodextrin, sucrose	Maltodextrin	Maltodextrin, sucrose
Protein source	Sodium and calcium caseinates	Sodium and calcium caseinates; soy protein isolate	Sodium and calcium caseinates; soy protein isolate	Sodium and calcium caseinates	Sodium and calcium caseinates	Sodium and calcium caseinates; soy protein isolate	Casein
Fat source (MCT:LCT)	Corn oil (NA)	Corn oil (NA)	Corn oil (NA)	Soy oil, MCT (30:70)	Partially hydrogenated soy oil (NA)	Corn oil, MCT (50:50)	MCT, Corn oil (48:52)
Carbohydrate (g/liter)	180	200	199.9	200	250	202	170.0
(% Kcals)	48	53.3	53.3	40	50	54	45.0
Protein (g/liter)	60	54.9	62.6	75	70	60	60.0
(% Kcals)	16	14.7	16.7	15	14	16	16.0
Fat (g/liter)	60	53.3	49.9	102	80	50	67.5
(% Kcals)	36	32.0	30.0	45	36	30	39.0
% Free water	77.8	76.9	76.9	71	69	(NA)	78
Volume (ml) for 100% RDA (adults)	1,000	1,420	947	1,000	1,000	1,000	1,000
mOsm/kg H$_2$O	410	690	650	690	590	610	410
Na (mEq/liter)	48	45.7	51.5	35	43.5	45	32.7
K (mEq/liter)	47	49.6	46.5	43	32.0	45	48.1
Cl (mEq/liter)	48	53.5	45.3	34	26.8	48	42.3
Ca (mg/liter)	1,000	705	1,056	1,000	1,000	1,000	1,050
Phos (mg/liter)	1,000	705	1,056	1,000	1,000	1,000	1,050
Mg (mg/liter)	400	282	423	400	400	400	510
Manufacturer	Sherwood Medical	Ross Labs	Ross Labs	Mead Johnson	Sherwood Medical	O'Brien/KMI[b]	Clintec Nutrition
Available flavors	Unflavored, vanilla; ready-to-use liquid; available in a closed system	Vanilla, chocolate, coffee, eggnog, strawberry; ready-to-use and closed delivery system	Vanilla, chocolate; ready-to-use liquid and closed delivery system	Unflavored; ready-to-use liquid	Mild vanilla; ready-to-use liquid	Unflavored; ready-to-use liquid; available in closed system	Unflavored, vanilla, chocolate; ready-to-use liquid
Description/features	Flavored variety contains sucrose	Fortified with chromium, selenium, and molybdenum	Fortified with taurine, carnitine, chromium, selenium, and molybdenum				

MCT = medium-chain triglyceride; LCT = long-chain triglyceride; NA = not available.
[a]Newtrition One and a Half is now called Ultrala.
[b]O'Brien/KMI is now called Elan.
Source: Reprinted with permission from Nashville District Dietetic Association, Inc. Manual of Nutrition and Dietetics (4th ed). Nashville, TN: Tennessee Hospital Association, 1991.

Table AVI-6. High-Caloric Density Formulas (1.5–2.0 Calories/ml) and Half-Strength Standard Formulas

	Nutren 2.0	Resource Plus	Sustacal HC	TwoCal HN	Introlite	Half-Strength Entrition	Pre-Attain
Calories (ml)	2	1.5	1.5	2	0.5	0.5	0.5
Carbohydrate source	Corn syrup solids, maltodextrin, sucrose	Maltodextrin, sucrose	Corn syrup solids, sugar	Hydrolyzed corn starch, sucrose	(NA)	Maltodextrin	Maltodextrin
Protein source	Casein	Sodium and calcium caseinates, soy protein isolate	Sodium and calcium caseinate	Sodium and calcium caseinates	(NA)	Casein	Sodium caseinate
Fat source (MCT:LCT)	MCT, Corn oil (73:27)	Corn oil (NA)	Corn oil (NA)	Corn oil, MCT (20:80)	(NA)	Corn oil (NA)	Corn oil (NA)
Carbohydrate (g/liter)	196	200	190	216.4	70.5	68	60
(% Kcals)	39	53.3	45	43.2	53	54.5	48
Protein (g/liter)	80	54.9	61	83.4	22.2	17.5	20
(% Kcals)	16	14.7	14.4	16.7	16	14	16
Fat (g/liter)	106	53.3	58	90.6	18.4	17.5	20
(% Kcals)	45	32.0	13.6	40.1	31	31.5	36
% Free water	70	70	78	71.2	92	(NA)	93
Volume (ml) for 100% RDA (adults)	750	1420	1200	947	(NA)	(NA)	1,600
mOsm/kg H_2O	710	600	650	690	(NA)	120	150.0
Na (mEq/liter)	43.5	49.6	36	56.8	40.4	15.2	15.0
K (mEq/liter)	64.1	59.3	38	62.4	40.1	15.4	15.0
Cl (mEq/liter)	56.3	56.9	36	46.3	40.6	14.1	15.0
Ca (mg/liter)	1,400	634	850	1,052	758	250	312.5
Phos (mg/liter)	1,400	634	850	1,052	758	250	312.5
Mg (mg/liter)	680	317	340	422	304	100	250.0
Manufacturer	Clintec Nutrition	Sandoz Nutrition	Mead Johnson	Ross Labs	Ross Labs	Clintec Nutrition	Sherwood Medical
Available flavors/forms	Vanilla; ready-to-use liquid	Vanilla, chocolate; ready-to-use liquid; instant crystals	Vanilla, chocolate, eggnog; ready-to-use liquid	Vanilla; ready-to-use liquid	Unflavored; ready-to-use liquid and closed delivery system	Unflavored; ready-to-use liquid; available in closed system	Unflavored; ready-to-use liquid; available in closed system
Description/features				Fortified with selenium, chromium, and molybdenum	Fortified with chromium, selenium, and molybdenum		

MCT = medium-chain triglyceride; LCT = long-chain triglyceride; NA = not available.

Source: Reprinted with permission from Nashville District Dietetic Association, Inc. Manual of Nutrition and Dietetics (4th ed). Nashville, TN: Tennessee Hospital Association, 1991.

Table AVI-7. Nutritional Supplements

	Carnation[a] Instant Breakfast	Carnation[b] Instant Breakfast: No Sugar Added	Citrotein	Delmark Instant Breakfast	Ensure Pudding[c]	Forta Shake[d]	Meritene Liquid
Calories (ml)	280/svg	188/svg	0.67	1.06	250/svg	290/svg	0.96
Carbohydrate source	Lactose, sucrose	Lactose	Sucrose, hydrolyzed corn starch	Maltodextrin, corn starch	Nonfat milk (lactose), sucrose, modified food starch	Nonfat milk (lactose), sucrose	Concentrated sweet skim milk (lactose, sucrose, corn syrup solids)
Protein source	Casein, egg white, whey	Casein, egg white, whey	Egg white solids	Partially skimmed milk, sodium caseinate	Nonfat milk	Nonfat milk	Concentrated sweet skim milk
Fat source	Milk fat	Milk fat	Partially hydrogenated soy oil	Corn oil	Partially hydrogenated soy oil (NA)	Milk fat	Corn oil
(MCT:LCT)	(NA)	(NA)		(NA)		(NA)	(NA)
Carbohydrate (g/liter)	35.9	20.7	120.6	139.2	34.0	37.0	110.4
(% Kcal)	51.0	44.0	73.0	52.0	54.2	51.4	46.0
Protein (g/liter)	15.2	15.0	40.9	50.6	6.8	17.0	57.6
(% Kcal)	22.0	32.0	25.0	19.0	10.9	23.6	24.0
Fat (g/liter)	8.3	5.0	1.6	33.8	9.7	8.0	32.0
(% Kcal)	27.0	24.0	2.0	29.0	34.9	25.0	30.0
% Free water	81.1	(NA)	93.0	(NA)	65.0	(NA)	84.0
Volume for 100% RDA (adults)	4 pkts	(NA)	1,100	(NA)	six/5-oz servings	four/8-oz servings	1,250
mOsm/kg	671/758	(NA)	480 (punch) 495 (orange) 515 (grape)	(NA)	(NA)	(NA)	510 (vanilla)
Na (mEq/liter)	11.1	10.9	32.6	35.0	10.4	10.4	38.4
K (mEq/liter)	18.9	17.4	19.2	51.2	8.4	20.7	41.0
Cl (mEq/liter)	12.3	(NA)	28.2	40.4	6.2	(NA)	45.2
Ca (mg/liter)	491	412	1,125	1,250	200	550	1,200
Phos (mg/liter)	408	327	1,125	1,250	200	450	1,200
Mg (mg/liter)	113	113	446	250	68	100	320

Table AVI-7. Continued

	Carnation[a] Instant Breakfast	Carnation[b] Instant Breakfast: No Sugar Added	Citrotein	Delmark Instant Breakfast	Ensure Pudding[c]	Forta Shake[d]	Meritene Liquid
Manufacturer Available flavors/forms	Clintec Nutrition Vanilla, chocolate, strawberry, chocolate malt; powder	Clintec Nutrition Vanilla, chocolate; powder	Sandoz Nutrition Orange, fruit punch, grape; powder	Delmark Ready-to-use liquid; powder	Ross Labs Vanilla, tapioca, chocolate, butterscotch; ready to serve	Ross Labs Vanilla, eggnog, Dutch chocolate; powder	Sandoz Nutrition Vanilla, chocolate, eggnog; ready-to-use liquid; powder
Description/ features			Appropriate for clear liquid diets				

[a]Contents of 1.23 oz powder in 8 oz of whole milk.
[b]Contents of 0.67 oz powder in 8 oz of 2% milk.
[c]Contents per 5-oz serving.
[d]Contents of 1.4 oz powder in 8 oz whole milk.

MCT = medium-chain triglyceride; LCT = long-chain triglyceride; NA = not available; sgv = serving.

Source: Reprinted with permission from Nashville District Dietetic Association, Inc. Manual of Nutrition and Dietetics (4th ed). Nashville, TN: Tennessee Hospital Association, 1991.

Appendix VII
Nutrition for Ostomies

Purpose

This diet provides general guidelines in food selection for individuals with a colostomy, ileostomy, or urostomy.[25]

Description

The nutritional needs of the ostomate are similar to those of the general population. The presence of an ostomy does not necessitate a change in eating habits; however, some nutrition-related problems may occur such as diarrhea, constipation, gas, and unpleasant odors. Individuals must learn by trial and error which foods cannot be tolerated. The following guidelines are suggested to help avoid these complications and to aid in food selection.

Adequacy

This diet will meet the Recommended Dietary Allowances.

Guidelines for Postoperative Period

After surgery, the diet generally progresses as follows:

1. Clear liquids
2. Bland, low residue diet for 6–8 weeks
3. High fiber foods added slowly at a rate of 1 per week to determine tolerance

Guidelines for Individuals with a Colostomy or Ileostomy

1. Choose foods carefully after surgery; gradually add foods for variety. Some foods may not be tolerated at first but after a few weeks may be included without difficulty.
2. Chew foods thoroughly because large pieces may cause a blockage. Chew slowly and with mouth closed as swallowed air may increase gas.
3. Eat in a pleasant, relaxed atmosphere. Emotional upsets and tension may cause bowel problems.
4. Eat on a regular schedule. Skipping meals may actually increase gas.
5. Eat in an upright position rather than lying down.
6. Eat a well-balanced diet and drink plenty of fluids. Fluids should not be restricted to try to control diarrhea.
7. If a food is poorly tolerated, it should be tried again in a few months.

Foods That May Produce Gas

1. Dried beans and peas, nuts
2. Vegetables of the cabbage family (broccoli, cauliflower, brussels sprouts, cabbage)
3. Asparagus, sweet potatoes, cucumbers, turnips, turnip greens, corn, and onions

4. Eggs
5. Fish
6. Certain cheeses (Roquefort, brie, and other strong cheeses)
7. Milk
8. Melons, raw apples
9. Excessive sugar, sweets, carbonated beverages
10. Beer
11. Whips and meringues

Other Factors That May Contribute to Gas

1. Chewing gum
2. Using straws
3. Constipation
4. Lack of exercise
5. Inadequate fluid intake
6. Excessive amounts of high-fiber foods

Foods That May Contribute to Diarrhea

1. Green leafy vegetables
2. Broccoli
3. Beans
4. Raw fruits
5. Beer
6. Highly seasoned foods

Foods That May Help Control Diarrhea

When diarrhea is a problem, drink plenty of fluids.

1. Bananas
2. Applesauce
3. Rice
4. Tapioca
5. Creamy peanut butter

Suggestions To Help Relieve Mild Constipation

1. Increase fluids
2. Increase fruit juices
3. Increase cooked fruits and vegetables
4. Moderate intake of whole grain breads and cereals

Large quantities of high-fiber foods may result in bowel blockage. The blockage could cause the ostomy to cease functioning.

Foods That May Produce Strong Odors

1. Asparagus
2. Fish
3. Chicken
4. Eggs
5. Onions
6. Baked beans and other legumes
7. Cabbage-family vegetables
8. Mustard
9. Some strong-flavored cheeses
10. Alcohol (especially beer)
11. Some antibiotics and vitamins

Foods That Help Reduce Odors

1. Cranberry juice
2. Yogurt
3. Buttermilk
4. Parsley

Guidelines for the Individual with a Urostomy

1. Urine should normally be odorless; urinary odor may be the first sign of an infection.
2. A diet with increased protein will help urinary acidity and may prevent urinary infection.
3. A diet containing an abundance of vegetables but low in protein foods (meat, poultry, fish, eggs) will promote an alkaline urine and may cause skin problems and alkaline crystal formation on the stoma.
4. Refer to the foods above that may produce and reduce strong odors.
5. Eat a well-balanced diet.

The following national organization may be contacted for additional information:

United Ostomy Association
2001 W. Beverly Boulevard
Los Angeles, CA 90057.

Chapter 30

Radiotherapeutic Techniques

Subir Nag

Introduction

Pain is the most common symptom experienced by cancer patients, occurring in 30–50% of cancer patients and in more than 75% of patients with advanced cancers.[1, 2] Radiotherapy plays a major part in palliation of pain and consequently in reduction of narcotic requirement in these patients.

History

In 1895 in Lyon, soon after the discovery of x-rays by Roentgen, Despeignes reported on the analgesic effect of radiographic therapy on a patient with cancer of the floor of the mouth and a patient with stomach cancer.[3] In 1896, Williams reported pain relief in a patient with breast cancer.[4] In the early days, only superficial x-ray was available; hence external beam radiation was not particularly effective in palliating pain originating in tumors of deep organs. However, with the advent of megavoltage radiation in the 1950s, more penetrating beams became available, extending the palliative usefulness of external beam radiation to deeper structures. Radiotherapy is now an important tool that is used in conjunction with analgesics to control cancer-related pain.

Mechanism of Pain Production in Cancer Patients

Tumors can cause pain in cancer patients either directly by a mass effect or indirectly by destroying bone or by causing inflammatory response. These mechanisms include those listed here:

1. Tumor infiltration of the periosteum causing an increase in interosseus pressure and irritation of the nociceptors present in the periosteal membrane[5]
2. Tumor mass causing expansion of the capsule, e.g., in the liver
3. Infiltrative tumor mass exerting pressure on the nerve plexus (e.g., lumbosacral and brachial plexi), nerve roots, spinal cord, and cranial nerves
4. Erosion of bone with resultant bony instability
5. Bony fragments from a pathologic fracture exerting pressure on the spinal cord
6. Infiltration of inflammatory cells and lymphocytes in the tumor and peritumoral area causing mechanical pressure
7. The chemical products of inflammation (prostaglandins, bradykinin) that irritate the nociceptors.[6]

Radiation Therapy

Principles

The relative indications for radiotherapy have changed over the years with the trend toward multidisciplinary and multimodal management of cancer. In addition to this trend, there have been rapid improvements in technology.[7] Most radiation oncology departments have developed technically but are often isolated from the rest of the medical community. Furthermore, both patients and other medical personnel have a fear of radiation. However, overexposure of medical personnel to radiation is uncommon. A brief review of the principles of radiotherapy is outlined to facilitate a better understanding of the role radiation therapy plays in cancer pain relief.

Radiation therapy deals with the treatment of malignant diseases using ionizing radiation. X-rays are electromagnetic radiation similar to visible light but of higher energy (or shorter wavelength). Electromagnetic radiation with wavelengths shorter than ultraviolet rays are ionizing radiation. The various modalities available to the radiation oncologist are summarized in Table 30-1.

The currently defined unit used in radiotherapy is the Gray (Gy), which represents 1 J per kg. However, many readers may be more familiar with the previously used unit of dose (the rad), which is equivalent to 0.01 Gy or 1 cGy.

Table 30-1. Classification of Common Radiotherapy Modalities

Teletherapy (external beam)
    X-ray beam (usually from a linear accelerator)
    Gamma beams (cobalt 60)
    Particle beams
        Electron
        Heavy particles (e.g., protons)
Brachytherapy
    Low-dose rate brachytherapy
        Permanent implants (iodine 125, palladium 103)
        Removable implants (iridium192, cesium 137)
    High-dose rate brachytherapy
    Pulsed-dose rate brachytherapy
Intraoperative radiation therapy
Systemic radionuclides

Fractionation

Radiation therapy is normally administered as a series of small, daily radiation doses usually given for 2–7 weeks. The delivery of radiation therapy as a number of small discrete doses is termed fractionation. Fractionation allows time between treatments so that the body can repair any sublethal damage to the normal cells. Another reason for fractionation is that x-rays are inefficient at killing hypoxic cells. Tumors generally have a hypoxic core that becomes reoxygenated when some of the peripheral cells are killed, allowing the core better access to oxygen available at the margins. Fractionation also allows redistribution of the tumor cells from the less sensitive "synthetic" phase of the cell cycle to the more radiosensitive "mitotic" phase, allowing a better cell kill.

It is important to realize that a specified dose of radiation kills a constant fraction of irradiated cells. Hence, the number of cells killed depends on the number of tumor cells initially present. Therefore, a specified dose of radiation will kill a large number of cells in a big tumor, e.g., even a small radiation dose will rapidly reduce tumor size, while a large radiation dose is required to eradicate the tumor.

compare the total dose in terms of the number of Gray given. The biological effects of radiation on tissue depend on the total dose, dose per fraction, the overall duration of treatment, and total volume radiated. The effects can be divided into early radiation damage, effects on tumor tissue, and late radiation damage. The larger the volume radiated, the lower the dose tolerated. The larger the dose per fraction given, the lower the total dose tolerated. Thus, the effect of 30 Gy in 10 treatments is not the same as the effect of 30 Gy in 15 treatments or in 5 treatments. The fraction size is probably the dominant factor in determining the late effects of radiation; a better late effect is obtained by using smaller fractions.

The conventional fraction size for curative radiation is 1.8–2.0 Gy per day, whereas 3 Gy per day is often used for palliative treatments. Hence, a standard curative regime may be 60 Gy in 30 fractions over 6 weeks of daily treatment given at 2 Gy per fraction; in comparison, a common palliative dose used is 30 Gy in 10 treatments over 2 weeks. In certain situations, 20 Gy in 5 fractions over 1 week or even a single large fraction of 6–8 Gy has been used. Common palliative doses are summarized in Table 30-2.

Dose, Time, and Volume Relationship

It is important to realize that a dose, time, and volume relationship exists in radiotherapy. One cannot

Morbidity

The morbidity resulting from radiotherapy depends on the dose and the volume radiated. The

Table 30-2. Examples of Palliative Dose Fractionation

Total dose (Gy)	40	30	20	8
Dose (Gy)/treatment	2	3	4	8
Number of treatments	20	10	5	1
Overall duration (days)	26–28	12–14	5–7	1

acute morbidity often seen with curative radiation therapy treatments can include nausea, vomiting, fatigue, skin reactions, diarrhea, mucositis, alopecia, and bone marrow suppression. Latent normal tissue damage occurs in slowly dividing normal cells; thus, organs such as the brain, spinal cord, lungs, and vasculature are especially sensitive to late damage. Late effects are often irrelevant for patients with very advanced malignancies because most of them do not live long enough to be at risk for developing those late complications.

The morbidity also depends on the volume of tissue treated. The larger the volume treated, the greater the morbidity. Treating only the tumor and the margin around the tumor is called involved field radiation therapy; treating the tumor, the surrounding margin, and the regional lymph nodes is termed regional treatment (often used in curative therapy). One may also give wide field treatments including half body (lower or upper) or whole body radiation therapy as discussed later. For palliative treatment, the volume treated is kept as small as possible and a moderate dose is chosen to minimize morbidity. The number of treatments is minimized to reduce the inconvenience to the patient.

Planning

Careful planning is essential for a successful radiotherapy course. After a complete clinical evaluation, one has to determine if the treatment is to be curative or palliative. Radiotherapy is used equally for curative purposes in about 50% of patients and for palliation in remaining the 50% of patients. A major palliative role of radiotherapy is pain control. In fact, of all patients treated by radiotherapy, about 40% are treated for control of pain.

Treatment Goals

Radical Radiotherapy Treatment

Radical radiotherapy treatment refers to the delivery of a course of radiation with the intent to completely eradicate the tumor. Larger volumes are radiated so as to include the tumor with sufficient margin and lymphatic drainage areas. Because the objective in radical radiotherapy is to achieve a cure or to prolong survival, a greater morbidity (toxicity or side effects) can be accepted when compared with that in palliative treatments. Patients with small, localized disease are generally treated with a curative intent. In these cases, the highest dose of radiation that normal tissues can tolerate is delivered, and the treatments are given over several weeks.

Palliative Radiation Therapy

The major indication for palliative radiotherapy is to relieve pain. It is also used to control bleeding (hemoptysis, hematemesis, hematuria, and rectal and vaginal bleeding, etc.) and to overcome obstructions (airway, spinal cord compression, brain metastasis).

The general principles of palliative radiation therapy include the establishment of diagnosis and extent of the tumor and confirmation that the disease is incurable. We must determine that the tumor is the cause of the symptoms and realistic treatment goals must be established. Should the patient be treated at all, and if so, which modality would best achieve this goal? The least morbid modality with minimal inconvenience to the patient should be chosen. The side effects should be minimal, and they certainly should not be worse than the symptoms being palliated. The Patterns of Care Study shows that the total dose used for palliative care varies widely across the United States from 10–50 Gy with fraction sizes from less than 2 Gy per fraction to greater than 3.5 Gy per fraction.[8] Usually, to minimize morbidity, a short course is given, with a high dose per fraction to a small field; however, even for palliation, high doses are sometimes required to achieve local control of incurable tumors.

The Mechanism of Palliation of Bony Pain

The mechanism by which radiotherapy achieves pain relief is not fully understood. Appreciable bone healing can occur after only moderate doses of radiation (radiographic evidence of recalcification being seen in 78% of patients with breast cancer, receiving 20–25 Gy).[9] The onset of pain relief after radiation often occurs within a few days of treatment and can be achieved with low-dose radiation.[10] However, small doses of radiation may result in considerable tumor cell killing with a survival fraction of 0.1–0.8 for a radiation dose of 2 Gy.[11]

However, it is unlikely that tumor shrinkage or even tumor cell kill can satisfactorily account for relief of bone pain, which may be seen within 24 hours of radiation.[12] Another proposed mechanism for bone pain relief by small doses of radiation therapy is destruction of lymphocytes. Lymphocytes are the most radiosensitive cells in the body. They secrete a variety of chemical mediators (cytokinins, interleukin 1 beta, interleukin 8, interferons) that modulate pain. These lymphocytes are killed by small doses of radiation, resulting in rapid pain relief.[13]

Modalities Used for Cancer Pain Relief

Radiotherapy can be used in many ways to obtain relief. The common radiotherapy modalities have been reviewed earlier (see Table 30-1). The various methods by which radiotherapy can be helpful in controlling cancer pain are summarized in Table 30-3 and are detailed below.

Localized Radiation Therapy

If the area of pain originates in a small area, localized radiation therapy is given. External beam radiation therapy (EBRT) is the most common type of radiotherapy used in most situations, although brachytherapy or intraoperative radiation therapy are also used, depending on the circumstances.

External Beam Radiation

EBRT is widely available and is generally given to the painful area for palliation of pain. It is most commonly used to treat bony pain, although it is also used in other circumstances causing pain. The results of localized EBRT have been reported in retrospective analysis and in randomized trials outlined in the following discussion.

Table 30-3. Modalities Used in Radiotherapy to Relieve Pain

Teletherapy
   Localized
   Hemibody irradiation
Brachytherapy
Intraoperative radiotherapy
Systemic radionuclides: phosphorous 32, strontium 89, samarium 153, rhenium 186, iodine 131
Indirect methods: radiotherapeutic ablation of ovaries, pituitary, thalamus

Hoskin[14] summarized the results of 16 nonrandomized studies.[15–29] Of 2,422 treatments for bone pain, there was a mean overall response rate of 86% (range, 73–100%) and mean complete response rate of 52% (range, 20–90%). The duration of response was difficult to define and the mean survival was less than 1 year. Patients treated with a single fraction did not seem to have any disadvantages over those treated with multiple fractions.[15–29]

Arcangeli found a straight correlation between the total dose given and complete pain relief ($P = 0.0002$).[30] In contrast, the fraction size was not significant. Total doses higher than 40 Gy may not add to complete pain control. The incidence of pain recurrence was also related to the total dose, regardless of the fraction size. They concluded that patients with primary tumors in the prostate, breast, or kidney (who may have a long expected life span) should be given a full course of protracted radiation therapy with doses from 40–50 Gy.

Hoskin reported on a randomized trial between 4 and 8 Gy single doses in the treatment of metastatic bone pain.[31] At 4 weeks, the actual response rates were 69% for 8 Gy and 44% for 4 Gy ($P < 0.001$), but there were no differences in complete response rates at 4 weeks and no difference in duration of response between the two doses. They concluded that 8 Gy gave a higher probability of pain relief than 4 Gy, but that 4 Gy could be an effective alternative in situations of reduced tolerance.

Madsen reported on a randomized trial comparing 24 Gy in six fractions versus 20 Gy in two fractions.[32] There was no difference in either treatment group, with satisfactory pain control in approximately 48% of the cases. He concluded that a short course of treatment using a moderate dose was preferred for the convenience of the patients.

Okawa et al. reported on a prospective randomized trial comparing small, large, and twice-a-day fraction treatment for relief of painful metastases.[33] Eighty patients with painful bony metastases at 92 sites received either a conventional treatment of 30 Gy in 15 fractions (group 1), 22.5 Gy in 5 fractions given twice weekly (group 2), or 20 Gy in 10 fractions given twice a day (group 3). There was also no difference in the response rate. Hence, they concluded that the fractionation regime was a minor consideration in the treatment of painful bony metastasis.

The Radiation Therapy Oncology Group (a multi-institutional cooperative group in the United States) reported that 90% of their patients experienced some pain relief and 54% achieved complete pain relief among a total of 1,016 patients treated with local EBRT.[34] Patients with solitary metastases were randomized to receive 40.5 Gy in 3 weeks or 20 Gy in 1 week. Patients with multiple metastases were randomized to receive one of the following treatment protocols: 30 Gy in 2 weeks, 15 Gy in 1 week, or 20 or 25 Gy in 1 week. There was no significant difference in the response to pain relief by the dose; however, patients with prostate and breast primaries had more frequent, complete pain relief than did those from lung or other primary lesions. More than 70% of patients who experienced some relief did not relapse before death. The median duration of complete relief was 12 weeks. In the solitary group, the patients treated with 14.5 Gy had a higher incidence of fracture at the treatment site than the group that received 20 Gy. Hence, they concluded that low-dose, short-schedule treatments were as effective as more aggressive protracted regimens.

A reanalysis of this data by Blitzer[35] showed that when patients with solitary and multiple metastases were grouped together and analgesic requirements were included in the pain score, a highly significant association between numbers of fractions and response became apparent. A complete response rate of 55% was seen after 40.5 Gy in 15 daily fractions, compared with a response rate of only 28% after 25 Gy in 5 daily fractions.

A study from the Royal Marsden Hospital in London with a prospective randomized trial comparing single fractions of 8 Gy with 30 Gy in 10 daily fractions found no difference in the onset or duration of pain relief between the two treatment regimens.[36]

Kagei et al. reported a randomized trial of a single fraction radiation treatment (8, 10, 12, and 15 Gy) compared with a multifraction dose schedule (20 Gy in 4 fractions; 25 Gy in 5 fractions; 30 Gy in 6 fractions) for bone metastasis.[37] There was no difference in the incidence of pain relief, speed of onset, or acute morbidity of the two groups.

Localized EBRT is also effective in relieving pain in extensive hepatic metastases. If the entire liver is involved, whole liver irradiation is given (e.g., 2,100 cGy in seven treatments), taking care not to exceed the normal liver tolerance. If the involvement is more limited, local irradiation to higher doses is given to the metastatic nodule.

EBRT is also used to treat infiltrative tumor masses to relieve pain caused by irritation or pressure on cranial nerves, nerve roots, plexus, spinal cord, or brain. A dose of 30 Gy in 10 treatments is commonly used. Large dose per fraction is generally not used if long-term tolerance of neural tissues is a consideration.

It is important to realize that the pain may not be due to metastasis in all cases. In fact, benign disease may be the cause of pain in almost one-third of the patients.[38] A needle biopsy may be required to confirm metastasis if there is only a single area of recurrence. Because the treatment of metastatic disease is palliative, radiation therapy is not advisable if the metastasis is asymptomatic, except if the suspected metastases occur in weight-bearing bone such as the femur and humerus.

If pain increases during radiation, one must be alert to other causes, including growth of the lesion outside the field of radiation and the development of fracture. Patients with severe cortical destruction in weight-bearing bones should be considered for limitation of weight-bearing activities or for orthopedic intervention (pinning, hip replacement). Radiation therapy can be given in the presence of a pathologic fracture, although initial surgical fixation is preferred. Reiden et al. reported pain improvement in 67% of patients treated with EBRT of 40–50 Gy after pathologic fracture even without surgical fixation.[39] Stabilization was observed in 55% and recalcification in 33%.

Multiple fields of localized EBRT are sometimes used to treat widespread metastases. Although this can achieve pain relief in some cases, there can be some associated problems. The localized EBRT may relieve pain in one area only to unmask new areas of pain. The treatments can be rather prolonged, which may be impracticable in those with a short expected life span. Difficulties in matching adjacent radiation fields can sometimes result in overlaps and increased reactions. In these situations, hemibody irradiation (HBI) or systemic radionuclide administration may be more appropriate and are discussed later in this chapter.

One can conclude that localized EBRT plays a major role in the palliation of cancer pain and the reduction of narcotic medications. There is some controversy about dose response to the pain palliation. The majority of the studies show little dose response effect in the short-term, whereas better long-term effects are obtained with higher doses at smaller dose per fraction. Hence, a short course of moderate dose of radiation is generally prescribed for patients who are not expected to be long-term survivors; more protracted, higher doses are prescribed for those who have a long expected life span.

Brachytherapy

Localized radiation therapy can also be delivered by using brachytherapy. Brachytherapy involves the implantation of radioactive material into or close to the tumor to deliver a high tumor dose while sparing normal tissues. Although brachytherapy is usually used with curative intent, it can also be used for pain palliation, most often in pancreatic carcinoma patients.[40–43]

Peretz et al. reported on 98 patients with iodine 125 brachytherapy at the Memorial Sloan Kettering Cancer Center. Pain relief was obtained in 37 of 57 patients (65%) presenting with pain. However, the median survival for the entire group was only 7 months.[40]

Syed et al. reported on 18 patients treated with 30–50 Gy EBRT and 100–150 Gy iodine 125 brachytherapy to the pancreas. They noted excellent palliation of pain and a median survival of 14 months.[41]

Dobelbower et al. reported their experience with precision high-dose photon EBRT, systemic 5 fluorouracil (FU), and 120–210 Gy of iodine 125 brachytherapy on 12 patients with carcinoma of the pancreas. There was satisfactory palliation of pain and a median survival of 15 months.[42]

Mohiuddin et al. reported on the Thomas Jefferson University experience in treating 81 patients with unresectable carcinoma of the pancreas with iodine 125 implantation, EBRT, and chemotherapy.[43] They obtained satisfactory palliation and a median survival of 12 months.

In summary, brachytherapy can achieve satisfactory pain relief in patients with pancreatic cancer in about 60–80% of cases. It is therefore appropriate for patients having an exploratory laparotomy. Because it is an invasive procedure, an exploratory laparotomy is usually not recommended solely for the purpose of implanting the pancreas. Although the pancreas is the most common site where brachytherapy is used in the palliation of pain, brachytherapy can be used in many other sites (e.g., head and neck).

Intraoperative Radiation Therapy

Another modality of localized radiotherapy is intraoperative electron beam radiation therapy (IOEBRT). In this method, the area of the tumor is surgically exposed, normal radiosensitive structures (e.g., bowel) are retracted out of the field or shielded with lead, and the area including the tumor is irradiated intraoperatively with electron beam from a linear accelerator. Exposure of 10–20 Gy is commonly given as a supplement to EBRT, or 15–30 Gy if given alone.[44–49]

Kawamura et al. reported on 37 patients treated with IOEBRT.[44] Patients with unresectable carcinoma treated by IOEBRT plus EBRT survived longer than patients treated with IOEBRT alone. Pain relief was obtained in 95% of the unresectable patients with pain. They concluded that IOEBRT proved effective in the relief of pain and improvement of survival in patients with localized pancreatic carcinoma.

Tepper et al. reported (in the RTOG study 85-05) on the results of 86 patients with pancreatic cancer who were treated with 50.4 Gy EBRT in combination with 5 FU chemotherapy and 20 Gy IOEBRT.[45] The median survival time was 9 months. Major postoperative complications occurred in 12% of the patients, and two patients had major late morbidity leading to death. They concluded that patients receiving IOEBRT did not obtain better results than those treated with external beam alone.

Nishimura et al. reported on 33 patients treated with IOEBRT with single doses of 20–40 Gy with

8–25 MeV electrons, obtaining excellent pain relief in 50% of patients who had complained of pain. An improvement in survival rate was also reported.[46]

Dobelbower et al. reported on the Medical College of Ohio IOEBRT experience in treating 17 patients with cancer of the pancreas with precision high-dose radiation therapy of 40–60 Gy and 20–30 Gy of IOEBRT.[47] Pain relief was obtained in 11 of the 12 patients (92%). Jaundice was relieved in all patients, but patient survival was not significantly different from the survival of patients treated with EBRT alone.

Thus, although it may not prolong survival, IOEBRT can be effective in palliation of pain, especially in patients with advanced pancreatic cancer. However, it must be re-emphasized that, because IOEBRT is an invasive procedure, an exploratory laparotomy is usually not recommended solely for the purpose of delivering this modality to the pancreas.

Wide-Field Radiation

Because most metastases are due to hematogenous spread, it would be unusual to have only one site of metastasis. Therefore, there are probably multiple sites of metastases that may not be immediately apparent. Localized radiation may control pain in one area but unmask pain at other sites. Accordingly, patients with metastatic disease sometimes should receive multiple courses of palliative radiation therapy.

Many of these patients are elderly, and it may be difficult for them to undertake a long course of daily treatment. It is sometimes difficult to justify a long treatment course, especially when the patient has a short expected life span. Furthermore, the difficulty of matching radiotherapy fields can lead to the problem of the fields overlapping critical radiosensitive structures when adjacent areas must be irradiated by separate fields.

The source of pain may sometimes be difficult to locate. For example, pain in the hip may be caused by involvement of the lumbosacral root, sacroiliac joint, or pelvic bones. HBI may be considered in these situations.[12, 50–64] Irradiation to half of the body, or sequentially to both halves, in the treatment of widespread metastatic disease has been termed "systemic radiation." It is an attractive alternative because single doses are given to the patient. The radiation is generally given using photons from a cobalt-60 machine or a linear accelerator at an ex-

tended distance with the patient lying on the floor. Lower and middle HBI is given on an outpatient basis with an antiemetic administered 1–2 hours before treatment. The lower hemibody usually extends from the iliac crest to below the knee joint. The midbody radiation extends from the diaphragm to below the ischium. Upper HBI is given with premedication of steroids, an antiemetic, and hydration the night before irradiation. The field for the upper HBI extends from the umbilicus to the scalp, with shielding of the parotid and eyes.

Although 6–8 Gy is the common dose given, Nag et al.[51] studied lower HBI of 16 Gy (8 Gy 1 week apart in two fractions) to the lower hemibody in 19 patients. Patients tolerated this treatment well, with 100% of the patients responding (53% complete response and 47% partial response). The mean duration of pain relief was 5 months, and 10 of the 15 patients (67%) who died were pain-free at the time of death. This study concluded that high-dose lower HBI produced prolonged effective palliation of pain with minimal morbidity, but that it did not prolong survival.

Salazar et al. reported on the Radiation Therapy Oncology Group study of increasing doses of HBI.[12] The most effective and safest doses were 6 Gy for upper HBI and 8 Gy for mid HBI. Increasing doses beyond these levels did not increase pain relief or duration of relief, but was associated with increase in toxicity. HBI was found to relieve pain in 73% of patients. Twenty percent of the patients had complete pain relief, with more than two-thirds achieving better than 50% pain relief. The pain relief was dramatic, with nearly 50% of all responding patients achieving relief within 48 hours and 80% within 1 week of HBI. The pain relief was long lasting and continued without retreatment for at least 50% of the patients' remaining life.[12]

A subsequent RTOG study (8206) reported by Poulter[58] explored the possibility that HBI added to local field radiation might delay the appearance of new metastases and decrease the frequency of further treatment. Four hundred ninety-nine patients were randomized to receive local field radiation alone (30 Gy in treatments) or local radiation plus HBI. The HBI was delivered as a single 8 Gy fraction to the predetermined hemibody area within 7 days of completion of local field radiation. The local field was shielded during HBI, and lung correction and thin lung shields were required to reduce the dose to the lung to 7 Gy. The survival data of the two patient groups were not significantly different. Time to disease progression at 1 year was significantly delayed for those receiving HBI (46% compared with 35% for those treated locally). Time to new disease in the targeted hemibody was also improved at 1 year (50% for HBI compared with 68% for local only). The median time to new disease within the HBI area was 12.6 months versus 6.3 months for patients receiving local treatment only. The time to new treatment within the hemibody segment was also delayed. Tolerance to HBI was excellent.

Salmon et al.[59] reported on the South West Oncology Group study with 614 patients with multiple myeloma. All patients underwent remission induction with chemotherapy and were then randomized to receive either vincristine, melphalan, prednisone, cyclophosphamide, and (VMPC) chemotherapy or sequential HBI with vincristine and prednisone (VP) chemotherapy. Patients receiving VMPC chemotherapy had a better relapse-free survival (26 months) and overall median survival (36 months) when compared with HBI (20 months and 28 months, respectively). Myelosuppression was also significantly worse after HBI. Hence, they concluded that chemotherapy was superior to HBI for remission consolidation in multiple myeloma.

Zelefsky et al. reported on a group of 15 patients with hormone refractory metastatic adenocarcinoma of the prostate who were treated with fractionated hemiskeletal radiation of 25–30 Gy in 9–10 fractions compared with a second group of 14 patients treated with a single dose of 6–8 Gy HBI.[57] All patients achieved complete or partial relief shortly after completing their therapy. Of the patients treated with single dose, 71% ultimately needed retreatment because of recurrent bone pain. In contrast, only 13% of patients receiving fractionated treatment courses needed retreatment. The median survival of both groups was similar (10 and 11 months); however, the median duration of palliation was greater for those patients receiving fractionated treatments (8.5 versus 2.8 months). The incidence of treatment-related toxicity was similar for both groups. They concluded that fractionated HBI was more effective as palliation compared with single-dose HBI.

Side effects resulting from the toxicity of HBI include nausea, vomiting, and diarrhea. These typically occur within a few hours of treatment in most patients. Premedication (antiemetics for lower HBI and hydration, steroids and antiemetics for upper HBI) reduces these side effects. Bone marrow depression occurs in less than 10% of cases if only one-half of the body is radiated. However, bone marrow depression occurs in most patients receiving sequential upper and lower HBI. These patients should therefore be carefully followed for bone marrow depression and symptomatically treated when necessary.

Patients with upper hemibody radiation also have problems with lung toxicity if doses of more than 6–7 Gy are used. The patients are usually hospitalized, and there is dose correction by lung transmission. Patients should not have received previous lung radiotherapy, or these areas should be shielded. An aggressive premedication program including steroids, hydration, and antiemetics is required. Fractionated radiation may reduce the toxicity of this treatment.

In summary, review of studies with hemibody radiation shows that HBI is a useful modality for palliation of pain from widespread metastasis. The pain relief occurs within 1–2 days in about 75–80% of the cases. The toxicity of lower HBI (mainly nausea and myelosuppresion) is acceptable. With upper HBI, a proper premedication program is essential, the dose must be limited, and lung toxicity can be a problem.

Systemic Radionuclides

The traditional treatment for painful bony metastases has been analgesics and local and wide-field EBRT. Localized radiation therapy is effective in treating limited areas of bony metastases. Although HBI can be used as a systemic treatment, its associated myelosuppression may be problematic. Bone-seeking radionuclide given systemically has been used to treat multiple areas of bony pain and to possibly increase survival. The bone-seeking radioisotope is selectively taken up by the tumor in bone so that a highly localized dose of radiation is delivered. Initially, phosphorous 32 (P-32) was used; however, strontium 89 (Sr-89) has been recently approved for clinical use. Likewise, samarium 153 (Sm-153) and rhenium 186 (Re-186) are being investigated.

Phosphorus 32

P-32 is a pure beta emitter with a maximum energy of 1.71 MeV, a mean energy of 0.7 MeV, and a half-life of 14.3 days. The average tissue penetration from P-32 beta particle is 2.5 mm, with a maximum range of 8 mm.[65] Intravenously administered P-32 is taken up mainly in the bone.[66-68] Kenney et al. initially reported, in 1941, the use of P-32 for treatment of bony metastasis for carcinoma of the breast and osteogenic sarcoma.[69]

Initially, testosterone derivatives were used to potentiate the uptake of P-32 at the site of bony metastasis.[70, 71] However, exogenous androgens may stimulate metastatic carcinoma of the prostate, and there can be transient increase of bone pain by androgens.[72–74] Therefore, parathyroid hormone has been used as the potentiating agent for P-32 therapy.[70–74]

Silberstein recently reviewed 28 studies of the use of P-32 to relieve bony pain in cases of primary breast or prostate tumors.[75] Eighty-four percent of the 342 patients with breast carcinoma and 77% of the 494 patients with prostate carcinoma responded to the P-32. A complete response to P-32 was noted in 20–50% of the patients. There was no dose–response relationship to the wide range of activity (4–24 mCi in single and divided doses) used.

The main toxicity of P-32 is bone marrow suppression, which occurs in more than 90% of patients.[76] Pancytopenia depends on the dose and usually occurs 4–5 weeks after injection, with recovery to near normal levels in 6–7 weeks. P-32 injection has also been associated with development of acute leukemia in patients with polycythemia vera.[77] This usually occurs 6–10 years after treatment. Because patients with extensive bony metastasis rarely have long survival times, this side effect is not a commonly observed morbidity of P-32 therapy for painful bony metastasis.

Moreover, varying doses of P-32 can reduce or relieve bony pain from bony metastases in approximately 50–80% of patients. This is similar to the effects of localized or wide-field radiation therapy. There was no dose–response relationship between the dose of P-32 and the degree of response. Thus, P-32 is not commonly used primarily due its severe hematologic toxicity.

Strontium 89

Because P-32 produced significant bone marrow toxicity, Sr-89 has recently been used for the systemic relief of bone pain.[78–92] It is a pure beta emitter with a maximum beta energy of 1.4 MeV and half-life of 50.6 days. As a calcium imitator, Sr-89 is not incorporated into the marrow and rapidly washes out of healthy bone, with a biological half-life of 14 days with retention of isotope at the site of metastasis.[78, 79] Approximately 2–20 Gy of absorbed dose is achieved per mCi of Sr-89 delivered.[78–81]

Firusian reported on 11 patients of carcinoma of the prostate with bony metastasis treated with 30 μCi of Sr-89 per kg.[92] They obtained a significant long lasting clinical improvement in 8 of 11 patients. A remarkable alleviation of pain was observed within a few days and in some cases within 24 hours after the intravenous injection.

Porter et al. reported on the randomized trans-Canada Sr-89 study.[88] In eight Canadian cancer centers, 126 patients with endocrine refractory metastatic prostate cancer were randomized to receive local field radiotherapy and placebo versus local field radiotherapy with 10.8 mCi of Sr-89. Patients were considered eligible for inclusion into the study if they had multiple bone metastases secondary to prostate cancer. The patients also had failed hormonal manipulation. The patients were excluded if they had extensive soft tissue involvement. Local radiation therapy was given (30 Gy in 10 fractions or 20 Gy in 5 fractions). Intake of analgesics was significantly reduced in patients treated with Sr-89. There was statistically significant reduction of new sites of pain or requirements for radiotherapy in these patients. Quality of life was improved, and prostatic acid phosphatase, alkaline phosphatase, and prostate-specific antigen levels were reduced in the group receiving Sr-89. Hematologic toxicity (reduction in platelets and white cells) was significantly greater in the group receiving Sr-89 compared with the group receiving placebo. Clinical bleeding, pneumonia, and hemorrhage were more common in the Sr-89–treated group. There was no significant statistical improvement in survival benefit with the Sr-89 treatment. It was concluded that Sr-89 was an effective adjuvant therapy to local field radiotherapy.[88]

The Radiation Therapy Oncology Group (a multi-institutional cooperative group in the United States) has a phase I study (RTOG 88-21) to evaluate the use of Sr-89 in metastatic prostate cancer. In this study, Sr-89 doses are escalated from 4.0–11.5 mCi to determine the maximum safe dose and to evaluate the efficacy and morbidity of Sr-89 therapy in endocrine resistant metastatic prostate cancer.

Intravenous administration of Sr-89 produces a response rate of 70–80% of patients treated (especially breast and prostate primary), with 10–25% of patients remaining pain free. The major toxicity (dose dependent) is hematologic. Sr-89 was recently approved for clinical use in the United States and is the radionuclide most commonly used for treating symptomatic, widespread bone pain.

Samarium 153

Sm-153 is a beta emitter with a maximum energy of 810 keV, with an average penetration range of 0.8 mm. It also emits 103 keV of gamma photons and has a half-life of 46 hours. The beta emission allows treatment, whereas the gamma emission allows imaging and estimation of radiation dose to bone marrow. Sm-153 has therefore been used in the systemic treatment of bone pain.[93–95]

Turner et al. treated 35 patients with 20 mCi (740 MBq) of Sm-153.[93] The radiation dose to bone marrow was restricted to 2 Gy. Symptomatic relief of bone pain was reported in 14 of 23 evaluable patients (61%), with a median duration of 8 weeks.[94] The major toxicity was myelosuppression occurring at 2–4 weeks. Fifteen patients were re-treated with Sm-153, and good control of pain was obtained in 13 (87%). The median duration of pain control (24 weeks) and median survival of 9 months were substantially greater in the re-treated group than in patients treated with a single dose. Nine of the 15 patients (60%) in the re-treated group required blood transfusion due to anemia. Sm-153 has the advantage of having a beta and gamma emission, thus making it suitable for both imaging and therapy. It is currently undergoing clinical trials and has a lower hematologic toxicity.

Rhenium 186

Re-186 is a radiolabeled biphosphonate that localizes in metastatic foci in bone and that emits beta particles suitable for therapy and a gamma ray suitable for diagnostic imaging. This allows the clinician to verify localization in areas that cause pain and to allow quantitation of the radiation dose to be delivered to the tumor site and to bone marrow. Re-186 has a beta energy of 1.07 MeV. This lower beta energy allows for less penetration.[96–99] The gamma energy of 138 keV is 9%, which allows for imaging but does not present a radiation hazard to surrounding tissue. The half-life of Re-186 is 3.8 days, which allows for shipment, processing, and convenient disposal.

Maxon et al.[98] administered single intravenous injection of 34 mCi (1258 MBq) of Re-186 in 43 patients. Pain improved significantly in 77% of the patients. The only adverse clinical reaction was a transient increase in pain in 10% of the patients. There was a decrease in total white blood cell count and total platelet count within the first 8 weeks after therapy.

Curley et al.[99] treated 18 patients with prostate cancer with metastases to the bone. They received a single administration of 35 mCi of Re-186. They noted a response rate in 67% of the patients, with a maximal response during the second week. There was reversible hematologic toxicity in 28% of the patients.

Iodine 131

I-131 has both gamma and beta emissions. The beta emission is suitable for imaging and the gamma emission is suitable for therapy. I-131 is easily available; however, its lower beta energy has a shorter penetration rate and may give shorter duration of pain relief. However, in the relief of bone pain, the response rates are similar to treatment with other radionuclides.[100]

The use of I-131 is well established for thyroid carcinoma. Because it is concentrated by the follicular thyroid cells, I-131 has been used for palliation of painful bony metastases in patients with this disease.[101]

Brown et al. treated 235 patients with thyroid ablation followed by 5.5 GBq of I-131. They reported good response in the treatment of lung metastases, but no objective improvement of bone metastases. Pain relief was seen in only 2 of 21 patients (10%). However, the authors reported better relief of pain by the use of EBRT. Hence, EBRT remains the treatment of choice for localized bone pain from metastatic thyroid cancer.[101]

Enhancement of Therapeutic Response to Systemic Radionuclides

It may be possible to increase the response rate and duration of pain relief by increasing the dose of radionuclide administered while supporting bone marrow suppression by the administration of colony-stimulating factors.[102] Biphosphonates may possibly increase radioisotope retention.[103] Low-dose infusion cisplatin has also been used to potentiate the action of Sr-89.[104] Another possibility is to combine HBI with systemic radionuclide therapy[83] so that systemically administered radionuclide could give a greater radiation dose to areas of bony metastases while hemibody radiation could also treat areas of soft tissue metastases not treated by the administered radionuclide. Further investigations are needed in this field.

Indirect Methods of Relief of Bone Pain by Radiotherapy

Although pain relief is obtained by directing the radiotherapy at the site of bone pain, in certain instances, relief of bone pain can be obtained by ablating endocrine functions. Although radiotherapy was used in the past to ablate endocrine functions, it is rarely used for that purpose presently and is mentioned mainly for its historical interest. The mechanism involved is unclear but may be due to tumor regression.

Ovarian function can be ablated by the use of whole pelvic EBRT of 15–20 Gy[3]; however, this treatment is usually performed using the antiestrogen drug tamoxifen.

Pain relief may also be obtained after hypophysectomy.[105–107] Pituitary ablation has been accomplished by EBRT, proton beam irradiation, or by interstitial brachytherapy using gold or iodine.[3] However, pituitary ablation can result in diabetes insipidus, cerebrospinal fluid leak, blindness, nerve damage, or meningitis[105, 106]; therefore, this technique is not currently used.

Another indirect method of pain relief is the use of stereotactic radiosurgery in the thalamus to ablate the neural tracts, obtaining response rates of 75–90%.[3, 108, 109] A single dose of 150–200 Gy delivered by the gamma knife technique with cobalt 60 has been used to relieve intractable and severe pain. This technique has not become popular because there is danger of brain damage.

Conclusion

Radiation therapy is an important way to achieve pain relief and reduce narcotic requirements for cancer patients. It is delivered mainly as localized EBRT, although HBI, brachytherapy, intraoperative radiotherapy, and systemic administration of radionuclides have also been used. Indirect methods (ablation of ovary, pituitary, or thalamus) are no longer used in routine clinical practice.

For localized pain, EBRT, IOEBRT, or brachytherapy provide relief in approximately 80% of the cases. For diffuse pain, wide-field radiotherapy or systemic administration of radionuclides would be a preferable choice, although hematologic toxicity is possible. These simple treatments can reduce analgesic requirements and produce long-term pain relief for patients with advanced cancers.

Acknowledgments

I would like to thank Dr. Richard Pieters for his valuable comments, Anne Brandt for her assistance in preparing this manuscript, and David Carpenter for reading and editing it.

References

1. Portnoy RK. Cancer pain: Epidemiology and syndromes. Cancer 1989;63:2298.
2. Bonica JJ. Treatment of Cancer Pain: Current Status and Future Needs. In HL Fields, R Bubner, F Cervero (eds), Advances in Pain Research and Therapy. New York: Raven Press, 1985;589.
3. Kuttig H. Radiotherapy of cancer pain. Recent Results Cancer Res1984;89:190.
4. Glasser O. Wilhelm Conrad Röntgen und die Geschichte der Röntgenstrahlen. Berlin: Springer-Verlag, 1958.
5. Hungerford DS. Bone Marrow Pressure and Intramedullary Venography. In R Owen, J Goodfellow, P Bullough (eds), Scientific Foundations of Orthopaedics and Traumatology. London: Heinemann, 1980;357.
6. Schaible H-G, Schmidt RF. Direct Observations of the Sensitization of Articular Afferents During an Experimental Arthritis. In R Dubner, GF Gehbart, MR Bond (eds), Pain Research in Clinical Management (Vol. 3). Proceedings of the 5th World Congress on Pain. Amsterdam: Elsevier, 1988;44.
7. Hellman S. Principles of Radiation Therapy. In VT DeVita, S Hellman, SA Rosenberg (eds), Cancer: Principles and Practice of Oncology (4th ed). Philadelphia: Lippincott, 1993;248.
8. Coia LR, Hanks GE, Martz K, et al. Practice patterns of palliative care for the United States 1984–1985. Int J Radiat Oncol Biol Phys 1988;14:1261.
9. Garmatis CJ, Chu F. The effectiveness of radiation therapy in the treatment of bone metastases from breast cancer. Radiology 1978;16:235.

10. Price P, Hoskin PJ, Easton D, et al. Low dose single fraction radiotherapy in the treatment of metastatic bone pain. Radiother Oncol 1988;12:297.

11. Deacon J Peckham MJ, Steel GG. The radioresponsiveness of human tumors and the initial stage of the cell survival curve. Radiother Oncol 1984;2:317.

12. Salazar OM, Rubin P, Hendrickson FR, et al. Single-dose half-body irradiation for palliation of multiple bone metastases from solid tumors. Cancer 1986;58:29.

13. Aitasalo K. Effect of irradiation on early enzymatic changes in healing mandibular periosteum and bone. Acta Radiol Oncol 1986;25:207.

14. Hoskin PJ. Scientific and clinical aspects of radiotherapy in the relief of bone pain. Cancer Surv 1988;7:69.

15. Allen K, Johnson T, Hibbs G. Effective bone palliation as related to various treatment regimens. Cancer 1976;37:984.

16. Ambrad AJ. Single dose and short, high dose fractionation radiation therapy for osseous metastases. Int J Radiat Oncol Biol Phys 1978;4:207.

17. Benson R, Hasam S, Jones A, Schilse S. External beam radiotherapy for palliation of pain from metastatic carcinoma of the prostate. J Urol 1982;127:69.

18. Gilbert H, Kagam A, Nussbaum H, et al. Evaluation of radiation therapy for bone metastases: Pain relief and quality of life. Am J Roentgenol 1977;129:1095.

19. Hendrickson F, Shehata W, Kirchner A. Radiation therapy for osseous metastases. Int J Radiat Oncol Biol Phys 1976;1:275.

20. Horwich A. The Role of Radiotherapy in Locally Advanced and Metastatic Breast Cancer. In RC Coombes, TJ Powles, HT Ford, J-C Gazet (eds), Breast Cancer Management. London: Academic Press, 1981;227.

21. Jensen N-H, Roesdahl K. Single dose irradiation of bone metastases. Acta Radiol Ther Phys Biol 1976;15:337.

22. Kumar P, Bahrassa F, Espinosa M. The role of radiotherapy in management of metastatic bone disease. J Natl Med Assoc 1978;70:909.

23. LeBourgeois JP, Casset JM. Irradiation concentree des metastases osseuses. J Radiol Med 1978;58:737.

24. Martin WMC. Multiple daily fractions of radiation in the palliation of pain from bone metastases. Clin Radiol 1983;34:245.

25. Penn CRH. Single dose and fractionated palliative irradiation for osseous metastases. Clin Radiol 1976;27:405.

26. Qasim MM. Single dose palliative irradiation for bony metastasis. Strahlentherapie 1977;153:531.

27. Schocker JD, Brady LW. Radiation therapy for bone metastasis. Clin Orthop 1982;169:38.

28. Trodella L, Ansili-Cefaro G, Turrisiani A, et al. Pain in osseous metastases: Results of radiotherapy. Pain 1984;18:387.

29. Vargha Z, Blicksman A, Beland J. Single dose radiation therapy in the palliation of metastatic disease. Radiology 1969;93:1181.

30. Arcangeli G, Micheli A, Arcangeli G, et al. The responsiveness of bone metastases to radiotherapy: The effect of site, histology and radiation dose on pain relief. Radiother Oncol 1989;14:95.

31. Hoskin PJ, Price P, Easton D, et al. A prospective randomized trial of 4 Gy or 8 Gy single doses in the treatment of metastatic bone pain. Radiother Oncol 1992;23:74.

32. Madsen LE. Painful bone metastasis: efficacy of radiotherapy assessed by the patients: A randomized trial comparing 4 Gy × 6 versus 10 Gy × 2. Int J Radiat Oncol Biol Phys 1983;9:1775.

33. Okawa T, Kita M, Goto M, et al. Randomized prospective clinical study of small, large, and twice-a-day fraction radiotherapy for painful bone metastases. Radiother Oncol 1988;13:99.

34. Tong D, Gillick L, Hendrickson FR. The palliation of symptomatic osseous metastases: Final results of the study by the radiation therapy oncology group. Cancer 1982;50:893.

35. Blitzer PH. Reanalysis of the RTOG study of the palliation of symptomatic osseous metastasis. Cancer 1985;55:1468.

36. Price P, Hoskin PJ, Easton D, et al. Prospective randomized trial of single and multifraction radiotherapy schedules in the treatment of painful bony metastases. Radiother Oncol 1986;6:247.

37. Kagei K, Suzuki K, Shirato H, et al. A randomized trial of single and multifraction radiation therapy for bone metastasis: A preliminary report. Gan No Rinsho 1990;36:2553.

38. Kagan RA. Radiation Therapy in Palliative Cancer Management. In CA Perez, LW Brady (eds), Principles and Practice of Radiation Oncology (2nd ed). Philadelphia: Lippincott, 1992.

39. Reiden K, Kober B, Mende U, zum Winkel K. Strahlentherapie pathologischer frackturen und frakkurge fahrdeter skelettlasionen. Strahlenther Oncol 1986;162:742.

40. Peretz T, Nori D, Hilaris B, et al. Treatment of primary unresectable carcinoma of the pancreas with I-125 implantation. Int J Radiat Oncol Biol Phys 1989;17:931.

41. Syed AM, Puthawala AA, Neblett DL. Interstitial iodine-125 implant in the management of unresectable pancreatic carcinoma. Cancer 1983;52:808.

42. Dobelbower RR, Merrick HW, Ahuja RK, Skeel RT. 125I interstitial implant, precision high-dose external beam therapy, and 5-FU for unresectable adenocarcinoma of the pancreas and extrahepatic biliary tree. Cancer 1986;58:2185.

43. Mohiuddin M, Roasato F, Barbor D, et al. Long-term results of combined modality treatment with 1-125 implantation for carcinoma of the pancreas. Int J Radiat Oncol Biol Phys 1992;23:305.

44. Kawamura M, Katoaka M, Fujii T, et al. Electron beam intraoperative radiation therapy (EBIORT) for localized pancreatic carcinoma. Int J Radiat Oncol Biol Phys 1992;23:751.

45. Tepper JE, Noyes D, Krall JM, et al. Intraoperative radiation therapy of pancreatic carcinoma: a report of RTOG-8505. Int J Radiat Oncol Biol Phys 1991;21:1145.

46. Nishimura A, Nakano M, Otsu H, et al. Intraoperative radiotherapy for advanced carcinoma of the pancreas. 1984;54:2375.

47. Dobelbower RR, Howard JM, Bagne FR, et al. Treatment of cancer of the pancreas by precision high dose (PHD) external photon beam and intraoperative electron beam therapy (IOEBT). Int J Radiat Oncol Biol Phys 1989;16:205.

48. Dobelbower RR, Bronn DG. Radiotherapy in the treatment of pancreatic cancer. Ballieres Clin Gastroenterol 1990;4:969.

49. Heijmans HJ, Hoekstra HJ, Mehta DM. Is adjuvant intraoperative radiotherapy (IORT) for resectable and unresectable pancreatic carcinoma worthwhile? Hepatogastroenterology 1989;36:474.

50. Fitzpatrick PJ, Garrett PG. Metastatic breast cancer: Ovarian oblation with lower half-body irradiation. Int J Radiat Oncol Biol Phys 1981;7:1523.

51. Nag S, Shah V. Once-a-week lower hemibody irradiation (HBI) for metastatic cancers. Int J Radiat Oncol Biol Phys 1986;12:1003.

52. Wilkins MF, Keen CW. Hemi-body radiotherapy in the management of metastatic carcinoma. Clin Radiol 1987;38:267.

53. Hoskins PJ, Ford HT. Hemibody irradiation (HBI) for metastatic bone pain in two histologically distinct groups of patients. Clin Oncol 1989;1:67.

54. Huttner J, Wiener N, Quadt C, et al. A randomized clinical trial comparing systemic radiotherapy versus chemotherapy versus local radiotherapy in small cell lung cancer. Eur J Cancer Clin Oncol 1989;25:933.

55. Kuban DA, Schellhammer PF, El-Mahdi AM. Hemibody irradiation in advanced prostatic carcinoma. Urol Clin North Am 1991;18:131.

56. Lombardi F, Rottoli L, Gianni C, et al. Advanced neuroblastoma: Results of two treatment programs including sequential hemibody irradiation. Int J Radiat Oncol Biol Phys 1989;17:485.

57. Zelefsky MJ, Scher HI, Forman JD, et al. Palliative hemiskeletal irradiation for widespread metastatic prostate cancer: A comparison of single dose and fractionated regimens. Int J Radiat Oncol Biol Phys 1989;17:1281.

58. Poulter CA, Cosmatos D, Rubin P, et al. A report of RTOG 8206: A phase III study of whether the addition of single dose hemibody irradiation to standard fractionated local field irradiation is more effective than local field irradiation alone in the treatment of symptomatic osseous metastases. Int J Radiat Oncol Biol Phys 1992;23:207.

59. Salmon SE, Tesh D, Crowley J, et al. Chemotherapy is superior to sequential hemibody irradiation for remission consolidation in multiple myeloma: A Southwest Oncology Group study. J Clin Oncol 1990;8:1575.

60. Itami J, Ogata H, Miura K, et al. Hemibody irradiation in the treatment of generalized metastases. Gan No Rinsho 1987;33:1751.

61. Nseyo UO, Fontanesi J, Naftulin BN. Palliative hemibody irradiation in hormonally refractory metastatic prostate cancer. Urology 1989;34:76.

62. Thomas PJ, Daban A, Bontoux D. Double hemibody irradiation in chemotherapy-resistant multiple myeloma. Cancer Treat Rep 1984;68:1173.

63. Tobias JS, Richards JDM, Blackman GM, et al. Hemibody irradiation in multiple myeloma. Radiother Oncol 1985;3:11.

64. Reed RC, Lowery GS, Nordstrom DG. Single high dose-large field irradiation for palliation of advanced malignancies. Int J Radiat Oncol Biol Phys 1988;15:1243.

65. Reinhard EH, Moore CV, Bierbaum OS, et al. Radioactive phosphorus as a therapeutic agent. A review of the literature and analysis of the results of treatment of 155 patients with various blood diseases, lymphomas, and other malignant neoplastic diseases. J Lab Clin Med 1946;31:107.

66. Tong ECK, Rubenfeld S. The treatment of bone metastases with parathormone followed by radiophosphorus. Am J Roentgenol 1967;99:422.

67. Friedell HL, Storaasli JP. The use of radioactive phosphorus in the treatment of carcinoma of the breast with wide-spread metastases to the bone. Am J Roentgenol Rad Ther 1950;64:559.

68. Lawrence JH, Scott KG. Comparative metabolism of phosphorus in normal and lymphomatous animals. Proc Soc Exp Biol Med 1940;40:694.

69. Kenney J, Marinelli L, Woodard H. Tracer studies with radioactive phosphorus in malignant neoplastic disease. Radiology 1941;37:683.

70. Hertz S. The modifying effect of steroid hormone therapy of human neoplastic disease as judged by radioactive phosphorus (P-32) studies [abstract]. J Clin Invest 1950;29:821.

71. Maxfield JR, Maxfield JG, Maxfield WS. Use of phosphorus and testosterone in metastatic bone lesions from the breast and prostate. South Med J 1958;51:320.

72. Joshi DP, Seery WH, Goldberg LG, et al. Evaluation of phosphorus-32 for intractable pain secondary to prostatic carcinoma metastases. JAMA 1965;193:621.

73. Johnson DE, Haynie TP. Phosphorus-32 for intractable pain in carcinoma of prostate. Analysis of androgen priming, parathormone, rebound, and combination therapy. J Urol 1977;9:137.

74. Parsons RL, Campbell JL, Thomley MW. Experiences with P-32 in the treatment of metastatic carcinoma of the prostate: A follow-up report. J Urol 1962;88:812.

75. Silberstein EB. The treatment of painful osseous metastases with phosphorus-32-labeled phosphates. Semin Oncol 1993;20:10.

76. Aziz H, Choi K, Sohn C, et al. Comparison of P32 and SHBI for bony metastases. Am J Clin Oncol 1986;9:264.

77. Landaw SA. Acute leukemia in polycythemia vera. Semin Hematol 1986;23:156.

78. Blake GM, Gray JM, Zivanovic MA, et al. Strontium-89 radionuclide therapy: A dosimetric study using impulse response function analysis. Br J Radiol 1987;60:685.

79. Blake GM, Zivanovic MA, McEwan AJB, Ackery DM. Strontium-89 therapy: Strontium kinetics in disseminated carcinoma of the prostate. Eur J Nucl Med 1986;12:447.

80. Breen SL, Powe JE, Porter AT. Dose estimation in strontium-89 radiotherapy of metastatic prostate cancer. J Nucl Med 1992;33:1316.

81. Robinson RG. Radionuclides for the alleviation of bone pain in advanced malignancy. Clin Oncol 1986;5:39.

82. Laing AH, Ackery DM, Bayly RJ, et al. Strontium-89 chloride for pain palliation in prostatic skeletal malignancy. Br J Radiol 1991;64:816.

83. McEwan AJB, Porter AT, Venner PM, et al. An evaluation of the safety and efficacy of treatment with strontium-89 in patients who have previously received wide field radiotherapy. Antibody, Immunoconjugates, and Radiopharmaceuticals 1990;3:91.

84. Robinson RG. Systemic radioisotope therapy of primary and metastatic bone cancer. J Nucl Med 1990;31:1326.

85. Robinson RG, Blake GM, Preston DF, et al. Strontium-89: Treatment results and kinetics in patients with painful metastatic prostate and breast cancer in bone. Radiographics 1989;9:271.

86. Tennvall J, Darte L, Lundgren R, et al. Palliation of multiple bone metastases from prostatic carcinoma with strontium-89. Acta Oncol 1988;27:365.

87. Lewington VJ, McEwan AJ, Ackery DM, et al. A prospective, randomized double-blind crossover study to examine the efficacy of strontium-89 in pain palliation in patients with advanced prostate cancer metastatic to bone. Eur J Cancer 1991;27:954.

88. Porter AT, McEwan AJB, Powe JE, et al. Results of a randomized phase-III trial to evaluate the efficacy of strontium-89 adjuvant to local field external beam irradiation in the management of endocrine resistant metastatic prostate cancer. Int J Radiat Oncol Biol Phys 1993;25:805.

89. Bolger JJ, Dearnley DP, Kirk D, et al. Strontium-89 (Metastron) versus external beam radiotherapy in patients with painful bone metastases secondary to prostatic cancer: preliminary report of a multicenter trial. Semin Oncol 1993;20(Suppl. 2):32.

90. Robinson RG, Preston DF, Baxter KG, et al. Clinical experience with strontium-89 in prostatic and breast cancer patients. Semin Oncol 1993;20(Suppl. 2):44.

91. Ackery D, Yardley. Radionuclide-targeted therapy for the management of metastatic bone pain. Semin Oncol 1993;20(Suppl. 2):27.

92. Firusian N, Mellin P, Schmidt CG. Results of 89 strontium therapy in patients with carcinoma of the prostate and incurable pain from bone metastases: A preliminary report. J Urol 1976;116:764.

93. Turner JH, Claringbold PG, Heatherington EL, et al. A phase I study of samarium-153 ethylenediaminetetramethylene phosphonate therapy for disseminated skeletal metastases. J Clin Oncol 1989;7:1926.

94. Turner JH, Claringbold PG. A phase II study of treatment of painful multifocal skeletal metastases with single and repeated does samarium-153 ethylenediamine-tetramethylene phosphonate. Eur J Cancer 1991:27:1084.

95. Collins C, Eary J, Nemiroff C, et al. Phase I trial of samarium (Sm) 153-EDTMP in hormone refractory D2 prostate carcinoma [abstract]. Proc Am Soc. Clin Oncol 1990;9:134.

96. Maxon HR, Beutch EA, Thomas SR, et al. Re-186(Sn)DEDP for treatment of multiple metastatic foci in bone: biodistribution and dosimetric studies. Radiology 1988;166:510.

97. Maxon HR, Schroder LE, Hertzberg VS, et al. Rhenium-186(Sn)HEDP for treatment of painful osseous metastases: results of a double-blind crossover comparison with placebo. J Nucl Med 1991;32:1877.

98. Maxon HR, Thomas SR, Hertzberg VS, et al. Rhenium-186 hydroxyethylidene biphosphonate for the treatment of painful osseous metastases. Semin Nucl Med 1992;22:33.

99. Curley T, Scher H, Thaler HM, et al. Rhenium for palliation of painful bone metastases from prostatic cancer [abstract]. Proc Annu Meet Am Soc Clin Oncol 1991;10:A1231.

100. Eisenhut M, Berberich R, Kimming B, Oberhause E. I-131-labeled biphosphonates for palliative treatment of bone metastases: Preliminary clinical results with iodine-131 BDP3. J Nucl Med 1986:27:1255.

101. Brown AP, Greening WP, McCready VR, et al. Radioiodine treatment of metastatic thyroid carcinoma: The Royal Marsden Hospital experience. Br J Radiol 1984;57:323.

102. Mertens WC. Radionuclide therapy of bone metastases: Prospects for enhancement of therapeutic efficacy. Semin Oncol 1993;20(Suppl. 2):49.

103. Fleisch H. Bisphosphonates: Pharmacology and use in the treatment of tumor-induced hypercalcemic and metastatic bone disease. Drugs 1991;42:919.

104. Mertens WC, Porter AT, Reid RH, et al. Strontium-89 and low-dose infusion cisplatin for patients with hormone refractory prostate carcinoma metastatic to the bone: A progress report [abstract]. Nucl Med Commun 1992;13:212.

105. Denoix P. Treatment of Malignant Breast Tumors. Berlin: Springer, 1970.

106. Piotrowski W. Hyopihysenausschaltung mit Radioisotopen bei Fortgeschrittenen Krebserkrankungen. In F Linder, G Ott, H Rufolph (eds), Diagnostische un Therapeutische Fortschritte in der Krebschirurgie. Berlin: Springer, 1971;70.

107. Forrest APM, Stewart HJ. Technical Problems and Results of Yttrium Hypophysectomy. In M Dargent, C

Romieu (eds), Major Endocrine Surgery for the Treatment of Cancer of the Breast in Advanced Stages. Lyon: Simap, 1967;89.

108. Dahlin H, Larsson B, Leksell L, et al. Influence of absorbed doses and field size on the geometry of the radiation-surgical brain lesion. Acta Radiol Ther Phys Biol 1975;14:139.

109. Leksell L, Meyerson BA, Forster DMC. Radiosurgical thalamotomy for intractable pain. Confinia Neurologica (Basel) 1972;34:264.

Chapter 31
The Nurse's Role

Debra Wujcik and Susan Utley

Introduction

Cancer is a significant health problem in the United States and worldwide. In 1993, an estimated 1,170,000 people were diagnosed with cancer and 526,000 died from cancer in the United States.[1] Pain is a common problem associated with cancer. Based on an analysis of published reports, the World Health Organization (WHO) found that 70% of patients with advanced cancer experienced pain as a major symptom, and that 50% of persons undergoing cancer treatment experienced pain.[2] Sadly, the WHO estimated that 50–80% of patients did not have satisfactory relief of cancer pain.

It is recognized that control of cancer pain is often inadequate, despite the fact that most cancer pain can be effectively managed. All clinicians involved in the care of patients with cancer pain need to be familiar with the available standards, guidelines, and recommendations. The nurse is integral in coordinating and evaluating the plan of care for the patient experiencing chronic cancer pain. The nurse can assess the pain, administer appropriate medication (scheduled or as needed) using expert clinical judgment, and provide feedback to the health care team. To perform that function effectively, a thorough understanding of the physiology of pain, action of analgesics, and knowledge of nonpharmacologic methods for treating pain are required.

Agencies

World Health Organization

Several agencies and organizations have addressed the issue of cancer pain at international, national, state, and local levels (Table 31-1).[3] The WHO is an international agency, which has delineated effective pain management as a major priority of its cancer program.[2] In its 1986 publication "Cancer Pain Relief," the WHO described the nature and extent of the worldwide problem of cancer pain and detailed its recommendations for comprehensive cancer pain management. The WHO guidelines included pain assessment, therapeutic strategy, and continuing care as components of cancer pain management. Recommendations for education and legislative issues were also proposed.

Agency for Health Care Policy and Research

Efforts are being directed to the issue of cancer pain on the national level as well. The Agency for Health Care Policy and Research (AHCPR) is an agency of the Health and Human Services of the United States government whose purpose is to enhance quality, appropriateness, and effectiveness of health care services and to improve access to these services. An AHCPR panel has developed and recently released guidelines for cancer pain. This publication presents specific guidelines for the management of cancer pain, developed by a multidisciplinary panel of experts.

American Pain Society

The American Pain Society (APS) is a scientific organization of clinicians, health professionals, and basic scientists with interest and expertise in pain management. Because advances in pain management often appear in specialty journals, the APS developed a booklet to disseminate current information and advances in analgesic treatment to a broad audience.[4] This publication details principles in the management of acute pain and cancer pain that were developed by a consensus panel of clinical investigators and consultants. The booklet is brief and concise, and serves as a handy reference for use by clinicians.

The issue of inadequately relieved pain has also prompted organizations to direct attention to quality assurance as it relates to pain management. The APS has published quality assurance standards that were developed with input from the Joint Commission for the Accreditation of Health Organizations (JCAHO).[5] These standards outlined five critical areas for quality assurance monitoring and evaluation relevant to pain management, including process and outcome standards. Recently, the JCAHO standards included a section on patients' rights in their standards, which emphasized effective pain and symptom management for the dying patient.[6] Because of the new JCAHO requirements, health care organizations are compelled to develop quality assurance programs focusing on the issue of pain management. The APS standards may provide a useful framework for the development of such programs.

Oncology Nursing Society

Professional organizations have also addressed the problem of cancer pain. In 1990, the Oncology Nursing Society (ONS) issued a position statement on cancer pain.[7] This paper pointed out that control of cancer pain overall is inadequate and emphasized the right of the patient to adequate pain control by having pain recognized and treated as a priority. The paper also described the role of the nurse in pain management as pivotal and stated that nurses should assume a leadership role in the area of pain management.

American Society of Clinical Oncologists

Recently, the American Society of Clinical Oncologists (ASCO) issued a formal statement on cancer pain.[8] This paper acknowledged the right of patients to adequate pain control and recommended including pain management in education of oncologists and oncology fellows. A curriculum was outlined emphasizing (1) assessment, (2) proficiency in prescribing opioids, nonopioids, and adjuvant analgesic medications, and (3) potential benefits of a variety of treatment approaches including a coordinated multidisciplinary approach.

State Pain Initiatives

The past several years have witnessed a trend toward the development of multidisciplinary organizations that address the problem of cancer pain at the state level. In 1985, the Wisconsin Cancer Pain Initiative was the first such organization. Since then, similar groups have been formed in other states, and, as of May 1996, 46 states have organized state cancer pain initiatives.[9] In addition, a resource center has recently been established in Wisconsin to serve as a clearinghouse of information for state cancer pain initiatives.

Documents described in the preceding discussion represent considerable work by recognized experts in the area of cancer pain and respected agencies and organizations. Despite the compelling evidence that cancer pain control is inadequate, most cancer-related pain can be easily managed. These principles, guidelines, and position papers provide clinicians with considerable information on which to formulate clinical decision-making procedures for optimal control of cancer pain. In all of the information reviewed, the concept of a multidisciplinary or team approach to care in the effective management of cancer pain is widely supported. The following discussion will highlight the team concept.

Table 31-1. Major Agencies and Organizations Involved with Cancer Pain

Abbreviation	Name	Description	Resources
AHCPR	Agency for Health Care Policy and Research	Multidisciplinary federal agency, committee by invitation	Clinical guidelines for acute and postoperative pain; guidelines for cancer pain
APS	American Pain Society	Multidisciplinary organization	Quality assurance standards; principles of analgesic use in the treatment of acute pain and cancer pain; APS Bulletin, APS Journal
ASCO	American Society of Clinical Oncology	Predominantly medical and radiation oncologists	Cancer pain assessment and treatment guidelines; Journal of Clinical Oncology
IASP	International Association for the Study of Pain	Multidisciplinary organization	Educational curriculum; taxonomy of pain syndromes
NCI	National Cancer Institute	Multidisciplinary federal agency	Funding for pain research
NIH	National Institutes of Health	Multidisciplinary federal agency	Consensus statement for integrated management of pain funding for pain research
NCNR	National Center for Nursing Research	Federal agency	Priority expert panel state-of-the-science document; funding for pain research
ONS	Oncology Nursing Society	Oncology nurses	Position paper on cancer pain; pain special interest group; Oncology Nursing Forum
WHO	World Health Organization	International agency	Multiple publications, e.g., Cancer Pain Relief and Palliative Care

Source: Reprinted with permission from DB McGuire, VR Sheidler. Pain. In SL Groenwald, MH Frogge, M Goodman, CH Yarbro (eds), Cancer Nursing: Principles and Practice (3rd ed). Boston: Jones & Bartlett, 1993;499.

Team Approach

Rationale

Cancer pain has been described as a multidimensional phenomenon consisting of sensory, affective, cognitive, and behavioral components.[10] The complex nature of cancer pain and the inadequacy of cancer pain relief have made multimodal treatment employing the skills of multiple professionals an attractive approach to cancer pain management. There is considerable support in the literature for a multidisciplinary, collaborative team approach to the management of pain.[2, 7, 11–16] In 1986, the National Institutes of Health (NIH) issued a consensus statement on the management of pain.[11] The NIH concluded that, although no single model is universally accepted, an integrated approach is indicated, and emphasized the importance of joint effort and communication among team members.

Team Members

The WHO stated that "teamwork is crucial for optimal care."[2] The team may be formal or informal. The composition and function of the team may vary, depending on the needs of the patient and the health care setting. Several authors advocated a patient-centered team.[2, 13, 15] In addition to the patient and family, other team members often include physicians, nurses, social workers, and clergy. The lines between role functions of team members are indistinct, and often overlap, which is appropriate within the context of the multidisciplinary team concept.[16] Table 31-2 summarizes the roles of various team members in cancer pain management.

Table 31-2. Roles of Health Team Members in the Care of Persons Experiencing Cancer-Related Pain

Patient/Family	Physician	Nurse	Social Worker	Clergy
Report pain Participate in plan of care Participate in pain relief methods (when appropriate)	Assess pain Diagnose and treat underlying cause (if appropriate) Order analgesic therapy Communicate treatment goals, plan, and progress with other team members Evaluate pain relief and modify analgesic therapy as necessary	Assess pain Carry out pain relief methods Use nonpharmacologic pain relief methods Teach patient/family about pain and pain relief methods Facilitate communication among patient, family, and other health team members Evaluate response to pain relief methods and identify need for and obtain modification	Assess impact of pain on patient/family system Provide psychosocial support Mobilize community resources for patient/family Facilitate continuity of care as patient moves among health care settings	Assess impact of pain on psychosocial and spiritual well-being Provide psychosocial support Address spiritual issues related to pain, life-threatening illness, and dying

Source: Adapted from World Health Organization. Cancer Pain Relief. Geneva: World Health Organization, 1986; and M McCaffery, A Beebe. Pain: Clinical Manual for Nursing Practice. St. Louis: Mosby, 1989.

Other professionals may make valuable contributions as members of the pain management team. Pharmacists have been advocated as invaluable team members because they provide expertise related to pharmacologic methods of analgesia.[17] Because of the anxiety and depression often associated with chronic pain, psychologists and other therapists may also serve as active members or as consultants to the team.

Although there is variation among the pain management teams described in the literature, several common themes emerge. In one report, six models for delivery of pain management services were examined, with the purpose of identifying these themes.[18] Three common elements for successful programs were identified: (1) team effort and coordination, (2) provision of education, and (3) accountability and administrative support. As health care providers strive to organize and improve services delivered to cancer pain patients, the team approach with these elements should be firmly anchored in pain management programs.

Role of the Nurse

The nurse has a substantial role in cancer pain management, especially by virtue of frequent interaction with the patient.[6, 16] In addition, an advanced practice nurse (one who is prepared at the masters' or doctoral level) can further enhance the effectiveness of the health care team. By identifying barriers and developing strategies for effective pain management, the nurse can not only improve pain relief at the individual patient level, but also have a broader impact at the unit or institutional level.[19]

Physiology of Cancer Pain

Types of Cancer Pain

There is nothing inherent in malignant cells that causes pain. Cancer pain is generally related to direct tumor infiltration (70–80%) or treatment (20%).[20] Tumor-related pain is frequently due to bone, nerve, or hollow viscus infiltration. Surgery, chemotherapy, radiation, and some diagnostic tests can induce treatment-related pain.[3] Incisional, phantom, and lymphedema pain are associated with surgery.[21] Chemotherapy may produce painful neuropathies, mucositis, and gastrointestinal or hematologic side effects. Radiation causes fibrosis, neuropathies, and skin reactions.

In addition, several types of pain have been described.[22] Somatic pain can be superficial or deep and is described as constant and aching and is usually well localized. Visceral pain is also a continual aching, but tends to be poorly localized. The pain may be referred to the skin. Neuropathic pain is both central and peripheral, with shooting, stabbing, and burning pain components.

The ability to effectively treat pain is based on understanding the different pain mechanisms in the body and the process of transduction, transmission, modulation, and perception in the central nervous system. In 1644, Descartes published the *Specificity Theory of Pain*. He asserted that body damage sends direct messages to the brain causing emission signals and the subsequent occurrence of responses. We now know that the process is more complex. A brief review of physiology of pain transmission and the sites of action of common drugs used in the management of chronic pain follows.

Chronic and Acute Pain

The objective signs of acute pain (grimacing, tachycardia, hypertension, diaphoresis, mydriasis, pallor) indicate an autonomic nervous system response. Patients with chronic pain that lasts longer than several months do not usually demonstrate these signs and symptoms.[22] Patients experiencing chronic cancer pain must often prove they are in pain to the health care provider. Chronic pain may be accompanied by changes in lifestyle, personality, functional abilities, and signs and symptoms of depression (hopelessness, helplessness, loss of libido and weight, sleep disturbances).

Pain Processes

Four processes must occur simultaneously to produce pain: transduction, transmission, modulation, and perception.[8, 23] The relay of the pain message begins with pain receptors or nerve endings found on skin surfaces. When the nerves are stimulated by mechanical, thermal, or chemical stimuli, biochemical transmitters are released. These include potassium, substance P, bradykinin, prostaglandin, and others. Of these, prostaglandin is significant. The pain message can be interrupted here by nonsteroidal anti-inflammatory drugs (NSAIDs), which block the formation of prostaglandin.[23]

Transduction

Transduction occurs when receptors are stimulated, biochemical transmitters are released, and the primary afferent fibers become depolarized. Calcium channels are opened, allowing the sodium to flow into the cell and the potassium to flow outward. This creates an action potential along the neuron and transmission of the impulse from the peripheral nerves to the dorsal horn of the spinal cord. Calcium channel blockers and other membrane stabilizers (anesthetics and anticonvulsants) can inhibit this process. Neuropathic pain, described as tingling, burning, or shooting is relieved by these agents.[24]

Transmission

When the pain impulse terminates in the dorsal horn of the spinal cord, substance P and other neurotransmitters such as somatostatin and vasoactive intestinal peptide are released. Substance P binds to receptors on other neurons, continuing the transmission of the pain message.

Modulation

The dorsal horn contains significant opiate receptors. The pain impulse is interrupted when opiates are administered or the body's own endorphins are released and bound to receptors, inhibiting the release of substance P. This is also the site of action of intraspinally administered opiates.[23]

Next, the impulse is transmitted via the spinothalamic tract to the thalamus and midbrain. From the thalamus, areas of the brain such as the parietal lobe (somatosensory and association cortices), frontal lobe, and the limbic system are stimulated.[23, 25] Pain is perceived once the transmission

Table 31-3. Assessment of History of Cancer Pain

Characteristic	Question
Location	Where is the pain?
	Can you point to the location of the pain?
	Does the pain move or remain in one place?
Onset	When did the pain begin?
Frequency	How often do you experience pain?
Duration	How long does the pain last?
	Is the pain intermittent or constant?
Quality	Can you describe the pain?
	Is it stabbing, burning, aching, throbbing, or piercing?
Precipitating factors	What starts the pain?
	Is the pain affected by movement, position, or certain activities?
Alleviating factors	What relieves the pain?
	Does medication, positioning, immobility, or massage relieve the level of pain?
	How has the pain affected your ability to eat, sleep, or participate in activities?

of the impulse terminates within these regions. If the midbrain is stimulated, certain descending projections send a modulatory impulse to the dorsal horn. Serotonin and norepinephrine may be released, blocking the impulses in the dorsal horn. Tricyclic antidepressants work at that level by decreasing neuronal reuptake of serotonin. This allows more free serotonin to be available and painful impulses are blocked.[26]

Perception

The perception of pain is more elusive. The perception is modified by past experience and meaning of the pain. These meanings are discussed further under assessment.

Assessment

History

A complete assessment of the cancer pain patient includes the history, cultural influences, and psychological factors. The history provides a full description of the experience of pain (Table 31-3).[8, 22, 27] However, there are times when the patient presents in acute, uncontrolled pain where a modification of the full assessment is more appropriate.[28]

Cultural Assessment

Cultural influences include age, sex, religious beliefs, location of pain, and the patient's view of the health care team.[29] For example, it is usually acceptable for children to cry when in pain, whereas adults are expected to be more stoic. Patients older than 55 years reported less intensity of pain.[30] Similarly, tears are more acceptable from women than from men. Depending on the religious beliefs and experience, a person's religion may be a source of comfort or distress. Some view the cancer and subsequent pain as punishment for sin. Pain in certain body parts, such as breasts or genitals, may be more embarrassing for the patient to discuss and, therefore, complaints may be minimal.

Psychological Factors

Psychological factors can also aggravate the experience of pain. Other concurrent or recent losses or traumatic life experiences can worsen pain. A patient can sometimes experience secondary gains of attention, affection, comfort, and physical contact with loved ones when the pain is severe or uncontrolled. The presence of pain may be a mechanism for the patient to maintain contact or a relationship with the team. If the patient's role within his or her

Table 31-4. World Health Organization and American Pain Society Guidelines for Managing Chronic Cancer Pain

World Health Organization Step	Type of Pain	Type of Analgesic	Specific Drug
1	Mild	Nonopioid ± adjuvant	Acetaminophen, ibuprofen
2	Mild to moderate	Opioid ± nonopioid ± adjuvant	Codeine, oxycodone
3	Moderate to severe	Opioid ± nonopioid ± adjuvant	Morphine, hydromorphone

family has been manipulative, it is difficult for the health care team to change that life-long behavior. The team should not reinforce the noneffective behavior. Likewise, the patient should be referred to a psychologist or psychiatrist if necessary.[21]

A previously good experience with pain control such as the use of breathing techniques during childbirth can convince the patient that the pain can be successfully controlled. The knowledge or understanding by the patient about the causes and meaning of the pain should be explored. Although a patient in pain is unlikely to welcome education about pain management strategies, it is important to determine the patient's understanding and beliefs in order to dispel misinformation. A patient who feels powerless and out of control is less likely to respond to pain control measures. Cancer and pain, can cause the patient to fear loss of life, financial status, family love and respect, a job, and the integrity of his or her body.

Obstacles to Pain Assessment

There are numerous obstacles to a proper assessment of the cancer patient in pain. The patient experiencing chronic pain usually does not appear to be in pain. Team members are encouraged to accept the patient's self-report of pain as the most reliable indicator of this symptom. Pain assessment is subjective. The use of pain scales (visual or verbal rating scales) encourage communication of the presence and severity of pain.[16] This documentation can facilitate communication between patient and the health care team. In addition, denial of pain by the patient may occur to avoid upsetting the physician or family. Again, the nurse is in an important position to explore this area with the patient and dispel fears of abandonment.

McCaffery[31] identified several other barriers that may hinder effective pain management:

1. Lack of education about pain control
2. Hindrances to appropriate pain assessment
3. Inappropriate use of pain-rating scales
4. Fears of opioid addiction
5. Reluctant upward titration of opioid doses

McCaffery advocated using the WHO guidelines and APS principles to counter these obstacles.[2, 5] These methods satisfactorily relieved pain in at least 75% of the patients. Furthermore, use of pain assessment flow sheets, pain-rating scales, equianalgesic charts, and education of physicians and nurses are strategies to overcome barriers to use of current available information about pain control.

Drug Therapy

Nonopioid Medications

The WHO and APS provide clear guidelines for managing chronic cancer pain using a three-step method (Table 31-4).[2, 4] Nonnarcotic analgesics are recommended to treat mild-to-moderate pain. Included in this class are over-the-counter preparations such as aspirin, acetaminophen, and ibuprophen. Prescription NSAIDs include naproxen and indomethacin. The nonnarcotic analgesics work at the peripheral nervous system level and do not produce tolerance or physical or psychological dependence. Along with antipyretic action, they inhibit cyclooxygenase, an enzyme that is necessary for formation of prostaglandin E_2. In general, however, they have a limited effect for increasing analgesia, and long-term use is limited by gastrointestinal and hematologic effects.

Aspirin provides satisfactory analgesia but causes gastrointestinal toxicity including vomiting, hematemesis, and some hypersensitivity reactions. Acetaminophen has no anti-inflammatory or antiplatelet effects. NSAIDs inhibit platelet aggregation by reversibly inhibiting prostaglandin synthetase. Although NSAIDs are particularly useful for bone metastases,[4, 22] they produce gastrointestinal side effects (dyspepsia, nausea, vomiting, ulcerations, bleeding, or perforation), renal insufficiency, and occasional central nervous system side effects.

Opioids

Narcotic analgesics, including agonists and antagonists, are recommended for moderate-to-severe pain. Agonists work by binding to opioid receptors at the central nervous system level.[22] Included in this category are morphine, hydromorphone, oxymorphone, and meperidine. The milder narcotics, codeine, hydrocodone, and oxycodone, have a short duration of action and lack flexibility in dosing schedules. Inadequacy in controlling severe chronic pain limits usefulness beyond mild-to-moderate pain.[21]

Morphine sulfate is the prototype opioid by which all analgesics are measured. It is especially useful in controlling cancer pain because it is available for administration in most routes, with a wide dosage range. The usual route is oral but other routes are used as indicated.[32, 33]

Rectal morphine is equivalent to oral morphine with available strengths from 5–30 mg. Analgesia lasts from 4–6 hours. Another common practice is the rectal administration of sustained-release oral tablets. Some data demonstrate slower absorption; however, the same total dose is absorbed.[21] This may be useful for patients who have been maintained on oral morphine sulfate until the terminal phase of care.

Hydromorphone, another opioid agonist, is available for oral, parenteral, and rectal administration. However, it has no particular advantage over morphine and there are no sustained-release preparations.[21]

Fentanyl is a short acting, synthetic opioid that is 80 times more potent than morphine. It is available as a transdermal patch that is replaced every 72 hours.[34] It is recommended for patients once a steady dose is established. It is important to note that the fentanyl continues to be absorbed from the skin for up to 17 hours after removal. If the patch is removed due to oversedation, the patient should be observed for hypotension or respiratory depression for up to 24 hours following removal.

Meperidine is contraindicated in chronic pain management.[35, 36] Although it is effective for short-term acute pain, it has no advantages for chronic pain management. Meperidine has a short half-life, thus making frequent dosing necessary. The accumulation of a toxic metabolite, 17-normeperidine, causes central nervous system excitability.

Narcotic agonists-antagonists have properties of narcotic analgesics but also may precipitate withdrawal in narcotic-dependent patients. Butorphanol, nalbuphine, and pentazocine are mixed agonist-antagonist opiates, but they are not recommended for routine cancer pain management.[16]

Administration

Route

The oral route is ideal for the typical cancer pain patient, providing consistent analgesia and peak effect at 1.5–2.0 hours.[2] If given as an intravenous bolus, onset of action peaks in 15–30 minutes. The patient frequently experiences recurrence of pain when this method is used. For stable chronic pain, it is preferable to use the oral route. A subcutaneous route is used if patients are unable to take oral medications.

Intravenous infusion produces steady blood levels to rapidly titrate relief in acute pain or an acute exacerbation of chronic pain. If using a continuous intravenous infusion, the effects of increasing the rate will usually not be felt for up to 12 hours. Therefore, an as needed intravenous bolus in an amount equivalent to 1 hour of drug infusion is recommended.

When converting from intramuscular or oral morphine to a continuous intravenous infusion, the starting dose is equivalent to a 24-hour dose.[2, 37] Clinical experience shows that the 24-hour intravenous dose is approximately the same as the intramuscular dose. However, research is inconclusive in this area and some clinicians recommend starting with one-half the intramuscular dose.[38]

When using other narcotics to manage cancer pain, an equianalgesic dosage is required (Table 31-5). When converting from oral to intravenous forms or switching from one medication to another, the

Table 31-5. Equianalgesic Table

Medication	IM Dose (mg)	PO/IM Potency	Usual Starting Dose (mg)
Morphine	10	3	30–60
Hydromorphone	1.5	5	4–8
Oxymorphone	10 (suppository)		
Meperidine	75	4	Not recommended

equianalgesic table will provide the conversion factor for a comparable dosage.

The rectal route is an alternative if the oral route is not possible due to nausea and vomiting, obstruction, or disorientation. Suppositories of sustained-release morphine can be administered through a colostomy stoma,[39] while the vaginal route for suppositories is useful. Oxymorphone suppositories (two 5-mg suppositories) are equivalent to morphine, 30 mg orally or 10 mg intramuscularly.[40]

Titration

Titration of drugs to effect is recommended. Satisfactory pain relief with manageable side effects is the desired goal. Some believe erroneously that increasing the dose contributes to development of tolerance. Studies show that advancing disease causes a need for increased analgesia.[41] There is no maximum dose of narcotics used to treat cancer pain. Increased dosages do not usually cause lethal respiratory depression because tolerance develops rapidly.

The initial calculation of the analgesic dosage is an educated guess based on established recommendations. The calculated dose is administered and the response to the analgesic is carefully assessed. The dose, time interval, route, and drug are adjusted accordingly.[39] The nurse is the health care team member who spends the most time with the patient and assesses response to changes in the analgesic regime. The nurse is in the ideal position to titrate medications and manage side effects. In general, nurses have a great deal of experience in this area and this experience should be used.[41] The use of a standardized pain assessment form is recommended. This form contains space for the medication dose and timing and the patient's response to the intervention.

In general, an adequate trial of the analgesic must be given, which may necessitate increasing the dose until the appearance of limiting side effects and then switching to another analgesic. Around-the-clock administration is established only after the optimal dose is determined.

Addiction

Nurses and physicians continue to fear contributing to addiction in patients despite strong evidence that addiction is not usually an issue for patients with cancer pain.[42] Opioid addiction is a behavioral pattern distinguished by the urge to use the drug for effects other than pain relief.[22] Many people have extensively reviewed the literature and concluded that addiction in cancer patients using opioids for cancer pain management is rare. It is well established that undermedication is more likely to lead to psychological dependence than to effective pain control.[21, 22, 33]

Tolerance and physical dependence are physiologic phenomena that occur separately from addiction.[2, 40, 43] Fewer than 0.1% of patients with cancer develop addiction after using opioids. As a result, use of opioids for cancer pain management is appropriate. The failure to prescribe or administer narcotics due to fear of contributing to addiction is called opiophobia.[44]

Tolerance

Tolerance is the state in which escalating dosages are required to maintain the desired analgesic effect.[22] If the patient becomes tolerant, switching to another narcotic can provide relief since cross-tolerance is not complete. The recommendation is to administer one-half the equianalgesic dose.[16, 28] In addition, nonnarcotics, neurosurgical, and anesthetic approaches may be considered in unresponsive patients.

Table 31-6. Etiology Interventions for Common Side Effects of Opioid Analgesia

Side Effect	Etiology	Interventions
Constipation	Opioids bind to receptors in smooth muscle	Stool softener with stimulant; osmotic laxative. Goal is bowel motility every 2–3 days; increase fluids to 2,000 ml; institute foods and fluids that support regular elimination
Nausea/vomiting	Stimulation of chemoreceptor trigger zone; inhibition of gastrointestinal motility; stimulation of vestibular nerve	Antiemetics (phenothiazines). Add dimenhydrinate if motion sickness. Add metoclopramide
Sedation	CNS depression	Stepwise reduction of dose or add stimulant. Assess sedation versus exhaustion; assess other etiology for sedation
Respiratory depression	Opioids bind to receptors in CNS	Physical stimulation. Administer diluted naloxone if respiration <8/min and unable to arouse

Physical Dependence

Physical dependence is defined as the onset of severe symptoms of withdrawal if the narcotic is discontinued.[22] Physical dependence may develop after several days of continued narcotic use. Physical dependence is not synonymous with addiction. Appropriate weaning of narcotics will diminish the uncomfortable effects of drug withdrawal. In general, the dosage can be reduced by 20% daily.

Management of Side Effects

Side effects are expected from opioid use. However, the clinician should devise a plan to prevent them. The patient should not need to choose between pain control and constipation or nausea. Table 31-6 describes the etiology and appropriate interventions to prevent expected side effects of opioids.[8, 45] Respiratory depression rarely occurs in patients receiving chronic opioid therapy. If respirations decrease to less than eight breaths per minute and the patient cannot be aroused, intravenous naloxone may be administered slowly. The addition of 0.4 mg naloxone to 10 ml normal saline, administered 0.5–1.0 ml every 2 minutes until the patient begins to arouse, will reverse respiratory depression without precipitating acute withdrawal symptoms.

Nonpharmacologic Pain Control

Many nonpharmacologic methods are used to support pain control either with or without opioid interventions.[8, 16, 46] Relaxation procedures reduce muscular tension, autonomic hyperarousal, and anxious and angry feelings. Hypnosis may enhance relaxation and help reinterpret noxious stimuli. Hypnosis is useful for short painful periods, but not chronic pain relief.

The physical therapist can recommend numerous methods to decrease pain such as heat, cold, electrical stimulation, massage, trigger point therapy, traction, mobilization, exercise, and ice massage. The patient is encouraged to use a variety of measures to control the pain. Due to multiple variables contributing to the pain response, many strategies may be incorporated to control the pain response. The nurse is in a position to constantly reassess the pain and the response to pain. The nurse provides a link between the patient, family, and physician, and makes appropriate referrals.

Issues

Legislative

Drug control regulations that were originally instated to reduce narcotic abuse and related illegal activities may have a deleterious effect on legitimate uses of opioids for pain relief.[2, 47] The "Just Say No to Drugs" campaign may foster within patients an attitude incongruent with achieving relief from pain. Collaboration among health care providers, drug regulators, and lawmakers, in state cancer pain initiatives, for example, is an essential way to promote a sociolegal environment that is conducive to the legitimate use of opioids to relieve cancer pain.

High-Tech Methods

The last decade has seen a substantial increase in technology in the treatment of pain as well as in the treatment of cancer. In 1991, Whedon and Ferrell, within an ethical framework, explored issues related to the use of high-tech methods of pain management.[48] These include subcutaneous, intravenous, and intraspinal routes of analgesia, and the use of ambulatory, implanted, or patient-controlled analgesia pumps. The authors purported that further study of the indications and outcomes of high-tech methods is urgent because the inappropriate application of such therapies may lead to increased cost, continued discomfort, or morbidity from invasive methods and associated side effects. As pain control has become a priority, it has also become a growing business. The authors suggested that ownership by health care organizations or professionals in these businesses may create a conflict of interest. Furthermore, they pointed out that the current system for reimbursement is often inconsistent with the needs of the patient. High-tech analgesia may be reimbursable, whereas less expensive oral analgesia is not often covered on an outpatient basis, thus giving the impression that oral analgesia is inferior and is therefore undesirable. These issues warrant a closer look, particularly within the context of clinical research comparing efficacy and cost outcomes of various methods.

Economic Considerations

In addition to quality, cost is a consideration of ever-increasing importance in the changing health care environment. Inadequate pain management may necessitate hospitalization and may extend the length of hospital stay. A study at a cancer center indicated that unrelieved pain at home resulted in 12% of hospital admissions, with an estimated cost of $5.1 million for 1 year.[49]

Although costs of pain control methods have not been reported extensively in the literature, some cost information is available to help make quality- and cost-conscious clinical decisions. It is widely recognized that oral analgesia is efficacious in most cases and is a cost-effective method of pain control. When the oral route is not feasible, administration of sustained-release morphine by the rectal route has been found to be safe and effective.[50] The transdermal route is another alternative to parenteral analgesia. The use of subcutaneous infusions for pain and other cancer symptoms is a safe and cost-effective alternative to therapies administered by intravenous and intramuscular routes.[51] In further support of the subcutaneous rote, one author reported that the cost to a hospice of maintaining subcutaneous analgesia was $100 per week, in contrast to a weekly cost of at least $450 for intravenous analgesia.[52]

Future

The effective relief of cancer pain must remain a health care priority. The following are recommendations for the future:

1. Efforts to improve the education of health care providers regarding pain management, especially physicians and nurses, should be begun. Clinicians with expertise in the area of pain should help educate their colleagues and help disseminate current information regarding pain management.

2. Cancer pain programs should integrate a multidisciplinary team approach (whether formal or informal) that incorporates current recommendations and guidelines for pain management. Quality assurance programs should monitor pain control outcomes.

3. Future research studies are needed to look at outcomes of analgesic methods that include combinations of nonpharmacologic and pharmacologic interventions. Cost effectiveness and quality of life should be addressed in these outcome studies. Collaborative research efforts among physicians, nurses, psychologists, pharmacists, and other researchers are indicated, given the complexity of cancer pain.

4. Clinicians alone cannot bear the burden of pain relief. Administrators, third-party payers, and lawmakers must also support efforts to promote quality and cost-effective care for persons experiencing cancer pain.

Conclusion

It is incumbent on all clinicians caring for persons with cancer pain to be knowledgeable and skilled in the area of pain management and to be accountable for adequate pain control. Pain management is not the sole responsibility of the physician, but must be a responsibility shared by all involved team members. Effective communication and collaboration across boundaries between the various health care disciplines will not only enhance cancer pain management in the 1990s, but will position health care providers to meet the challenges of the twenty-first century.

References

1. American Cancer Society. Cancer Facts & Figures, Atlanta: ACS, 1993;1.
2. World Health Organization. Cancer Pain Relief. Geneva: World Health Organization, 1986.
3. McGuire DB, Sheidler VR. Pain. In SL Groenwald, MH Frogge, M Goodman, CH Yarbro (eds), Cancer Nursing Principles and Practice (3rd ed). Boston: Jones & Bartlett Publishers, 1993;499.
4. American Pain Society. Principles of Analgesic Use in the Treatment of Acute Pain and Cancer Pain (3rd ed). Skokie, IL: American Pain Society, 1993.
5. American Pain Society Subcommittee on Quality Assurance Standards. Standards for monitoring quality of analgesic treatment of acute pain and cancer pain. Oncol Nurs Forum 1990;6:952.
6. Joint Commission for the Accreditation of Health Organizations. Accreditation Manual for Hospitals. Oakbrook Terrace, IL: JCAHO, 1992.
7. Spross JA, McGuire DB, Schmitt R. Oncology Nursing Society position paper on cancer pain. Oncol Nurs Forum 1990;17:595, 751, 825, 944.
8. Ad Hoc Committee on Cancer Pain of the American Society of Clinical Oncologists. Cancer pain assessment and treatment curriculum guidelines. J Clin Oncol 1992;10:1976.
9. Wineke J. Wisconsin Cancer Pain Initiative. Personal communication, May 1996.
10. Ahles TA, Blanchard EB, Ruckdeschel JC. The multidimensional nature of cancer-related pain. Pain 1983;17:277.
11. National Institutes of Health Consensus Development Conference Statement. The Integrated Approach to the Management of Pain. 1986;6(3):1.
12. Acute Pain Management Guideline Panel. Acute Pain Management: Operative or Medical Procedures and Trauma. Clinical Practice Guideline. AHCPR Publication No. 92-0032. Rockville, MD: Agency for Care Policy and Research, Public Health Service, US Department of Health and Human Service, 1992.
13. Ventafridda V, Selmi S, Di Mola G, et al. A new model of continuing care for advanced cancer pain treatment. Hospice J 1987;3:85.
14. Walsh D. Continuing care in a medical center: The Cleveland Clinic Foundation Palliative Care Service. J Pain Symptom Manage 1990;5:273.
15. Coyle N. A model of continuity of care for cancer patients with chronic pain. Med Clin North Am 1987;71:259.
16. McCaffery M, Beebe A. Pain: Clinical Manual for Nursing Practice. St. Louis: Mosby, 1989.
17. Ferrell BR, Wenzl C, Wisdom C. Evolution and evaluation of a pain management team. Oncol Nurs Forum 1988;15:285.
18. Williams A, Kedziera P, Osterlund H, et al. Models of health care delivery in cancer pain management. Oncol Nurs Forum 1992;19(Suppl.):20.
19. Whedon M, Shedd P, Summers B. The role of the advanced practice oncology nurse in pain relief. Oncol Nurs Forum 1992;19(Suppl.):12.
20. Foley KM. Pain Syndromes in Patients with Cancer. In JJ Bonica, V Ventafridda (eds), Advances in Pain Research and Therapy (Vol. 2). New York: Raven, 1979:59.
21. Ogle KS, Warren W, Plumb JD. Pain management in advanced cancer. Primary Care 1992;19:793.
22. Foley KM. The treatment of cancer pain. N Engl J Med 1985;313:84.
23. Paice JA. Unraveling the mystery of pain. Oncol Nurs Forum 1991;8:843.
24. Maciewicz R, Bouckoms A, Marin JB. Drug therapy for neuropathic pain. Clin J Pain 1985;1:39.
25. Sundaresan N, DeGiacinto GV. Antitumor and antinociceptive approaches to control cancer pain. Med Clin North Am 1987;71:329.
26. Walsh TD. Antidepressants in chronic pain. Clin Neuropharmacol 1983;6:271.
27. Levy MH. Pain management in advanced cancer. Semin Oncol 1985;12:394.
28. Coyle N, Folwy KM. Alterations in Comfort: Pain. In B Baire, R McCorkle, M Grant (eds), Cancer Nursing: A Comprehensive Textbook. Philadelphia: Saunders, 1991;782.
29. Bohnet NL. Assessment of Pain. In MO Amenta, NL Bohnet (eds), Nursing Care of the Terminally Ill. Boston: Little, Brown, 1986;81.
30. McMillan S. The relationship between age and intensity of cancer-related symptoms. Oncol Nurs Forum 1989;16:237.
31. McCaffery M. Pain control: Barriers to the use of available information. Cancer 1992;70:1438.
32. Goodman L, Gilman A. The Pharmacological Basis of Therapeutics. New York: Pergamon, 1990.
33. Walsh TD. Prevention of opioid side effects. J Pain Symptom Manage 1990; 5:362.
34. Miaskowski C. New approaches to cancer pain management. Curr Issues Cancer Nurs Pract 1992, 1:1.
35. Kaiko RF, Foley KM, Grabinsky PY, et al. CNS excitatory effects of meperidine in cancer patients. Ann Neurol 1983;13:180.

36. McCaffery M. Giving meperidine for pain—Should it be so mechanical? Nursing 1987;17:61.

37. Foley KM. The practical use of narcotic analgesics. Med Clin North Am 1982;6:1091.

38. McCaffery M, Beebe A. Giving narcotics for pain. Nursing 1989;19:161.

39. Kinzbrunner BM, Policzer J, Miller B, Neiber L. Non-invasive pain control in the terminally ill patient. American Journal of Hospice and Palliative Care 1989;6:34.

40. World Health Organization. Cancer Pain Relief and Palliative Care. Geneva: The World Health Organization, 1990;1.

41. McCaffery M. Pain management: Nurses lead the way to new priorities. Am J Nurs 1990;90:45.

42. McCaffery M, Ferrell BR. Opioid analgesics: Nurses' knowledge of doses and psychological dependence. J Nurs Staff Dev 1992;8:77.

43. American Pain Society. Principles of Analgesic Use in the Treatment of Acute Pain and Chronic Cancer Pain (3rd ed). Slokie, IL: American Pain Society, 1992.

44. Morgan JP. American opiophobia: Customary underutilization of opioid analgesics. Adv Alcohol Subst Abuse 1985;5:163.

45. McCaffery J, Beebe A. Managing your patients' adverse reactions to narcotics. Nursing 1989;19:166.

46. Evans WD. Psychological, social and physical interventions for cancer pain. Indiana Med 1991;82:524.

47. Angarola RT. National and international regulation of opioid drugs: Purpose, structure, benefits, and risks. J Pain Symptom Manage 1990;5(2 Suppl):S6.

48. Whedon M, Ferrell BR. Professional and ethical considerations in the use of high-tech pain management. Oncol Nurs Forum 1991;18:1135.

49. Ropchan R, Ferrell BR, Grant M, Fleming I. Pain management as a nursing administration concern. Oncol Nurs Forum 1992;19:317.

50. Maloney C, Kesner RK, Klein G, Bockenstette J. The rectal administration of MS Contin: Clinical implication of use in end stage cancer. Am J Hospice Care 1989;6:34.

51. Storey P, Hill HH, St. Louis RH, Tarver EE. Subcutaneous infusions for control of cancer symptoms. J Pain Symptom Manage 1990;5:33.

52. Johanson GA. IV versus SQ opioid infusions for cancer pain. Am J Hospice Palliat Care 1991;84:6.

Chapter 32

Group Support

Patricia M. Way

There are many citations in the literature[1-10] to support the general conception that confirmation of a diagnosis of cancer is one of the most feared events that can happen in a person's life. Presently, only the acquired immune deficiency syndrome is considered to be a more dreaded diagnosis.[9] Not only is the diagnosis of cancer a major life stress, but the therapeutic treatment modalities such as chemotherapy, surgery, and radiation used to treat it can produce ongoing stressors that patients must adapt to over time. The cancer pain patient must also adjust to the possibility of recurrence or of a fatal outcome.[10]

My own experiences as an oncology nurse have validated these concerns. Patients have told me how they felt when they were told by their physician that they indeed had cancer. Listed below are a few of their stories.

An 18-year-old man with metastatic Ewing's sarcoma said, "You can't believe at first that [the physician] is talking to you. You almost feel as if you are removed from your body, that you are another person and that you are watching the whole thing from up on the ceiling." A 28-year-old man with acute myelogenous leukemia said, "I felt as if I had been punched in the stomach and that I couldn't breathe. An overwhelming fear came over me and I felt totally paralyzed. I didn't hear much after he told me I had leukemia." A 53-year-old man, also with acute leukemia, described how the diagnosis had intruded on his self-concept and his role as the provider in his family: "I felt as if I had been served a death sentence. All I could think about was my wife and children and how all of this would affect them. I knew life would never be the same."

In her classic paper on communication and the cancer patient,[11] Abrams states that a basic assumption contributing to the feeling of panic that most people experience on hearing the initial cancer diagnosis is that cancer is the one disease that they feel they have no control over. Unlike the cardiac patient who may alter stress patterns to prevent another cardiac event, or the diabetic patient who can change dietary intake and curb the diabetes with insulin, cancer patients view their disease as a purely medical one, in which control of one's physical or emotional activity cannot alter its progression.

Patients may confront feelings of alienation, mutilation, mortality, and loss of control[1] during the diagnosis and treatment of cancer. Alienation can be related to fears of abandonment and isolation once the diagnosis is confirmed. Patients fear that certain treatment modalities may cause a degree of mutilation, even though in many instances this may not be the case. It is fairly evident that a diagnosis of cancer can make one confront the possibility of mortality, even when the diagnosis is treatable and remission is possible. Loss of control refers to the vulnerability and loss of autonomy that often accompanies a malignant diagnosis, in as much as the nature and treatment of the disease contributes to one's sense of loss of control.[1]

There is also support in the literature for the belief that cancer not only affects patients themselves, but also their immediate family and others with whom they have had meaningful relationships.[1, 5, 12] Even those families that may possess adequate coping skills may feel powerless when confronted with this diagnosis. Koocher and Sallen, in describing how a cancer diagnosis in a child affects the family, state that even the basically sound family will confront an inordinate amount of stress that they are powerless to control. These authors further state that even the most well-adjusted family will be "unable to escape reactive emotional difficulties linked to powerful reality events," in the context of the diagnosis.[13]

Many patients report that with the diagnosis of the disease comes an awakening of their perceptions of themselves, their relationships with others, and a re-ordering of life's priorities. Blumberg et al. assert that coping with cancer does not begin when the diagnosis is made. Coping begins with patterns of adaptation to stress in general that people have integrated into their personalities over a period of time. These authors believe that people have established methods for maintaining psychic equilibrium before disease confronts them.[11] Bolund describes the first 2 years after the initial cancer diagnosis as a process of learning and adaptation involving adjustment to uncertainty, anxiety, dependence on medical care, and loss of and changes in bodily function and roles.[9] In addition to adapting to the shock of the initial diagnosis, coping with cancer also involves a reordering of one's thinking to incorporate the belief that cancer itself may be a chronic disease that needs to be reckoned with over an uncertain period of time. The therapeutic options used to treat a malignancy support this concept. It is the rare type of cancer that can be treated in a short time. Most oncologic diagnoses require prolonged treatment. Moos and Tsu advocate that adaptation in response to illness consists of two tasks: (1) the individual must cope with illness and attendant problems such as pain or paralysis, and (2) the individual must learn to cope with life as it is altered by illness. These tasks must be accomplished by patients and their significant others if successful coping is to occur.[14]

Cancer is frequently conceptualized as a chronic disease accompanied by physical, psychologic, emotional, and social problems.[1] The American Cancer Society reports that 1,359,150 new cases of cancer will be diagnosed in 1996, and that 4 out of 10 patients who were diagnosed will be alive 5 years later for a 40% "observed" survival rate. Adjusted for normal life expectancy (i.e., death from heart disease, accidents, and diseases of old age), a relative 5-year survival rate of 56% can be expected.[15] The impact of a cancer diagnosis is still inexorable in many cases, yet cancer today does not quite have the connotation of a death sentence as in previous years. Today, more people are living with and coping with cancer than ever before. Survivorship and quality-of-life issues have become important most likely because of the emergence of more effective treatment strategies, better supportive care, and improved outcomes for many of the differing cancer diagnoses. Consequently, the needs of cancer patients and their families, and of the responses relative to those needs have changed in the past decade. The improved chances for long-term survival have shifted the emphasis from short-term prognosis, immediate survival, and religious concerns to concerns relative to the cancer treatment and resultant side effects, and the potential for full recovery.[16]

The use of support groups as an effective psychotherapeutic tool for coping with a cancer diagnosis has been well documented.[17–23] Cancer support groups are an effective way to augment the necessary coping skills that allow cancer patients and their significant others to remain in the mainstream of life.

The Concept of Social Support

Support groups are based on the concepts of mutual aid and social support theory. Mutual aid, simply stated, is the art of people organizing to help one another. Those patients facing a common stress need and provide social support to each other in the hopes of finding a solution to a common problem.[24] Taylor et al. define social support as an interpersonal transaction involving emotional concern, instrumented aid (i.e., goods and services), information, and appraisal. These authors further state that it is possible to receive one or more of the preceding concepts from a social support group.[25] A social support group is defined as a group that incorporates face-to-face interaction in small groups with special emphasis given to personal participation, voluntary attendance, and an acknowledged purpose for coming together.[25] Most examinations of social support groups relate to the methodology by which these groups lessen or buffer the effect of stress in a positive way.[26–28]

Information sharing is another important construct in understanding the positive consequences of social support. Bloom asserts that social support on the part of the health care system in relation to communicating information on specific health care issues may determine adaptation or adjustment to illness.[28]

In her review of social support as it relates to the cancer patient, Wortman believes that the uncertainties and fears that accompany a cancer diagnosis are likely to lead to an "enhanced" need for social support.[26] The need for social support may grow stronger as cancer patients deal with treatment, and the outcome of that treatment. Wortman cautions that it is important to recognize that differing types of support may be needed at different stages in the cancer trajectory. Newly diagnosed patients for instance may have more of a need for information specific to their type of cancer and its treatment, whereas terminally ill patients may have needs related to comfort, pain control, or palliative care.

The availability of emotional support—usually a powerful component of social support groups—has been shown to effect positive outcomes for the person diagnosed with cancer. Bloom defines emotional support as behavior that ensures the individual that he or she is loved and valued as a person regardless of achievement.[28] The continual need for emotional support is crucial during any phase of a cancer diagnosis. The giving and receiving of emotional support implies an implicit sense of caring, positive regard, and affirmation that discussion of the myriad feelings surrounding a cancer diagnosis is permissible. Opportunities to discuss feelings, particularly negative ones, are important. The verbalization of personal concerns, clarification of feelings, the development of effective coping strategies, and actual problem solving can help alleviate stress.[26]

Types of Support Groups

Neuman describes support groups as being the oldest method of dealing with human problems, whether they are designed for treating psychological ills, social and interpersonal maladaptations, or for the purpose of learning, training, awareness, or action.[29] She describes the support group as a natural forum for bringing about change and for learning to deal with other human beings.

There are basically three types of support groups: psychotherapy groups, self-help or peer groups, and professionally led health-oriented support groups.

The psychotherapy group is a formal group process that involves a therapist working in an interpretive fashion.[30] Changes in personality or behavior are sought in these groups.

Self-help or peer groups, a more informal type of group support, are run by lay people without the assistance of a professional facilitator. As defined by Katz and Bender, self-help groups are voluntary, small group structures for mutual aid and the accomplishment of a special purpose.[31] These authors further state that self-help groups are usually formed by peers who have come together for mutual assistance in satisfying a common need, overcoming a common handicap or life-threatening problem, and bringing about desired social and personal change. Self-help groups are usually organized for battling isolation, depression, and other conditions related to social stigmatization. Members of self-help groups bond together, give each other emotional support, and unify to gain acceptance from a larger community.[32] Self-help and peer support groups usually have three basic goals: the imparting of information, the giving of hope, and the sharing of feelings with people in similar situations.[33]

Self-help groups can also be formed out of necessity. Health care professionals in a community may have failed to provide a forum to address the needs and concerns of a particular population.[32] The self-help or peer support group is decisive when its members are undergoing active cancer treatment such as chemotherapy, surgery, radiation therapy, or biological therapy. "Specialists" can share effective coping strategies for dealing with some of the more practical elements of cancer treatment.

Yalom asserts that patients themselves are an untapped source of information and should be deferred to and respected for their experiences.[30] Wortman also suggests that there is convincing evidence that when people are in a crisis, or experiencing extreme distress, those who have had similar experiences may be in a unique position to provide effective support.[26] Cancer survivorship groups are based on this premise.

Professionally led support groups are usually created by health care professionals for a specific population. The formation, process, and composition of these types of support groups depend on professional leadership and guidance.[32] These types of groups are formed with specific purposes and goals in mind. In cancer support groups, the purpose is to assist patients and their families in coping with the physical and psychological sequelae of a cancer diagnosis. In specifically addressing group support as it relates to cancer patients, Vachon identifies a common purpose of both the professionally led group and the self-help group: giving support to patients and their families during the difficult "psychosocial transition" of adjusting to a life-threatening illness.[34]

Some authors believe that the purpose and direction of a support group for cancer patients should be clearly distinguished at the start.[24, 28, 32] Obviously, the common thread running through a support group for this population is the commonality of a cancer diagnosis, yet controversy exists regarding the inclusion of patients in the same group who are in different phases of their illness. For example, is it appropriate or therapeutic for a newly diagnosed patient and family to attend the same group with a patient who is experiencing distressing side effects from cancer therapy, or with a patient who is in the terminal phase of his or her illness? Some studies have suggested that including patients in different phases of illness does not create barriers to the communication of feelings of empathy within a group.[35, 36] One method to assess potentially problematic situations concerning the intermixture of patients in different phases of the cancer experience is to conduct a screening interview by telephone to determine the specific needs of an individual or family member seeking group support.

Who Joins Cancer Support Groups?

Bolund, quoting Derogatis et al. and Plumb and Holland, states that most cancer patients cope with their illness without specific psychosocial interventions.[9]

However, the group setting is used by many as a vehicle for seeking support and enhancing coping skills relative to a cancer diagnosis. There are several reasons why cancer patients and their family members join support groups. The first is fairly obvious and involves the need for belonging and relating to others who have encountered similar experiences, i.e., people join support groups to feel supported. They wish to validate their own cancer experience by sharing this experience with others in a similar situation. Other reasons to join support groups that have been evaluated include the need to seek information about a specific cancer diagnosis

and its treatment, relief from fear and depression caused by cancer itself, relief from the stigma of being a cancer "victim," exploration with other members on methods to control treatment side effects such as pain, examining role changes due to the disease, investigation concerning loss of control, defined as the inability to manage or influence events, and spiritual inquiries relative to the notion of cancer as a fatal illness (existential concerns).[16, 18, 24, 25, 37] Cella identifies the concept of hope and the search for inspiration relative to survival and quality of life as two important reasons why some patients seek group support.[16]

Women use cancer support groups more than men—at a ratio of almost 4 to 1. This may be because women are more comfortable than men in asking for and receiving support.[16] Men tend to seek out groups that are related specifically to information sharing and specific skill training.[25] Gordon et al., in studying the concept of who joins cancer support groups and the reasons why, have found that such groups are disproportionately used by white, middle-class to upper middle-class women, and are disproportionately underused by men, minorities, and individuals with low socioeconomic status.[38] Among people of color, the poor, and the elderly, the use of cancer support groups is very low.[39] This area deserves more study, as these groups are most often diagnosed with cancer.[15]

Several authors have validated positive outcomes related to participation in cancer support groups,[19, 40–42] but there exists a paucity of well-designed controlled studies to augment their findings.

Successful Support Groups

Initiating and sustaining successful support groups for cancer patients and their families is often a daunting task. Cancer support groups may take a long time to get established. Barriers to their success may range from such logistical concerns as location, timing of meetings, transportation, group size, and child care issues, to more philosophical concerns such as differing disease stages for group members, heterogeneous cancer diagnoses, or the inexperience of group facilitators in group process.

A typical time frame from the first planning session to the first group meeting may be about 6 months. The first task of the group facilitators is to define the group's focus. [43] A mission statement should be developed that clearly states the group's purpose and its goals. For example, the Leukemia Society of America's mission statement for their network of Family Support Groups is as follows:

> The concept of a Family Support Group is based on the idea that open communication about the illness is critical to coping with all the feelings that arise. With appropriate professional guidance, patients and family members discuss anxieties with each other and with other patients and families who share the same burden. This sharing of ideas and feelings serves to strengthen the family unit, thereby enhancing their ability to cope with the disease. [44]

When identifying the purpose of the group, it is important to identify whether the stress confronting the members is acute, amelioratory, or permanent. [24] For example, a support group for parents of newly diagnosed pediatric oncology patients will have a different focus and purpose than a group for terminally ill patients in a hospice setting. Those patients, in turn, would have different concerns than would a postmastectomy breast cancer support group who meet to discuss concerns relative to adaptation in having a breast removed.

Vugia [24] identifies four important issues that should be discussed when planning the composition of a support group for cancer patients:

1. What cancer diagnosis will the group encompass?
2. What stages of illness will the group cover?
3. Will the group target cancer survivors, spouses, parents, siblings, friends, or all of these people?
4. Will membership be open or closed?

Ideal group size is usually 10–12 participants, yet most cancer support groups maintain open fluid membership. [24]

The Role of Group Facilitator

There are citations in the cancer support group literature that suggest that the union of a mental health professional with formal training in family-centered therapy with a medical professional well versed in the disease process of cancer and its treatment is the most beneficial approach to successful group facilitating. [4, 24, 44] The contributions of two committed facilitators is advantageous to group process and content. Wasserman and Danforth [32] have outlined six recommendations that constitute successful facilitating of support groups in general.

1. Promote cohesion, i.e., the facilitators recognize the participants preexisting homogeneity. The facilitators encourage interaction, attempt to minimize social distance, and use consensus in decision making.
2. Develop a safe climate. The facilitators avoid demands for self-disclosure, help members accept one another's differences, focus on the goal of support, avoid interpretation and transference, maintain control, and use humor to modulate intensity.
3. Help support evolve. The facilitators introduce the concept of mutual aid, empower individual group members, model empathy as a support-building process, and model support via group interaction.
4. Be generous with reinforcement. The facilitators focus on positive and productive behaviors, and promote the building of members' self-esteem.
5. Foster reduction of stress. The facilitators provide refreshments to foster comfort, provide a structure to give the group direction and support, and plan enjoyment to balance the seriousness of the situation.
6. Give information. The facilitators impart information by being well informed, and explore ideas as a group, i.e., the leaders do not always have to be the experts.

These six constructs can be applied to the successful facilitation of a cancer support group. Pragmatic concerns, such as maintaining consistency in regards to the meeting place, time, and even seating arrangement should not be overlooked by the facilitators. Attention to these details promotes a harmonious environment. It is also advantageous to maintain the same format for starting and ending the group meeting times. For instance, many groups begin with an informal period of talking and socializing, move into a more structured format for discussion, and then allow time for members to network with one another at the end of the meeting.

Many successful groups use the concept of a contract to establish and maintain the tone of the group. [43] A contract is defined as an agreement or a stipulation that lends structure to group process, and the terms of the contract should be mutually acceptable to the facilitators and the members. Effective contracts define group behavior and may be used to discourage inappropriate actions by group members.[43] Contracts are often thought of as "ground rules." Ground rules that facilitate appropriate or therapeutic group dynamics are beginning and ending the group on time, respect for one another's feelings, allowing only one person to speak at a time, and respecting the group's confidentiality.

Schnaper et al. believe that listening to a patient's concerns can be the most important and demanding task for those providing support to cancer patients. These authors define actual listening as the "quintessence of emotional support." The following is a list of positive active listening steps for the support group facilitator.

1. Put yourself in the other person's place to understand what the person is saying and feeling.
2. Show understanding and acceptance of nonverbal behavior.
3. Restate the person's most important thoughts and feelings.
4. Be aware that to interrupt, offer advice, or give suggestions may impede successful group dynamics.
5. Recognize the importance of remaining neutral and of not taking sides.[44]

The Concept of Loss

Because cancer often brings with it an uncertain prognosis, some patients feel that the very word *cancer* connotes a sense of loss. This loss can be defined in many ways, such as a loss of previous good health, role and function, independence, or loss of a spouse, partner, parent, child, sibling, or friend. Loss is a recurrent theme in cancer support groups.[43] This may be due to the fact that for some the eventuality of death from the disease is an ever-present reality.

One of the most difficult losses to discuss is the loss of a group member. When individual group members are confronted with bereavement situations that other members are experiencing, the tendency to reflect on and personalize those experiences is great. This is especially true when members are confronted with issues of grief and loss relative to death.[45]

For example, in one cancer support group, a very dynamic and treasured member named Joan died

rather suddenly after appearing stable at the previous meeting. Her medical condition became steadily worse during the month and she died unexpectedly before the group could meet again. Other members with the same diagnosis and similar treatment courses became extremely introspective and were forced to consider the real possibility of developing the same complications and perhaps succumbing to the disease as well. Many of the members reflected their thoughts and cried as they remembered Joan and her valiant struggle with leukemia. There was much praise and admiration expressed for her courage and stamina in dealing with a disease that eventually took her life. By encouraging a reflective and caring discussion concerning Joan's death, the facilitators allowed the members to come to terms with not only their extreme sadness over the death of their friend, but also enabled them to share their own sense of pain and loneliness associated with the possibility that they also may die due to their disease.

McEvoy, in examining Flynn's framework of responses to dying, describes "death in the second person" as an identification with the dying person as a loved one. When we let ourselves experience death in the second person we truly can grieve that person's death and death becomes a shared experience. Experiencing death in the second person implies that the person who died is as dear to us as we are to ourselves. McEvoy describes relationships as making people human, and believes that a part of us is dying when we participate in dying in the second person. She describes a most intense experience.

Participation in support groups can let the cancer patient feel that he is actively coping with his disease. His efforts at interaction with other patients and their families may lead him to feel that at least he has some control over a disease that indiscriminately picked him as its victim. In the face of overwhelming odds, most people still have both desire and energy to reach out to others. Perhaps this reaching out and caring is the unique human gift that a cancer patient leaves as his legacy. Cancer caregivers can provide supportive services, yet it is the patients themselves that sometimes have the most to offer. They are able to share with others that in those dark, despairing moments when all seems lost, a ray of hope almost always can be found. They share practical methods of dealing with cancer day to day. They share funny anecdotal situations related to their treatment, because even with cancer, a sense of humor is almost never lost.[46]

Alexander Solzhenitsyn in an excerpt from *The Cancer Ward* sums it up very succinctly.

Where he lived no one understood him, not a soul in his apartment or his building or his block. They were healthy people who ran about from noon till night thinking of successes or failures—things that seemed terribly unimportant to him. It was only here, on the steps of the cancer clinic, that the patients listened to him for hours and sympathized. They understood what it means to a man when a small triangular area grows bone hard and the irradiation scars are thick on the skin where the x-rays have penetrated.[47]

References

1. Blumberg BD, Ahmed P, Flaherty M, et al. Living with Cancer—An Overview. In P Ahmed (ed), Living and Dying with Cancer. New York: Elsevier, 1981;3.

2. Kubler-Ross E. Death—The Final Stage of Growth. Englewood Cliffs, NJ: Prentice-Hall, 1975.

3. Weisman AD. Coping with Cancer. New York: McGraw-Hill, 1979.

4. Whitman HH, Gustafson JP. Group therapy for families facing a cancer diagnosis. Oncol Nurs Forum 1989;16:539.

5. Farrow JM, Cash DK, Simmons G. Communicating with Cancer Patients and Their Families. In A Blitzer, AH Kutscher, SL Klagsrun (eds), Communicating with Cancer Patients and Their Families. Philadelphia: Charles Press, 1990;1.

6. Telch CF, Telch MJ. Group coping skills instruction and supportive group therapy for cancer patients: A comparison of strategies. J Consult Clin Psychol 1986;54:802.

7. Ahmed P (ed). Living and Dying with Cancer. New York: Elsevier, 1981.

8. Goldberg RJ (ed). Advances in Psychosomatic Medicine (Vol. 18). Basel: Karger, 1988.

9. Bolund C. Crisis and Coping: Learning to Live with Cancer. In JC Holland, R Zittoun (eds), Psychosocial Aspects of Oncology. New York: Springer, 1990;13.

10. Linn MW. Psychotherapy with Cancer Patients. In RJ Goldberg (ed), Advances in Psychosomatic Medicine (Vol. 18). Basel: Karger, 1988;55.

11. Abrams RD. The patient with cancer: His changing pattern of communication. N Engl J Med 1966;274:317.

12. Slaby AE. Cancer's Impact on Caregivers. In RJ Goldberg (ed), Advances in Psychosomatic Medicine (Vol. 18). Basel: Karger, 1988;134.

13. Koocher JP, Sallen SE. Psychological Issues in Pediatric Oncology. In PR Magrab (ed), Psychologic Management of Pediatric Problems (Vol. 1). Early Life Conditions and Chronic Disease. Baltimore: University Park Press, 1978; 283.

14. Moos RH, Tsu VD. The Crisis of Physical Illness: An Overview. In RH Moos (ed), Coping with Physical Illness. New York: Plenum, 1977;3.

15. American Cancer Society. Facts and Figures. Atlanta: ACS, 1993.

16. Cella DF, Yellen SB. Cancer support groups. The state of the art. Cancer Pract 1993;1:56.

17. Nerenz DR, Love RR. Types of Supportive Therapy. In BA Stoll (ed), Coping with Cancer Stress. Dordrecht: Martinus Nijhoff, 1986;95.

18. Vugia HD. Support groups in oncology: Building hope through the human bond. J Psychosoc Oncol 1991;9:89.

19. Cullinan AL. Existential Group Therapy with Mastectomy Patients. In A Blitzer, AH Kutscher, SL Klagsrun (eds), Communicating with Cancer Patients and Their Families. Philadelphia: Charles Press, 1990;150.

20. Schnaper N, Legg-McNamara C, Dutcher J, Kellner T. Emotional Support of the Patient and His Survivors. In P Viernik (ed), Supportive Care of the Cancer Patient. Mount Kisco, NY: Futura, 1983;1.

21. Morgenstern H, Gellert G, Walter S, et al. The impact of a psychosocial support program on survival with breast cancer: The importance of selection bias in program evaluation. J Chronic Dis 1984;37:273.

22. Spiegel D, Bloom J, Yalom I. Group support for patients with metastatic cancer. Arch Gen Psychiatry 1981;38:527.

23. Ferlic M, Goldman A, Kennedy BJ. Group counseling with adult cancer patients. Cancer 1979;43:760.

24. Vugia HD. Support groups in oncology: Building hope through the human bond. J Psychosoc Oncol 1991;9:89.

25. Taylor SE, Falke RL, Shoptaw SJ, Lichtman RR. Social support, support groups, and the cancer patient. J Consult Clin Psychol 1986;54:608.

26. Wortman CB. Social support and the cancer patient. Conceptual and methodologic issues. Cancer 1984;53(Suppl. 10):2339.

27. Turner RJ. Social support as a contingency in psychological well-being. J Health Social Behav 1981;22:357.

28. Bloom JR. Social Support Systems and Cancer: A Conceptual View. In J Cohen, J Cullen, LR Martin (eds), Psychosocial Aspects of Cancer. New York: Raven, 1982;129.

29. Neuman R. Group Psychotherapies. In GU Balis (ed), Psychiatric Clinical Skills in Medical Practice. Boston: Butterworth, 1978;253.

30. Yalom ID. The Therapeutic Factors in Group Therapy. In The Theory and Practice of Group Psychotherapy. New York: Basic Books, 1985;3.

31. Katz AH, Bender EI. The Strength in Us: Self Help Groups in the Modern World. New York: New Viewpoints, 1976.

32. Wasserman H, Danforth H. The Human Bond. Support Groups and Mutual Aid. New York: Springer, 1988.

33. Kopel K, Mock LA. The use of group sessions for the emotional support of families of terminal patients. Death Education 1978;1:409.

34. Vachon ML, Lyall WA. Applying psychiatric techniques to patients with cancer. Hospital Community Psychiatry 1976;27:582.

35. Johnson EM, Stark DE. A group program for cancer patients and their family members in an acute care teaching hospital. Soc Work Health Care 1980;5:335.

36. Block LR. On the potentiality and limits of time: The single session group and the cancer patient. Social Work Groups 1985;8:81.

37. Van Den Borne HW, Pruyn JFA, Meij K. Help Given by Fellow Patients. In B Stoll (ed), Coping with Cancer Stress. Dordrecht: Martinus Nijhoff, 1986;103.

38. Gordon WA, Freidenbergs I, Diller L, et al. Efficacy of psychosocial intervention with cancer patients. J Consult Clin Psychol 1980;48:743.

39. Deans C, Bennet-Emslie GB, Weir J, et al. Cancer support groups: Who joins and why? Br J Cancer 1988;58:670.

40. Spiegel D, Bloom J, Yalom I. Group support for patients with metastatic cancer. Arch Gen Psychiatry 1981;38:527.

41. Ferlin M, Goldman, A, Kennedy BJ. Group counseling with adult cancer patients. Cancer 1979;43:760.

42. Morgenstern H, Gellert G, Walter S, et al. The impact of a psychosocial support program on survival with breast cancer: The importance of selection bias in program evaluation. J Chronic Dis 1984;37:273.

43. Hieney SP, Wells LM. Strategies for organizing and maintaining successful support groups. Oncol Nurs Forum 1989;16:803.

44. Leukemia Society of America. Family Support Group Guidelines (3rd ed). New York: LSA, 1992.

45. Schnaper N, Legg-McNamara C, Dutcher J, Kellner T. Emotional Support of the Patient and His Survivors. In P Wiernik (ed), Supportive Care of the Patient. Mount Kisco. NY: Futura, 1983;1.

46. McEvoy M. When Your Dying Becomes My Dying: Aspects of Caregivers' Grief. In A Blitzer, AH Kutscher, SL Klagsurn (eds), Communicating with Cancer Patients and Their Families. Philadelphia: Charles Press, 1990;206.

47. Solzhenitsyn AI. The Cancer Ward. New York: Dial Press, 1968.

Appendix

Organizations with Support Group Programs in the United States

American Brain Tumor Association
2720 River Road, Suite 146
Des Plaines, IL 60618
800-886-2282
Offers free services including publications about brain tumors, support group lists, referral information, and a pen-pal program.

American Cancer Society (ACS)
1599 Clifton Road N.E.
Atlanta, GA 30329
800-ACS-2345
Dedicated to eliminating cancer as a major health problem through research, education, and service. Several service and rehabilitation programs are available at the state and local level for many types of cancer diagnoses.

Bone Marrow Transplant Family Support Network
PO Box 845
Avon, CT 06001
800-826-9376
Enables families to feel "connected" when coping with the decision, daily routines prior to and following the transplant, and with follow-up care after a transplant.

Candlelighters Childhood Cancer Foundation
7910 Woodmont Avenue, Suite 460
Bethesda, MD 20814
301-657-8401
800-366-2223
Provides information, support, and advocacy to families of children with cancer, survivors of childhood cancer, and professionals who work with them.

Chemocare
231 North Avenue West
Westfield, NJ 07090
800-55-CHEMO (outside NJ)
908-233-1103 (inside NJ)
Offers support to people undergoing chemotherapy and radiation treatment by trained and certified volunteers who have survived the treatment themselves.

Encore Plus
YWCA of the USA
624 91st St. N.W.
Washington, D.C. 20001
800-95-EPLUS
Office of Women's Health Initiative offering peer support and exercise information, among other services related to women's health.

International Myeloma Foundation
2120 Stanley Hills Drive
Los Angeles, CA 90046
800-452-CURE
Promotes education and research regarding the treatment and prevention of myeloma and informs patients about available treatments and provides knowledge and support to community-based services and patient support groups.

Leukemia Society of America
600 Third Avenue
New York, NY 10016
800-955-4LSA
Dedicated solely to seeking the cause and eventual cure of leukemia and its related diseases. The society offers a Family Support Group Program for patients diagnosed with leukemia and related diseases and their families.

Make Today Count
c/o Connie Zimmerman
Mid-America Cancer Center
1235 E. Cherokee
Springfield, MO 65804-2263
800-432-2273
A mutual support organization that brings together those persons affected by a life-threatening illness so they may help each other.

National Alliance of Breast Cancer Organizations
(NABCO)
9 East 37th Street, 10th Floor
New York, NY 10016
212-719-0154.

National Brain Tumor Foundation
785 Market Street, Suite 1600
San Francisco, CA 94103
800-934-CURE
Pursues two major goals: providing support and education for brain tumor patients, and finding a cure through research.

National Breast Cancer Coalition
1707 L Street N.W., Suite 1060
Washington, D.C. 20036
202-296-7477
A grass roots advocacy effort whose goal is to work to eradicate breast cancer through research, access, and influence.

National Cancer Institute (NCI)
Building 31, Room 10A16
9000 Rockville Pike
Bethesda, MD 20892
800-4-CANCER
Provides a nationwide telephone service for cancer patients and their families and friends, the public, and health care professionals that answers questions and sends booklets about cancer.

National Coalition for Cancer Survivorship
1010 Wayne Avenue, 5th Floor
Silver Spring, MD 20910
301-650-9127
Exists to enhance the quality of life for cancer survivors and to promote an understanding of cancer survivorship.

National Hospice Organization (NHO)
1901 N. Moore Street, Suite 901
Arlington, VA 22209
800-658-8898
A resource for hospice professionals, volunteers, and the general public for terminally ill patients and their families.

The Chemotherapy Foundation
183 Madison Avenue, Suite 403
New York, NY 10016
212-213-9292.
Supports research to develop more effective methods of diagnosis and therapy for the control and cure of cancer. Conducts education programs and provides free patient and public information booklets.

The Wellness Community
2716 Ocean Park Blvd., Suite 1040
Santa Monica, CA 90405
310-314-2555
Provides free psychosocial support to cancer patients, as an adjunct to conventional medical treatment. Seventeen facilities nationwide.

Y-Me National Organization for Breast Cancer Information and Support
212 West Van Buren Street, 5th Floor
Chicago, IL 60607-3908
800-221-2141
Hotline counseling, educational programs and self-help meetings for breast cancer patients, their families, and friends. Peer counseling is available.

Chapter 33

Assessment of Quality of Life

Nancy Wells

Pain is a pervasive symptom associated with cancer. It is estimated that 50% of all patients with cancer experience pain and that the prevalence of pain increases to 70–90% in terminally ill patients.[1] Adequate pain management has become a national issue with the development of clinical guideline panels by the Agency of Health Care Policy and Research. One primary task of the clinical guideline panels is to determine the most effective methods of pain management for acute[2] and cancer-related[3] pain. Cancer pain management has relied on analgesic therapies that, if managed properly, can adequately control pain in most patients.[4] Analgesic therapies, both opioid and nonopioid, can produce distressing side effects, however. Pain resistant to analgesic therapies may require more invasive techniques, e.g., neuroablative and implantable pump procedures. Although relief of pain is the major goal of these interventions, quality of life has been suggested as an essential outcome measure of pain control interventions.[5, 6] This chapter reviews the concept of quality of life, discusses measurement issues related to quality of life, and presents an argument for using quality of life as an outcome measure for pain control interventions.

Quality of Life

Quality of life has become an important issue for cancer patients because treatments have been developed with the potential to substantially prolong life. Patients may be faced with living longer with a variety of sequelae from both the cancer and its treatment. This has forced health care providers and patients to examine not just the quantity of life, but also the quality of prolonged survival.[5, 7] This advancement and success of cancer therapies has led the Food and Drug Administration to recommend that quality of life measures be included in clinical trials of cancer therapies with multiple treatment arms.[8] In this way, quality of life becomes one aspect on which policy decisions can be made.

The definition of quality of life has important implications for the measurement of it. The World Health Organization (WHO) laid the foundation for measurement with their definition of health as "a state of complete physical, mental, and social well-being and not just the absence of disease and infirmity."[9]

Traditional measures of treatment outcomes—clinical indicators—are familiar to most health care providers. Tumor size, biological markers of treatment response, toxicity, performance status, and survival have been used for many years to evaluate patient response to treatment. These measures make sense to the clinician as a means of determining successful treatment, mainly because of their objectivity. If we return to the WHO definition of health, it is apparent that these clinical indicators focus on the physical dimension of health, but provide no information on the mental or social dimensions. A different approach is necessary to determine the impact of interventions on psychological and social well-being in patients with cancer.

Research has consistently demonstrated the multidimensional nature of quality of life and indicates

Table 33-1. Attributes of Quality of Life

Function	Physical Symptoms	Emotional Well-Being	Social Concerns
Physical independence	Pain	Life satisfaction	Emotional support
Activities of daily living	Nausea and vomiting	Happiness	Interpersonal interaction
Strength	Fatigue	Enjoyment	Affection
Ability to work	Sleep	Adjustment to disease	Appearance
		Ability to concentrate	
		Anxiety, depression, fear	

there are a minimum of four core dimensions or domains: functional status; physical status, including disease symptoms and treatment side effects; psychological well-being; and social well-being.[10–14] Table 33-1 displays the core dimensions of quality of life and their attributes. *Functional status* reflects the patient's ability to meet both self-care and role demands.[13] The functional dimension is most consistent with the clinical indicators (e.g., performance status), and, not surprisingly, is most highly correlated with physician ratings of function and well-being.[14] The *physical symptoms* dimension taps changes in somatic sensation that are perceived as disruptive to body function.[13, 14] Pain, nausea and vomiting, and fatigue are commonly experienced by patients with cancer who are undergoing treatment. The impact of these physical discomforts on overall quality of life is largely unknown, but may be great.[14] Obviously, somatic sensations are not as observable as functional status, and, therefore, not as easily detected by outside observers. *Psychological well-being* reflects positive and negative affect related to current health status.[13] Positive affective states, such as happiness and joy, have not been as closely examined as negative affective states in patients with cancer. Common negative affective states included in quality of life measures are anxiety, depression,[14, 15] and fear.[14] A pattern of emotional responses has been identified as patient disease progresses. Anxiety and depression occur at the time of diagnosis; an increase in anxiety occurs with each new assessment of disease progress, and fear predominates during periods of diagnostic and treatment uncertainty.[14] Negative mood also has been found to fluctuate with pain[16] and correlate highly with fatigue.[17] Psychological well-being correlates most highly with global assessments of quality of life.[6] *Social well-being* is the ability to

interact with others to maintain social relationships.[13] Social relationships take on many forms, and may be considerably influenced by the patient's functional status and psychological state. Adequate social support has been positively related to psychological well-being and adjustment to illness.[18] According to Schipper and colleagues,[14] the importance of social well-being during illness has been underestimated.

Cognitive function, which may influence not only quality of life but the way in which measures are completed, has been largely ignored.[19] However, areas such as the ability to concentrate and memory are commonly included in quality of life definitions and measures within the psychological dimension. Inclusion of the meaning of disease and symptoms to the individual, and the degree of uncertainty experienced are less commonly found in quality of life measures. Of greater concern, however, is the lack of screening for changes in mental status that may seriously compromise quality of life self-reports.

Additional domains have been suggested by various authors, e.g., spirituality,[13, 20, 21] sexuality,[13, 22] and financial concerns.[20, 23] Arguments have been made that financial concerns and work status are influenced by many factors aside from health status and therefore do not add meaning to quality of life related to illness.[24]

Quality of life, in addition to its multidimensional nature, is a subjective phenomenon, which requires the individual's assessment of well-being.[6, 10, 11, 13, 25] Although the validity of self-report is sometimes viewed with skepticism, research has demonstrated that there is a modest relationship between patient self-report and proxy (i.e., health care provider or significant other) measures of quality of life.[26] Based on the attributes described, any measure of quality of life should contain multiple dimensions of well-being, including physical symptoms and functional, emotional, and social dimensions, and should be obtained from the patient. These characteristics of multidimensionality and subjectivity are shared with the concept of pain.[27]

Measurement Models

Two basic models have been used to measure quality of life. Each serves a different purpose. Table 33-2 reviews the models and purposes. The first model of measurement is the psychometric, which uses multi-item questionnaires to assess day-to-day function. Psychometric measures provide specific information about progression of the disease process and patient response to treatment. Psychometric measures provide assessment data for the clinician that may be used to guide interventions to alleviate the negative effects of disease and treatment. Clinical experience and research suggest that different treatment regimens affect different aspects of quality of life.[28, 29] The psychometric measures reveal the patterns of change that occur with various treatment regimens. The Functional Living Index-Cancer[30] is an example of a psychometric measure of quality of life in patients with cancer. A variant of the psychometric model, the "gap theory," posits that the critical aspect of quality of life is the discrepancy or gap between aspirations and reality.[12, 23, 31, 32] Measures using the gap theory provide specific information about the dimensions of quality of life by weighing satisfaction with quality of life by importance to the individual. Ferrans and Powers[23] used the gap theory to develop their Quality of Life Index (QL Index).

Utility models based on economic and decision theory provide the second model of measurement. Utility models combine quantity and quality into a single summary score.[33, 34] In effect, utility models weight quantity of life by quality. The quality component (i.e., utilities) is judgments about the worth or value of specific health states.[19, 33] Utilities can be determined through a variety of techniques. For example, the Quality-Time With and Without Symptoms and Toxicity (Q-TWIST) technique uses a statistical estimation technique to determine the weights of time with symptoms and relapse.[33] Utility values can also be obtained using reference

Table 33-2. Models of Quality of Life Measurement

Model	Purpose
Psychometric	Assess day-to-day function
Standard	Assess response to treatment
Disparity	Design interventions for patient and family
Utility	Assess health outcomes
	Cost analysis
	Policy decision making

groups (e.g., patients, healthy individuals, health care providers), as was used in developing the Quality of Well-Being Scale.[34] Patient preferences provide another method to determine utilities for various health states.[35] This method requires, however, a substantial amount of time and concentration, and therefore may not be appropriate for patients who are ill. As patients tend to adjust their preferences to current health states,[36] different values will operate over time.[19, 37] For example, Gelber et al.[38, 39] used the Q-TWIST methodology in women with positive node breast cancer to compare short- (single cycle) and long-term (6–7 months) chemotherapies. Analyses at a 5-year endpoint revealed that long-term therapy resulted in 2.2 months more time without symptoms or toxicity than the short-term therapy. Thus, utility models take complex data and reduce it to a single "marker," commonly termed, quality adjusted life years. Utility models provide useful data for policy decisions and cost analyses.[40] They are not as useful in tracking patient response to the disease and treatment protocols because the complexity of quality of life is lost in the summary score. In addition, sensitivity is reduced with utility models.[41]

Types of Psychometric Measures

A wide variety of instruments have been developed to measure the functional, physical, emotional, and social dimensions of quality of life. Aaronson[11] has suggested a taxonomy of quality of life measures, based on their generality and applicability to specific patient populations. Table 33-3 displays examples of instruments within each level of measurement. This is not meant to be a comprehensive list of quality of

Table 33-3. Examples of Pyschometric Measures

Instrument	No. of Items	Dimensions	No. of Pain Items	Sensitivity
Generic				
Sickness Impact Profile[44, 45]	136	fx, em, soc	0	Moderate
Nottingham Health Profile, Pt 1[46–49]	38	fx, phy, em, soc	8	Moderate
McMaster Health Index[50, 51]	59	fx, em, soc	0	?
Medical Outcomes Survey-Short Form[52]	20	fx, phy, em, soc	1	?
Cancer Specific				
Functional Living Index-Cancer[30]	22	fx, phy, em, soc	2	?
QL Index[6, 53]	14	fx, phy, em	1	High
EORTC QLQ30[54]	30	fx, phy, em, soc	2	Moderate
LASA[55]	31	fx, phy, em, soc	1	High
LASA[56]	4–6	fx, phy	1	Moderate
Functional Assessment Cancer Therapy General[57]	33	fx, phy, em, soc	1	High
QLI-Cancer Version[20]	64	fx, phy, em, soc	1	Moderate
Symptom Distress Scale[58–60]	13	phy	2	High
Rotterdam Symptom Checklist[61]	35	fx, phy, em	5	High
Brief Pain Inventory[62, 63]	23	fx, phy, em, soc	6	High
Brief Pain Inventory-Short Form[63]	8	fx, phy, em, soc	6	High
Diagnosis or Treatment Specific				
QL Index-Colostomy[6]	23	phy, em, soc	2	High
QL Index-Radiation Therapy[22]	21	fx, phy, em	1	?
EORTC-Lung[64]	13+30	phy core	2	?
EORTC-Head & Neck [65, 66]	13+30	phy	1	?
Lung Cancer Symptom Scale [67]	9	fx, phy	1	?

QL Index = Quality of Life Index; EORTC = European Organization for Research and Treatment of Cancer; LASA = Linear Analogue Scale Assessment; fx = function; phy = physical symptoms; em = emotional well-being; soc = social concerns; ? = unknown in this patient population or not well established.

life measures; excellent reviews of measures can be found in Cella and Tulsky,[12] Moinpour et al.,[42] and Donovan et al.[43]

Generic measures of quality of life have been developed to reflect patient response to illness, and therefore do not typically tap all of the physical symptoms and responses related to cancer and its treatment. Generic measures frequently used in patients with cancer include the Sickness Impact Profile [44, 45] and the Nottingham Health Profile.[46–49] Additional generic measures of single dimensions of quality of life, such as the Profile of Mood States,[68] also are commonly used in assessing quality of life. Generic measures of quality of life, such as the three mentioned, have undergone rigorous testing during development and standardization in various patient populations. In addition, both measures used a reference group to determine weights for individual items on their questionnaires. When generic measures are used, comparisons to healthy and ill populations can be made.

Disease-specific measures are developed to closely match the dimensions of quality of life affected by a specific disease, such as cancer. Generally, disease-specific measures are more sensitive to changes in quality of life dimensions than generic instruments, but may lack some of the rigor in development found in the generic instrument.[11] Examples of disease-specific instruments with good psychometric properties include The Functional Living Index-Cancer[30] and the European Organization for Research and Treatment of Cancer (EORTC) QLQ-C30.[54] Because cancer does not reflect a single disease entity, and treatment adverse effects vary greatly, diagnosis- and treatment-specific instruments also have been developed. These instruments are highly specific to anticipated changes related to diagnosis or treatment, and therefore provide a high level of sensitivity to change in the patient's quality of life. However, their specificity does not allow comparison across different diagnoses or treatments. The Quality of Life Index-Radiation Therapy[22] and the Lung Cancer Symptom Scale[67] are examples of diagnosis- and treatment-specific instruments.

Few instruments will contain all of the dimensions affected by cancer and cancer treatments; therefore, a modular approach has been recommended[11, 32, 64] that includes either a generic or disease-specific core, supplemented with diagnosis- or treatment-specific modules. The EORTC has adopted this approach, and currently has seven core quality of life dimensions, to which diagnosis- or treatment-specific modules can be added. Currently, specific EORTC modules are available for lung[64] and head and neck[65, 66] cancers. Other diagnosis- and treatment-specific instruments may require development by investigators with a high level of clinical knowledge about their patient population.[25] Selection of quality of life instrument(s) should balance the critical aspects of quality of life in the identified patient population and the need for brief but sensitive measures. In addition, an overall measure of quality of life, typically a single item, is recommended to gain information about the totality of the patient's experience.[11, 25]

Criteria for Instrument Selection and Administration

With the wide variety of quality of life instruments available at present, selection of appropriate instruments has become more difficult. Instruments selected should be brief and easily completed.[10, 32] Attrition in clinical trials where quality of life has been monitored is high because as the treatment progresses patients become too ill to complete complex questionnaires.[69] The items on the questionnaire should "make sense" to the patient, as repetitive or irrelevant items may reduce initial participation and increase attrition. Categorical response formats, e.g., five to seven response selections, are less confusing to patients than continuous response formats, such as visual analog scales.[42, 43] Continuous response formats also require more time for scoring, thus increasing time and effort by the clinician or researcher in interpretation. To be useful in monitoring patient progress,

instruments must be sensitive to changes in health status and quality of life dimensions.[10, 43] Donovan et al.[43] recommend a minimum of five items per dimension to maintain adequate sensitivity to change. Because of the subjective nature of quality of life, instruments need to be patient-based; for maximum understanding of the patient's responses, written questionnaires should be supplemented with clarifying interviews when necessary.[13] Although patient self-report provides the best estimate of quality of life, proxy measures from a health care provider and significant other may be used to supplement patient-based data.[13, 25] When using proxy measures, it is important to realize that health care providers and significant others tend to underestimate both pain and impact of disease and treatment on quality of life.[26] To improve the reliability of proxy measures, patients may select their own proxy measure, or ratings from a number of proxies can be obtained.[70] Finally, instruments selected should have demonstrated reliability and validity to ensure that quality of life is being assessed.[42] Standardized instruments are preferable, as they allow comparison across patient samples and disease states.[10]

The Southwest Oncology Group has recommended using several quality of life instruments in their cooperative clinical trials.[42] These include a generic measure of function, social, and psychological well-being (Medical Outcome Survey-Short Form),[52] a 13-item physical symptom instrument specific to cancer (Symptom Distress Scale),[58–60] and a global measure of quality of life (LASA Uniscale).[55] The Cancer Unit of the WHO has recently recommended using the Brief Pain Inventory (BPI)[62] to measure outcomes of pain management programs in patients with cancer.[71] The BPI is a pain-specific instrument, which includes items on pain intensity, quality, location, and relief, in addition to activity interference. Activity interference includes functional (e.g., ability to walk and work), emotional (mood, enjoyment in life), and social (interaction with others) items. A short form of the BPI also is available, with emphasis on pain, pain relief, and activity interference.[63] This is a particularly useful instrument for a brief assessment of patients with pain.

Timing of measures is important to capture the patterns of change in quality of life dimensions as treatment progresses. Moinpour et al.[42] recommend a minimum of three measurement points: prior to starting treatment, during treatment (when changes are most likely to occur), and on completing treatment. Timing of measures becomes more problematic when treatment arms are different in onset, peak action of treatment, and overall duration. This leads to multiple endpoints and poses difficulties for statistical analyses of endpoint data. Clinically, individual patient data can be plotted over time, which will provide an indication of disease and treatment response. Aggregated data may suggest patterns of response to various interventions. Alternatives to discrete measurement points include brief, daily measures of highly relevant aspects of quality of life. Examples of brief daily measures that have been used in patients with cancer include the Qualitator[72] and the daily diary card.[73]

Impact of Pain on Quality of Life

Pain is one of several symptoms included in quality of life measures (see Table 33-3 for pain items in selected quality of life measures). It is not surprising to find that pain is a critical attribute in patients' assessment of their quality of life,[36] and that pain interferes with functional status, psychological, and social well-being.[25] It is interesting to note that pain fluctuates differently from other quality of life dimensions when monitored daily,[73] and is not predictive of survival in patients in breast cancer trials.[74] Even factor analysis of quality of life items shows different configurations in cancer patients with and without pain.[5, 21] Physical symptoms, which are typically combined into one factor or scale, may not produce the high level of internal consistency desired in multi-item scales. For example, Ringdal and Ringdal[15] reported poor internal consistency of EORTC items tapping gastrointestinal disturbances, fatigue, and pain. Each symptom complex was more psychometrically sound when used alone. Pain has been consistently, if moderately, related to functional, physical, psychological, and social dimensions of quality of life.[15, 54, 62, 65]

To determine the impact of pain on quality of life, Strang and Qvarner[75] measured quality of life in 84 patients with cancer-related pain using a nine-item scale. They found that 76% of the patients reported that pain interfered with function, 56% were awakened from sleep by pain, 56% felt pain interfered with concentration, and 20% felt they had no or partial social support. Consistent with previous research,[16] greater anxiety and depression were associated with a higher level of pain.[75] Disruption in activity has been related to inadequate analgesic use in patients with cancer-related pain[71] and level of pain.[62] In a sample of 667 patients with cancer, a substantial increase in activity disruption was noted when pain increased from 4–5 on a scale of 0–10.[76] Pain can thus have a substantial impact on the functional, emotional, and social dimensions of quality of life.

Quality of Life as an Outcome for Pain Control Interventions

It is apparent that the multiple dimensions of pain overlap considerably with the multiple dimensions of quality of life. Use of well-developed and psychometrically sound quality of life instruments as measures of outcome in pain intervention research best uses our current knowledge base. For example, Ferrell et al.[77] used the QL Index to compare patient response to short-acting and controlled-release oral opioids in 83 patients with cancer-related pain. Findings suggested that controlled-release opioids were beneficial in terms of adjustment to disease, physical strength, social interaction, and pain relief while leading to more constipation and nausea early in treatment. The benefit may be related, at least in part, to better patient compliance with controlled-release oral opioids than with short-acting oral opioids. These data suggest that patients may benefit from controlled-release oral opioids, particularly if management of constipation and nausea are adequately addressed early in the treatment regimen.

A wide variety of interventions are available for managing cancer pain, as has been discussed in other chapters. Evaluating their effect in terms of pain relief is essential. However, if different interventions produce equal pain relief, knowledge of effects on quality of life may help the health care provider and patient select the best pain control strategies. For example, the sedative effects of opioid analgesics may affect function and social interaction to a degree that distresses the patient. Would the addition of nonopioid analgesics or adjuvant medications reduce opioid requirements to the point that the patient can complete role responsibilities and interact with family and friends? The impact of invasive pain control interventions on quality of life may be particularly relevant in decision making. Can the patient tolerate the numbness and loss of function associated with neuroablative procedures? Will spinal administration of opioids lead to uncomfortable and distressing physical symptoms that interfere with psychological well-being and social interaction? The use of a quality of life framework may broaden the type of intervention(s) used for a particular patient, including analgesic, invasive, and more psychologically based therapies.[14] Utility measures, although still in early development, may be applied when testing various pain management interventions.

The addition of brief, comprehensive quality of life instruments in research may help us improve pain control in patients with cancer. Clinically, quality of life assessment may provide critical information that can guide interventions and allow patients and health care providers to make informed decisions about pain management.

References

1. Portenoy RK. Cancer pain: Epidemiology and syndromes. Cancer 1989;63:2298.
2. Acute Pain Management Guideline Panel. Acute Pain Management: Operative or Medical Procedures and Trauma. Rockville, MD: AHCPR Pub. No. 92-0032, 1992.
3. Management of Cancer Pain Guideline Panel. Management of Cancer Pain. Rockville, MD: AHCPR, Publication No. 94-0592, 1994.
4. Ventafridda V, Tamburini M, Caraceni A, DeConno F. A validation study of the WHO method for cancer pain relief. Cancer 1987;59:850.
5. Ferrell BR, Wisdom C, Wenzl C. Quality of life as an outcome variable in the management of cancer pain. Cancer 1989;63:2321.
6. Padilla GV, Grant MM. Quality of life as a cancer nursing outcome variable. Adv Nurs Sci 1985;8:45.
7. Loewy JW, Kapadia AS, Hsi B, Davis BR. Statistical methods that distinguish between attributes of assessment: Prolongation of life versus quality of life. Med Decis Making 1992;12:83.
8. Johnson JR, Temple R. Food and Drug Administration requirements for approval of new anticancer drugs. Cancer Treat Rep 1985;69:1155.
9. World Health Organization. The First Ten Years of the World Health Organization. Geneva: WHO, 1958.
10. Aaronson NK. Quality of life research in cancer clinical trials: A need for common rules and language. Oncology 1990;4:59.
11. Aaronson NK. Assessment of quality of life and benefits from adjuvant therapies in breast cancer. Recent Results Cancer Res 1993;127:201.
12. Cella DF, Tulsky DS. Measuring quality of life today: Methodological aspects. Oncology 1990;4:29.
13. Cella DF, Tulsky DS. Quality of life in cancer: Definition, purpose, and method of measurement. Cancer Invest 1993;11:327.
14. Schipper H, Clinch J, Powell V. Definitions and Conceptual Issues. In B Spilke (ed), Quality of Life Assessments in Clinical Trials. New York: Raven, 1990;11.
15. Ringdal GI, Ringdal K. Testing the EORTC quality of life questionnaire on cancer patients with heterogeneous diagnoses. Quality Life Res 1993;2:129.
16. Shacham S, Reinhart LC, Raubertas RF, Cleeland CS. Emotional states and pain: Intraindividual and interindividual measures of association. J Behav Med 1983;6:405.
17. Blesch KS, Paice JA, Wickham R, et al. Correlates of fatigue in people with breast or lung cancer. Oncol Nurs Forum 1991;18:81.
18. Wortman C. Social support and the cancer patient. Cancer 1984;53:2339.
19. Williams JI, Wood-Dauphine S. Assessing Quality of Life: Measures and Utility. In F Mosteller, J Falotico-Taylor (eds), Quality of Life and Technology Assessment. Washington, DC: National Academy Press, 1989;65.
20. Ferrans CE. Development of a quality of life index for patients with cancer. Oncol Nurs Forum 1990;17 (Suppl. 3):15.
21. Ferrell B, Grant M, Padilla G, et al. The experience of pain and perceptions of quality of life: Validation of a conceptual model. Hospice J 1991;7:9.
22. Padilla GV, Grant M, Lipsett J, et al. Health quality of life and colorectal cancer. Cancer 1992;70:1450.
23. Ferrans CE, Powers MJ. Quality of life index: Development and psychometric properties. Adv Nurs Sci 1985;8:15.
24. Falotico-Taylor J, McClelland M, Mosteller F. Use of Quality-of-Life Measures in Technology Assessment. In F Mosteller, J Falotico-Taylor (eds), Quality of Life and Technology Assessment. Washington, DC: National Academy Press, 1989;7.
25. Moinpour CM, Chapman CR. Pain Management and Quality of Life in Cancer Patients. In KA Lehmann, D Zech (eds), Transdermal Fentanyl. London: Springer, 1991;42.
26. Sprangers MA, Aaronson NK. The role of health care providers and significant others in evaluating the quality of life of patients with chronic disease: A review. J Clin Epidemiol 1992;45:743.
27. Melzack R, Wall PD. The Challenge of Pain (2nd ed). London: Penguin, 1988.
28. Fraser SC, Dobbs HJ, Ebbs SR, et al. Combination or mild single agent chemotherapy for advanced breast cancer? CMF vs epirubicin measuring quality of life. Br J Cancer 1993;67:402.
29. Holmes S. Preliminary investigation of symptom distress in two cancer patient populations: Evaluation of a measurement instrument. J Adv Nurs 1991;16:439.

30. Schipper H, Clinch J, McMurray A, Levitt M. Measuring the quality of life of cancer patients: The Functional Living Index-Cancer (FLIC). Development and validation. J Clin Oncol 1984;2:472.

31. Oleson M. Subjectively perceived quality of life. Image 1990;20:187.

32. Olweny CL. Quality of life in cancer care. Med J Aust 1993;158:429.

33. Gelber RD, Goldhirsch A, Cole BF. Evaluation of effectiveness: Q-TWIST. Cancer Treat Rev 1993;19 (Suppl. A):73.

34. Kaplan RM. Quality of life assessment for cost/utility studies in cancer. Cancer Treat Rev 1993;19(Suppl. A):85.

35. Torrance GW. Measurement of health status for economic appraisal: A review. J Health Econ 1986;5:1.

36. Padilla GV, Ferrell B, Grant MM, Rhiner M. Defining the content domain of quality of life for cancer patients with pain. Cancer Nurs 1990;13:108.

37. Fries JF, Spitz PW. The Hierarchy of Patient Outcomes. In B Spilker (ed), Quality of Life Assessments in Clinical Trials. New York: Raven, 1990;25.

38. Gelber RD, Goldhirsch A, Cavalli F. Quality-of-life-adjusted evaluation of adjuvant therapies for operable breast cancer. Ann Intern Med 1991;114:621.

39. Gelber RD, Cole BF, Goldhirsch A. How to compare quality of life of breast cancer patients in clinical trials. International breast cancer study group. Recent Results Cancer Res 1993;127:221.

40. Morris J, Goddard M. Economic evaluation and quality of life assessments in cancer clinical trials: The CHART trial. Eur J Cancer 1993;29A:766.

41. Guyatt GH, Jaeschke R. Measurements in Clinical Trials: Choosing the Appropriate Approach. In B Spilker (ed), Quality of Life Assessments in Clinical Trials. New York: Raven, 1990;37.

42. Moinpour CM, Feigel P, Metch B, et al. Quality of life end points in cancer clinical trials: Review and recommendations. J Natl Cancer Inst 1989;81:485.

43. Donovan K, Sanson-Fisher RW, Redman S. Measuring quality of life in cancer patients. J Clin Oncol 1989;7:959.

44. Bergner M, Bobbitt RA, Carter WB, et al. The Sickness Impact Profile: Development and final revision of a health status measure. Med Care 1981;19:787.

45. Bergner M. Development, Testing, and Use of the Sickness Impact Profile. In SR Walker, RM Rosser (eds), Quality of Life Assessment: Key Issues in the 1990's. Boston: Kluwer, 1993;95.

46. Hunt SM, McKenna SP, McEwen J, et al. A quantitative approach to preceived health status. J Epidemiol Community Health 1980;34:281.

47. Hunt SM, McKenna SP, Williams J. Reliability of a population survey tool for measuring perceived problems. A study of patients with osteoarthrosis. J Epidemiol Community Health 1981;35:297.

48. Hunt SM, McKenna SP, McEwen J, et al. The Nottingham health profile: Subjective health status and medical consultations. Soc Sci Med 1981;15A:221.

49. McEwen J. The Nottingham Health Profile. In SR Walker, RM Rosser (eds), Quality of Life Assessment: Key Issues in the 1990's. Boston: Kluwer, 1993;111.

50. Chambers LW, MacDonald LA, Tugwell P, et al. The McMaster Health Index Questionnaire as a measure of quality of life for patients with rheumatoid disease. J Rheumatol 1982;9:780.

51. Chambers LW. The McMaster Health Index Questionnaire: An Update. In SR Walker, RM Rosser (eds), Quality of Life Assessment: Key Issues in the 1990's. Boston: Kluwer, 1993;131.

52. Stewart AL, Hays RD, Ware JE. The MOS short-from general health survey: Reliability and validity in a patient population. Med Care 1988;26:724.

53. Padilla GV, Presant G, Grant MM, et al. Quality of life index for patients with cancer. Res Nurs Health 1983;6:117.

54. Aaronson NK, Ahmedzai S, Bergman B, et al. The European Organization for Research and Treatment of Cancer QLQ-C30: A quality of life instrument for use in international clinical trials in oncology. J Natl Cancer Inst 1993;85:365.

55. Selby PJ, Chapman JAW, Etazadi-Amoli J, et al. The development of a method for assessing the quality of life in cancer patients. Br J Cancer 1984;50:13.

56. Coates A, Dillenbeck CF, McNeil DR, et al. On the receiving end. II. Linear analogue self-assessment (LASA) in evaluation of aspects of the quality of life of cancer patients receiving therapy. Eur J Cancer Clin Oncol 1983;19:1633.

57. Cella DF, Tulsky DS, Gray G, et al. The functional assessment of cancer therapy scale: Development and validation of the general measure. J Clin Oncol 1993;11:570.

58. McCorkle R, Young K. Development of a symptom distress scale. Cancer Nurs 1978;1:373.

59. McCorkle R, Benoliel JQ. Symptom distress, current concerns and mood disturbance after diagnosis of life-threatening disease. Soc Sci Med 1983;17:431.

60. McCorkle R. The measurement of symptom distress. Semin Oncol Nurs 1987;3:248.

61. de Haes JC, van Knippenberg FC, Neijt JP. Measuring psychological and physical distress in cancer patients: Structure and application of the Rotterdam Symptom Checklist. Br J Cancer 1990;62:1034.

62. Daut RL, Cleeland CS, Flanery RC. Development of the Wisconsin Brief Pain Questionnaire to assess pain in cancer and other diseases. Pain 1983;17:197.

63. Cleeland CC. Measurement of Pain by Subjective Report. In CR Chapman, JD Loeser (eds), Issues in Pain Measurement. New York: Raven, 1989;391.

64. Aaronson NK, Bullinger M, Ahmedzai S. A modular approach to quality of life assessment in cancer clinical trials. Recent Results Cancer Res 1988;3:231.

65. Bjordal K, Kaasa S. Psychometric validation of the EORTC core quality of life questionnaire, 30-item version and a diagnosis-specific module for head and neck

cancer patients. Acta Oncol 1992;31:311.

66. Jones E, Lund VJ, Howard DJ, et al. Quality of life of patients treated surgically for head and neck cancer. J Laryngol Otol 1992;106:238.

67. Hollen PJ, Gralla RJ, Kris MG, Potanovich LM. Quality of life assessment in individuals with lung cancer: Testing the lung cancer symptom scale (LCSS). Eur J Cancer 1993;29A(Suppl. 1):S51.

68. McNair DM, Lorr M, Droppleman LF. Manual for the Profile of Mood States. San Diego, CA: Educational Testing Service, 1971.

69. Finkelstein DM, Cassileth BR, Bonomi PG, et al. A pilot study of the Functional Living Index-Cancer (FLIC) scale for the assessment of quality of life for metastatic lung cancer patients. Am J Clin Oncol 1988;11:630.

70. Barofsky I, Sugarbaker KT. Cancer. In B Spilke (ed), Quality of Life Assessments in Clinical Trials. New York: Raven, 1990;419.

71. Ward SE, Goldberg N, Miller-McCauley V, et al. Patient-related barriers to management of cancer pain. Pain 1993;52:319.

72. Fraser SC, Ramirez AJ, Ebbs SR, et al. A daily diary for quality of life measurement in advanced breast cancer trials. Br J Cancer 1993;67:341.

73. Geddes DM, Dones L, Hill E, et al. Quality of life during chemotherapy for small cell lung cancer: Assessment and use of a daily diary care in a randomized trial. Eur J Cancer 1990;26:484.

74. Coates A, Gebski V, Signorini D, et al. Prognostic value of quality of life scores during chemotherapy for advanced breast cancer. Australian New Zealand breast cancer trials group. J Clin Oncol 1992;10:1833.

75. Strang P, Qvarner H. Cancer-related pain and its influence on quality of life. Anticancer Res 1990;10:109.

76. Daut RL, Cleeland CS. The prevalence and severity of pain in cancer. Cancer 1982;50:1913.

77. Ferrell B, Wisdom C, Wenzl C, Brown J. Effects of controlled-release morphine on quality of life for cancer patients. Oncol Nurs Forum 1989;16:521.

Chapter 34

Surgical Approaches

William O. Richards and Steven P. Key

Chronic pain syndromes can dramatically affect the patient's quality of life and can lead to long-term suffering and disability.[1] The effective operative management of chronic pain depends on the timely execution of a multidisciplinary approach to the syndrome, which usually involves physiotherapeutic and psychological interventions in addition to the operative procedure. Like other disease processes, chronic pain syndromes are more amenable to therapy when treated early in their course. The surgeon can surgically remove the tumor, thus removing the underlying cause of pain. However, oftentimes the surgeon must deal with a patient who has an unresectable primary or recurrent tumor whose severe pain must be addressed. This chapter discusses surgical resection and other surgical procedures (palliative and therapeutic) for the cancer patient.

Surgical Resection

There are several procedures that can be used for operative intervention to relieve chronic pain. Operative resection, even palliative resection, often gives the best and longest lasting relief of pain. Because of tremendous advances in surgical and anesthetic care, major operative procedures once associated with prohibitive perioperative morbidity and mortality can be performed with relatively low risk to the patient. Thus, palliative resection of the esophagus,[2] stomach,[3] pancreas,[4] small intestine,[5] and other organs can often be the most effective

therapy. Recurrent rectal cancer locally invasive in the pelvis can cause severe debilitating pain. Patients with large, bulky rectal neoplasms who undergo total pelvic exenteration will prevent the occurrence of intestinal obstruction and will also receive palliation for pain syndrome.[6] Indeed, many tumors of the alimentary tract may become resectable after a course of radiation therapy and chemotherapy. Multimodality treatments not only enhance the chance for cure, but also produce long-term effective palliation, especially from pain.[7]

Intraoperative Celiac Plexus Block

Despite advances in diagnostic modalities, 90% of patients with pancreatic carcinoma present with advanced regional or metastatic involvement at the time of diagnosis. The dominant symptom is usually pain, which occurs in 80–95% of patients with advanced stages of pancreatic carcinoma and is thought to correlate directly with shortened survival.[8] Therefore, both as a palliative and therapeutic measure, pain control is vitally important in the management of the patient with cancer of the pancreas.

Cancer of the pancreas produces chronic midepigastric pain that radiates to the back. Pain occurs as a result of obstruction of the pancreatic duct, inflammation, and infiltration of the pancreatic connective tissue, capillaries, and afferent nerves. The intensity of this pain usually parallels the severe progressive nature of this disease. The pain experienced with chronic pancreatitis is thought to be from hypertensive main pancreatic duct and pseudocyst formation. Pancreaticoduodenectomy may provide satisfactory pain relief with a low incidence of reoperation for pain control. Postoperative mortality is usually less than 2%.[4, 9]

Although some surgeons believe that obstruction of the pancreatic and common bile duct is responsible for most of the chronic abdominal pain associated with pancreatic cancer, biliary bypass and gastrojejunostomy procedures have failed to alleviate the pain in most patients.[10] Even in those patients who experience some improvement in their pain, symptoms usually worsen within a few weeks to a few months after operation. Additional procedures to drain the obstructed pancreatic duct are not routinely performed because of the increased morbidity and mortality associated with pancreatic anastomoses. In the past, many surgeons have performed palliative procedures that did not address the pain associated with the disease.

Percutaneous celiac plexus block with alcohol or phenol is the most commonly used modality for chronic abdominal pain caused by pancreatic carcinoma. Chemical splanchnicectomy for the treatment of chronic abdominal pain from cancer has been known about since the early 1900s. Adequate pain control may last for many months after the injection. Additional benefits include decreased need for narcotic analgesics, decreased nausea and vomiting, increased food intake, and improved bowel motility.[8] Anticipated side effects of chemical celiac plexus blockade include orthostatic hypotension, dizziness, increased gut motility, and urinary retention. The percutaneous technique involved a transaortic, transcrural, or a bilateral puncture with the patient in the prone position.

Chemical splanchnicectomy may also be performed under direct vision at the time of operation for surgical palliation of biliary obstruction and gastric outlet obstruction. Injection of the neurolytic agent into the junction area of the splanchnic nerves with the celiac ganglia also decreases nausea and vomiting by interfering with branches of the vagus nerve that innervate the pancreas. In patients with unresectable pancreatic cancer who underwent operative splanchnicectomy, Sharp[11] reported *complete* relief of pain in 83% and partial relief of pain in the remaining 17%. Furthermore, no adverse effects of intraoperative nerve blocks were noted in that series. The complications resulting from percu-

taneous celiac blocks are related to inadvertent injection of alcohol into the aorta and include bleeding, hypotension, and pancreatitis. Because intraoperative celiac plexus blocks (Figure 34-1) are performed under direct vision, there is minimal chance for inadvertent intravascular injection and resultant complications.

Lillemoe et al.[12] undertook a prospective randomized blinded study of plexus (saline) injection versus alcohol celiac plexus blocks in 137 patients with unresectable pancreatic cancer. No complications were related to the celiac plexus block when the celiac plexus was directly visible. When compared with placebo, patients receiving intraoperative chemical splanchnicectomy with alcohol resulted in significantly lower pain scores (Figure 34-2). Those patients with preoperative pain who underwent alcohol splanchnicectomy demonstrated a significant improvement in survival when compared with controls (Figure 34-3).[12] This prolongation in life from pain relief after surgical splanchnicectomy would be hailed as one of the most important advances of the decade if it resulted from traditional chemotherapy. This improvement in actuarial survival is thought to result from improved psychological well-being and nutrition. Splanchnicectomy and celiac axis blocks are less effective when the cancer has spread beyond regions supplied by the splanchnic nerves. Nevertheless, a strong argument can be made for intraoperative celiac plexus blocks in all patients undergoing exploration for surgical bypass, because most patients are relieved of their pain usually until death.

Thoracoscopic Splanchnicectomy

Thoracoscopic splanchnicectomy involves resection of the greater and lesser splanchnic nerves around the sympathetic chain (Figure 34-4), rather than injection of neurolytic agents.[13] This technique offers improved visualization of the splanchnic fibers because the splanchnic chain is readily identified through the parietal pleura. Following splanchnicectomy, regardless of technique, 70% of patients are relieved of pain for at least 1 month or until death. This technique can be performed in patients with intractable pain and who have failed or are unsuitable for celiac plexus block. The site of greatest pain, either the right or left side, is set up first. McKernan and Laws[14] estimate that 30% of pa-

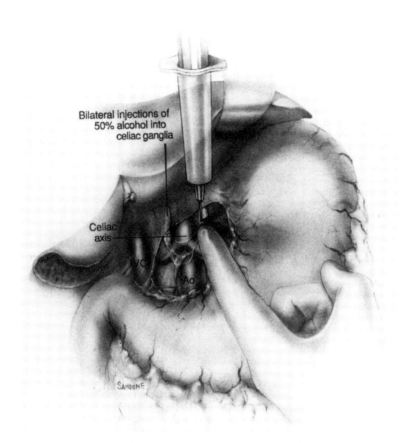

Bilateral injections of
50% alcohol into
celiac ganglia

Celiac
axis

IVC

Ao

SANDONE

Figure 34-1. Operative chemical splanchnicectomy performed by the operating surgeon with injection of 20 ml of absolute alcohol on each side of the aorta at the level of the celiac axis. (IVC = inferior vena cava; AO = aorta.) (Reprinted with permission from KD Lillemoe. Chemical splanchnicectomy: An unresectable pancreatic cancer. Ann Surg 1993;217:447.)

tients will require resection of the splanchnic nerves on the other side of the chest. Because the actual nerves are resected, pain relief usually is long-term (years) after the procedure. This procedure, which at one time required thoracotomy, can now be performed using minimally invasive techniques requiring a reduced hospital stay and decreased recovery time, which is more acceptable to the patients.

Recurrent Mechanical Obstruction Secondary to Cancer

Practitioners are often faced with patients who have previously undergone curative or palliative surgery for abdominal malignancy and who present with signs and symptoms of mechanical bowel obstruction. Because of abdominal distention and cramps associated with mechanical obstruction, these pa-

tients are usually in a great deal of discomfort and pain. Nevertheless, because of the concern of widespread metastatic disease, many surgeons are reluctant to operate for fear they may face unresectable metastatic disease and that they may be unable to alleviate the mechanical obstruction or provide any other palliation for these patients. Unfortunately, nasogastric tube decompression provides little palliation to these patients and consideration of operative therapy to alleviate the obstruction or bypass should be encouraged. Gallick et al.[15] identified 50 patients with intra-abdominal malignancies who, after primary treatment, subsequently developed small bowel obstruction. Thirteen of those patients had obstruction secondary to nonmalignant causes. Thus, a significant proportion of patients with previous surgical resection for abdominal malignancy did present with mechanical obstruction that was not due to malignancy. Obviously, it would be wise

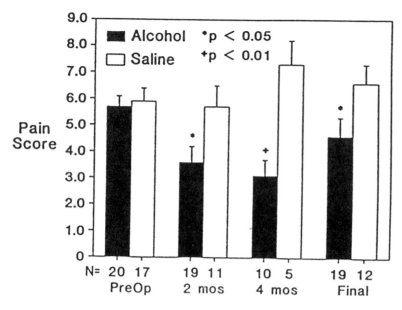

Figure 34-2. The impact of operative splanchnicectomy with alcohol injection on pain score compared with the control group (saline). Operative splanchnicectomy profoundly affects postoperative pain, with a nadir at 4 months. Patients with saline injection experienced even more pain postoperative to a peak at 4 months postoperatively. (Reprinted with permission from KD Lillemoe. Chemical splanchnicectomy: An unresectable pancreatic cancer. Ann Surg 1993;217:447.)

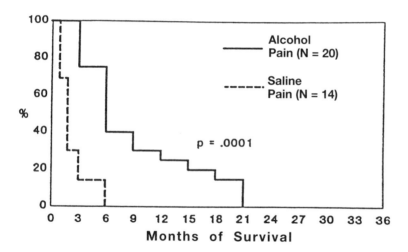

Figure 34-3. Kaplan-Meier survival cures demonstrating profound impact on survival in patients treated with operative splanchnicectomy with alcohol injection as compared with survival achieved by the saline (central) group. Here, operative splanchnicectomy not only profoundly affects pain control, but improves survival. (Reprinted with permission from KD Lillemoe. Chemical splanchnicectomy: An unresectable pancreatic cancer. Ann Surg 1993;217:447.)

to subject these patients to an appropriate diagnostic workup that, in many cases, includes exploratory laparotomy. Alleviation of the mechanical obstruction restores the patient's sense of well-being and alleviates pain associated with mechanical intestinal obstruction. Many patients with mechanical obstruction secondary to malignant disease are able to have either a bypass or localized resection of the tumor performed, thus alleviating the mechanical obstruction. This patient group resolved their pain

and discomfort from the mechanical obstruction once an appropriate bypass was performed.

What about other forms of treatment? Some clinicians have used nonoperative methods, such as nasogastric tube decompression, intravenous fluids, and increasing doses of narcotics to treat patients. Unfortunately, a large number of patients (41%) who initially responded to this nonoperative management were readmitted with the same symptoms within 30 days of discharge. Thus, the delay of exploratory laparotomy only increases morbidity and mortality and does not provide pain control or palliation.[15]

Laparoscopy

Laparoscopy will define the etiology in 55% of patients with chronic abdominal pain. In some cases, therapeutic interventions via the laparoscope will prove definitive in patients with known cancer, but with continued abdominal pain.[16] Diagnostic laparoscopy provides an opportunity to exclude other causes of chronic abdominal pain including endometriosis, inflammatory bowel disease, tumor, ovarian cyst, and adhesions, as well as providing an opportunity for concurrent therapeutic intervention. The use of a minimally invasive technique such as laparoscopy to identify the etiology of chronic abdominal pain has dramatically decreased the morbidity associated with the procedure and has helped improve the quality of life for these patients.

Laparoscopy is instrumental in the evaluation and treatment of chronic pelvic pain (CPP). Pelvic pathology can be identified in 60% of patients with CPP. Endometriosis is diagnosed most frequently (38.3%).[17, 18] Approximately 40% of all laparoscopic procedures performed by gynecologists in the United States are done to evaluate pelvic pain. Laparoscopy may reveal a cause for the pain in more than 50% of cases.[19] In the primary care setting, as many as 84% of patients with CPP may be helped by laparoscopic lysis of an adhesion.[20] Surgical therapy includes removal of endometrial implants, presacral neurectomy, and lysis of adhesions. Hysterectomy is often performed as a last resort. Although lysis of adhesions is beneficial in most cases, investigation of organic disease should not exclude evaluation of any psychosocial factors that may play a significant part in the patient's disease process.

Presacral neurectomy, or transection of the hypogastric plexus, performed via laparotomy has been used successfully to control pelvic pain since 1899.[21] This modality, which is performed laparoscopically in the outpatient setting as the laparoscopic uterine nerve ablation procedure, has become an effective and convenient way to evaluate and treat CPP.[21, 22] Approximately 2–3 cm of the superior hypogastric plexus and the initial segments of the inferior hypogastric plexuses are resected. The average operating time is 90 minutes. Uterosacral ligament

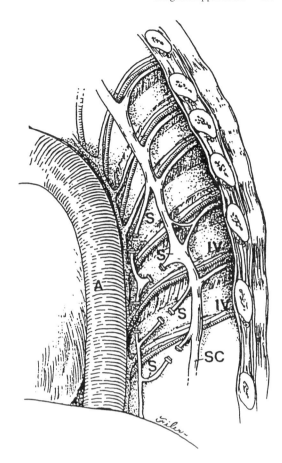

Figure 34-4. Diagram demonstrates operative splanchnicectomy as depicted from the left thoracic cavity. Splanchnic nerves are divided along several intercostal spaces. The sympathetic chain (SC) is readily visible through the pleura. (IV= intercostal vessels; A= aorta; S = splanchic nerve branches.) (Reprinted with permission from J Worsey. Thoracoscopic pancreatic denervation for pain control in irresectable cancer. Br J Surg 1993;80:1051.)

transection offers no greater success. Unfortunately, less than half the patients treated by laparoscopic uterine nerve ablation experience adequate pain relief 12 months following therapy.

Vascular Access Procedures

Surgeons now implant a large number of long-term central venous catheters for administration of medication, parenteral nutrition, chemotherapy, as well as access to chronic blood drawing. These have revolutionized the outpatient treatment of many patients with tumors for chemotherapy administration, malnutrition with treatment of total parenteral nutrition, and also for patients with intractable pain syndromes for chronic administration of narcotics. The Hickman catheter, which can have up to three lumens, is the catheter most frequently inserted in the United States. The concept behind the Hickman catheter is that contamination with skin flora is inhibited by a long subcutaneous tunnel and the ingrowth of tissue into a fibrous pledget just underneath the skin at the exit site. In addition, the catheter itself is made of a nonthrombogenic material that is soft enough to prevent erosion of the catheter through the vascular structure, usually the subclavian vein, superior vena cava, or right atrium. However, Hickman catheters require meticulous care because they require an exit site. Also, daily flushing of the ports with a heparinized saline solution is essential to prevent thrombosis. Generally speaking, it is thought that the more ports that a catheter has, the more likely catheter sepsis will occur due to the number of times it must be handled and flushed. Furthermore, an operative morbidity to the procedure is related to complications from puncture of the lung or pleural cavity during insertion of the catheter, which results in a pneumothorax and sometimes requires treatment using a chest tube until the air leak seals. Long-term complications related to catheter use include venous thrombosis and superior vena cava syndrome. Other types of vascular access include port-a-caths, which are accessed via a needle inserted into the port through the overlying skin. The advantages of the completely covered port are reduced infection rate because the port is completely covered with skin and increased patient acceptance because the port is cosmetically appealing and requires less care (i.e., skin cleansing and sterile dressing changes).

Feeding Gastrostomy Tubes

While long-term intravenous access can be obtained for administration of total parenteral nutrition, if the gastrointestinal tract can be used for feeding it is generally much more physiologic, cheaper, and less likely to develop infections or thrombotic complications related to long-term placement in the superior vena cava. Most tubes placed now are percutaneous endoscopic gastrostomy tubes. The placement of these tubes can be done under intravenous sedation and local anesthesia and is generally much better tolerated in patients with tumors because they are minimally invasive procedures. In patients with severe anorexia, placement of a feeding gastrostomy tube can help supplement the oral intake of protein and calories. Similarly, for patients with head and neck tumors, esophageal tumors, or other tumors that make it difficult or painful for the patient to swallow, placement of tubes into the stomach can be extremely beneficial to the overall well-being of the patient.

There are a wide variety of surgical approaches for alleviating cancer pain. Of great importance is the realization that surgeons can provide tremendous postoperative pain relief, specifically directed to patients with cancer pain. It is hoped that surgeons will adopt many of the techniques discussed in the chapter.

References

1. Ashburn MA, Fine PG. Evaluation and treatment of chronic pain syndromes. Compr Ther 1990;16:37.
2. Stewart JR, Hoff SJ, Johnson DH, et al. Improved survival with neoadjuvant therapy and resection for adenocarcinoma of the esophagus. Ann Surg 1993;218:571.
3. Scott HW, Adkins RB, Sawyers JL. Results of an aggressive surgical approach to gastric carcinoma during a 23 year period. Surgery 1985;97:55.
4. Cameron JL, Pitt HA, Yeo CJ, et al. One hundred and forty-five consecutive pancreaticoduodenectomies without mortality. Ann Surg 1993;217:430.
5. Richards WO Jr. Obstruction of the Large and Small Intestine. In JL Sawyers, LF Williams (eds), The Acute Abdomen. Philadelphia: Saunders, 1988;355.
6. Williams LF, Huddleston CB, Sawyers JL, et al. Is total pelvic exenteration reasonable primary treatment for rectal carcinoma? Ann Surg 1988;207:670.
7. Kahn PJ, Skornick Y, Inbar M, et al. Surgical palliation combined with synchronous therapy in pancreatic carcinoma. Eur J Surg Oncol 1990;16:7.
8. Lebovits AH, Lefkowitz M. Pain management of pancreatic carcinoma: A review. Pain 1989;36:1.
9. Howard JM, Zhang Z. Pancreaticoduodenectomy (Whipple resection) in the treatment of chronic pancreatitis. World J Surg 1990;14:77.
10. Singh SM, Reber HA. Surgical palliation for pancreatic cancer. Surg Clin North Am 1989;69:599.
11. Sharp KW, Stevens EJ. Improving palliation in pancreatic cancer: Intraoperative celiac plexus block for pain relief. South Med J 1991;84:469.

12. Lillemoe KD, Cameron JL, Kaufman HS, et al. Splanchnicectomy in patients with unresectable pancreatic cancer. Ann Surg 1993;217:447.
13. Worsey J, Ferson PF, Keenan RJ, et al. Thoracoscopic pancreatic denervation for pain control in irresectable pancreatic cancer. Br J Surg 1993;80:1051.
14. McKernan JB, Laws HL. Thoracoscopic vagotomy, sympathectomy, and splanchnicectomy. Laparoscopic Surg 1994;2:71.
15. Gallick HL, Weaver DW, Sachs RJ, et al. Intestinal obstruction in cancer patients. Am Surg 1986;8:434.
16. Salky BA. Laparoscopy for Surgeons. New York: Igaku-Shoin, 1990;152.
17. Vercellini P, Fedele L, Arcaini L, et al. Laparoscopy in the diagnosis of chronic pelvic pain in adolescent women. J Reprod Med 1989;34:827.
18. Kames LD, Rapkin AJ, Naliboff BD, et al. Effectiveness of an interdisciplinary pain management program for the treatment of chronic pelvic pain. Pain 1990;41:41.
19. Hurt WG. Outpatient gynecologic procedures. Surg Clin North Am 1991;71:1099.
20. Steege JF, Stout AL. Resolution of chronic pelvic pain after laparoscopic lysis of adhesions. Am J Obstet Gynecol 1991;165:278.
21. Perez JJ. Laparoscopic presacral neurectomy. Results of the first 25 cases. J Reprod Med 1990;35:625.
22. Nezhat C, Nezhat F. A simplified method of laparoscopic presacral neurectomy for the treatment of central pelvic pain due to endometriosis. Br J Obstet Gynecol 1992;99:659.

Chapter 35

Neurosurgical Approaches

Bennett Blumenkopf

Pain represents the most common presenting complaint of people to their physician. Pain generally subserves a "protective usefulness" to the organism. However, many times its usefulness is lost, at which time it becomes a debilitating effect.

The cause and duration of pain often has a significant impact on the medical management. The two broad etiologic categories are benign pain and malignant pain. The former includes pain due to a multitude of causes, whereas the latter is pain associated with cancer, generally widespread metastatic disease. One may also consider the physiologic causes of pain: somatic pain due to ongoing tissue injury with the resultant release of a variety of neurohumoral agents, and neurogenic or deafferentation pain resulting from injury to either the peripheral or central nervous system (CNS). Pain is considered acute if it has been relatively short-lived, and if one has an expectation of its imminent resolution. Chronic pain, on the other hand, is persistently present with no foreseeable resolution.

Malignant pain generally is somatic in nature, but may have a neurogenic or deafferentation component. Involvement of osseous structures leads to pathologic fractures with pain resulting from soft tissue damage, mechanical or structural instability, and peripheral nervous system and CNS compression. In addition, direct infiltration of neural structures results not only in functional deficits, but also significant discomfort. Deafferentation pain involves the perception of painful sensations such as burning, tearing, throbbing, and so forth, in a region of the body that is partially or totally sensorially deprived.

Thus, all or some of the peripheral nociceptors are physically disconnected from the central centers. Finally, the pain of cancer may frequently have an acute onset. The pain may become chronic, however, depending on the extent of the underlying disease.

Neurosurgeons are frequently involved in the management of painful disorders, particularly in the context of malignant disease. This involvement may directly address the underlying mechanism for the pain, such as in the case of spinal instability from a pathologic compression fracture treated by stabilization and fusion. However, the neurosurgical approach can only attempt to achieve palliation of the pain. This chapter reviews some aspects of malignant pain management from a neurosurgical standpoint. A review of the basic anatomy and physiology involved in pain transmission is presented initially. With this basic understanding, we then discuss several of the neurosurgical procedures used to alleviate malignant pain.

Neuroanatomy and Neurophysiology of Pain

One must understand the anatomy and physiology of pain transmission in order to understand the many causes of pain and also the procedures used to alleviate it.[1-3] The nervous system involves the peripheral nerves that convey the important sensory information about the organism to the central centers: the spinal cord, brain stem, and the brain. The skin, mucous membranes, and periosteum may be considered the most peripheral expanse of the nervous system because these structures contain the sensory receptors. Some receptors are very specific for a single modality whereas others are polymodal.

When considering the perception of pain, free nerve endings are generally thought to represent the receptor. The impulses generated by these free nerve endings are then conveyed to the central centers by the peripheral nerves. Among the various subtypes of peripheral nerve fibers, two appear especially concerned with nociceptive transmission—the nonmyelinated C fibers and the thinly myelinated A-delta fibers—and seem to subserve different types of pain experience. The A-delta fibers are faster conducting fibers and reflect a sharp, localized pain. The unmyelinated C fibers are slower conducting fibers and thus convey a poorly localized dull, burning, aching sensation.

The cell bodies or neurons of all the nociceptive afferent fibers are located within the dorsal root ganglia of each spinal root or the gasserian ganglia of the trigeminal roots. These neurons are bipolar, with their central connections in the spinal cord or brain stem. The central fibers of the primary nociceptive afferents—the A-delta and C fibers—terminate in the superficial regions of the dorsal aspect of the spinal cord, specifically laminae I, II, III of Rexed. It is in this region, the dorsal root entry zone (DREZ), that the first integration of pain information occurs.

The neurons in the DREZ project their fibers—the secondary nociceptive afferents—to the thalamus. These fibers constitute the lateral spinothalamic tract, which decussates within a segment or two of its segmental level and traverses the anterolateral column of the spinal cord. An additional pathway of secondary afferents projects to the brain stem reticular formation. Both the direct spinothalamic tract and the indirect spinoreticulothalamic tract terminate in the thalamus, especially the ventrobasal complex. From the thalamus, tertiary projections go to the cerebral cortex, specifically the primary and secondary somatosensory areas.

There are other neural systems that attempt to modify pain. In the peripheral nerves, the large myelinated A-alpha and A-beta fibers have an inhibitory effect on the spinothalamic neurons. This effect is probably mediated by inhibitory interneurons locally at each level of the dorsal horn laminae II and III. Also, the dorsal column nuclei and other brain stem locations project caudally to laminae I,

IV, and V and, with direct stimulation, inhibit the activity in the nociceptive thalamic cells.

Several compounds appear to be involved in the processing of nociceptive information at the DREZ level. These compounds include the "classical neurotransmitters," such as the excitatory and inhibitory amino acids and catecholamines. The recent discovery of several previously described gastrointestinal tract peptides in the CNS has significantly advanced the understanding of neural transmission, especially of pain signals. When considering pain signals, the concept of a neuromodulator, a compound that modifies the responses of neurons to other transmitters and, thereby, modulates synaptic transmission, has been proposed. Neuropeptides have been identified in the small ganglia cells mentioned previously, in the axons of the dorsal roots, and in axon terminals in the superficial dorsal horn laminae (I and II). This group includes substance P, somatostatin, cholecystokinin, calcitonin gene-related product, vasoactive intestinal polypeptide, neurotensin, and the endogenous opiates or endorphins. Substance P, somatostatin, cholecystokinin, calcitonin gene-related product, and vasoactive intestinal polypeptide are important products of the primary sensory neurons. Endorphins reduce the responsiveness of dorsal horn neurons to noxious stimulation both through interneurons at a segmental level and through a descending inhibitory system. Intracisternal neurotensin produces a potent antinociceptive response that is insensitive to naloxone.

Neurosurgical Pain Procedures

Peripheral Procedures

Based on this knowledge, several neurosurgical procedures can be performed to alleviate malignant pain (Table 35-1). Most peripherally, the peripheral nerve carrying the pain fibers from the periphery can be addressed. One may suppose that cutting a nerve (peripheral neurectomy) would abolish future pain impulses conveyed from the periphery and, thereby, abolish pain. However, there are several problems associated with this approach that limit its applicability. There is a significant overlap in the distribution of innervation among the peripheral nerves. Thus, rarely is pain limited to the zone of a single peripheral nerve. Furthermore, most periph-

Table 35-1. Neurosurgical Pain Procedures

Peripheral
    Peripheral neurectomy
    Rhizotomy
    Selective posterior rhizotomy
    Ganglionectomy
Central
    Spinal cord
        Cordotomy
        Midline myelotomy
        Spinal stimulator
        Intraspinal narcotic analgesia
        Dorsal root entry zone lesion
    Brain
        Mesencephalotomy
        Brain stimulator
        Hypophysectomy

eral nerves are mixed motor and sensory. A peripheral neurectomy procedure could, therefore, incur an unacceptable neurologic deficit. Accordingly, this procedure is rarely done to control malignant pain. Peripheral nerve stimulation has also frequently been used to manage chronic pain. This approach attempts to selectively stimulate the large myelinated fibers, which inhibit the nociceptive pathway at the level of the dorsal horn. This may be performed with either a transcutaneous or implanted device, but has not been commonly applied to the pain of cancer.

The next most proximal approach involves sectioning of the sensory fibers that comprise the peripheral nerves. This procedure (rhizotomy)[4–6] may be performed extradurally or intradurally. In the former, the entire dorsal root is sectioned, whereas in the latter the multiple rootlets are cut. Selective posterior rhizotomy[7] has also been described; this procedure limits the involvement to the ventrolateral aspect of the rootlet, where the small fibers are organized. Rhizotomy has proved useful in the management of pain due to malignant involvement in a restricted or segmental distribution such as the brachial plexus (Pancoast's syndrome), the chest wall, and, occasionally, the pelvis.

Excision of the sensory ganglia (ganglionectomy)[8] has also been proposed for segmentally restricted pain of malignant origin. This procedure removes the dorsal root ganglia at multiple levels. A suggestion has been made that this procedure has an advantage over sensory rhizotomy because a percentage (up to 20%) of the nociceptive afferents traverse the ventral root.

Central Procedures

Spinal Cord

Several procedures are performed on the spinal cord itself in an attempt to palliate malignant pain. These procedures include a destruction of the lateral spinothalamic tract (cordotomy)[9] through either a formal hemilaminectomy, usually in the thoracic region, with sectioning of the tract, or, more recently, through a percutaneous approach performed at C-1 to C-2 level using a radiofrequency electrode. Cordotomy results in a contralateral analgesia below the level of the procedure and is remarkably effective for malignant pain that is predominately one-sided, e.g., a metastasis in the femur. Bilateral cordotomies are generally not performed due to a high risk of respiratory complications, thus essentially eliminating the applicability of this procedure for widespread metastatic involvement.

A procedure that simultaneously divides the decussating nociceptive fibers from both sides of the body at the level of the anterior commissure (midline commissurotomy or myelotomy)[10] has been used in cases of midline perineal, pelvic, and rectal pain of malignant etiologies. Through a single cord incision, bilateral effects are thereby produced, provided the site of the pain is limited. This procedure does, however, have a significant morbidity risk of paraplegia or visceroplegia and is not generally popular.

Stimulation of the spinal cord particularly through the dorsal columns (dorsal column stimulator or spinal cord stimulator)[11] has been applied generally to cases of chronic benign pain. The stimulation current presumably activates the descending inhibitory pathways to provide pain relief. Paresthesias are perceived with the stimulation, which should also be in the distribution of the pain. The success of spinal stimulation for pain relief has generally been modest at best. This factor, coupled with the expenses for the device and its implantation, have severely limited its usefulness in malignant pain syndromes.

Finally, an approach to pain relief at a spinal level that takes advantage of the basic neurochemistry of pain (intraspinal narcotic analgesia)[12, 13] has gained widespread popularity. When instilled directly into the cerebrospinal fluid or into the epidural space, small doses of morphine or other opiates provide profound and prolonged analgesia and thus have been used for cases of metastatic malignancy. A variety of pump devices have been designed for chronic therapy. Tolerance to the opiate remains a problem and a long-term concern. In addition, the economic costs suggest that this approach be used in those cases with a reasonable (e.g., 4–6 month) life expectancy.

Brain

As is the case at the spinal cord level, both stimulation and ablation procedures for malignant pain have been described. Regions in the mesencephalon and diencephalon are approached using stereotaxic techniques. Stereotaxic mesencephalotomy[14] is indicated for cephalobrachial pain due to carcinoma that may involve the skull base or proximal upper extremity. A radiofrequency lesion is made after placement of the electrodes in the rostral midbrain (Figure 35-1). This procedure relieves not only the pain itself but also the suffering associated with it. Stimulation of areas in the midbrain and thalamus (deep brain stimulation)[15, 16] has also been used in cases of malignant pain. The stimulating electrode(s) are placed using stereotactic coordinates and a trial phase of stimulation is performed. The analgesia following midbrain stimulation appears to be opiate mediated, whereas that following thalamic stimulation does not. Midbrain stimulation in the region of the periaqueductal gray has been proposed primarily for somatic type pain, whereas thalamic stimulation may be more useful for neurogenic pain.

A central procedure that is particularly effective in palliating the pain of metastatic (especially osseous metastases) cancer is hypophysectomy.[17] The pituitary gland may be surgically excised by the transsphenoidal route or chemically ablated using absolute ethanol injections (Figure 35-2). In cases of hormonally responsive malignancies, such as breast or prostate, a remarkable, long-lasting pain relief is often achieved. The mechanisms responsible for this effect of hypophysectomy are not clearly understood.

As mentioned, the pain of metastasis may involve a deafferentation component. Most of the aforementioned neurosurgical approaches have

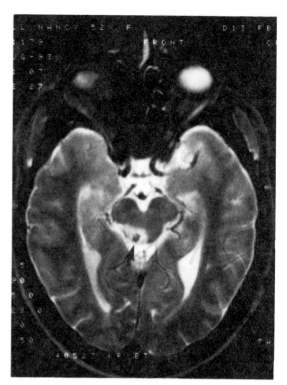

Figure 35-1. T_2-weighted magnetic resonance imaging of the brain reveals stereotactic lesion in the right midbrain. The lesioning was performed for brachial plexopathy pain consequent to metastatic breast carcinoma.

limited success regarding deafferentation pain, with the exception of thalamic stimulation. It has been suggested that deafferentation results not only in the loss of sensory input from the periphery, but also that the disconnected central spinal sensory neurons behave in a pathologic way. This abnormal neuronal activity is then perceived as pain. The neurophysiologic explanations for this activity include (1) a hypersensitivity of the deafferented central neuron—an epileptic-like pain phenomenon, (2) a release from the influences of powerful central inhibitory systems, and (3) an effect due to a change in the local concentrations of some of the classical neurotransmitters or of the recently described peptide neuromodulators.

Using the anatomic knowledge of the dorsal horn region and its neurophysiologic importance, especially with regard to nociceptive transmission and pain, Nashold created the DREZ operation.[18] He thought that a nonfunctional or destroyed patho-

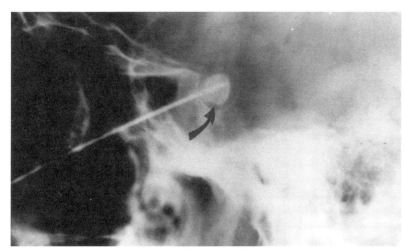

Figure 35-2. A transsphenoidal removal of the pituitary gland (hypophysectomy) provides excellent pain relief in those cases with osseous metastases from endocrine-sensitive cancers, e.g., breast and prostate. The pituitary gland can also be chemically ablated with an injection of absolute alcohol through a needle placed within the sella turcica.

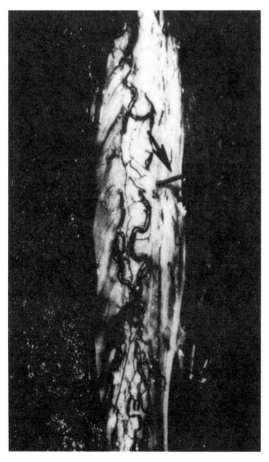

Figure 35-3. The dorsal root entry zone lesion procedure is designed to treat deafferentation pain. The treatment attempts to destroy the abnormally active dorsal horn neurons in the spinal cord at each segmental level of the pain. A small electrode is advanced into the spinal cord and radiofrequency lesions approximately 1 mm in diameter are then created in a serial fashion.

logic central neuron was better than a sick one. Thus, the placement of radiofrequency lesions in the DREZ sought to convert partially injured central neurons (i.e., "hyperactive") into quiescent scars (Figure 35-3).

The DREZ procedure was initially performed in a group of patients with brachial plexus avulsion pain[19] and other benign deafferentation syndromes. Recently, it has been applied to deafferentation pain associated with malignancy with good results. In addition, a trigeminal nucleus caudalis DREZ procedure has been developed for pain from carcinoma of the orbit. These latter results are only preliminary.

References

1. Albe-Fessard D, Berkley KJ, Kruger L, et al. Diencephalic mechanisms of pain sensation. Brain Res Rev 1985;9:217.
2. Basbaum AI, Fields HL. Endogenous pain control systems: Brainstem spinal pathways and endorphin circuitry. Annu Rev Neurosci 1984;7:309.
3. Fields HL, Heinricher MM. Anatomy and physiology of a nociceptive modulatory system. Phil Trans R Soc Lond 1985;B308:361.
4. Esposito S, Bruni P, Delitala A, et al. Therapeutic approach to the Pancoast pain syndrome. Appl Neurophysiol 1985;48:262.
5. Loeser JD. Dorsal rhizotomy for the relief of chronic pain. J Neurosurg 1972;36:745.
6. Onofrio BM, Campa HK. Evaluation of rhizotomy. J Neurosurg 1972;36:751.
7. Sindou M, Goutelle A. Surgical Posterior Rhizotomies for the Treatment of Pain. In H Krayenbuhl (ed), Advances and Technical Standards in Neurosurgery (Vol. 10). Wien, Germany: Springer, 1983;147.

8. Smith FP. Trans-spinal ganglionectomy for relief of intercostal pain. J Neurosurg 1970;32:574.

9. Spiller WG, Martin E. The treatment of persistent pain of organic origin in the lower part of the body by division of the anterolateral column of the spinal cord. JAMA 1912;58:1489.

10. Sindou M, Daher A. Spinal Cord Ablation Procedures for Pain. In R Dubner, GF Gebhart, MR Bond (eds), Proceedings of the Vth World Congress on Pain. New York: Elsevier, 1988;477.

11. De La Porte C, Siegfried J. Lumbosacral spinal fibrosis (spinal arachnoiditis): Its diagnosis and treatment by spinal cord stimulation. Spine 1983;8:593.

12. Auld AW, Maki-Jokela A, Murdoch DM. Intraspinal narcotic analgesia in the treatment of chronic pain. Spine 1985;10:777.

13. Penn RD, Paice JA, Gottschalk W, Ivankovich AD. Cancer pain relief using chronic morphine infusion. J Neurosurg 1984;61:302.

14. Nashold BS Jr. Brainstem Stereotaxic Procedures. In G Schaltenbrand, AE Walker (eds), Stereotaxy of the Human Brain. New York: George Thieme Verlag, 1982;475.

15. Adams JE, Hosobuchi Y, Fields HL. Stimulation of internal capsule for relief of chronic pain. J Neurosurg 1974;41:740.

16. Hosobuchi Y. Subcortical electrical stimulation for control of intractable pain in humans. J Neurosurg 1986;64:543.

17. Levin AB, Katz J, Benson RC, Jones AG. Treatment of pain of diffuse metastatic cancer by stereotactic chemical hypophysectomy: Long term results and observations on mechanism of action. Neurosurgery 1980;6:258.

18. Nashold BS Jr. Deafferentation pain in man and animals as it relates to the DREZ operation. Can J Neurosci 1988;15:5.

19. Nashold BS Jr, Ostdahl RH. Dorsal root entry zone lesions for pain relief. J Neurosurg 1979;51:59.

Chapter 36

Cancer Pain Emergencies

Richard B. Patt and Paolo L. Manfredi

Although the "pain emergency" is not a well-defined disorder, it can be considered operationally as an acute condition characterized by rapidly escalating pain that, in the absence of prompt intervention, poses a significant threat to psychological and physiologic well-being.

Oncologic Emergencies

Oncologic emergencies (Table 36-1) have been described that, although relatively uncommon, require prompt identification and treatment to limit morbidity and mortality. Because the nononcologist pain specialist may see the patient with advanced cancer more frequently than the primary oncologist,[1] the pain specialist must be familiar with the presentation of these syndromes, especially because their presentation sometimes mimics slowly progressive neoplastic disease. With the exception of epidural spinal cord compression, the identification and early management of other oncologic emergencies is discussed elsewhere.[2, 3] This chapter deals predominantly with the generic pain emergency.

Factors Distinguishing Cancer Pain Emergencies

Several features of cancer pain distinguish urgent complaints from those typically associated with other medical conditions.

The Pain Emergency as an Expression of Undertreatment

It is widely accepted that cancer pain is globally undertreated.[4, 5] As a result, the so-called "pain emergency" is often not a new problem at all, but rather a longstanding problem that has been chronically undertreated. Thus, the consultant may not observe features typically associated with an emergency (i.e., recent onset, rapid progression) but instead may encounter chronic symptoms that have progressed in severity. The apparent cancer pain emergency may simply reflect a failure of the system to identify what would, under other circumstances, be viewed as a straightforward problem.

This characterization of chronic problems as emergent does not negate the seriousness with which such complaints should be regarded. A chronic problem that has presented as emergent is a signal of heightened distress, which can often be eased when effective pain treatment is rapidly instituted. Paradoxically, pain may be difficult to control in this setting if anticipation and memory of unrelenting pain are well established.

Pain as a Multiply Determined Experience

Pain is a subjective symptom, and as such, is the sum of tissue injury and an individual's ability, willingness, or predisposition to tolerate a noxious stimulus.[6] Thus, urgent complaints of pain may reflect (1) new or progressive tissue injury, (2) a sud-

Table 36-1. Oncologic Emergencies

Epidural spinal cord compression
Raised intracranial pressure
Cardiac tamponade
Pleural effusion
Superior vena cava syndrome
Gastric outlet obstruction
Bowel obstruction
Biliary obstruction
Ureteral obstruction
Hypercalcemia
Neutropenic fever
Acute thrombocytopenia
Acute anemia
Leukostasis
Tumor lysis syndrome and uric acid nephropathy

den decrease in pain threshold associated with deterioration of an individual's coping mechanisms, or (3) a combination of these factors.

This potpourri of potential causes should not be viewed as a basis for determining a complaint's authenticity or for gauging the appropriate intensity of response. The relative contribution of physiologic versus psychological causes often cannot be ascertained, and, even when one determinant is prominent, a patient's statement that the pain is much worse is inarguably a cry for help.[7] While an inappropriate determinant of intensity of response, the degree to which increased pain can be distinguished from increased distress does, however, influence the nature of the therapeutic response. As a result, assessment must be sufficiently comprehensive to capture information that suggests new progression of disease, as well as psychosocial influences on the expression of pain.[8]

The presence of historical factors that suggest a prominent influence of psychosocial factors (e.g., recent disclosure of a poor prognosis or discontinuation of antitumor therapy) should always be sought. Such factors may call for consultation from a mental health care professional to interview family members and obtain a more comprehensive psychosocial history.[9] Ultimately, a therapeutic approach that includes counseling and psychopharmacology may be indicated.[10] Features that suggest a predominantly physiologic basis for increased pain (new physical findings, measurable increase in tumor bulk) should elicit a therapeutic response that relies on new antitumor therapy when appropriate, and symptomatic management with analgesics.[11]

Psychological distress and increased nociception are often inextricably linked, and the degree to which one mechanism predominates often cannot be determined with meaningful accuracy. In such cases, to the degree that is possible, both the physiologic and psychological determinants of pain should be identified and managed. The inconstant correlation between new complaints of pain and easily measurable, objective changes emphasizes the central role of a careful history and physical examination.[12-15]

Empirically Based Expedient Pain Relief

Acute pain has been characterized as a "biologic red flag" that, by signaling the need to seek medical attention, serves a useful, protective purpose.[16] Although new complaints of pain warrant careful assessment, their warning function does not imply that treatment should be withheld while diagnostic studies are undertaken. The breadth of the contemporary pharmacologic armamentarium ensures that reversible and titratable pain relief can be achieved during assessment. The intent of early intervention is to render the patient comfortable, usually with careful titration of intravenous opioids. Because pain serves as an antagonist to opioid-mediated respiratory and sedative effects, pain relief can be achieved safely in this fashion, especially in a supervised setting. Opioid-mediated pain relief is not an "all-or-none" phenomenon, and therefore, a modicum of pain relief can be achieved while still preserving signs that would suggest progression of an acute process.[17]

The Value of Providing Expedient Pain Relief

Independent of the moral imperative to relieve suffering, the protean value of relieving severe pain early in the therapeutic encounter is often underappreciated.

Psychological Value

A demonstration that the health care provider is capable of inducing pain relief is reassuring to patients with low expectations regarding the prognosis for controlling pain. The health care provider's willingness to take the time to relieve the pain communicates empathy and helps establish a relationship of trust that will encourage the patient to communicate honestly during assessment. Early development of a sound therapeutic alliance may also lend added weight to subsequent treatment recommendations. In this regard, the health care provider should be aware of the potential value of personally administering the first dose of rapidly acting analgesic.[18]

Diagnostic Value

Despite the value of the pain history in helping establish a diagnosis, severe pain may confound assessment. Unrelieved pain and distress may interfere with the completion of an adequate history and physical examination, both on the basis of their effects on compliance and by obfuscating distinctions between findings related to pain and those that are secondary to neurologic injury. The intravenous administration of a rapidly acting opioid analgesic titrated to comfort is recommended. Once the patient is more comfortable and relaxed, efforts to obtain a more detailed history may be more productive. Establishing a baseline level of comfort is particularly important for an adequate physical examination, especially when pain on movement is prominent. A thorough neurologic examination requires a patient who is cooperative and who can concentrate. The detection of early signs of neurologic compromise is especially important when evaluating unexplained pain, since early intervention may limit neurologic morbidity, as in the case of epidural spinal cord compression.

Therapeutic Value

Expedient pain relief has potential therapeutic value. Neurohumoral responses to escalating pain may be associated with their own morbidity.[19, 20] The activation of spinal reflexes and the stimulation of hypothalamic nuclei, adrenal medulla, or both may result in increased sympathetic tone, cardiac output, peripheral resistance, blood pressure, cardiac workload, and myocardial oxygen consumption.[21] Although under some circumstances this "flight or fight" response empowers the organism to withstand threats to its homeostatic balance, such changes may be deleterious in the setting of coexisting systemic illness and limited cardiorespiratory reserves.

Another response to pain that is teleologically protective but can, under some circumstances, contribute to morbidity is immobility or splinting. Unrelieved chest or abdominal pain promotes shallow breathing and suppression of cough, factors that contribute to retention of secretions, atelectasis, and pneumonia. The degree to which back, pelvis, and lower extremity pain limit ambulation may increase risks of depression, deep venous thrombosis, and pulmonary emboli. Mouth opening and swallowing are often inhibited by cervicofacial pain, which may consequently trigger a reluctance to communicate, depression, and even malnutrition. In these settings, aggressive management of pain is an important determinant of functional restoration.[22–24]

Delayed or insufficient pain treatment may result in chronic pain that is more refractory to conventional therapies. This may occur on the basis of learned pain behavior, reflex muscle spasm, spreading sympathetically mediated pain, and central neuronal plasticity.[25–27] Finally, preliminary experimental evidence that untreated pain compromises the cytotoxic activity of natural killer T-lymphocytes and promotes tumor growth suggests a possible influence of adequacy of pain treatment on survival.[28]

Fiscal Considerations

As a result of health care reform and more widespread acceptance of the concept that pain should be regarded as a legitimate medical complaint, economic consequences of unrelieved pain are increasingly appreciated. Such consequences range from the sobering example of a recent $15,000,000 award for damages related to a nursing home's failure to relieve pain,[29] to a sharp increase in research evaluating the effects of adequacy of pain control on length of hospitalization and associated costs.[30, 31]

Treating the Pain Emergency

The axiom that management decisions must be predicated on careful assessment is particularly pertinent in the emergency setting. When the urgent complaint is of uncontrolled pain, it is essential to distinguish between (1) preliminary therapies that are initiated to relieve acute suffering, establish a therapeutic alliance, and facilitate assessment, and (2) long-term treatment decisions.

Initial Encounter

The first encounter with the patient is ideally complemented by information obtained from the medical record and observations of triage personnel. A brief history and pertinent examination are undertaken to exclude the presence of life-threatening conditions, as well as obvious manifestations of an oncologic emergency (see Table 36-1). The attributes that influence the urgency of response to a complaint of cancer pain include its rapidity of onset, severity, location, and associated symptoms and signs. Many patients with cancer pain benefit from treatment that, though palliative in nature, targets the disease process.[1]

Cancer pain assessment has been described elsewehere in detail.[13] A host of cancer pain syndromes has been described,[12, 32, 33] familiarity with which is essential. Assessment should include an evaluation of the disease, person, and pain. In the emergency setting, it is particularly important to seek information about recent events (e.g., a fall, recent treatment) and changes in the patient's condition (loss of appetite, vomiting, incontinence). When appropriate, the interview may be supplemented by standardized questionnaires, although this is often impractical in the setting of an urgent consultation. The patient should, however, be taught to use a pain intensity and pain relief scale to determine the effectiveness of treatment administered on site. In this regard, many clinicians prefer a verbal 0–10 scale, with 0 signifying an absence of pain and 10 signifying the most severe pain the patient can imagine. A categoric scale (none, mild, moderate, severe, or intolerable) may be more appropriate for patients who are confused or anumeric.

Once it has been established that the patient's condition is stable, a preliminary conversation should occur among the representatives of the treatment team and the patient and family. It should be communicated that the patient's complaints of pain will be taken seriously, and that the prognosis for treatment is, overall, favorable. The need for a care-

ful assessment is conveyed, along with a general sense of requirements for tests and the time they may take.

Considerations for Initiating Empiric Opioid Therapy

Preliminary evaluation should determine the necessity for expedient symptomatic treatment. When appropriate, this will most often involve the intravenous administration of a rapidly acting opioid analgesic, titrated to comfort.

Allergy

Few absolute contraindications exist to opioid therapy. A detailed history of untoward reactions to medications should be sought. True allergic reactions to the opioid analgesics are rare.[34, 35] Most often such histories represent unrecognized side effects, especially for nausea, vomiting, or dysphoria.[36] A history of untoward reactions to an opioid warrants a careful explanation of the distinction between allergy and side effects, and the infrequent occurrence of untreatable side effects in a closely supervised setting. In the presence of a history suggestive of a true allergic reaction, an alternate opioid may be selected and administered in small doses under careful observation, with consideration of pretreatment with an antihistamine.[35]

Dyspnea

Because opioids reduce subjective reports of dyspnea,[37] breathing difficulties rarely contraindicate their administration, especially in a supervised setting. Although a history of dyspnea, primary or metastatic lung cancer, or chronic lung disease warrant more careful monitoring, these conditions should not be regarded as contraindications to the administration of carefully titrated doses of opioids.

Abdominal Pain

Severe abdominal pain may be due to actual or impending obstruction, perforation, hemorrhage, or infection of intra-abdominal structures. Traditional teaching dictates that opioids be withheld because they may mask symptoms of progression of an underlying pathologic condition. This viewpoint originates from the misconception that opioid effects are binary (all or none) in nature, and that analgesia is invariably associated with sedation. Clinical experience in hospitalized patients with progressive terminal illness and in patients undergoing diagnostic procedures, however, suggests that, when carefully titrated, incremental pain relief can be achieved without profound sedation.[38] Experimental work demonstrates that opioids relieve the "tonic" pain that follows tissue injury, but have little effect on the "phasic" pain associated with new injury.[39]

Most opioids raise biliary pressure, although clinical signs of colic are rare.[40] A history of abdominal pain does not represent a contraindication to opioid therapy. If new or worsening right upper quadrant colic occur after an opioid has been administered, spasm of the sphincter of Oddi can be excluded by administering 2 mg of glucagon intravenously or minute doses of naloxone.[38]

Abdominal pain in patients already being treated with opioids or other obstipating drugs, together with the results of a physical examination and a flat plate of the abdomen may suggest constipation as the underlying cause for abdominal pain. In these cases, the judicious use of opioids may still be required as an interim solution while bowel cleansing is initiated. Laxatives, enemas, and disimpaction are usually adequate, although endoscopic procedures and even surgery are sometimes required. Chronic management may be problematic, especially when gastrointestinal function is compromised by ileus induced by tumor spread, or adhesions due to surgery or radiotherapy. In confirmed "narcotic bowel syndrome," the use of nonopioid analgesics such as ketorolac or methotrimeprazine, or approaches such as neural blockade or intraspinal analgesia should be considered.

Substance Abuse

Patients should be questioned for a history of substance abuse, which, if present, should elicit a more comprehensive interview.[41] A history of substance abuse should not be regarded as a contraindication to opioid therapy.[11] Such a history, however, is an important predictor of both clinician stress and undertreatment of pain.[38] Ongoing substance abuse creates difficulties in distinguishing medical use from addictive behavior, and warrants a specialized treatment plan.[42, 43] In contrast, patients with a distant history of addiction, or who are in a twelve-step recovery program, may resist opioid therapy, fearing readdiction or criticism from their peers.[44]

Treating the Pain Emergency Empirically

Once a preliminary assessment has been completed, empiric therapy is usually indicated to provide comfort during the conduct of diagnostic studies and observation. This treatment may be of a finite duration when the results of assessment identify a treatable etiology. Often, only symptomatic treatment is warranted; in which case, the initial therapy serves as the basis for developing an ongoing pain treatment plan. When initial treatment has successfully reduced pain, intravenous therapy can be converted to an oral regimen for ambulatory treatment. If sufficient stability has not been achieved or if interventional therapy is required, hospitalization for further diagnostic studies and medication titration or preparation is indicated.

Initiating Treatment

Given their overall favorable risk-to-benefit ratio, intravenously administered opioid agonist drugs form the basis for the initial treatment of the uncomplicated cancer pain emergency. The clinician should select a drug with which he or she is familiar, and it should be administered based on its pharmacokinetic and pharmacodynamic properties. Morphine is most commonly selected, based on clinician familiarity; hydromorphone and fentanyl are reasonable alternatives. Methadone and levorphanol are poor first choices because of their potential to accumulate over time.[45] Meperidine should be avoided because of the potential for metabolite-induced convulsions.[46, 47] Agonist-antagonist agents should be avoided because analgesia is limited by so-called "ceiling effects." In addition, these agents may interact unfavorably with pure agonists, and may be associated with a high incidence of dysphoria.[48]

The fundamental principle for treating the cancer pain emergency with intravenous opioids initially involves the sequential administration of increasing aliquots of drug until pain diminishes, using the patient's self-report as a guide. A 10-mg dose of intravenous morphine is the standard of comparison for most analgesic regimens and usually represents a reasonable starting dose, especially for the opioid-naive patient. After the intravenous administration of a therapeutic dose of morphine, patients typically appreciate the onset of analgesia within 5 minutes, and experience peak analgesia at 10–15 minutes. In practice, the initial dose of intravenous morphine may be followed by repeated doses every 10 minutes, ranging from 20–100% of the original dose.

The optimal starting dose for opioid-tolerant patients depends mainly on the magnitude of their regular dose. Maintenance doses of oral morphine often exceed 1 or more grams daily.[49] Long-acting around-the-clock agents are usually supplemented with as needed "rescue" or "escape" doses, each of which are usually given as 5–15% of the total (around-the-clock) daily dose.[11] The calculation of a starting intravenous dose for the opioid-tolerant patient commences by summing the usual 24-hour dose of around-the-clock opioid. If necessary, this dose is converted to morphine equivalents by employing a standard drug equivalency table.[11] If the conversion has been to oral morphine equivalents, the sum is divided by three to account for oral to parenteral bioavailability (first-pass effect) to achieve the 24-hour intravenous morphine dose equivalent. Depending on the level of pain, the starting dose of intravenous morphine is then estimated at 5–15%. Patients chronically maintained on high doses of opioids are likely to require increases of a greater magnitude to achieve relief from a pain emergency. Selection of the proper dose and tempo of titration are guided by careful monitoring and reports of relief versus side effects.

If side effects limit upward dose titration before pain relief is achieved, aggressive symptomatic treatment, usually with antiemetics, should be instituted. Naloxone should be immediately available, although the risk of clinically significant respiratory depression is small if titration is implemented gradually.

Maintenance Opioid Therapy

Once a reasonable level of comfort has been achieved, continued interim management is ide-ally achieved by establishing a basal infusion of opioid supplemented by either patient-controlled or nurse-administered boluses.[50, 51] If assessment reveals no need for other than symptomatic management, the efficacy of the prescribed management is assessed, and if adequate, the intravenous dose is converted to an oral regimen using standard conversion tables.[11] Depending on the patient's prior drug regimen and the degree of difficulty encountered in establishing an adequate dose, the patient may be discharged on a regimen consisting of either controlled-release oral or transdermal preparations supplemented by as needed rescue doses, or may rely entirely on immediate release preparations until greater stability is achieved. If adequate pain control has not been established in a reasonable time frame, hospital admission is indicated.

Other Considerations

Assessment should take into account the variety of conditions capable of producing rapidly escalating complaints of pain in the cancer patient. Psychological distress, evolving abdominal processes, and obstipation have already been discussed, and references describing other cancer pain syndromes have been provided.[12, 32, 33]

Epidural Spinal Cord Compression

Rapid and accurate assessment of new or worsening back pain is essential. Metastatic cord compression is preceded by new back pain, often initially in the absence of gross neurologic changes in 90% of cases.[52, 53] However, because back pain is an exceedingly common symptom in the general population, and is even more ubiquitous in cancer patients due to uncomplicated vertebral metastases, symptoms are sometimes disregarded. New back pain, however, is an important clinical sign because the onset of progressive neurologic symptoms is often insidious and may go unrecognized until late signs are already established, particularly in patients who are already multisymptomatic.

In most instances, mechanical compression of the spinal cord is caused by extension of vertebral body metastases. Lesions that extend posteriorly into the epidural space transmit pressure across the dura to the cord and its vascular supply that, if unchecked, leads to mechanical injury, ischemia, venous stasis, and infarction.[2] Extradural tumor growth is responsible for about 95% of cases of cord compression with intramedullary metastases and paraspinal extension of soft tissue tumors accounting for the remaining cases.[54] The thoracic spinal cord is involved in about 70% of cases, the cervical cord in 15%, and the lumbosacral cord in the remaining cases.[14] Because the spinal cord is the common pathway for the transmission of sensory and motor impulses to and from the periphery, compression leads to progressive loss of sensation and muscle strength and autonomic deregulation below the site of the lesion.

Patients with epidural spinal cord compression (ESCC) usually present with back pain in the absence of neurologic signs.[55] If symptom progression goes unrecognized and intervention is consequently delayed, paraplegia, numbness, and bowel and bladder dysfunction result. Added disability adds hardship to patients and families who are already struggling with the difficulties of cancer and its concomitant symptoms. With cord compression in the cervical or high thoracic region, patients are at further risk for quadriplegia and respiratory death.

Breast and lung cancer are the most common primary malignancies associated with the development of spinal cord compression, followed by prostate cancer, lymphoma, and multiple myeloma.[55] Any neoplasm that metastasizes to bone may produce cord compression, including renal cell cancer, melanoma, unknown primaries, and more rarely, gynecologic and gastrointestinal malignancies. While there is usually initial involvement of the vertebral bodies, lymphoma can give rise to paraspinal nodal masses that infiltrate through neural foramina to compress the cord.

The early diagnosis of ESCC requires maintenance of a high degree of clinical suspicion and careful serial neurologic examinations, coupled with appropriate diagnostic imaging. The differential diagnosis includes simple back strain, degenerative disk disease, referred pain from retroperitoneal processes, and osseous metastases. Localized paraspinal, radicular, or referred pain are usually the first sign of metastases to the bony vertebral column. Uncomplicated vertebral metastases tend to produce dull, steady, aching pain that increases gradually over time. Pain may be elicited by palpation or percussion of the spinous processes of the involved segments, may be exacerbated when lying down, and partially relieved by sitting or standing. Neurologic evaluation for cord compression should include inquiry about symptoms of weakness, radicular pain, alterations in gait, numbness, urinary retention or incontinence, and constipation. The examination should include testing of reflexes, muscle strength, sensation to light touch and pinprick, and Babinski's response. When practical, the patient's gait and ability to heel-walk and toe-walk should be observed. A rectal examination is performed to assess sphincter tone and sensation, and the abdomen is palpated to determine if the bladder is enlarged.

When spinal cord compression is suspected, multidisciplinary assessment involving an oncologist, neurologist, neurosurgeon, and radiologist is desirable. Urgent radiologic evaluation is undertaken. The choice of the most appropriate investigation is somewhat controversial.[14] While the traditional "gold-standard" study has been myelography, magnetic resonance imaging is now widely accepted. If ESCC is confirmed, treatment is with the immediate administration of intravenous dexamethasone in doses of up to 100 mg, followed by specialist consultation for consideration of external beam radiotherapy, surgery, or both.[56]

Pathologic Fracture

Pathologic fractures are a frequent cause of sudden, severe, localized pain and should be especially suspected after a history of a fall, sudden pain on movement, or the rapid and sudden onset of immobility.[56] A diagnosis can usually be confirmed with plain radiographs, after which an orthopedic consultation is indicated. External beam radiotherapy or, if the patient is sufficiently fit, surgery are indicated since spontaneous healing is unusual.[57] If movement-related pain is severe, epidural analgesia should be considered.

Infection

Localized infection may cause rapidly escalating pain. Although usually heralded by systemic or local signs, these may be modest or absent in the presence of bone marrow depletion or a sequestered abscess. Anecdotal evidence suggests that an empiric course of antibiotics may significantly reduce pain, especially in patients with fungating lesions or in patients with advanced head and neck or pelvic cancer.[58, 59] New back or trunk pain in patients with in-dwelling epidural catheters should be carefully evaluated to exclude epidural abscess or subcutaneous tract infections.[60]

Breakthrough Pain Versus the Pain Emergency

Emerging Methodologies

Clinicians have only recently recognized the cancer pain emergency as a distinct entity that warrants therapy, and consequently investigators have only recently begun to prospectively investigate specific methodologies for treatment. It is important to recognize that these interventions have been conducted under controlled, monitored circumstances. Before endeavoring to treat a cancer pain emergency it is essential to undertake a careful history and physical examination to exclude a cause of pain that requires urgent treatment. In addition, protocols for administering intravenous and novel analgesics in increasing doses should be carried out in a monitored setting.

The Morphine Test

Using the "morphine test," Hill[61] has described a method for attaining rapid pain relief for cancer patients experiencing uncontrolled pain. The results of the morphine test form the basis for prescribing maintenance therapy to achieve sustained pain relief and may have additional value in helping to distinguish between pain that is predominantly nociceptive or neuropathic in origin. Ambulatory cancer patients with poorly controlled pain were administered intravenous boluses of morphine sulfate, initially in 5- to 15-mg doses, followed every 10–15 minutes with similar doses until pain relief or an unacceptable side effect occurred. Using test doses of 8–400 mg of intravenous morphine (median, 20 mg), Hill reported on 108 tests performed in 102 subjects. Eighty-one percent of patients had

positive responses (> 75% reduction in pain), 11% had a partial response (> 50% relief), and 8% had a negative response (< 50% relief). Eighty-one of the 94 positive and partial responders were started on around-the-clock oral morphine in doses that corresponded to the intravenous test dose converted to oral drug using a 1 to 3 ratio (60–5280 mg/day; median, 270 mg/day). Of the 79 patients available for follow-up, 52 (66%) achieved immediate and sustained pain relief, and 14 (18%) required treatment with an alternate opioid or route of administration. This procedure appears to be equally effective when hydromorphone is substituted for morphine, and is the subject of more carefully controlled ongoing trials at M.D. Anderson Cancer Center (D Thorpe, R Payne, RB Patt, unpublished data, 1996).

Hagen et al.[62] have recently described their successful experience with a similar technique that uses more aggressive upward titration. They treated nine patients with ten cancer pain emergencies, defined as recent history of 8/10 pain persisting for more than 6 hours. Patients underwent intravenous titration with either their usual or an alternate opioid, depending on whether they described dose-limiting side effects with their chronic oral regimen. An initial dose of intravenous opioid equal to 10–20 mg of intravenous morphine was administered over 15 minutes, after which each successive dose was doubled and administered every 30 minutes until pain control was achieved. The final dose was repeated on an as needed basis during the first 24 hours of follow-up, after which around-the-clock parenteral or oral therapy was initiated based on the outcome of each patient's test. With only minor modifications of the protocol in two patients, all achieved satisfactory relief in a mean of 58 minutes (range, 4–215 minutes), which was maintained during their hospitalization.

Sublingual and Transmucosal Opioids

In virtue of the vascularity of the oral and nasal mucous membranes, the administration of drugs by these routes may be associated with rapid uptake and onset of analgesia, as well as profound analgesia, since hepatic first-pass metabolism is bypassed.[63, 64] Although there is considerable anecdotal evidence from the hospice literature that liquid preparations of sublingual and buccal morphine may provide acceptable analgesia,[65] morphine is a relatively inappropriate drug for administration by these routes due to its hydrophilicity. The recent introduction of a lozenge-based oral transmucosal preparation of fentanyl citrate is a promising approach for temporizing cancer pain emergencies in a noninvasive fashion. Although currently approved for limited indications (management of pain and anxiety prior to a painful procedure),[66] this preparation is an extremely effective method for treating breakthrough pain in cancer patients (RB Patt, R Payne, unpublished data, 1996),[67, 68] and by extension will undoubtedly find applications for the management of cancer pain emergencies.

Kunz et al.[69] described the management of severe episodic pain in a cancer patient using sublingual sufentanil. Gardner-Nix[70] has recently described her experience with the use of sublingual sufentanil and fentanyl drops for incident pains that closely resembled pain emergencies in six patients, three of whom had pain due to cancer, and three of whom had pain of nononcologic origin. Sufentanil or fentanyl were administered in doses ranging from 2.5–15 μg every 2 hours as needed, and was found to be relatively free of side effects, safe, effective, and cost-effective compared with other methods.

Other Interventions

This section has focused on the pharmacologic management of the cancer pain emergency because drug therapy is most practical in this setting. Treatment with analgesics is effective for most pain problems, including multifocal and diffuse pain, because it is reversible, titratable, and does not require specialized or sophisticated resources. Further, similar principles can be applied to adults and children, as well as across cultures.

When available, anesthetic interventions may be considered for pain that is refractory to conventional management. Local anesthetic nerve blocks may be especially valuable, at least as a temporizing measure, for pain that is well localized or precipitated by movement. Temporary epidural catheterization can now be more regularly considered as a treatment option because of the development of more sophisticated home care support.

References

1. Gonzales GR, Elliott KJ, Portenoy RK, Foley KM. The impact of a comprehensive evaluation in the management of cancer pain. Pain 1991;47:141.
2. Smith JL. Oncologic Emergencies. In RB Patt (ed), Cancer Pain. Philadelphia: Lippincott, 1993;527.
3. Kramer ZB, Keller JW, Rubin P. Oncologic Emergencies. In P Rubin (ed), Clinical Oncology (7th ed). Philadelphia: Saunders, 1993;147.
4. Bonica JJ. Cancer pain: A major national health problem. Cancer Nurs 1978;1:313.
5. Swerdlow M, Stjernsward J. Cancer pain relief: An urgent problem. World Health Forum 1992;3:325.
6. Twycross RG, Lack SA. Therapeutics in Terminal Cancer. Edinburgh: Churchill Livingstone, 1984;11.
7. Cleeland CS. The impact of pain on the patient with cancer. Cancer 1984;54:2643.
8. Derogatis LR, Marrow GR, Fetting J, et al. The prevalence of psychiatric disorders among cancer patients. JAMA 1984;249:751.
9. Millard RM. Behavioral Assessment of Pain and Behavioral Pain Management. In RB Patt (ed), Cancer Pain. Philadelphia: Lippincott, 1993;85.
10. Breitbart W. Diagnosis and Treatment of Psychiatric Complications. In RB Patt (ed), Cancer Pain. Philadelphia: Lippincott, 1993;209.
11. Jacox A, Carr DB, Payne R, et al. Management of Cancer Pain. Clinical Practice Guideline No 9. Rockville, MD: AHCPR Publication No. 94-0592, March 1994.
12. Patt RB. Cancer Pain Syndromes. In RB Patt (ed), Cancer Pain. Philadelphia: Lippincott, 1993;3.
13. Rowlingson J, Hammill RJ, Patt RB. Assessment of the Patient with Oncologic Pain. In RB Patt (ed), Cancer Pain. Philadelphia: Lippincott, 1993;23.
14. Longmire DR. The pain history. Pain Digest 1991;1:28.
15. Longmire DR. The physical examination: Methods and application in the clinical evaluation of pain. Pain Digest 1991;1:136.
16. Sternbach RA. Acute Versus Chronic Pain. In PD Wall, R Melzack (eds), Textbook of Pain (2nd ed). Edinburgh: Churchill Livingstone, 1989;242.
17. Beerle BJ, Rose RJ. Lower extremity compartment syndrome not masked by epidural bupivacaine and fentanyl. Reg Anesth 1993;18:189.
18. Griner P. Pain and symptom control in patients with advanced cancer. Am J Hospice Palliat Care 1990;7:8.
19. Taff RH. Pulmonary edema following a naloxone administration in a patient without heart disease. Anesthesiology 1983;59:576.
20. Prough BS, Roy R, Bumgarner J, et al. Acute pulmonary edema in healthy teenagers following conservative doses of intravenous naloxone. Anesthesiology 1984;60:485.
21. Canon WD. Bodily Changes in Pain, Hunger, Fear and Rage (2nd ed). New York: Appleton, 1929.

22. Patt RB, Jain S. Management of a patient with osteoradionecrosis of the mandible with nerve blocks. J Pain Symptom Manage 1990;5:59.

23. Engberg G, Wiklund L. Pulmonary complications after upper abdominal surgery: Their prevention with intercostal blocks. Acta Anaesthesiol Scand 1988;32:1.

24. Toledo-Pereyra LH, DeMeester T. Prospective randomized evaluation of intrathoracic intercostal nerve block with bupivacaine on postoperative ventilatory function. Ann Thorac Surg 1979;27:203.

25. Zimmerman M. Peripheral and central mechanisms of nociception, pain and pain therapy: Facts and hypothesis. Adv Pain Res Ther 1979;3:3.

26. Woolf CJ. Preemptive analgesia: Treating postoperative pain by preventing the establishment of central sensitization. Anesth Analg 1993;77:362.

27. Weinstein SM. Phantom pain. Oncology 1994;8:65.

28. Liebeskind JC. Pain can kill. Pain 1991;44:3.

29. Angarola RT. Opioids, cancer and the law. APS Bull 1991;9.

30. Kehlet H. Modification of Responses to Surgery by Neural Blockade: Clinical Implications. In MJ Cousins, PO Bridenbaugh (eds), Neural Blockade (2nd ed). Philadelphia: Lippincott, 1988;145.

31. Yeager MP, Glass DD, Neff RK, Brinck-Johnsen T. Epidural anesthesia and analgesia in high risk surgical patients. Anesthesiology 1987;66:729.

32. Foley KM. Cancer pain syndromes. J Pain Symptom Manage 1987;2:S13.

33. Foley KM. Pain Syndromes in Patients with Cancer. In JJ Bonica, V Ventafridda (eds), Advances in Pain Research and Therapy (Vol 2). New York: Raven, 1979;59.

34. Levy JH, Rockoff MA. Anaphylaxis to meperidine. Anesth Analg 1982;61:301.

35. Stoelting RK. Allergic reactions during anesthesia. Anesth Analg 1983;62:341.

36. Ellison NM. Opioid Analgesics: Toxicities and Their Treatments. In RB Patt (ed), Cancer Pain. Philadelphia: Lippincott, 1993;185.

37. Bruera E, Macmillan K, Pither J, MacDonald RN. Effects of morphine on the dyspnea of terminal cancer patients. J Pain Symptom Manage 1990;5:341.

38. Kanner RM, Foley KM. Patterns of narcotic use in a cancer pain clinic. Ann N Y Acad Sci 1981;362:161.

39. Melzack R. The tragedy of needless pain. Sci Am 1990;262:27.

40. Stoelting RK. Pharmacology and Physiology in Anesthetic Practice. Philadelphia: Lippincott, 1987;79.

41. Foley KM. The treatment of cancer pain. N Engl J Med 1985;313:84.

42. Stimmel B. Adequate analgesia in narcotic dependency. Adv Pain Res Ther 1989;11:131.

43. Portenoy RK, Payne R. Acute and Chronic Pain. In JH Lowinson, P Ruiz, RB Millman (eds), Substance Abuse: A Comprehensive Textbook. Baltimore: Williams & Wilkins, 1992;691.

44. Fultz JM, Sonay EC. Guidelines for the management of hospitalized narcotic addicts. Ann Intern Med 1975;82:815.

45. Portenoy RK. Clinical Application of Opioid Analgesics. In RS Sinatra, AH Hord, B Ginsberg, LM Preble (eds), Acute Pain: Mechanisms and Management. St. Louis: Mosby, 1992;93.

46. Kaiko RF, Foley KM, Grabinski PY, et al. Central nervous system excitatory effects of meperidine in cancer patients. Ann Neurol 1983;13:180.

47. Inturrisi CE, Umans JG. Meperidine Biotransformation and Central Nervous System Toxicity in Animals and Humans. In KM Foley, CE Inturrisi (eds), Opioid Analgesics in the Management of Clinical Pain. New York: Raven, 1986:143.

48. Martin WR. Pharmacology of opioids. Pharmacol Rev 1984;35:283.

49. Hill CS. Oral Opioid Analgesics. In RB Patt (ed), Cancer Pain. Philadelphia: Lippincott, 1993;129.

50. Portenoy R. Continuous intravenous infusion of opioid drugs. Med Clin North Am 1987;71:233.

51. Bruera E, Ripamonte C. Alternate Routes of the Administration of Narcotics. In RB Patt (ed), Cancer Pain Management: A Multidisciplinary Approach. Philadelphia: Lippincott, in press.

52. Rodiochock LD, Harper GR, Ruckdeschel JC, et al. Early diagnosis of spinal epidural metastases. Am J Med 1981;70:1181.

53. Posner JB. Back pain and epidural spinal cord compression. Med Clin North Am 1987;71:200.

54. Willson JKV, Masaryk TJ. Neurologic emergencies in the cancer patient. Semin Oncol 1989;16:494.

55. Gilbert RW, Kim JH, Posner JB. Epidural spinal cord compression from metastatic tumor: Diagnosis and treatment. Ann Neurol 1978;3:40.

56. Galasko CSB. Orthopaedic Principles and Management. In D Dolye, GWC Hanks, N MacDonald (eds), Oxford Textbook of Palliative Medicine. Oxford: Oxford University Press, 1993;274.

57. Rosier RN. Orthopedic Management. In RB Patt (ed), Cancer Pain. Philadelphia: Lippincott, 1993;461.

58. Bruera E, MacDonald RN. Intractable pain in patients with advanced head and neck tumors: A possible role for local infection. Cancer Treat Rep 1986;70:691.

59. Colye N, Portenoy RK. Infection as a cause of rapidly increasing pain in cancer patients. J Pain Symptom Manage 1991;6:266.

60. DuPen SL, Peterson DG, Williams A, Bogosian AJ. Infection during chronic epidural catheterization: Diagnosis and treatment. Anesthesiology 1990;73:905.

61. Hill CS, Thorpe DM, McCrory L. A method for attaining rapid and sustained pain relief and discriminating nociceptive from neuropathic pain in cancer patients. Pain 1990;(Suppl. 5):S498.

62. Hagen NA, Elwood T, Ernst S. Cancer pain emergencies: A protocol for management. J Pain Symptom Manage, in press.

63. Motwani JG, Lipworth BJ. Clinical pharmacokinetics of drugs administered buccally and sublingually. Clin Pharmacokinet 1991;21:83.

64. Ripamonti C, Bruera E. Rectal, buccal, and sublingual narcotics for the management of cancer pain. J Palliative Care 1991;7:30.

65. Davis T, Miser AW, Loprinzi CL, Kaur JS, et al. Comparative morphine pharmacokinetics following sublingual, intramuscular, and oral administration in patients with cancer. The Hospice Journal 1993;9:85.

66. Schechter NL, Weisman SJ, Rosenblum M, Bernstein B, et al. The use of oral transmucosal fentanyl citrate for painful procedures in children. Pediatrics 1995;95:335.

67. Fine PG, Marcus M, De Boer AJ, der Oord BV. An open label study of oral transmucosal fentanyl citrate (OTFC) for the treatment of breakthrough cancer pain. Pain 1991;45:149.

68. Ashburn MA, Fine PG, Stanley TH. Oral transmucosal fentanyl citrate for the treatment of breakthrough cancer pain: A case report. Anesthesiology 1989;71;615.

69. Kunz KM, Theisen JA, Schroeder ME. Severe episodic pain: Management with sublingual sufentanil. J Pain Symptom Manage 1993;8:189.

70. Gardner-Nix J. Sublingual fentanyl and sufentanil for management of incident pain. J Pain Symptom Manage (in press).

Chapter 37

The Hospice Movement: A Practical Approach

James C. Pace and Emma Lee Ann Meffert

An Introduction: The Hospice Concept

The hospice concept is one that attempts to give cancer patients and their families the necessary care, education, and support needed for the journey that lies ahead. This journey captures the time period prior to the patient's death (usually the patient's prognosis is 6 months of life or less, with an average of 3 months in our agency), the phase of active dying, the death event itself, and the first year of bereavement. The patient's family and significant others are a vital part of care planning and delivery and are given all the support and encouragement possible during the hospice experience. The relief of the patient's pain is one of the primary objectives of hospice care and has a variety of perspectives and applications that are explored briefly in this chapter. From the hospice perspective, the relief of pain requires multidisciplinary collaboration, constant evaluation and follow-up, a keen sense of the need to be proactive and creative rather than reactive and static, and as broad an understanding of the human condition as is humanly possible. In addition, it is crucial to the hospice concept of care that one understands that certain ways of life and methods of coping with life (and death) can never be changed nor should they. Sometimes the best that one can do is simply to be present with the patient and family and experience the passion of life along with another—this, after all, is the very root meaning of the word *compassion*. This is the challenge, joy, and the privilege of hospice care.

Pain and Suffering

The words pain and suffering are commonly used by most people associated with the hospice setting: patient, family, medical director, nurse, social worker, home health aid, and chaplain. The differences in the two terms present an important dimension in the concept of hospice care. Before a specific discussion on pain and its relief in the hospice community is presented, it is appropriate to review the concept of suffering from the authors' perspective.

Suffering

According to Benedict,[1, 2] the concept of suffering involves four essential features. For a person to suffer:

1. She or he must have had an experience or an event that was negative or unpleasant. These events or experiences can include but are not limited to physical pain, cognitive experiences or losses, real, potentially real, or imagined.
2. Suffering occurs only when the person perceives the event or experience as being negative or unpleasant.
3. When the event is perceived as such, some type or manner of distress results.
4. The negative event endures for some time, or, the event is expected to endure or to recur.

Anticipation of a negative event may cause one to suffer more than the actual experience of the event itself.

Pain, when present, is only one component of suffering. Pain is a physiologic response. It is "an unpleasant sensory and emotional experience associated with actual or potential tissue damage, or described in terms of such damage."[3] Suffering may include painful stimuli but is not limited to such stimuli. Pain is usually thought of as more of a physiologic response whereas suffering is more of a product of experiences with life, more often than not, unpleasant. Psychological pain—to be distinguished from physiologic pain—can be thought of as synonymous with suffering. Anguish and agony are subclasses of suffering. The patient who is in either state undoubtedly suffers, but the converse may not necessarily be true. Thus, suffering is an unpleasant mental state resulting from an event or situation that is perceived to be harmful, uncomfortable, unpleasant, or psychologically or physically painful.[1] Suffering contains the essential elements of event, perception, distress, and time. Suffering is always of a unique nature and can only be inferred by others. Suffering and pain are not synonymous. Suffering is a much broader concept than is pain. However, when one is in pain, not only is the suffering compounded in many ways, but the pain makes it virtually impossible to address the wider issues involved with the suffering. The hospice concept can really help patients and their family deal with this dilemma.

One of the primary tasks of a hospice care professional is to provide relief of the patient's pain. Once the physical pain is relieved, then the suffering that may be present can be approached in a multidisciplinary manner. All too often, the cause(s) of suffering cannot be adequately addressed until the physical pain has been eliminated or reduced to the point that the patient can begin to concentrate on other issues causing distress.

Pain

Pain is always subjective.[4] Objective observations such as grimacing, limping, groaning, crying, wincing with movement, irritability, apathy, and tachycardia may be useful at times and may indicate acute pain states, but these signs and symptoms are often absent in the hospice patient who suffers from chronic pain. In the hospice setting, the professional must accept the patient's report of pain and then labor to relieve that pain, using every available channel and mechanism. An operational definition of pain that has gained acceptance in the literature is as follows: "Pain is whatever the experiencing person says it is, existing whenever that person says it does."[5]

Chronic pain may be acute, chronic, or intermittent. It has usually been described as that which lasts beyond 3 months, is poorly localized, and is most often described as dull, aching, diffuse, constant, nagging, and often intractable, affecting patients with symptoms of listlessness, depression, withdrawal, and a feeling of helplessness.[6] In the hospice population, the lack of objective signs of pain should *never* dissuade the professional from believing the patient's report of pain. The World Health Organization "analgesic ladder" serves as the model for choosing among the three steps of analgesic treatment.[7] Some types of cancer pain respond to nonopioid drugs alone, which are listed in Table 37-1.[8]

Pain of an increasing intensity may be relieved by combining a weak opioid (Table 37-2)[8] with the nonopioid. Pain of increasing intensity may require a stronger opioid and, in selected cases, analgesic adjuvants may also be found useful.

Nonopioid Analgesics

Nonsteroidal anti-inflammatory drugs are useful for treating cancer pain of mild intensity and also musculoskeletal pain, especially when associated with inflammatory lesions (see Table 37-1).[8, 9] Nonopioids differ from opioid analgesics in that they (1) have a ceiling effect to pain control, (2) do not produce psychological or physical dependence, (3) are antipyretic, and (4) the primary mechanism of action is inhibition of the enzyme cyclo-oxygenase, thus preventing the formation of prostaglandin. Some of these drugs are available for parenteral and rectal administration. There are many health care professionals who believe that every analgesic regimen should include a nonopioid drug for the previously mentioned reasons.[8]

Opioids

When nonopioids alone cannot control a hospice patient's pain, weak opioids and subsequently

Table 37-1. Selected Nonopioid Analgesics

Drug	Proprietary Drug Names (Not All-Inclusive)	Average Analgesic Dose (mg)	Dose Interval (hrs)	Maximum Daily Dose (mg)
Acetaminophen	Numerous	500–1,000 PO	4–6	4,000
Salicylates				
Aspirin	Numerous	500–1,000 PO	4–6	4,000
Diflunisal	Dolobid	1,000 PO initial, 500 PO subsequent	8–12	1,500
Choline magnesium trisalicylate	Trilisate	1,000–1,500 PO	12	2,000–3,000
Nonsteroidal anti-inflammatory drugs				
Propionic acids				
Ibuprofen	Motrin, Rufen, Nuprin, Advil, Medipren	200–400 PO	4–6	2,400
Naproxen	Naprosyn	500 PO initial, 250 PO subsequent	6–8	1,250
Naproxen sodium	Anaprox	550 PO initial, 275 PO subsequent	6–8	1,375
Fenoprofen	Nalfon	200 PO	4–6	800
Ketoprofen	Orudis	25–50 PO	6–8	300
Indolacetic acids				
Indomethacin	Indocin	25 PO	8–12	100
Pyrrolacetic acids				
Ketorolac	Toradol	30 or 60 mg IM initial, 15 or 30 mg IM subsequent	6	150 first day, 120 thereafter
Anthranilic acids				
Mefenamic acid	Ponstel	500 PO initial, 250 PO subsequent	6	1,500

Source: Reprinted with permission from MB Max, R Payne, WT Edward, et al. Principles of Analgesic Use in the Treatment of Acute Pain and Cancer Pain (3rd ed). Stokie, IL: American Pain Society, 1992.

strong opioid analgesics are then added. The only opioids that have dose limitations are those that are marketed in combination with a nonopioid—the nonopioid serves to limit the dose. For example, with Tylenol No. 3 or oxycodone (e.g., Percocet), it is the acetaminophen that causes 24-hour dose limitations. Table 37-3[8] details the medications that are most commonly used in cancer patients with severe pain who are treated in a hospice program.

Dosage, Route, and Schedule for the Hospice Patient's Pain

Usually, the oral route is desirable for cancer pain treatment because of its convenience, flexibility, and the relatively steady blood levels produced. For those patients who find it difficult to swallow pills, many opioids are available in liquid formulations. After oral administration, most opioids (with exception of time-released tablets), peak in approximately 1.5–2.0 hours. Thus, after 2 hours, if the side effects are minimal, and if the pain is not relieved, the patient may be administered another opioid dose safely.[8]

Intramuscular administration of pain medication should be avoided whenever possible. Such injections are painful, often inadequately absorbed, inconsistently metabolized, and possess variable blood levels when compared with oral opioid administration. Because of decreased muscle in that patient population, intramuscular injections are relatively contraindicated in most hospice situations.

Table 37-2. Opioid Analgesics Commonly Used for Mild-to-Moderate Pain

Name	Starting Dose* Adults (mg)	Precautions and Contraindications
Morphine-like agonists		
Codeine	30–60	Caution in patients with impaired ventilation, bronchial asthma, increased intracranial pressure, liver failure
Oxycodone	5	Same as for codeine
Meperidine (Demerol)	50	Normeperidine accumulates with repetitive dosing, causing central nervous system excitation; avoid in patients with impaired renal function or who are receiving monoamine oxidase inhibitors; avoid any chronic use
Propoxyphene (Darvon)	65–130	Propoxyphene and metabolite accumulate with repetitive dosing; overdose complicated by convulsions
Mixed agonist-antagonists		
Pentazocine (Talwin)	50	May cause psychotomimetic effects; may precipitate withdrawal in narcotic-dependent patients

*Starting doses are approximately equianalgesic to aspirin 650 mg (adults). The optimal dose for each patient is determined by titration.
Source: Reprinted with permission from MB Max, R Payne, WT Edward, et al. Principles of Analgesic Use in the Treatment of Acute Pain and Cancer Pain (3rd ed). Stokie, IL: American Pain Society, 1992.

Intravenous bolus doses of opioid medication provide rapid onset of activity and are useful in a therapeutic analgesic concentration that provides pain relief to be followed by maintenance infusion. Such continuous infusions provide for steady blood levels that provide effective analgesia with relatively few side effects. When intravenous opioid analgesia is necessary for extended periods in the hospice environment, patient-controlled analgesia (PCA) is often the modality of choice. Maximum safe usage is set at an upper limit that is programmed as a total dose over a given time. Standard infusion pumps allow either a 1-hour or a 4-hour cumulative dose limit. Once the nurse observes the actual hourly consumption of pain medication, this limit can be adjusted upward or downward. This objective can usually be accomplished in 24 hours. Guidelines for PCA administration for adults with acute pain are found in Table 37-4.[8] Dosages and lockouts and limits are determined and adjusted based on the patient's age, health status, required loading dose, and presence of opioid tolerance. It should be stressed to the hospice patient and family that there is no upper limit to the amount of drug that can be given with the PCA pump, provided that there is attending physician accountability and comprehensive nursing supervision.

Transdermal Patches

The fentanyl patch has become an important modality in the hospice pain relief arsenal. Fentanyl is readily absorbed through the skin and offers continuous opioid infusion without pumps or needles. Transdermal fentanyl possesses a 72-hour dosing interval reservoir and comes in 25-, 50-, 75-, and 100-μg per hour packages. The manufacturers suggest that a 25-μg per hour patch is approximately equal to oral morphine, 30 mg every 8 hours, i.e., approximately 90 mg of oral morphine in a 24-hour period. However, many clinicians have found that higher dosages of fentanyl are needed to replace this morphine dosage. When changing to the patch, it takes 12–16 hours to observe any therapeutic effect and 48 hours to achieve a steady-state blood concentration. When that change is about to be implemented, it is suggested that the hospice patient's pain be controlled with a short-acting opioid that can be titrated to relief during the initial period of

Table 37-3. Opioid Analgesics Commonly Used for Severe Pain

Name	Equianalgesic Dose (mg)		Starting Oral Dose Adults (mg)	Comments
	Oral	Parenteral		
Morphine-like agonists				
Morphine	30	10	15–30	Standard of comparison for narcotic analgesics; sustained-release preparations (MS Contin, Oramorph-SR) release drug over 8–12 hours. For all opioids, caution in patients with impaired ventilation, bronchial asthma, increased intracranial pressure, liver failure
Hydromorphone (Dilaudid)	7.5	1.5	4–8	Slightly shorter duration than morphine
Oxycodone	30	—	15–30	—
Methadone (Dolophine)	20	10	5–10	Good oral potency; long plasma half-life (24–36 hours). Accumulates with repetitive dosing, causing excessive sedation (on days 2–5)
Levorphanol (Levo-Dromoran)	4	2	2–4	Long plasma half-life (12–16 hours). Accumulates on days 2–3
Fentanyl	—	0.1	—	Transdermal fentanyl (Duragesic). Because of skin reservoir of drug, 12-hour delay in onset and offset of transdermal patch; 25–50 μg/hr roughly equivalent to 30 mg sustained-release morphine q8h; fever increases dose rate
Oxymorphone (Numorphan)	—	1	—	5 mg rectal suppository = 5 mg morphine IM; like IM morphine
Meperidine (Demerol)	300	75	Not recommended	Slightly shorter acting than morphine. Normeperidine (toxic metabolite) accumulates with repetitive dosing, causing central nervous system excitation; avoid in patients with impaired renal function or who are receiving monoamine oxidase inhibitors.
Mixed agonist-antagonists				
Nalbuphine (Nubain)	—	10	—	Not available orally; not scheduled under the Controlled Substances Act; incidence of psychotomimetic effects lower than with pentazocine; may precipitate withdrawal in narcotic-dependent patients
Butorphanol (Stadol)	—	2	—	Like nalbuphine
Dezocine (Dalgan)	—	10	—	Like nalbuphine. May precipitate withdrawal in narcotic-dependent patients; SC injection irritating
Partial agonist				
Buprenorphine (Buprenex)	0.4	—	—	Not available orally; sublingual preparation not yet in United States; less abuse liability than morphine; does not produce psychotomimetic effects; may precipitate withdrawal in narcotic-dependent patients; not readily reversed by naloxone; avoid in labor

Source: Reprinted with permission from MB Max, R Payne, WT Edward, et al. Principles of Analgesic Use in the Treatment of Acute Pain and Cancer Pain (3rd ed). Stokie, IL: American Pain Society, 1992.

Table 37-4. Guidelines for Patient-Controlled Intravenous Opioid Administration for Adults with Acute Pain

Drug*	Usual Starting Dose After Loading (mg)	Usual Dose Range (mg)	Usual Lockout Range (min)
Morphine (1.0 mg/ml)	1.0	0.5–2.5	5–10
Meperidine (10 mg/ml)	10	5–25	5–10
Hydromorphone (0.2 mg/ml)	0.2	0.05–0.40	5–10

*Standard concentrations for most patient-controlled analgesia machines are listed in parentheses.
Source: Reprinted with permission from MB Max, R Payne, WT Edward, et al. Principles of Analgesic Use in the Treatment of Acute Pain and Cancer Pain (3rd ed). Stokie, IL: American Pain Society, 1992.

dosing with fentanyl. As usual, a short-acting opioid (oxycodone, hydromorphone, or immediate-release morphine) should be available to the patient for breakthrough pain even when the steady state of fentanyl has been reached. If the patient begins to take more and more of the rescue doses, then the transdermal dose should be increased based on the 24-hour total of rescue opioid taken.

Rectal Route

The rectal route of opioid medication administration is especially helpful in those hospice patients who are unable to swallow or who do not have access to PCA systems or the ability to begin the transdermal route of dosing. There are many creative ways that a pharmacist can prepare rectal administrations of opioids combined with adjuvants for effective pain relief. The presence of diarrhea, chronic or intermittent, must always be assessed and monitored. Inconclusive evidence exists as to the effectiveness of pain medications given vaginally in suppository form.

Epidural and Intrathecal Routes

Intraspinal opioids are used in some hospice situations where the supervision of such a regimen can be closely monitored. When an indwelling spinal catheter is present in a patient admitted to hospice care, usually that catheter is connected to a continuous infusion pump. A local anesthetic can also be added with the opioid; this combination produces analgesia at dosage levels that are lower than if the drugs had been administered individually. Tolerance

to this delivery system does not appear to develop any more rapidly than with systemic opioid delivery.

Hospice "Rules of Thumb"

The following principles may be applied to the control of pain in cancer patients in a hospice environment.

1. It is always appropriate to have dosage leeway written into the orders given by the attending physician, i.e., the nurse can titrate the amount of drug as needed to control pain without having to constantly call the physician for a higher dosage. This flexibility in titration is especially helpful during the night or on weekends. Along with this leeway is also the possibility for a change in route of administration when necessary (e.g., from tablet form to liquid, from liquid to suppository) along with the related dosage equivalencies. This flexibility is predicated on the training, experience, and cooperation of the permanent nursing staff in the hospice facility.

2. Pain medications are to be administered regularly. This does not mean as needed or as little as possible. One of the hospice nurse's major roles is to convince the patient and family that pain medications are to be taken on a scheduled basis when pain is present during most of the day, evening, and night. When pain medication has been ordered on a regular basis, (such as continuously released morphine [MS Contin], 30 mg every 12 hours), an "as needed" order of a supplemental opioid for breakthrough pain that can be administered between regular doses of pain medication is an essential backup in the hospice pharmacologic arsenal as well. Even when pain occurs just during certain times of the

day (or night), a regularly scheduled analgesic dose should be established with the patient or primary caregiver. Such dosing has the possibility of eliminating the pain altogether.

3. The hospice nurse must be skilled in "prescribing" stool softeners and laxatives, e.g., senna (Senokot, Senokot DS). Few pain regimens exist that do not require an accompanying laxative dosage. These dosages can also be titrated according to patient response.

4. Patient and family communication are important in the hospice environment. Patients have to be followed closely for pain control response, and it is not always possible to implement nurse visitation in the home care environment as often as may be desirable. The nurse must monitor pain relief and side effects frequently, always adjusting the regimen as necessary. When a new analgesic regimen is started, the nurse should initiate telephone follow-up at least once daily until pain is satisfactorily controlled.

5. When changing to a new analgesic dosage, it is absolutely imperative that the nurse consult equianalgesic tables to make sure the new dosage will adequately control pain. This is usually best accomplished under the direction of the attending physician responsible for the patient's care, or an appropriate pain specialist.

6. It is important for the hospice nurse to be a tactful and responsive team player. In many situations, the hospice nurse has had years of experience with pain regimens whereas a new primary physician may lack such skills. Physicians and nurses alike work best in an environment where mutual respect, cooperation, and positive attitudes are associated with professional behaviors.

7. The hospice nurse must be ever alert to side effects of pain medications and be skilled in their treatment. The most common side effects of opioid analgesics include sedation, constipation, nausea, vomiting, itching, and respiratory depression. The possibility of drug interactions and synergism are always possible when sedative, hypnotic, or tranquilizer drugs are combined with opioids. Opioid-related nausea and vomiting can often be controlled with the use of the scopolamine patch and an oral phenothiazine antiemetic. Tetrahydrocannabinol (THC) is used in some hospice facilities in either tablet form or by "cigarette or joint." However, the use of THC is controversial and, in some states, is illegal. Itching may necessitate the

use of an antihistamine. Although respiratory depression is rare in hospice patients who are used to relatively high dosages of pain medication, the nurse must be aware of such side effects and provide teaching related to the importance of avoiding the possibility of airway obstruction by the tongue during sleep. If the patient does succumb to respiratory depression or coma, the nurse must be aware that the hospice patient may be highly sensitive to narcotic antagonists. Dosages of such antagonists, e.g., naloxone, should be titrated to avoid profound withdrawal, seizures, and severe pain. It is also helpful to remember that meperidine (Demerol) often produces anxiety, tremors, myoclonus, and generalized seizures with chronic usage due to the formation of the active metabolite normeperidine. For this reason, Demerol is usually a poor choice for pain control in the hospice patient. In addition, pentazocine (Talwin) has been known to cause confusion and hallucinations.

8. The hospice nurse must be always aware of the development of tolerance to opioid analgesics. Tolerance is a phenomenon that occurs when increasing amounts of opioid analgesics are necessary to maintain the initial effect of the drug. Tolerance is common in all age groups taking opioid analgesics on a scheduled basis. The first sign of tolerance is a decrease in the duration of effective analgesia. To delay or minimize tolerance, opioids may be combined with nonopioids or changed to an alternate opioid using standard equianalgesic principles.

9. If, for some reason, the patient fails to receive pain medication after chronic usage, the nurse must be aware of the following symptoms of withdrawal: anxiety, irritability, chills that alternate with hot flashes, salivation, lacrimation, rhinorrhea, diaphoresis, piloerection, nausea, vomiting, abdominal cramps, and insomnia. With long half-life drugs (e.g., methadone and levorphanol), these symptoms are often delayed for several days. Weaning the hospice patient off pain regimens is rarely indicated, and as a result, is usually never an issue. The informed and empathetic nurse and physician should always avoid using terms such as "addicted" and "drug user or abuser." Physical dependence on pain medication is not the same as addiction. Fears of opioid addiction in the hospice population should not be an issue for patients or their families. The effective hospice nurse will educate all parties to the fact that the hospice patient

takes such medications because of a physiologic need and not due to a psychological need or craving. The treatment of chronic pain in the hospice population is usually not associated with issues of addiction. However, in some isolated cases, family members, who are generally healthy and pain free, may abuse the opioid medications prescribed for the patient. This particular problem necessitates the work of the entire team to ensure pain relief for the patient and some type of treatment for the offending family member.

Noninvasive Methods of Pain Control and Treatment

Health professionals and family caregivers, alike, may participate in pain relief measures using certain cutaneous modalities rather than or alongside systemic medications. Employing positioning, movement, massage, and application of heat, cold, or menthol may be overlooked, yet they still offer low-risk techniques for pain relief for hospice patients. A diversity of noninvasive approaches for the treatment of pain also includes such approaches as therapeutic touch, cognitive behavioral therapy, music therapy, biofeedback, body positioning, and range of motion exercises, among others. These modalities are simple and inexpensive and are often welcomed by patients because they are nondrug-related means of achieving some measure of pain control.[10] Additionally, the use of transcutaneous electrical nerve stimulation may provide acceptable pain relief that is commonly associated with musculoskeletal dysfunction including decreased mobility and poor positioning.

Another noninvasive modality, hypnosis, has been shown to be a valuable tool in controlling pain in terminally ill patients. Doody et al.[11] describe hypnosis as an altered state of consciousness accompanied by feelings of relaxation involving intense focal concentration and decreased peripheral awareness of the actual surroundings.

Spira and Spiegel[12] state that the successful use of hypnosis depends on the patient's cognitive style, his or her hypnotizability, the level of cognitive functioning, and the motivation to participate in the hypnotic process. The patient's ability to visualize abstract concepts helps him or her separate from the physical experience of pain. Depending on the patient's inherent capability, self-induced hypnosis, as well as therapist-guided experiences, have produced positive results in controlling mild-to-moderate pain.

Nurses can help family members understand ways to assess the pain of their loved ones. Activities that increase pain should be noted, as well as the medications, dosages, and times of administration that diminish the pain's effects. The use of a diary or pain flow chart can be helpful for family members to serve as a memory aid in discussing the patient's needs with his or her medical or nursing practitioners.

Ahles and Martin[13] believe that educational programs on cancer pain should include individualized information about the causes and expected course of the pain as well as strategies for patients to discriminate between changes in pain status related to disease progress versus nondisease etiologies. Fishman[14] advocates that patients should be taught ways to change their attitudes about pain through cognitive modification techniques. For example, patients with lifelong unrealistic or distorted attitudes (e.g., pessimism, self-blame, catastrophizing, poor self-control) appear to be predisposed to excessive suffering when faced with terminal illness and pain. Thus, teaching the patient and family members more effective ways to cope is one method to improve the patient's and family member's quality of life. The use of a professional psychologist may be necessary to facilitate or implement that process.

From the nursing perspective, interventions related to pain management may be delineated according to specific nursing diagnoses, including chronic pain, knowledge deficit, ineffective individual coping, ineffective family coping, spiritual distress, grieving, altered family processes, sleep pattern disturbance, social isolation, altered bowel elimination, activity intolerance, high risk for altered respiratory function, altered nutrition, impaired tissue integrity, self-concept disturbance, and high risk for self-harm, among others. As one might expect, the physiologic effects of terminal illness and their emotional ramifications are exceedingly broad based.

Working with terminally ill patients, whether they are treated in hospital environments or within the more personalized home or inpatient hospice settings, may present health care providers with considerable ethical dilemmas during the course of their association. Ferrell et al.[15] reported in their findings on clinical decision making that nurses experienced many ethical dilemmas related to overmedication as well as undermedication. Most commonly cited was a concern regarding inadequate pain relief and the related problem of undermedication. Three-fourths of nurses surveyed listed ineffective pain relief as an ethical concern. "Decisions made regarding pain treatments carry significant outcomes such as potential physical harm from oversedation or respiratory depression and psychological harm of suffering from unrelieved pain."[16] The study by Ferrell et al. recommends continued nursing research as a means of achieving the goal established in the original standards of oncology nursing: comfort for the person with cancer. Another goal is freedom from pain for all patients who are experiencing issues related to dying as a result of terminal illnesses.

Warner[17] advocates that those who help terminally ill patients with pain relief should explore the religious and spiritual beliefs held by the patient and family. Through careful listening and empathetic discussions of the meaning of pain and suffering to the involved individuals, the caregiver can help the parties understand feelings of anger toward or abandonment by a higher being. Whether such exploration into the patient's spiritual domain is initiated by the health provider or the clergy depends on the training and comfort level of all persons involved. The goal, however, is to turn conflicts over differences in beliefs about the meaning of illness into potential sources of mutual support.

Optimal treatment of pain in the terminally ill may be conceptualized and administered from a family perspective. The methods for helping families of terminally ill patients are organized around a theme of enhancing feelings of control and self-efficacy, especially from the patient's perspective. Control over pain and related problems may be maximized by providing education, improved decision-making and assertiveness skills, and by teaching specific techniques for pain and stress management. Such teaching may include such topics as proper analgesic use, progressive relaxation, imagery, distraction techniques, and time management.[17] With the improvement of psychologic variables to include expectancy of pain, fear, anxiety, perceived controllability of pain, self-efficacy (coping mastery), and preoccupation with physical symptoms, the severity of reported pain can indeed be modulated.

Pain abatement is thus a planned, collaborative effort to bring a peaceful transition to the mind, body, and spirit of the individual experiencing a terminal illness. In such cases, although the individual's life may be threatened, ultimately his or her quality of life will be enhanced. When the symptoms of pain have been relieved, the hospice professional is then able to explore other issues that lead to the relief of suffering, reconciliation needs, growth needs, and can initiate further exploration in regard to end-of-life issues. This is the joy and the honor of being a caring health care professional in the hospice movement.

References

1. Benedict S. A linguistic analysis of the concept of suffering. Unpublished paper. Alabama: University of Alabama at Birmingham School of Nursing, 1981.
2. Benedict S. The suffering associated with lung cancer. Cancer Nurs 1989;12:34.
3. Merskey H (ed). Classification of chronic pain: Description of chronic pain syndromes and definitions of pain terms. Pain 1986;(Suppl. 3):S217.
4. Wild L. Pain management. Crit Care Nurs Clin North Am 1990;2:537.
5. Meinhart NT, McCaffery M. Pain: A Nursing Approach to Assessment and Analysis. Norwalk, CT: Appleton-Century-Crofts, 1983;11.
6. Whipple B. Neurophysiology of pain. Orthop Nurs 1990;9:21.
7. World Health Organization Expert Committee. Cancer Pain Relief and Palliative Care. Geneva, Switzerland: World Health Organization, 1990.
8. Max MB, Payne R, Edward WT, et al. Principles of Analgesic Use in the Treatment of Acute Pain and Cancer Pain (3rd ed). Skokie, IL: American Pain Society 1992.
9. Sunshine A, Olson N. Non-narcotic Analgesics. In PD Wall, R Melzack (eds), Textbook of Pain (2nd ed). New York: Churchill Livingstone 1989;670.
10. McCaffery M, Wolff, M. Pain relief using cutaneous modalities, positioning, and movement. Hosp J 1992;8:121.
11. Doody SB, Smith C, Webb J. Nonpharmacologic interventions for pain management. Crit Care Nurs Clin North Am 1991;3:69.
12. Spira JL, Spiegel D. Hypnosis and related techniques in pain management. Hospice J 1992;8:89.
13. Ahles TA, Martin JB. Cancer pain: A multidimensional perspective. Hospice J 1992;8:25.
14. Fishman B. The cognitive behavioral perspective on pain management in terminal illness. Hospice J 1992,8:73.

15. Ferrell BR, Eberts MT, McCaffery M, Grant M. Clinical decision making and pain. Cancer Nursing 1991;14:289.

16. Ferrell BR, Eberts MT, McCaffery M, Grant M, et al. Clinical decision making and pain. Cancer Nursing 1991;14:296.

17. Warner JE. Involvement of families in pain control of terminally ill patients. Hospice J 1992;8:155.

Chapter 38

The Hospice Movement: A Philosophical Approach

Denise L. Dunlap

A hospice is "a place of meeting. Physical and spiritual, doing and accepting, giving and receiving, all have to be brought together . . . The dying need the community, its help and fellowship . . . The community needs the dying to make it think of eternal issues and to make it listen . . . We are debtors to those who can make us learn such things as to be gentle and to approach others with true attention and respect."

Dame Cicely Saunders, M.D., Founder, St. Christopher's Hospice, London, England, 1967[1]

Any discussion of symptom relief in terminal cancer patients would be incomplete without mentioning hospice care. Hospice has come to represent an invaluable asset in the care of patients in the last days to months of their lives. Hospice's strengths lie not only in the skilled application of the hospice principles but also in the emotional, spiritual, and practical aspects of care that represent what good care of the dying really means.

Hospice is a concept of caring that originated in medieval times, where it symbolized a place where travelers, pilgrims, and the sick, wounded, or dying could find rest and comfort. The contemporary hospice offers a comprehensive program of care to terminally ill patients and their families. Hospice is primarily a concept of care, not a specific place of care.

Hospice emphasizes palliative rather than curative treatment; quality of life rather than quantity of life. It is where dying patients are comforted, professional medical care is given, and sophisticated symptom relief is provided. The patient and family are both included in the care plan and emotional, spiritual, and practical support is given based on the patient's wishes and family's needs. Trained volunteers can also offer respite care for family members as well as meaningful support to the patient.

Hospice affirms life and regards dying as a normal process. Hospice neither hastens nor postpones death. Hospice provides personalized services and a caring community so that patients and families can attain the necessary preparation for a death that is satisfactory to them.

The first hospice in the United States was established in 1974 in New Haven, CT. Shortly, thereafter, several hospice programs were initiated across the country. By June 1996, there were more than 2,700 hospices in the United States (Figure 38-1).

The initiation and growth of the hospice movement is the result of nurses, physicians, social workers, clergy, terminally ill patients and their families, and volunteers getting together to bring humane, quality care to persons with limited life expectancies who hope for comfort, control, dignity, and quality of life until death.

In the early days of hospice care, there was no source of reimbursement, other than community support and an enormous amount of volunteer time. In the early 1980s, the Health Care Finance Administration conducted a study in cooperation with Brown University to assess the cost effectiveness and quality of hospice services in preparation for the potential Medicare reimbursement.

In 1983, the hospice Medicare benefit was added to the Social Security Act. Though the hospice

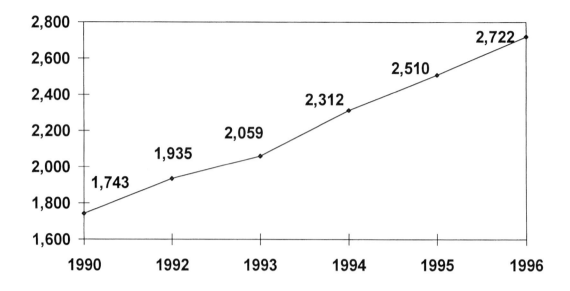

Figure 38-1. Growth of number of hospices in the United States from 1974 through June 1996. (Reprinted with permission from the National Hospice Organization, Arlington, VA, 1996.)

movement was still relatively small compared with other health care delivery systems, it had made its mark in getting the attention of legislators and policy makers, and had tremendous bipartisan support.

At the time of its legislative approval, the hospice Medicare benefit was a revolutionary concept in reimbursement. It was based on a prospective payment methodology, with capitation (i.e., restricted reimbursements). The benefit covered all services, supplies, equipment, and drugs that were related to the terminal illness. The hospice was both a provider of care and an insurer of care, very much like managed care organizations of today. Hospices were identified as being professionally responsible for the management of the care of their terminally ill patients at home, in hospitals, and in nursing homes.

Over the years, there have been many subjective and anecdotal accounts of hospice care's cost effectiveness and quality. In 1994, the National Hospice Organization published a comprehensive report of the results of a number of independent studies that had been conducted in recent years related to cost effectiveness and quality.[2]

These studies indicated that the substitution of home care for more costly inpatient care does not occur outside the framework of the hospice program. Analysis of the data showed that patients who received traditional home care services incurred approximately 30% more expense during the last 24 weeks of life than hospice home care beneficiaries. The studies also found that hospice care saves Medicare dollars, especially during the last month of the patient's life. Data also indicated that hospice patients had fewer out-of-pocket costs than conventional patients.

Most benefits managers in the public and private sectors also indicated their satisfaction with hospice benefits. Cost savings, improved quality, and the organizational capacity of hospices to coordinate care across all settings were identified as the advantages that hospice care offers compared with conventional care.

Quality of care is more difficult to measure in an objective and scientific manner. The research that has been done, and is described in the National Hospice Organization's report, does demonstrate statistically significant ways in which hospice patients and their caregivers experience a higher quality of life during the dying process than patients and families receiving conventional care. Working closely with the patient's primary physician, the hospice team of nurses, social workers, chaplains, home health aides, and volunteers strive to ensure adequate pain control, an improved social environment and interpersonal relationships, involvement in care, and less anxiety on the part of caregivers.

The Role of the Hospice Nurse, Medical Director, and Home Health Aide

The hospice nurse's role is a pivotal one as the advocate of the patient and his or her family, as well as being part of the professional hospice team.

Traditionally, nursing focuses on delivering individualized care to patients in order that their health status will improve so that they might carry on with the process of living. Hospice nursing, on the other hand, focuses on helping hospice patients live each day as fully and autonomously as possible until their death. This type of care enables patients to maintain control over their treatment and to live their last months in an environment that is familiar and comfortable.

A patient's physician must have diagnosed a disease process, malignant or nonmalignant, that will probably result in death in 6–7 months or less. In addition to cancer pain patients, hospice serves individuals with a variety of terminal nonneoplastic illnesses including amyotrophic lateral sclerosis, end-stage heart disease, respiratory and lung disease, and end-stage Alzheimer's disease. Although most hospice patients are cancer patients, care is provided regardless of the patient's type of disease. The last few years have seen an increasing number of patients with acquired immunodeficiency syndrome (AIDS) who have been using hospice care.

The hospice nurse's first visit involves making a complete physical assessment of the patient as well as evaluating the environment and the caregiver situation. Nurses explain hospice philosophy and services to both the patient and the family and clearly communicate what the family can expect from hospice.

Based on this initial visit, the hospice nurse determines the number of visits that will be made to the home each week. During each visit, the nurse assesses the patient's physical condition. The hospice nurse must draw on expertise gained through experience to provide control of pain and other symptoms that may occur in the advanced disease process as well as to maintain bowel function and nutritional intake. In order to provide the best physical care to each patient, a hospice nurse must stay updated on all of the latest medical and technical advances that might provide possible comfort to the patient. The nurse also alerts the family to possible symptoms that should be communicated to the hospice nurse as soon as possible. These symptoms include problems with pain, vomiting, bowel function, and shortness of breath.

A fundamental goal of the hospice nurse is to develop a close relationship with the patient and family. This is accomplished by becoming more acquainted during each home visit. By getting to know the family and taking the best possible care of symptoms, a nurse may establish a closeness that enables a family to be more open with issues and concerns about their loved one's approaching death. Nursing services are available to patients 24 hours a day, 7 days a week. As the patient deteriorates and is very close to death, the hospice nurse prepares the family by discussing the signs and symptoms they may observe in their loved one. If death occurs during the weekday, the primary nurse immediately goes to the home. If death occurs after hours or on the weekends, the on-call nurse goes to the home. The hospice nurse comforts and supports the family and makes any arrangements that are necessary related to the office of the coroner, funeral home, and police.

Throughout the time that the patient is under the care of hospice, the nurse keeps the patient's primary physician informed of the patient's changing condition. Due to their extensive and varied experience with these situations, hospice nurses can frequently make suggestions to the physician. The referring physicians rely on the hospice nurses to be their "eyes and ears" in the homes of the patients.

The hospice nurse meets with the other members of the interdisciplinary team once a week. The entire hospice team works together to coordinate the best possible care for the patient and family during this difficult time. At team meetings, patients and any problems or issues that patients or their family may have are evaluated. The patients who have passed away during the past week are also discussed and the bereavement needs of their family and friends are addressed.

Another member of the hospice team is the medical director. This is a physician who is either employed or volunteers his or her services to the hospice. When needed, the medical director acts as a liaison between the hospice nurse and the patient's primary physician. Medical directors attend team meetings and are available for consultations with the hospice nurse regarding pain control, disease process, or a particular patient's situation.

The home health aides provide assistance with the personal care of the patient. They lift and turn the patient, change the bed sheets, and provide hair, skin, and nail care. The home health aide is most often the team member who has the most contact with the patient and family and spends a great deal of time providing education to the patient and his or her family.

The experience of a hospice nurse is different from other nurses in that most of their patients die while under their care. Becoming a hospice nurse is an adjustment for every nurse regardless of his or her background. It can be difficult to maintain an average load of ten patients who are at different stages of their disease process and of various socioeconomic backgrounds. Frequently, a hospice nurse will lose four or five patients in 1 week. As with other areas of nursing, burnout can be a problem. Team meetings and support groups provide an outlet to discuss feelings. Family gratitude also imparts an added source of strength.

Role of the Hospice Social Worker

Social workers provide emotional support and counseling to hospice patients and their families as well as bereavement services after the patient's death. The hospice social worker has been educated and trained to address social and emotional needs by listening, counseling, supporting, problem solving, enhancing communication, and accessing community resources. Hospice social workers focus on quality of life and the unique needs of the patient and family rather than the disease.

Social workers assess patient and family needs; assist with financial and practical concerns; link patient and family with community resources; develop individualized care plans; assist with preneed planning; help caregivers cope; affirm the dignity of all patients; offer bereavement support; and evaluate the need for volunteers and other support services needed by the family.

One way hospice differs greatly from home health care is through the extensive attention given to grief and bereavement by the hospice social workers. They keep in contact with a patient's family for at least 1 year after the patient's death. Volunteers can also be enlisted to supplement the social worker's contact with the family by making telephone calls, personal visits, and correspondence through the mail.

Other helpful services provided by hospice social workers include assistance in a nonthreatening way, being a caring presence, listening in a nonjudgmental way, suggesting coping strategies to reduce stress, providing support to patient and family, relieving anxieties and emotional fears, giving honest, compassionate answers to questions, and helping the patient and family express emotions.

Role of the Hospice Chaplain

People faced with a life-threatening illness face the same religious and spiritual needs as everyone else. The role of the hospice chaplain is to provide palliative care but neither to change nor to judge the spiritual life of the hospice patient. Hospice chaplains take a spiritual approach to care rather than a religious or denominational approach. The goals of a hospice chaplain center around meeting the patient wherever they are on their spiritual path and walking with them to the end of the patient's life.

The hospice chaplain acknowledges that there are many pathways and, along the way, that each individual does the best she or he is able. Religion is only one such pathway. Those patients for whom religion and the religious community have been a resource are expected to make the fullest possible use of the resource. The purpose of the hospice chaplain is to bring whatever resources the patient has available into play in the current situation as effectively and expertly as possible.

When the patient is actively related to a worshipping community and the relationship provides the type and level of care and support the patient desires, the worshipping community is viewed as the primary provider of spiritual care and counsel. The role of the chaplain in this situation is as liaison to the worshipping community, informing them about hospice care, updating them regarding the patient's change in status, and providing support to their continuing care for the patient and family.

When the patient has been actively related to a worshipping community in the past but is now inactive, the chaplain assesses the situation in order to identify limitations and to work with the worshipping community to restore the kind and level of support the patient desires, thereby linking the patient to a nearby worshipping community.

When the patient has no relationship with a worshipping community and desires none, the role of the chaplain is to assess the spiritual needs and problems of care and to provide appropriate follow-up. As an attentive guide and listener, the hospice chaplain provides the patient opportunities to talk about God, spiritual issues, and the meaning and purpose in the changed and ever-changing situation.

In understanding the role of the chaplain it is important to remember that not all patients and not all families are religious. Many do not engage in religious practices and have not for many years. Religion has not been a part of their recent history. Religion is not a resource they use in coping with the changing seasons and circumstances of their life. Therefore, they are not expected to be religious in the last stages of their life.

Role of the Volunteer

Hospice volunteers are often the most direct link between the patient and the hospice agency. The volunteer maintains communication with patients and family members on a weekly basis and is sometimes the person who is the most sensitive to the unique needs of each individual. One who gives time and talents as a volunteer will receive much in return.

There are many ways to be a hospice volunteer. Most volunteers choose to work directly with patients and families, and hospice provides an opportunity for volunteers to contribute to the comfort of terminally ill patients and their families. A volunteer spends 3–4 hours a week providing companionship, help in the home, emotional support, and relief for the caregiver. Volunteers are usually assigned one patient at a time.

Volunteers are not expected to be nurses. They are companions (actually more like friends) during a time of need. In fact, volunteers provide important services beyond medical care such as running errands, reading to a patient, or simply holding a caregiver's hand.

Bereavement volunteers work with grieving family members or friends and make contact by telephone, mail, or personal visits. Volunteers also help in the office by providing assistance with special projects, mailings, reception, and clerical support.

Assistance with memorial services, fund raising projects, special events, community education, and public speaking is also often provided by a pool of volunteers. Some volunteers choose to share their professional expertise by serving as a member of the board of directors for a nonprofit hospice or on other board committees.

Bereavement Support

When someone we love has died, our world changes. Grief is a natural and necessary process of reacting to significant loss in our lives. Normal grief has no calendar or timetable. Many people are uncomfortable with the emotional pain of grief. Friends and family are sometimes unsure of what to say or how to be helpful. Grieving persons can feel isolated, abandoned, and easily overwhelmed by their situation.

Because there are such individual differences in how people experience grief, many hospices offer a wide variety of bereavement services from support groups to individual counseling. These services are designed to provide a safe environment to explore issues during the grieving process and are usually available to anyone in the community who has experienced the loss of a loved one.

Common experiences of grief include shock, confusion, panic, guilt, hostility, depression, aimlessness, fatigue, loss of appetite, sleep disturbances, crying spells, loss of past interests, weight loss or gain, and neglect of appearance.

Social workers often suggest that the bereaved express their feelings, ask for help when needed, be patient, keep healthy, be alert to physical needs, learn more about grief and its effects, and trust their ability to heal.

For those who care about the bereaved family or friend, it is helpful to be present and available during this difficult time, be a good nonjudgmental listener, be patient and let the person cry, respect the pain of loss, and continue to provide support after the initial shock of the loss has worn off. In addition to the group and individual counseling offered

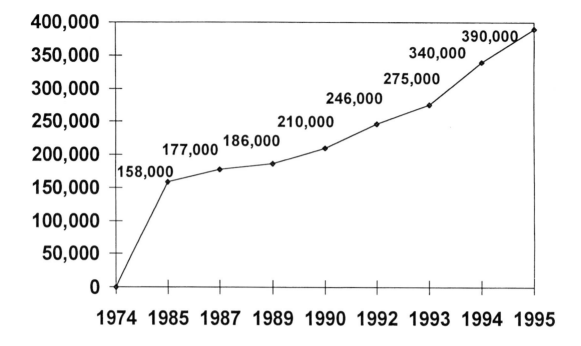

Figure 38-2. Growth of number of hospice patients in the United States from 1974 through 1995. The first hospice in the United States opened in 1974. (Reprinted with permission from the National Hospice Organization, Arlington, VA, 1996.)

by most hospices, there is often a memorial service held at least once a year. This memorial service provides an opportunity for families, hospice staff, volunteer, and friends to remember those persons who have died in the recent past. Memorial services are another support for the mutual grief felt by those close to the patient and his or her family.

Conclusion

More Americans are turning to hospice than ever before, according to survey data released by the National Hospice Organization. The survey indicated that 390,000 patients and their families were served by hospices in 1995 (Figure 38-2). Other data released by the National Hospice Organization in 1992 showed the following information[3]:

- Fifty-three percent of hospice patients were men and 47% were women.
- Most patients (68% of the men, 72% of the women) were older than age 65, although 9% of the male patients and 7% of the female patients ranged in age from infancy to 44.
- Seventy-eight percent of hospice patients were diagnosed with cancer, 10% had heart-related diagnoses, and 4% had AIDS.
- There was an increase in average length of patients stay in hospice to 64 days from 59 in 1990.
- Volunteerism continued to be a major personnel resource of hospice, with approximately 960,000 volunteers providing some 5.25 million hours of service during 1992.
- Fifty-nine percent of volunteer hours were spent in direct support of patients and families; the remainder went to assisting administrative aspects of the hospice program.

From the humble beginnings of many hospices in back rooms and church basements, hospice programs are now also being run by large home care organizations and hospital systems. Hospice has come into its own as a part of the continuum of health care delivery. The growth of hospice is exciting because it means more and more patients and their families who need this kind of service will be able to have access to it. Growth can also be an area of concern, if hospice philosophy and quality of care are not guaranteed to this population.

Regardless of the type of program or where it is housed, there are standards of care that are important for consumers and health care providers to know about in order to ensure that when patients and their families choose hospice, they are getting that choice in terms of quality. The following are important indicators of hospice philosophy and quality:

1. The hospice identifies the patient and the family as the unit of care, and provides services to both.
2. The hospice delivers care through an interdisciplinary team composed of nurses, physicians, social workers, home health aides, chaplains, and volunteers.
3. Volunteers are available for patients and families to provide respite, companionship, emotional support, errands, and transportation. (Medicare-certified hospices must demonstrate that volunteer hours represent at least 5% of the direct patient care hours delivered by the hospice program.)
4. The focus of care is to alleviate the physical, emotional, social, and spiritual pain related to death and dying.
5. Care is available on an on-call basis 7 days a week, 24 hours a day. This means that a nurse can come by in the middle of the night to provide comfort and to be there at the time of death to help the family with arrangements. This also means that oxygen or a pain prescription can be obtained over the weekend, if needed.
6. Care is provided regardless of ability to pay or reimbursement source.
7. Care is provided to the family after the death of the patient for at least 1 year. These bereavement services can take many forms including follow-up phone calls and visits with a social worker or bereavement counselor; written material sent on a regular basis to provide education and resources for dealing with grief; support groups facilitated by hospice staff and volunteers to provide support and education on the grief process and how to integrate the loss; phone calls and visits from trained hospice volunteers to provide social contact and emotional support; and hospice-sponsored memorial services to acknowledge the special memories and to honor loved ones.

Hospice care in this country will continue to grow. As many who were in this movement from the beginning had hoped, hospice is now integrated into the health care delivery system in the United States. The challenge for hospices is to maintain the customary high quality and integrity that has been achieved in the past.

References

1. Saunders C. And from sudden death . . . (reprint). Frontier, Winter, 1961.
2. Manard B, Perone C. Hospice Care. An Introduction and Review of the Evidence. The National Hospice Organization, January 13, 1994.
3. National data released by the National Hospice Organization at its 15th Annual Symposium, Salt Lake City, UT, October 13–16, 1993.

Chapter 39

Spirituality and Suffering

Jeanne Maguire Brenneis

The unexamined life is not worth living.

Socrates[1]

The chaplain has just made rounds on the hospice inpatient unit. No one is complaining of pain. Several patients are listening to soft music. Many are sleeping peacefully. Others are talking quietly with family members. One is sitting outside in a wheelchair, breathing deeply of the flower-scented May air. Another is sitting on the side of his bed going through insurance papers with his wife. (Actually, that does seem to be an uncomfortable experience, judging by his comments to me as I pause by his bed. But that "pain" is not physical.) Most of these patients are in the advanced stages of cancer or acquired immunodeficiency syndrome (AIDS). Many have experienced severe pain at one time or another. None is in pain now. But that does not mean that no one is suffering.

Jane is angry at God, according to a conversation with her nurse, and will not speak to me today. She has said that she is not ready to die and does not understand why this is happening to her. She has always been "a good person, a faithful church-goer."

Kathy is very short of breath and is grieving that the doctor has just told her that she is still too sick and too unstable to go back home. She tells me again that she blames herself for smoking. I comment on the fragrance of her beautiful yellow roses (she is too short of breath to sniff them herself), and

she tells me that they are from the bush that she planted on the grave of her son, who died 2 years ago in his thirties of cancer. As I pray with her she starts to cry, mourning her son, but cannot let the tears come freely because they interfere with her breathing. She says that the unshed tears "feel like a bowling ball" in her chest, as I hold her silently.

Chris is worried about his wife. They have had many quarrels about money through their 50-year marriage, and he fears that she will be unable to manage without him, that she is making poor investments, and will not trust their son to guide her. I know from visiting her that she is fearful of becoming destitute, although Chris is leaving enough to keep her more than comfortable. His anxiety increases his restlessness and his physical discomfort. I recognize that his concern for his wife as a survivor goes far beyond the financial concerns, but this is what he is willing to express at this time.

Ron is trying to die. He has lived with AIDS for several years. He has been deeply reflective about his life, his circumstances, his relationships, and, more recently, his spiritual growth. Two weeks ago I visited him at home, and, as we listened to Bach and Gregorian chants, he talked about his attempts to make sense of his illness, of his efforts to say goodbye to his family and all who are important to him, of a beloved cousin who is terminally ill with cancer and his hopes of seeing her in heaven, and of his grief at leaving behind his long-term lover.

Today he is sad because he believes he is ready to die and he can't understand why "it hasn't happened" yet. He is tired, and he wants to move on into death and is worrying that he is somehow holding himself back.

None of these people is in physical pain. Yet each of them is suffering. *Because* they are not in physical pain, they have the strength and energy to give their attention to the things that concern them most. They are all participating in the work of preparing for their death.

Ironic as it may seem, some clinicians believe that controlling a person's pain is essential for many reasons, one of which is so that she or he can be free to suffer existentially. This chapter (1) explains the rationale for that belief, (2) touches briefly on why so many patients come to hospice care in great pain or in fear of great pain, and (3) talks about the spiritual tasks of dying. I will also discuss the good and bad reasons why patients may deliberately choose to be undermedicated or in poor pain control, thus thwarting our earnest attempts to act in what we perceive to be the patient's best interests, and the importance of respecting the patient's autonomy in choosing his or her desired level of pain control.

I am writing this chapter from the viewpoint of both an ethicist and a Christian theologian. Therefore, my writings are set within the framework of a Christian belief in an afterlife and a higher power. While most major faith traditions also presume an afterlife, and while the reports of near-death experiences and nearing-death awareness confirm this belief for me, it is beyond the scope of this chapter to offer "proof" of an afterlife or to argue with those who disclaim such beliefs. However, the tasks of the dying that I shall be discussing remain the same for all—regardless of one's religious tradition or belief in an afterlife. Obviously, one's culture and tradition shape the way in which these tasks are faced and experienced. For those who do not believe in an afterlife, the developmental work associated with dying is crucial for achieving a full and meaningful life in the present.

Cancer patients usually experience pain. This phenomenon is not surprising to patients, their family, or their caregivers. Frequently, cancer pain is not well managed, which is no surprise to those who have experienced cancer in themselves or in their loved ones. According to Marcia Angell, "the treatment of severe pain in hospitalized patients is regularly and systematically inadequate."[2] Studies

in leading medical journals, including those cited in Dr. Angell's editorial, indicate that two-thirds or more of cancer patients with advanced disease experience significant pain. This occurs despite the fact that most pain, even the most severe, can be effectively relieved by narcotic analgesics,[2] supplemented by other techniques such as visualization, guided imagery, and nerve blocks. We have a duty to eliminate pain; this should be "at the core of a health care professional's commitment."[3] We should not only treat pain but also should eliminate it because, "Pain is soul destroying. No patient should have to endure intense pain unnecessarily. The quality of mercy is essential to the practice of medicine; here, of all places, it should not be strained."[2]

Pain is physical and unpleasant; an uncomfortable sensory experience connected with illness, injury, or tissue damage. It is a "complex, subjective response with several quantifiable features, including intensity, time-course, quality, impact, and personal meaning."[3]

Pain is hard to describe accurately, perhaps because our first experience of it comes in infancy, when we are preverbal and prelingual. The experience of pain is subjective, and exacerbated or mediated by many factors, such as fatigue, previous experience of pain, support (or lack of it) from those around us, and expectation of the cessation of the pain. Pain can make us feel isolated, angry, helpless, and vulnerable. It can paralyze our thought processes, force us into regression and frustrated dependency, and narrow our ability to search for coping mechanisms or resources.[4] Pain is not the same thing as suffering, although the two are often linked together. However, the experience of protracted pain and, even more, the fear of uncontrollable pain can play a primary part in causing suffering in patients with cancer and other serious illnesses. The pain endured by cancer patients is aptly described as "the agonies that invade, dominate, and shrivel their consciousness, that leave them no psychic space to be present to themselves and their loved ones, that rob them of even the briefest last moments of tranquility and equanimity."[5]

Yet I would not equate the worst, most intense pain with suffering. Pain is only a component, not the whole. One can experience severe pain, as in childbirth, yet be able to integrate it as a component of great joy. The physical nature of pain usually differentiates it from suffering; suffering is an experience of the whole person, something that may include the physical being but oftentimes goes beyond it.

Suffering, as Eric Cassell has said, "occurs when an impending destruction of the person is perceived."[6] He goes on to write:

> People in pain frequently report suffering from the pain when they feel out of control, when the pain is overwhelming, when the source of the pain is unknown, when the meaning of the pain is dire, or when the pain is chronic. In all these situations, persons perceive pain as a threat to their continued existence—not merely to their lives, but to their integrity as persons. . . . Suffering can be relieved, in the presence of continued pain, by making the source of the pain known, changing its meaning, and demonstrating that it can be controlled and that an end is in sight.[6]

This is true for some forms of suffering, or for some suffering patients. I would contend, however, that for many patients the elimination of physical pain is a desirable, ethical, and necessary objective *because* it releases one's energy, creativity, and spirit for the greater task of encountering one's mortality and for finding one's place in the universe; in other words, we should be freed from physical pain to assume the necessary task of exploring our existential or spiritual condition, even though suffering may be (and often is) a significant component of that ultimate exploration.

As humans, we are much more than the complex anatomic connections of tissue, organ systems, brain cells, and so forth, that we inhabit. In the Judeo-Christian tradition, we consider the person as being merely inanimate clay, of the very dust from the ground, until God "breathed into his nostrils the breath of life; and man became a living being" (Gen. 2:7). God thus created an interplay of the physical, emotional, intellectual, and spiritual elements that we can describe as our ego-self. In the story of Genesis, God went on to create woman as well (Gen. 1:27, 2:18, 21-23). It is in this ancient story of creation that we find the three most important components of humanity: one's relationship with one's own self and soul, one's relationship with other human beings, and one's relationship with God, with a higher power, with the creative force, with the universe, with whatever name we use for that sense of ultimate and profound relatedness that the theologian Paul Tillich has termed the "ultimate ground of being."[7]

Suffering results when we experience a threat to the integrity of any of these relationships: to our relationship with our physical, psychological, or emotional selves, to our relationship with others, or to our relationship with God. For patients who are experiencing physical pain, the suffering may indeed be mitigated or eliminated when the pain is relieved. The threat to the physical self is gone. If the pain is not related to something life threatening, if it is in fact due to kidney stones or a broken limb or any cause that we can heal quickly to regain wholeness, then pain relief may cure the suffering as well.

In cancer patients, however, pain relief will not "make everything better," because it is an intimation of mortality. The experience of pain when it occurs, especially severe pain, is a deep distraction from everything that is happening. It interferes with the patient's ability to relate to others and to God. It demands all of the patient's concentration and demoralizes, depresses, and causes the patient to turn inward. Cancer pain that is untreated, or undertreated (especially when the undertreatment or mistreatment results from "good" or "best available" medical care), deprives patients of all hope that things will ever be better. Even worse, however, is that it deprives them of their ability to focus their attention to the crucial, fearful, and fascinating task that is connected with the pain: the task of examining their own mortality. For cancer patients, pain is not a transient thing; a moment forgotten in the business of life continued on as before. Cancer pain is a harsh reminder that the body and self are under attack, and that death lurks. Even a cancer that goes into remission is always present in the back of one's mind, a reminder that as humans we are finite, and that cancer brings us one step closer to experiencing that finitude. Furthermore, many (perhaps most) cancer patients fear that the pain itself will reappear and will be unmanageable and unrelenting. They frequently believe that clinicians will be unable to keep them free from pain. As a result, anticipated pain may be more torturous and may cause more anguish and suffering than does actual pain. As physicians, we owe it to our patients to help them alleviate their pain, educate them about what pain relief technologies are available, listen to their fears, and promise them that we will take their fears seriously. We must communicate to them clearly that we want them to report any pain or discomfort and that we can, indeed, in almost all cases, relieve the pain and ensure their comfort.

But what happens when the pain is controlled? What happens when the clenched fist opens, the tension goes out of the body, and the mind can believe that the pain is indeed gone? The cancer patient knows that the illness has not disappeared. Death is still a reality to be dealt with.

Yet how can we believe that we will die? Seasons pass. The very rocks will be transformed by winds and time. Other people, even the most dearly beloved, do die, and although we may feel our very hearts are rent in grief, we do go on. In our experience, everything else in nature dies, ends, stops; we survive. So we manage to deny that our own physical existence will also die, end, stop. For how can we anticipate, how can we survive the stopping of *ourselves*? How can I imagine the radical transformation of a world that goes on without *me*?[8] How can I imagine my family, my husband, my wife, or my daughter, my friends and colleagues, continuing life without me? My death will destroy in this known universe the "me" that exists, my ego-self, and it will destroy my relationships with others, all those human relationships that are the framework and structure of my life. We try very hard to understand this, to fight against it, objectively to integrate the knowledge that death will come, both in a generalized way and then, with shock, in a very personal, subjective, and immediate way. We may have stages of acceptance. We may "rage against the dying of the light."[9] It is interesting how poignant that line is, in that it claims not that the person will no longer exist, but that light itself—the known world—will pass. Much great literature has been written about human attempts to comprehend human finitude. Recently, I was moved by a novel written by Elizabeth Goudge, in which she describes a child's first apprehension and realization of death:

> It meant that at one moment the person you loved best in the world was alive and warm beside you and the next there was no one there. She was stunned by the terror of this reversal. . . .Why should this happen to John Shepherd? He was a good old man and he had been trying to help save (others' lives). . . .When she looked back again John Shepherd had ceased to breathe. She could not believe it at first and she knelt on, still holding his hand. Then she knew. John Shepherd had gone through the door and this time he would not come back. She would never talk to him again. Some disasters could be righted but not this one. Yesterday she had feared without knowledge, as men fear pain who have never felt it burn into their own flesh, but now knowledge struck into her soul, not like burning but like the frost of winter. She no longer cried but shivered from head to foot. If this could happen at any moment to those one loved then all peace of mind was gone forever, and John Shepherd was gone forever. There was no foothold anywhere.[10]

Faced with the destruction of the self and with the knowledge that death is inevitable, we experience the same feelings that the child does. We are stunned and terrified. We argue the unfairness of it. We cling to our disbelief. We feel numb and powerless, and there is "no foothold anywhere." Perhaps the inability to change this truth, to ultimately defy death and put it off forever, is particularly poignant for "first world" humanity in the twentieth century, for we who have learned to take miraculous technology for granted. We have "conquered" so many diseases that, at some nonrational level, it seems incomprehensible that death still defeats all our medical wisdom. I remember an 83-year-old woman, never sick a day of her life (by her own report), who asked me indignantly and angrily why "this" (her dying) was happening. Her grandmother would probably not have asked the same question.

> For the wise men [sic] of old, the cardinal problem of human life was how to conform the soul to objective reality, and the solution was wisdom, self-discipline, and virtue. For the modern mind, the cardinal problem is how to subdue reality to the wishes of man, and solution is a technique.[11]

In discussing the above passage from C.S. Lewis' *The Abolition of Man*, Peter Kreeft observes that, "This new ideal of human power over nature means that suffering is a scandal, a problem to be conquered rather than a mystery to be understood and a moral challenged to be lived."[12]

Theologian Dorothee Soelle, in her classic text on suffering, says that two important components of suffering are perceived powerlessness and perceived meaninglessness. Indeed, we are powerless to prevent death. The physical pain may be relieved, the cancer may even go into remission, death may be put off for a while, but deep in the night, in our sleeplessness, we know that death will eventually come. Faced with the disintegration of the self, we wonder if any of this has any meaning. We despair. We are angry. We are depressed. We claim, like Keats in his poignant epigraph, that our lives are "writ on water."[13] And for what? How can God give us so much and then take it away? Like Christ on the cross, we cry, "My God, My God, why has thou abandoned me?" (Matt. 24:46; Mark 15:34.)

This is the true suffering I see in the hospice patients I have known: the struggle against powerlessness, the struggle to find meaning in having lived, the struggle to come to terms with death. This struggle can be very difficult for all the reasons mentioned previously. However, I believe that this struggle is a necessary and important part of dying, a developmental task just as important as teething, learning to walk, leaving the parental home, or assuming the responsibilities of adulthood.[14] It is difficult because life is precious, even when life is filled with physical, emotional, or spiritual pain. It is necessary to face the loss of one's physical life because finitude itself gives meaning to life. Death is the frame that completes the portrait, the boundary that makes the "road not chosen"[15] so poignant. Because of death, our choices, our mistakes, our chosen roads are real and meaningful; we cannot go back and have it both ways at the same point in life. The regret we experience in assessing the meaning of our lives comes from claiming both the things done and the things left undone, the unfinished business that we all must leave behind when we can no longer plan on another year, another month, even another day. If we believe that only through death can we be born into the next life, then these pains are like the pains of childbirth: real, sometimes harsh, but forgotten when the job is completed.

Therefore, spirituality does not eliminate suffering. Persons of faith still grieve the coming end of life. Spirituality does play an important role, however. Spirituality includes a sense of an "extrahuman presence" in the universe, a sense of "ultimate relatedness" to that presence, and a sense of "special significance" for one's life, of being "called to something beyond" oneself.[16] For some people this includes a belief in the incarnate deity in Christ; for others it might be a sense of being a part of a creation that transcends oneself. For many, it means being part of a great plan for our lives. Through our sense of a powerful presence beyond the human, of Tillich's ultimate ground of being, we can learn to view our lives as having future, meaning, and purpose beyond our time on earth. Our awareness of the spiritual transforms the task of coming to terms with dying, as we slowly recognize that death is not only a closing door but also an opening one, a passageway either into a new existence or to liberation

(moksha). The journey that is my life will not suddenly stop but will take me the rest of the way home, to a more complete experience of God's loving presence.

Thus, the ultimate task of dying is *to let go*, to allow oneself to be stripped of all the things one has worked so hard to achieve throughout one's life. As the old saying goes, you can't take it with you. How difficult a lesson that is to learn. Great spiritual leaders—from Moses to Buddha to Mohammed to the most peace-filled elderly woman I know—have all struggled to understand this. As the Dalai Lama has written, "When the time comes to carry the load of life through death's door, one can take neither relatives, friends, servants, nor possessions . . . [Therefore] Abandon attachment."[17] How hard it is to relinquish all that we have worked so hard to achieve: professional respect, a personal sense of identity, individuality, possessions, relationships, even control of the functioning of our own bodies. Yet that is the task. For me, this is epitomized by a story told by Peter Kreeft in *Love Is Stronger Than Death* (the best theology of death that I have ever read):

> In the Latin rite for the burial of an Austrian emperor, the people carry the corpse to the door of the great monastic church. The door is locked. They strike the door and say "Open!" The abbot inside says, "Who is there?" "Emperor Karl, King of X and Y and Z." "We know no such person here." Strike again. "Who is there?" "Emperor Karl." "We know no such person here." Strike a third time. "Who is there?" "Karl." The door is opened. You can't take it with you—any "it." You can only take you.[8]

Willingly or unwillingly, we must let go of the things that tie us to this life before we can go on to the next life. It is only when we have freed ourselves from the things of earth that we can encounter heaven, spiritual transcendence, moksha, or nirvana. This observation is not limited to the teachings of Christianity. Each major faith tradition has some way of describing what comes after death, but each makes it clear: You have to die to get there. Only in being released from the anchor that the body has become do we move into the Light. As Paul says, "now we see in a mirror dimly, but then (after death) face to face. Now I know in part; then I shall understand fully, even as I have been fully understood" (by God) (I Cor. 13:12).

Every human must die, and every human must come to terms with it in some way, whether by acceptance or by complete denial, by faith or without it, alone or within the loving support of his or her own community. Both the greatest hardship and the greatest gift of a lingering death through cancer or other disease, as opposed to a sudden death, is the opportunity and the time to live through the identified stages or faces of grief—anger, denial, despair, bargaining, and acceptance[18]—as one grieves one's own mortality. This experience of grief is an invitation to an exploration of this part of one's lifelong journey. For myself, I hope that when my time comes I can be fully open to this experience just as I have tried to be open to all the emotions, painful as well as joyful, of the other major experiences of my life, such as marriage, bereavement, the birth of a healthy child, and the loss of another child. All such major life experiences offer us the opportunity and the challenge to reevaluate our lives, examine them from a new angle, acknowledge loss as well as gain, and to continue to grow.[19] A terminal prognosis should not be a signal to stop learning and growing; quite the contrary. For me, this is a primary component of being fully alive. Personally, I intend to wrestle spiritually, emotionally, and psychologically with death (as perhaps my chosen vocation has continually called me to do anyway).

But what of the person who refuses this wrestling match, who chooses denial or avoidance as a response to the process of dying? This very denial is a part of the process. The invitation to explore the meaning of one's life and death is just that, an invitation and an opportunity, not a forced march. Each will undergo this task in his or her own way. For some who are in a stage where they consciously want no part of this process, pain can serve as a powerful distraction, necessary to the psyche at that time. For others, experiencing pain and finding meaning in it can be an important part of the developmental task.

Thus, the refusal to use the methods or treatments that can offer good pain control stem from three recognizable spiritual and psychological causes. One is the avoidance of the developmental task, which the patient will start when he or she is ready. For some people, that time never comes. This is their choice, and as such should be recognized and the patient still supported. The second cause is a perceived value and integration of the experience of the pain itself. The third cause is the desire to be totally lucid and alert, a condition that may be threatened by the side effects of opioids. Once the clinician or caregiver has provided good education and counseling concerning the realistic aspects of pain management, discussing such issues as fear of addiction, fear that tolerance will reduce the efficacy of the opioid later on when it is "most needed," alternative treatment modalities, and predictable side effects, the clinician or caregiver must respect the patient's right to refuse pain management treatment, even if that means accepting a higher level of pain than the practitioner thinks is in the patient's best interests, while providing the best palliative care possible. In other words, it is just as much the informed patient's right to refuse pain management as it is his or her right to refuse any other treatment or therapy.

Some patients find it preferable to tolerate pain than to give up control or mental acuity. If a method cannot be found that is appropriate for that patient's pain etiology and also guarantees mental clarity, the patient's wishes must be respected. As has been suggested throughout this article, mental clarity is very important to some people when they are engaged in the tasks of reflecting on their condition and on finishing unfinished business.

For some people, there is a perceived value in the experience of pain itself that can provide great comfort. One may judge the patient's reasons for valuing pain to be psychologically healthy or unhealthy, but in either case, one must respect the patient's choice. There is a tradition among some Christians to value pain as a means by which one can achieve a closer bond with God or an identification with Jesus Christ. (In my own professional experience, this tends to have validity among some Roman Catholics raised in the pre-Vatican II church.) I recall one gentleman who confounded the nursing staff by refusing his pain medications, while confiding to me, "How could I complain about pain when my Lord suffered so much on the cross? My pain is nothing compared to His." For this man, a lifelong daily Communicant, his faith had shaped his life and continued to give his life meaning. His face lit up when he talked about Jesus, and about his belief that his pain gave him some empirical insight into Jesus's suffering and allowed him to share in that suffering. He expressed biblical support for his beliefs in the writings of St. Paul: "We rejoice in our sufferings, knowing that suffering produces endurance, and endurance produces character, and character produces hope, and hope does not disappoint us, because God's love has been poured into our hearts through the Holy Spirit which has been given to us" (Rom. 5:3-5).

For him, physical pain and the attending suffering were a means of grace and the receiving of the Holy Spirit. What chaplain would ever want to deny that experience for a patient?

Others may find in physical pain an expiation for old guilts or old sins, a way of paying back or making amends for old wrongdoings. Such expiation can provide great physical and psychological relief, similar to that felt by a small child who has been punished for something she knows she has done and about which she feels guilty. The punishment leads to a clear conscience and a clean slate, and a renewed intimacy and peacefulness with the person the child has wronged (usually the parent). Theologians call this atonement, and it is a powerful therapy for the person who is in spiritual conflict. For example, a woman in her thirties was experiencing severe physical pain from uterine cancer. Her nurse was trying to bring her pain under control but had not yet succeeded. The patient confided in the nurse that she had had an abortion when she was 14 years old, that she believed that this was a sin, that she had never told anyone about the abortion, and that she had felt guilty about it ever since. The patient was convinced that the cancer pain she was experiencing was directly and physiologically related to that abortion 20 years earlier, and that somehow it was her duty to endure the pain. Through pastoral intervention, the patient came to believe that she had paid for her sin through her pain, that she was now forgiven and that she had atoned for committing that which she believed to have been a major wrongdoing. "Coincidentally," her pain was relieved at about this time. I suggest that the spiritual and emotional healing that occurred was just as important as the skilled application of analgesics, and that for her, that experience of pain was psychologically necessary for her healing. One would certainly not deliberately cause her to have pain to bring about that healing, but one would also support her interpretation of that pain and the meaning it had in her dying.

A third type of patient may cling to pain due to the attention it brings from family members or friends. For this person, the emotional comfort of that attention is more important or more necessary

than pain relief. One may deplore what can be interpreted as manipulation within a poorly functioning family system, and intervention can be made to try to meet the patient's emotional needs without the physical pain. However, the ensuing dynamics may be truly important in working out unfinished business within family relationships. This may add geometrically to the difficulty of this period for this family, but may also have discernible positive outcomes. Thus, while providing support, understanding, facilitative counseling, and the setting of limits for the family members involved in this dynamic, one must still respect the patient's choice to forego pain management, rather than rendering the patient unconscious for the family's comfort.

In all these examples, one can find again the three major areas of concern in the dying patient: exploring the meaning of one's own life, working for the healing of relationships and the finishing of unfinished business with others, and reconciliation and renewal in the relationship with the God of one's understanding. Some people approach these tasks with a continued intent to maintain control, whereas others recognize that such control may cease to become either possible or desirable. Daniel Callahan warns that through the *need* for control:

> The dying self can be deformed by allowing the fear of death, or the fear of what dying may do to our ideal self, itself to corrupt the self. Obsessions with a loss of control, or with a diminishment of the idealized optimal self, or with the prospect of pain, are other ways this can happen. . . . Anxiety, even terror, is to be expected as we approach our death, because of the physical threats of dying and also because of its challenge to our sense of self-worth and self-coherence. It is the preoccupation with those evils that introduces the potential deformity, the feeling that we cannot be worthy human beings if they are our fate, and the inability to think of anything but our losses, our failures, our diminution.[20]

How can we, as clinicians, as caregivers, or as the community surrounding the dying patient, help make the process meaningful and peaceful for that patient? How can we facilitate his or her continued growth? How can we provide support that reduces the sense of powerlessness, and enables the non-threatening relinquishing of the obsession or delusion of control? Turning again to a definition of suffering in which there is a threat to one's self, one's relationship with others, and one's relationship with God, one can define the task of providing support and intervention in these three areas. First, we can offer pain and symptom management to palliate the threat to the self, to make the experience physically more gentle, while recognizing that it is beyond our power to change the underlying circumstance. Second, we can offer ourselves, our fully committed and intentional presence. John Maes claims that "suffering is always interpersonal for human beings, that at the core of suffering is the sense of being cut off from normal human relationships."[16] Much has been written about the isolation of the dying, the avoidance by friends who don't know what to say, or professionals who think they no longer have anything to offer. Our greatest gift is our presence, our willingness to listen and to try to understand. Some people need to verbalize about what is happening to them, sometimes telling the same story over and over. Some seem to ask for only a silent but fully engaged presence, a hand held by the bedside when no outside intervention can change the direction of the illness (which is often the most difficult of tasks). The most profound response may be the sharing of tears. We can also pay attention to the patient's need to heal relationships and to say the things that have been unsaid. Maes recognizes that:

> In the long turnings of the world there are moments of grace and justice. . . . How often we who care for sufferers are conveyers of acceptance, grace and forgiveness. Often we are stand-ins for deceased, unresponsive, or overly terrifying figures who cannot be approached by those who suffer. Our faithful willingness to work with sufferers when they feel unlovely, even repulsive, may be the beginning of a spiritual healing that includes forgiveness, acceptance, and heightened self-esteem.[16]

Third, there is the similar task of helping the patient toward spiritual healing. Listening, facilitating the discussion of the patient's spiritual life, and sometimes just being there as a representative of the worshiping community can help the patient reconcile himself or herself to God (or to Creation, the universe, the ultimate ground of being beyond oneself), and to explore anticipations and fears of the life beyond. Scripture readings, prayer, sacraments, and symbols are powerful tools in helping the patient to be aware of God's presence in his or her dying as well as in living, and of the place of his or her own death in God's providence. As Paul has written: "None of us lives to himself, and none of us dies to himself. If we live, we live to the Lord, and if we die, we die to the Lord; so then, whether we live or whether we die, we are the Lord's" (Rom. 8:7–8).

I will never forget the elderly man in a state psychiatric hospital, hospitalized for dementia and organic brain syndrome, who had not been heard to utter a word in a least 5 years. Yet, when I sang "Jesus Loves Me" to him he sang along. The religious and spiritual symbols of our childhood may be the most powerful instruments of comfort and assurance when we are beyond the reach of the spoken or the rational intervention.

Ultimately, as Callahan states, "we must find our own meaning for death and die our own deaths."[20] But we do this within the human community. Just as the physical task of physical birth can be experienced only by the mother, no one can experience the process of dying for us. However, we need not go through the process entirely alone. Just as the birthing mother is surrounded by clinicians and caregivers, professionals and family and friends, so should the dying be supported, upheld, and coached. To continue the analogy, the difficulties and pains and suffering of childbirth are minimized by the delivery of a healthy child. That is not to say that the pains are not real, or should not be palliated, but that they are overwhelmed by the joy of the birth. Likewise, the pains and the sufferings of the dying are overwhelmed and forgotten in the successful completion of this life and the "delivery" into the next life. St. Theresa is reputed to have said that, from the perspective of heaven, the worst life is ultimately no more than the inconveniences of a night in a bad hotel. It is still up to us to do all we can to make the experience of the bad hotel a little better.

References

1. Plato. Apology. In AJ Ayer, J O'Grady (eds), Dictionary of Philosophical Quotations. Oxford, England: Blackwell, 1992;428.
2. Angell M. The quality of mercy. N Engl J Med 1982;306:98.
3. Acute Pain Management Guideline Panel. Acute Pain Management: Operative or Medical Procedures and Trauma: Clinical Practice Guideline. Rockville, MD: Agency for Health Care Policy and Research. Publication No. 92-0032. Public Health Service, U.S. Department of Health and Human Services, 1992.
4. Kleinman A, Brodwin PE, Good BJ, Good MJD. Pain

as Human Experience: An Anthropological Perspective. Berkeley and Los Angeles: University of California Press, 1992;1.

5. Roy DJ. Relief of suffering: The doctor's mandate. J Palliat Care 1991;7:3.

6. Cassell EJ. The nature of suffering and the goals of medicine. N Engl J Med, 1982;306:640.

7. Tillich P. Systematic Theology (Vol. I). Chicago: University of Chicago Press, 1971;passim.

8. Kreeft PJ. Love Is Stronger Than Death. New York: Harper & Row, 1979.

9. Thomas D. "Do Not Go Gentle Into That Good Night." In R Ellmann, R O'Clair (eds), The Norton Anthology of Modern Poetry. New York: Norton, 1973.

10. Goudge E. The Child from the Sea. New York: Pyramid Books, 1971;81, 83, 84.

11. Lewis CS. The Abolition of Man. New York: Macmillan, 1947.

12. Kreeft PJ. Making Sense Out of Suffering. Ann Arbor, MI: Servant Books, 1986;168.

13. Lord Houghton. Life of Keats. In The Oxford Dictionary of Quotations. Oxford: Oxford University Press, 1959.

14. Erikson E. Identity and the Life Cycle: Selected Papers. In Psychological Issues. New York: International Universities Press, 1959.

15. Frost R. The Road Not Taken. In Robert Frost's Poems. New York: Washington Square Press, 1946.

16. Maes JL. Suffering: A Caregiver's Guide. Nashville, TN: Abingdon Press, 1990.

17. Levine S. Who Dies? An Investigation of Conscious Living and Conscious Dying. New York: Doubleday, 1982;28.

18. Kubler-Ross E. On Death and Dying. New York: Macmillan, 1969.

19. Viorst J. Necessary Losses. New York: Simon & Schuster, 1986.

20. Callahan D. The Troubled Dream of Life: Living with Mortality. New York: Simon & Schuster, 1993.

Chapter 40

Nuances of Patient Interaction by a Physician–Patient

Stephanie M. Mouton

Cancer pain has many dimensions: physical, emotional, intellectual, and spiritual. Although physicians tend to specialize in the physical components, it is only after a personal experience with cancer that a physician realizes the depth of the illness.

Once the medical student learns the physical elements of illness, the other dimensions become evident as he or she continues to practice medicine. Yet, when a physician is stricken with a serious illness, it accelerates his or her understanding of how an illness can pervade all aspects of living. When illness strikes a physician personally, the idea of living takes on a whole new meaning.

Physicians as patients have produced significant works regarding patient care and ways to live. Most notable of these are by Bernie Siegal and Brugh Joy; both widely known for their efforts to "empower" patients.[1, 2] A motion picture, *The Doctor*, featuring the experience of a prominent surgeon's brush with laryngeal cancer is a popular tool for helping medical students experience some of the feelings that their patients experience. When a physician becomes a patient, the perception of having lost control of the situation can be shocking enough to precipitate an emotional crisis.

Control is an important ingredient in the personality makeup of most physicians. The need to be in control, to control situations, to control others, and to have self-control are all characteristics that are often necessarily present in physicians. This often stems from a lack of control that was perceived at an early age. Individuals who sense a lack of control overcompensate in later life by attempts to control everything and everyone near to them. Such people often can be excellent students and good candidates for the best medical schools. When serious illness occurs, however, an abrupt change in life-style and attitudes occurs. This perceived loss of supremacy over one's existence can add to the difficulty of managing cancer pain.

Although control is a factor for all patients to face, it can be even more challenging for physicians to accept the control forced on them by conventional medical practice. Having been in charge of medical decisions as a vocation, the physician may feel anger, resentment, hostility, and denial as he or she assumes the role of patient. Initially, there can be a narcissistic attempt to avoid other patients, such as in group therapy, as the physician denies the physical and emotional aspects of the illness. The physician may also choose to continue working, thus helping continue the denial of his or her position as a patient. Attempts to continue practice are admirable, yet the illness is a sign that change is necessary. Life is change, and old habits and attitudes may be contributing to illness. Illness challenges one to explore life in new directions. One can experience such stressors as losing a job or experiencing a divorce or separation and know that it is possible to rebuild a life. However, facing cancer creates a different person. Physicians may find themselves facing long-forgotten issues that have a significant effect on relationships with others.

Overall, the author's opinion is that current medical practice is just beginning to appreciate the multidimensional aspects of healing and living.

The experience of being a physician–patient has greatly expanded my understanding of medical treatment. Fortunately, it is not necessary for all physicians to sustain a life-threatening illness in order to practice medicine. However, insight into these processes can help physicians better care for patients with cancer pain.

The progression of physical, emotional, intellectual, and spiritual healing is a lifelong process for cancer patients, commencing with the onset of disease. Biochemical therapy will arrest cancer growth, yet healing occurs on many levels. Tissue damage resulting from radiation therapy, surgery, and chemotherapy persists indefinitely, and cancer patients are faced with sequelae that may require them to adjust to a different appearance of their body. Cancer patients always live with the threat of progressive disease or recurrence of cancer. These fears manifest in many ways; chronic and emotional pain in particular are an expression of such deep-rooted fears and anxiety.

The word *doctor* derives from the Greek term for teacher (*doktor*). Physicians caring for cancer patients may find that they are faced with patients' demands and need for healing that are beyond the training received in medical school. In reality, physicians serve as teachers in helping patients develop resources within themselves to live a healthy life. Physicians can help terminally ill patients accept the value of life even at its most difficult stage. Drugs and medical interventions, while life-saving or life-preserving, do not provide the solace and reassurance so often sought by cancer patients. Physicians may be unable to answer patients' questions such as, "What can I do to prevent progression or recurrence of disease?" or "How should I live now?" Cancer patients often seek some means to control their destiny, and nonmedical practices and techniques are within their grasp of reality, thus giving them active involvement in the process. The physician as teacher can help patients pursue these resources.

The patient's increased participation in the decision-making process has resulted in active programs that encourage patients to gain control or acceptance of their situation. The Exceptional Cancer Patient (ECAP) group at Yale University, under the direction of Dr. Bernie Siegal, is an example of such an organization.[1] Often, patients who desire guidance with regard to nontraditional therapies may feel afraid to reveal such activities to the physician.

Likewise, the physician can feel uncomfortable at not having been trained in such methods, and may discourage patients from seeking relief by other methods. Patients feel frustrated in their attempts to pursue adjunctive therapies if they do not have the counsel of a knowledgeable and willing physician.

The onset of serious illness necessitates a change in life-style for the cancer patient, which requires serious adjustments in attitudes toward life. Strategies for coping can take many different forms. The idea of a "balanced life-style" comes to the fore, as patients attempt to understand why they fell victim to illness and how to prevent it in the future. Joseph Campbell writes of the idea of myth in regard to how one understands the story of life as it pertains to one's personal interpretation of life: "The material of myth is the material of our life, the material of our body and the material of our environment."[3]

He encouraged each person to develop a myth in order to make sense of his or her own life and death. A myth is a way to show what a person has accomplished in life. Even short lives reveal accomplishment and impact. We are changed by the story of a life. Children stricken with disease evoke emotional responses from those around them that in turn affect the way others live. Adults can better understand their life because they understand how one has lived. For example, stress from an unsatisfactory marriage or job can result in an illness that provides exit from a distressing situation. One does not need to identify with Hercules or Odysseus to create myth. It is simply an explanation of one's life. This process is ancient. In the modern world, humans have less contact with the natural world and community, thus neglecting their roles in life. For example, many tribal cultures give names to members as a reflection of who one is or what one has accomplished. The significance of the name reveals the history of the community and of the individual, i.e., a role in life. Religion in modern times is separate from everyday life, while ancient civilizations such as the American Indians had no word for religion because life was lived in the context of spirit close to nature. The interpretation of life events in other cultures results from the forces of the natural world as applied to the individual. A major tenet of these civilizations is to live in harmony with nature.

The modern physician is not as far removed from the shaman of other civilizations as was formerly thought. The physician is the link to the pa-

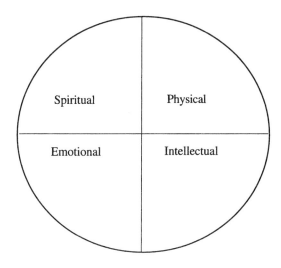

Figure 40-1. Health results from a balance of spiritual, physical, emotional, and intellectual aspects in daily living. (Reprinted with permission from E Kübler-Ross. Children and Death. New York, Macmillan, 1983;63.)

tient's physical survival. Yet, on every level—spiritual, emotional, and intellectual—the patient seeks healing. In tribal cultures, it is the shaman who provides this healing by including the patient in ceremonial practices of the culture, thus affirming the patient's role in the life of the community. Perhaps the modern physician, while healing the patient physically, provides the opportunity for the patient to continue healing on other levels. It is the wise physician who can counsel the patient to pursue other resources or communities.

Elizabeth Kübler-Ross writes that a balanced life is healthy, and is lived on four levels: spiritual, intellectual, emotional, and physical (Figure 40-1).[4] In the modern world, intellectual and physical activities predominate, leaving very little to the spiritual and emotional aspects. Other civilizations, such as the American Indians, included all four levels of existence in daily activities: Family provided emotional support, living close to nature was a spiritual effort, and survival techniques resulted in physical and intellectual development. The modern physician treating the cancer patient should be aware of these life requirements and should encourage the patient to reconcile life on all four levels. This may require nontraditional medicine to be used in conjunction with allopathic medicine.

The idea of balance in regard to health is thousands of years old. Chinese, Hindu, and Oriental philosophies believe that the life force, which, when unbalanced, results in disease.[5] Can a physician trained in the twentieth century provide "balance" to a patient? All efforts aimed at combating disease on a biophysical level may be useless if the emotional, physical, and spiritual aspects of the individual are unattended. Is it the modern physician's responsibility to oversee these aspects of patient care? The answer is yes, and the physician's understanding of these elements is essential to the health of the individual. The physician can facilitate healing by awareness of these requirements of health, and encourage the patient to seek development in these areas. This usually requires knowledge of nontraditional medicine and resources not commonly taught in medical schools. It may also require acceptance from the physician of nonphysician health care providers. Gone are the days when the shaman provided total care of the individual. Modern medicine is complex and specialized, and many consultants are called on to provide health care. It is also ultimately the individual's responsibility to be healthy, which requires self-discipline and control. The physician must not delude the patient into believing that all ills may be cured with modern medicine. The physician serves as a guide and supporter of balanced, healthy living in addition to his or her role as a provider of physical healing.

Physical healing can go beyond the medical treatment to cure disease. It is not uncommon for patients to explore different avenues of healing once the freedom that illness implies is realized. Interest in alternative medicine has increased.[6] The January 28, 1993 issue of the *New England Journal of Medicine* published a survey revealing that U.S. citizens spend an estimated $10–14 billion annually on nonconventional health care, or one-sixteenth of the total U.S. health care market.[6] Approximately one in four Americans who see their medical doctors for a serious health problem may be using unconventional therapy in addition to conventional medicine for that problem, and 7 of 10 encounters occur without patients telling their medical doctors that they use unconventional therapy (Figure 40-2). Unconventional therapies are often used as adjuncts to conventional therapy, rather than as replacement for it. Approximately 20 million Americans use these therapies without the supervision of a provider of unconven-

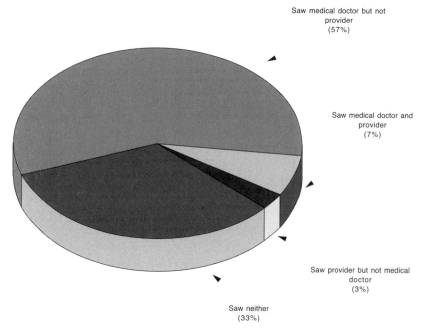

Saw medical doctor but not
provider
(57%)

Saw medical doctor and
provider
(7%)

Saw provider but not medical
doctor
(3%)

Saw neither
(33%)

Figure 40-2. One in three responders to a questionnaire regarding the use of unconventional therapy use it without the supervision of a care provider. (Reprinted with permission from DM Eisenberg, RC Kessler, C Foster, et al. Unconventional medicine in the United States: Prevalence, costs, and patterns of use. N Engl J Med 1993;328:246.)

tional therapy. The odds are greater than 1 in 3 that a patient is simultaneously using unconventional therapy without disclosing this fact to a physician.[6]

The lack of communication between patient and physician regarding unconventional therapy is a hindrance to good clinical care. Medical doctors need to question patients about such therapies because, if totally unsupervised, they may be harmful.

For the physician, the first step is to understand what patients are doing to help themselves. An adequate medical history including nonjudgmental inquiries about the use of unconventional therapies is necessary. Attempts to condemn such practices can further inhibit communication. If the patient feels humiliated by the physician, he or she may conclude that the alternative practitioner is less judgmental and more understanding.[7] The physician can be honest about possible risks without frightening the patient. The physician can concur with the patient's goal while admitting the lack of scientific evidence supporting most therapies. Another study in the *New England Journal of Medicine* reported, however, that patients who received unconventional therapy often suffered more than their conventionally treated counterparts.[8] This could be due to the patient's refusal to accept conventional medicine when needed after having rejected it. Physicians' attitudes could also play

a role. It is advantageous for the patient to have the support of a physician while exploring such therapy. The physician should retain the patient's trust and try not to feel threatened, because the patient will continue to rely on the physician to diagnose, treat, and deliver effective preventive and primary care for the disease.[7] Open-mindedness about new or even old-fashioned remedies is appreciated by patients. There are very few cures for any medical condition, so the exploration of new ideas can result in growth for both the patient and the physician. It is optimal for physicians to be familiar with alternative medicine.

The British Medical Association has recently published a broad-minded book, *Complementary Medicine: New Approaches to Good Practice,* following a study conducted by the Association's Board of Science and Education. It reveals that organized medicine in Britain no longer dismisses the contributions of nonconventional therapies.[9] Osteopathy, chiropractic, acupuncture, homeopathy, and herbalism are discussed. These disciplines are often used by British patients without rejection of conventional medical practice.

The physician in the United States may be confronted with inquiries from patients regarding a host of unconventional therapies including shiatsu, rolfing, vegetarianism, kinesiology, reflexology, crystal therapy, colonic irrigation, yoga, lymphatic drainage massage, Japanese mud baths, thermal baths, macrobiotic diet, vitamins, breathwork, aromatherapy, transcendental meditation, fasting, and many more. Whatever therapy is accepted by the patient, the physician can help support the belief system of the patient. It is important to be aware of what therapies are acceptable to the patient.

Treatments that are within the boundaries of the patient's belief system will be of greater healing benefit. A physician who is aware of the psychological, emotional, spiritual, and intellectual state of the patient can help guide the patient to a useful therapy. For example, it is not useful to encourage vegetarianism in a patient who is a confirmed meat eater or vice versa, or to suggest Eastern techniques such as yoga for relaxation to patients who are firmly grounded in fundamentalist religion. Some of the unconventional therapies involve an emotional release of one sort or another, such as in rolfing, shiatsu, reflexology, or kinesiology. Patients who are in denial of the emotional process of their illness will not derive much benefit from these experiences.

Group therapy, psychotherapy, and psychiatry are of great benefit to the patient when he or she is ready to explore issues surrounding the illness. At best, these disciplines are a way for the patient to discuss chronic concerns freely without the worry of shocking or creating distance between friends and family. The patient can establish a safe relationship to allow forward growth and development to make necessary changes. The value of a safe relationship during a time of crisis is inestimable. This is when the patient can be honest, try new behaviors, and make mistakes with the knowledge that no harm will be done. Confidences will be kept, feelings will not be ignored, and well-being will be valued. Such a relationship allows new ways of interacting with others and a realization that one's safest relationship is with oneself.[10] There are several emotional aspects of cancer patients that must be addressed by the physicians who care for them.

Fear is a central issue in the lives of all cancer patients. It can manifest from pervasive worry to panic. Or, a sense of loss of everything known and experienced can prevail, resulting in profound depression. Isolation results as the patient accepts a private reality that continually occupies the waking hours and is not shared by healthy friends. Health is usually taken for granted, and unnoticed most of the time until a serious illness occurs. A cancer patient forgets about the illness only in the morning after waking and just before remembering his or her condition.

The physician can ameliorate the fear and isolation experienced by cancer patients by being available for consultation or by providing resources as needed. Nothing is worse for the cancer patient than to be unattended by the physician at a time when physical or emotional crisis is present. A support system of many people is necessary to provide the care needed by patients at such a critical time in their lives. A support system for the support system may also be necessary. Physicians can encourage patients to seek support within the family or community. Traditional religious hospitals may be beneficial at such a time, because the emphasis on spirituality is present and another aspect of healing can occur.

It is important for the cancer patient to realize, however, that healing and victory can occur *with* the disease. Illness can make one wish to add to the myth of one's life; to attempt significant accomplishments in order to make the highest use of one's time. Empowerment does not imply that the patient is responsible for getting rid of the disease. Rather, the patient is empowered with a sense of contributing to the whole of humanity. The connection each person makes with others is vital and contributes to the myth of one's life, whether one has an illness or not. Illness can be treated as another path along the journey of life rather than the end of the road. Even after death a person's life continues as he or she is appreciated for the effect their life had on others as well as things that are left behind for others to appreciate. Patients' plans concerning family and friends following death relieve a loss as transition occurs.

A relationship exists among hope, fear, reality, and illusion in the cancer patient. Hope is the impetus for continued survival. The lack of hope shatters the will to live. On the other hand, a patient living in denial of the severity of the disease lives a life of illusion, based on the hope that things are different or that they may change. Denial may be effective initially for some patients, but true denial is devoid of hope because there is no illness. Acceptance of illness leaves room for hope, which can transcend denial, anger, and acceptance. Care providers must be cognizant of this process and be attentive not to disturb the patient's belief system. The patient may understand the reality of the disease process yet choose to deny it and proceed to create a reality that he or she can accept. A physician can unwittingly crush a patient's will to live by the announcement of further progression of the disease process at a time when the patient is not willing to accept such news. Of course, the physician has the responsibility of informing the patient; yet it may be beneficial to disclose such information in a manner that will be acceptable to the patient's belief system. For instance, a mother with a young family in the throes of metastatic disease may not desire to admit the circumstances to herself or to her family. She may decide to continue living with the idea that she *can* overcome the illness. She may shut out the thoughts of disease to live bravely with her children at her side. Everyone is aware of the grave nature of the situation, yet a decision has been made to ignore it. Life continues without mention of disease progress. The sensitive physician will be aware of such denial and can guide the patient to make choices beneficial for the course ahead. In addition, it is important when disclosing difficult information to be certain that the patient does have immediate support (family and friends) available in order to help deal with the issues. It is always difficult for the physician to be the bearer of bad news, yet some gleam of hope can be left with the patient.

Physicians are frequently asked to comment on life expectancy, which can be another means to deny hope to the patient. It is impossible to predict when someone may die, and expectancy information can add gloom to a person already consumed with disease. However, to others, it may add urgency to the remaining time. It is difficult to predict what an effect such information will have. The decision to give such information is controversial. Overall, it is the author's opinion that such information is not useful. Patients know by the changes in their personal medical condition how they feel and how much time is left. M. Scott Peck, a prominent psychiatrist, writes that we "choose to die," just as we choose to live. Choices regarding living such as smoking, fat consumption, exercise, and so forth, all affect the way one lives one's life. If family members or the patient insist on life expectancy information, the physician can make a judgment based on his or her own experience how and when to disclose the information. It is always possible to admit that one simply *does not know* when death will occur.

Patients can become preoccupied with the intellectual aspect of the disease, zealously harboring data and statistics. Patients can "become their own doctor" after researching the matter. Such individuals can be bothersome, yet their interest must be appreciated as empowerment on a personal level, resulting from involvement with the process. The physician may feel reluctant to care for these patients as they become demanding regarding care. For instance, in university hospitals, patients may reject care from individuals in training and insist on only attending physician interaction. If the patient's disease course is aggressive, the attending physician may feel overwhelmed by a protracted illness in an angry depressed individual and attempt to avoid interaction with the patient. This further isolates the patient, contributing to deepening depression and loss.

The physician can avoid such circumstances by establishing a relationship with the patient that is not exclusive of intervention from other professionals or resources, e.g., group therapy. Initially, patients may reject such suggestions, but options for the patient as well as the physician can exist. Also, encouraging the patient to pursue healing on other levels induces responsibility on the patient's part to become involved in fulfilling needs that are not met by traditional medicine. By embarking on this path, the patient becomes involved in a growth process that results in new relationships and ideas that can be helpful throughout the medical treatment. In addition, the physician who is aware of the supportive therapy can access the process to provide pertinent care to the patient and enhance his or her myth or belief system regarding the illness. This can be tremendously reassuring to the patient, thus allaying fear.

It is important to remember that fear is pervasive, and attempts to reassure the patient, or at best to confront fear and discuss it, are the best medicine. Physicians underestimate the power of their reassurance in even minor patient interactions. As a physician encounters each patient, the physician's awareness of fear in each individual is foremost. Sometimes just directly asking a patient "What are you afraid of?" can provide a valuable exchange between patient and physician that will go a long way in making the patient feel comfortable with the proposed medical therapy. When the physician takes the time to ask and hear the answer to such a question, it lets the patient know that the physician's presence is considered a valued expenditure of treatment resources. The fast paced life of medical training may inadvertently teach physicians that the only efficient use of time is administering a complex visible procedure or evaluating diagnostic information. Being present with a patient's fear can also be worthwhile and efficient. Physicians may be reluctant to investigate things for which there is no activity other than to listen. At each turning point in the treatment, however, fear will be a continual factor to confront, often on a daily basis. This is when the patient's personal support system can be invaluable to both the patient and the physician.

The daily encounter with cancer patients and crisis situations can render a physician insensitive to the demands of patients, especially those who are expected to have a poor prognosis or outcome. It is not uncommon for physicians to attend reluctantly to these patients as the medical therapy and tests become of no use. The physician feels powerless to change the course of the disease and thus avoids contact with the emotionally charged issue of imminent death, loss, and perceived failure. It is not uncommon at these times to find that consultations or diagnostic procedures from other professionals are aggressively sought to ward off contact with death. This is the time when physicians who have encouraged the patient to heal on other levels can appreciate that *death is healing,* not only for the patient, but for those left behind. The physician's role as doctor–teacher is to elicit the lesson learned from the life that was cared for. "We are here to learn," writes M. Scott Peck, "Everything that happens to us helps our learning. And nothing helps us to learn more than death."[11] Death is part of life, and by encouraging or teaching the patient to live spiritually, emotionally, physically, and intellectually, the physician guides the patient to acknowledge that death is not the end of a life. Having fully lived, the patient leaves a legacy of life, a myth that remains for others to know. The physician can encourage the patient to live fully and to accept circumstances as lessons to be learned in living. In his book *Further Along the Road Less Traveled,* M. Scott Peck aptly quotes Nobel Prize–winner Albert Schweitzer:

> We must all become familiar with the thought of death if we want to grow into really good people. We need not think of it every day or every hour. But when the path of life leads us to some vantage point where the scene around us fades away and we contemplate the distant view right to the end, let us not close our eyes. Let us pause for a moment, look at the distant view, and then carry on. Thinking about death in this way produces love for life. When we are familiar with death, we accept each week, each day, as a gift. Only if we are able thus to accept life—bit by bit—does it become precious.[11]

For a patient, death may be considered the end of suffering—a source of solace and consolation that offers peace after the turmoil of illness. Hindu and Buddhist religions welcome death because these religions subscribe to the notion of reincarnation theory that advocates the notion of continual rebirth until one has learned what it is on earth one is supposed to learn; after achieving this knowledge, one may finally die for good. It is not necessary, however, for one to subscribe to religion at the end of one's life. But, it is important to understand that death is as much a part of life as birth. It is a process experienced by all. It is not necessary to mystify death with religious allusion. The physician can teach the patient to understand death by the physician's efforts to guide the patient to accept the process. In addition, the physician's awareness of the *spiritual* aspects of the patient, i.e., those characteristics of the spirit, not religion, are essential in guiding the patient to a peaceful transition. It is bad medicine for the physician to impose his or her religious views on the patient at such a time. The realm of spirit is all that matters.

When physicians find themselves frantically searching for means to save a life, after exhausting all possibilities, they must not overlook the peace that can be attained by acknowledging and accepting death's finality. To accept the terminal phase of life as another aspect of living can add a new dimension to the process. Reverent acknowledgment of this final life phase by the physician is an example for those left behind to prepare for another life and to prepare for healing by allowing the process of grief to commence. Just as birth occurs with suffering, a passage to a new life can commence after the awareness of loss has been realized.

To quote M. Scott Peck again, it is important to "face death as early as possible and overcome fear of death." To do these things, one must outgrow one's narcissism and seek a more spiritual mode of life. For people who succeed at this, the prospect of death becomes a magnificent stimulus for psychological and spiritual growth.[7] To persist with technology (i.e., the ordering of tests) and procedures on dying patients, and to avoid this final dimension of life denies the patient and loved ones the occasion to understand the lesson of the life lived on earth.

The balanced doctor lives life on all four levels, too, in order to teach his or her patients how to live. This concept is not taught in medical schools, yet it is clear that the good doctor takes on an added role of teacher and compassionately helps patients discover in themselves deep resources to cope with illness. However, physicians can only discover these resources after living within the realm of spirituality and morality. Physicians may consider using the ideas presented in this chapter to develop awareness of these concepts. Myth making and analysis of one's life provides a means to develop compassion and understanding that are necessary in helping others.

Compassion means literally "to suffer with."[12] Compassion allows complete involvement with the patient's needs and inhibits the remoteness and reluctance to confront the most difficult issues in patient care such as the terminally ill condition. Compassion is the most important virtue in the development of a physician. "The essence of compassion is understanding, the ability to recognize the physical, material, and psychological suffering of others, to put ourselves 'inside the skin' of the other. The mind of compassion is truly present when it is effective in removing another person's suffering."[11]

In a chapter of the book *Living Beyond Limits* by David Spiegal, a cancer patient listed for her physician what she felt would make her feel comfortable. They are as follows:

1. Sit down with me.
2. Look at me.
3. Discuss your thinking about my treatment with me.
4. Acknowledge that you have heard my concerns.

The patient is encouraged to find a physician who will not only work with the patient to reduce the discomfort of disease, but will also treat the patient like a partner in health care.[11] It is acknowledged by Spiegal that an aggressive if impersonal physician may be necessary for the early stages of disease, but a more compassionate and less active physician may be more suitable for the later stages of illness. It is obvious that both types of medical care have benefits, but it is up to the physician to accept and provide such a balance in care. Again, physicians should not feel thwarted as patients search for second opinions or other therapies for disease. This is not a reflection of the physician's failure to provide care, but is a function of the patient's adaptation to the changes induced by the illness or therapy. En-

couragement to the patient by the physician to follow such pursuits is welcomed by most patients.

The advice given to patients in *Living Beyond Limits,* can be well taken by physicians to pass on to patients. If you or someone you love is ill, use it as an occasion to reassess your life, strengthen the ties that matter, and eliminate the ones that don't. "Look hard at what you and your body are facing, deal with the feelings of fear and sadness, and put it into perspective. Take charge of your treatment, allocate your time the way you want to, and savor every moment you have." By living better, you are living longer. You are living beyond limits.[11, 13]

In conclusion, the physician has the fortunate opportunity to provide care for cancer patients in a unique way. The physician is the only person who has the prerogative to address health issues on physical, emotional, intellectual, and spiritual levels. No physician can be equally competent in all dimensions. The challenge to the physician is to continue to be open to other methods of care. Unconventional medicine is here to stay because it plays a legitimate role in patient care. The role of teacher in guiding the patient to a higher level of understanding of these issues in regard to living is a sacred honor. Cancer pain management is multifaceted, and the patient benefits from integration of the four aspects of health.

Summary

The following list summarizes the key points of this chapter.

1. Control is an issue that is faced by all patients, but it may be more difficult for the physician.
2. Healing occurs on four levels: physical, emotional, intellectual, and spiritual.
3. Myth making is a process to understand the meaning of one's life. It can be encouraged to facilitate healing on all levels.
4. Unconventional therapies are frequently sought by patients. Physicians can help by providing information regarding the relevancy of such therapies to the patient's condition.
5. Fear is a pervasive reality for the cancer patient. It must be confronted daily. Physicians must acknowledge patient's fears openly. Human support systems are beneficial to the patient and the physician.

6. Fear of death must be overcome as early as possible. This requires a spiritual approach to life.
7. As physicians, we are here to learn.
8. Compassion removes another person's suffering.
9. Encourage patients to be active in their care and to savor every moment of life.

References

1. Siegal B. Love, Medicine and Miracles. New York: Harper & Row, 1986.
2. Joy B. Joy's Way. New York: Putnam, 1979.
3. Campbell J. Transformations of Myth Through Time. New York: Harper & Row, 1990;1.
4. Kübler-Ross E. Children and Death. New York: Macmillan, 1983;63.
5. Reid D. The Tao of Health, Sex, and Longevity: A Modern Practical Guide to the Ancient Way. New York: Simon & Schuster, 1989.
6. Eisenberg DM, Kessler RC, Foster C, et al. Unconventional medicine in the United States: Prevalence, costs, and patterns of use. N Engl J Med 1993;328:246.
7. Campion EW. Why unconventional medicine? N Engl J Med 1993;328:282.
8. Casselith BR, Lusk EJ, Guerry D, et al. Survival and quality of life among patients receiving unproven therapy as compared with conventional cancer therapy. N Engl J Med 1991;324:1180.
9. Research Council for Complementary Medicine: An International Collaborative Research Project. COST Project B4, RCCM, 1992.
10. Hazelden H. A Moment to Reflect: Accepting Ourselves. San Francisco: Harper & Row, 1989.
11. Peck MS. Further Along the Road Less Traveled. The Unending Journey Toward Spiritual Growth. New York: Simon & Schuster, 1993;47.
12. Hanh TN. Peace Is Every Step: The Path of Mindfulness in Everyday Life. New York: Bantam Books, 1991;81.
13. Spiegal D. Living Beyond Limits: New Hope and Help for Facing Life Threatening Illness. New York: Random House, 1993;240.

Chapter 41

Perspectives of a Pastor–Patient

Benjamin W. Johnson, Sr.

A pastor is a man called on by God to spend his life leading people to God. A pastor also spends much time in prayer for people and their problems. In addition to spending much time preparing messages for worship services, pastors are also active with other activities in the church and other engagements and activities in the community. A pastor is supposed to encourage people to trust God in difficult times. He is able to encourage people to pray, read, and study the Bible for hope and assurance in their daily lives.

It is part of a pastor's duties to visit ill church members in the hospital or at home. His presence signifies the presence of God, and his prayers are expected to work. His prayers are supposed to defy the final word of the doctors, even if the physical condition of the patient is terminal. If the pain does not stop while the pastor is praying, people tend to ask, "Why?" Even as pastors, we don't always know the answer.

Pastors have the same strengths and weaknesses as other human beings. They experience the same fears, doubts, denials, and moral challenges as others. An honest pastor will acknowledge his inner struggles, tensions, inabilities, shortcomings, and failures. He or she also experiences unfulfilled goals, objectives, and plans. He or she needs to be encouraged just like other people.

My Experience as a Pastor and as a Patient

I began to experience increasing weakness that was very noticeable to my family doctor. My doctor told me to bring three samples of my stool to his office in order to check for blood. He told me that I had a low iron count and that I was losing blood. He emphasized very strongly that I go to the hospital in order to have a computerized tomographic scan performed. It revealed a tumor in my left kidney that was probably cancerous. My doctor thought that it would have to be removed through surgery. What a shock! All my life I have taken very good care of myself, because of my dreadful fear of cancer and surgery. However, now I was being told that I was not going home, but rather was being admitted to have a transfusion of several units of blood, because my blood count was only 4.5, whereas it should be around 13 or 14. I was shocked and fear gripped me, when they informed me that I needed a series of blood tests and that they were going to take blood samples from me a number of times for the next few days. I have a dreadful fear of needles, but I did not want anyone to know it. I tried to ignore the pain of my swollen knees caused by cancer.

I have prayed for other people, not knowing whether they were Christians or not. God did heal some of those people miraculously.* Couldn't I be healed miraculously also? I felt that I too deserved to be healed, because I was a man of God dedicated to serving people.

---

* ". . . and people brought to him all who were ill with various diseases, those suffering severe pain, the demon-possessed, those having seizures, and the paralyzed, and he healed them." (Matt. 4:24; The Holy Bible: New International Version (NIV). Michigan: Zondervan Publishers, 1985.)

I asked myself several questions: Am I guilty? Am I being chastised? Is God permitting this to happen to teach me some truths that I will only learn through this forthcoming painful experience? Have I done all that I could do? Must I really experience the pain that I feared so much? Did people sense that I was a pastor in bed with the possibility of cancer? Did I resent people praying for me, and telling me, "just say that you are healed, and you will be healed?" Yet I was not healed? Yes, I did resent it. Was I rejoicing that I had the opportunity to tell others in the hospital that although I had cancer, I was rejoicing for the opportunity to witness about Jesus Christ? No! As a pastor, did I pray strong and courageously, or did I daydream about the possible pain? Did I pray for others in pain, or realize that others were in pain while I was in the hospital? No! Had I been faithful as a pastor? Yes!

It was very difficult for me to let my daughter drive me to the airport and to let my wife push my wheelchair: Oh, the feeling of helplessness, as my wife and the stewardess helped to seat me on the plane.

On September 26, 1994 I met the internist who was going to coordinate my care before and after the surgery. I also met the urologist, who would be my surgeon for the operation to remove my diseased kidney. He was very frank, kind, and sensitive as he took time to explain the serious possibilities that could occur during the surgery. I wanted to deny the necessity of the surgery; I wanted to believe that surgery could be bypassed with a miracle. It didn't happen. The internist and urologist told me that it would take a week to build me up for surgery, because I was so weak. The surgery was scheduled for October 3, 1994.

During the week before the surgery, my son, who is an anesthesiologist, told me that he and two of his colleagues would come to visit me. One of his colleagues would be my anesthesiologist, and the other was the director of the Pain Control Center.

These three doctors will never know the comfort that they gave me that evening. I experienced a peace that helped prepare me for surgery the next day. Doctors can bring much therapeutic healing to their patients, when they take a little of their time to say a few words to them. It means so much when the patient feels and believes that the doctor really cares for them. Patients need the encouragement that only a doctor can give before and after surgery, particularly the anesthesiologist.

I felt frightened as my wife, and my son's wife left me, as I was being prepared to enter the operating room for surgery. During the preparation, I felt numb, with a mixture of deep settled peace. I remember going into the operating room. The next thing I remember was that I heard voices saying that it was over. But, in a moment of inner confusion, I thought that I was going in for surgery, and wanted to scream, no! Then I looked at the clock, it was 6:00 P.M.; it was over.

About 12:30 A.M., October 4, 1994, I was awakened with a feeling of agonizing, excruciating pain in the right side of my back. With a catheter in my back, the intravenous lines in my left arm and left hand, and the bladder catheter, it was confusing, irritating, and uncomfortable, as I attempted to move, trying to escape the pain in my back. The pain felt like a sharp needle and spread all over the right side of my back, or as if a large knife was pressing into the right side of my back. The needle also felt like the point was pressing in and out, causing a sensation of intense agonizing pain. My reaction to the pain was a mixture of fear and desperation. I was startled out of a deep sleep and was bewildered, wondering if I would have to have to experience this pain throughout the night. I called for someone to come and give me some medication to help with the pain; but the pills didn't relieve the pain. About 3:00 A.M., I called for help again to relieve the pain, but the nurse stated that she had given me all that the doctor had ordered. I asked if there was a doctor available, and she said that she would call her. The pain was so intense that I got up out of the bed and sat on the side of the bed. I stood up and bowed down, twisted and turned, trying to obtain some relief. After I returned to the bed, I tried to lay down, but there was more pain in my midsection around the site of the surgery. My whole torso was full of pain. The slightest movement from side to side or bending forward intensified the pain in my torso as well as the pain in the right side of my back. I felt helpless and trapped in this situation. I wanted to scream, yell, and holler. I forgot to pray. My theology was not working for me now!* Finally I set-

---

* "He came to a broom tree, sat down under it and prayed that he might die. 'I have had enough Lord,' he said. 'Take my life; I am no better than my ancestors.'" (I Kings 19:4; The Holy Bible: New International Version (NIV). Michigan: Zondervan Publishers, 1985.)

tled down, and pushed myself to thank God that the surgery was over and that the pain was not going to last forever. The anesthesiologist said that he would increase the strength of the medicine in my epidural catheter. While I heard him talking softly to himself, calculating the strength of the medicine, I found it very hard to be patient. He went away and returned, and told me to turn over on my right side so that he could replace the epidural catheter. He talked to me and encouraged me as he was replacing the catheter in my back. I could feel him kneading the vertebrae in my back in order to put the needle back into the right place. Though the pain was almost unbearable, the touch of his fingers on my back was so gentle, that the intensity of the pain seemed to subside even before the medicine had taken effect. As the anesthesiologist left the room, I became less aware of the pain, and awakened later in the morning without any pain in my back.

If I have felt the tender touch of God,* I wonder if it was that morning, through the fingers of the anesthesiologist? I hope that other anesthesiologists are as comforting to their patients as this physician was to me. As a pastor and patient, my experience with cancer has given me a deeper appreciation for doctors, especially anesthesiologists. People do need more skilled doctors, who are also tender as they touch apprehensive patients.

What an experience I had on this day. I didn't know what a urinary catheter was. I thought I didn't need that thing hanging out of my "you know what." I tried to pull it out until it began to hurt, and then I left it alone! Then a male and female nurse gave me a bath—all over. I felt shocked and ashamed but I didn't tell anyone. What joy, pride, and comfort I felt when my son came in the room!

I also experienced episodes of anticipated, imagined pain: after the removal of the urinary catheter—no pain; bowel elimination—no pain; removal of staples by the nurse—no pain. What awful, dreaded thoughts patients can experience, even when the patient is informed that there would be no pain. I had my eyes closed and was very tense waiting for the removal of the skin staples. The

nurse said, "Mr. Johnson, I am pulling out staple number nine." There were 35 more staples to be removed, and I felt no pain.

Through this experience with cancer surgery, I have observed and experienced the sensitivity of doctors. It was a blessing and a comfort to see the number of doctors who came in to check on me and to spend time talking with me. I was able to ask questions and not feel that I was unwanted or unimportant. The Pain Center sent me a large basket of fruit, flowers, and other goodies. I cried like a baby and could not stop. The card was signed by the "Pain Gang." It is this expression from the Pain Unit, and the anesthesiologists, that helped me realize the sensitivity of their care for a fellow coworker and his father. This reveals their care as well as their feeling for each other. Not only were my emotions touched, but also my heart. This magnificent expression of mutual care will help me encourage many people that anesthesiologists are some of the most caring doctors in the medical profession.

It is a wonderful feeling to have several doctors come into your room morning and evening to visit. The questions that they ask, and the amount of time that they take to listen gives you a strong, positive feeling that they have concern for you. I have been educated and enriched as a pastor, and as a patient, by the doctors, especially the anesthesiologists.

Cancer, like many other scourges of humankind, is widespread and is associated with much pain. Oftentime, the pain associated with the treatment of cancer can be at times more painful than the original cancer. It is gratifying to know that our Lord Jesus Christ, although he did not have a cancer, suffered a great deal and eventually died on the cross to save the world. Thus, in dying, the world was saved. I have just described my experience with cancer, which was quite painful. The good news is my cancer has been controlled and, it is hoped, cured. My spiritual growth has been immense over that period and, perhaps, the final message I can give is that beyond the pain and the cancer, there is a force that is strengthening and that can provide inner peace. I am not advocating that pain is good and should be sought. Fortunately, my pain was well controlled by my doctors but, overall, the experience with cancer and the severe pain have provided significant positive experiences for me and my family.

---
*"Filled with compassion, Jesus reached out his hand and touched the man. 'I am willing,' he said. 'Be clean!' . . . and he was cured." (Mark 1:41; The Holy Bible: New International Version (NIV). Michigan: Zondervan Publishers, 1985.)

Chapter 42
Ethical Issues

Richard M. Zaner

Introduction

Although relief of pain is a primary clinical issue, it is widely reported that pain management for cancer patients has often been inadequate. Most of these studies only briefly mention ethical issues associated with pain management. The few studies that do address these issues typically take a standard approach. Critical analysis of this approach discloses serious shortcomings, thus prompting a closer look into the experience of pain and suffering in the context of the physician–patient relationship. The concept of *respect* is especially intriguing, and is proposed as the core of that relationship to shed light on the well-recognized need to establish sensitive communication and on how a moral awareness can best be awakened.

Overview

Most people manifest deep-seated fear of cancer, and that "the fear of cancer is the fear of pain."[1] Although relief of pain is a primary clinical issue, it is also widely reported that pain management for cancer patients is often inadequate.[2, 3] An estimated 80% of patients are believed to be undertreated,[4] even though there have been remarkable advances in pain management, with better drugs and newer routes for administration being developed (subcutaneous, epidural, or intrathecal), as well as improved surgical procedures and innovative instruments.

In contrast to the obvious importance of pain management, Morris et al. note that there have been few careful studies of the debilitating pain that is most often associated with cancer. Their review of the literature[5–13] revealed that "in only one study[13] was some explicit instrument or scale used to measure the presence and level of pain,"[1] while the other studies relied on indirect measures and reports (staff impressions, inference based on analgesic usage, etc.). The study by Morris et al., in contrast, queried patients in a variety of settings and institutions, used well-standardized questions to elicit information about the level of pain from the patient and a familial informant, and compared the prevalence and severity of pain among terminal cancer patients. Based on the largest sample to date, this helpful study noted shifts in prevalence and severity as patients approach death in different settings, and addressed the issue of the medical and demographic correlates of pain. Even so, none of these studies, including that by Morris et al., addresses ethical issues more than tangentially.

Nevertheless, there have been some efforts to examine the ethical issues specific to the experience and treatment of pain in cancer patients.[14–22] As with much of the literature in medical ethics, these share the same approach. It is uniformly emphasized that the "principles" of autonomy, beneficence, nonmaleficence, and justice should be taken as governing pain management, as well as all other ethical issues in health care,[23] whether those dealing with these problems are physicians[24–26] or clinical ethics consultants.[27, 28] Central to appropriate pain management for cancer patients is "an overriding moral duty to relieve pain and suffering"[2]—a duty that, however, often seems in conflict with the equally imperative duty "to avoid harm."[15] The conflict can be acute in treating terminally ill cancer patients, since relieving pain and suffering may seem equivalent to hastening death—either by directly killing the patient by using barbiturates or by using opioids for sedation, which also repress respiratory efforts and can allow death to occur.

The ethical question that then inevitably arises, as Truog et al. recognize, is whether "relevant criteria" can be identified for relieving pain and suffering while at the same time respecting "the prohibition against killing."[2] Most commentators argue that these issues should be governed by the right to self-determination, specifically to make decisions for oneself (autonomy), and balancing the duties of helping patients (beneficence) and not causing harm (nonmaleficence). Although appreciating this approach, Truog et al. argue its inadequacy (as discussed in the following section) and appeal to the principle of double effect: Distinguishing between "intended" and "unintended but foreseen" effects of an action, they argue that "since the caregiver's first responsibility is to relieve pain and suffering, the potential for hastening death is tolerated as a necessary evil."[2]

Unresolved Questions

Both approaches face serious problems that impact directly on the clinical management of pain. The main reason for regarding the first standard approach as inadequate lies in its requirement that the patient be informed of options.[15] Genuine informed consent often cannot be achieved because many patients are severely compromised by pain or medication, or both, and, with the development of new pain-relief technologies and medications, many patients lack necessary knowledge about side effects, for instance.[2] There is also an absence of randomized clinical trials to indicate the percentage of patients benefiting from a particular technology.[14] The appeal to autonomy, beneficence, nonmaleficence, and justice—in other words relying on the presence of a competent patient (or an appropriately signed directive)—is inadequate for any patient whose competence may be reasonably suspected and who

has left no such directive, and where conflict among family members, legal surrogate, and providers is present. As this type of situation is, at least at present, the most frequently encountered in hospital care for terminally ill cancer patients, an appeal to such principles simply gives no guidance for how best to manage acute pain.

There are, however, ethical difficulties even in situations involving patients who are either capable of making their own decisions or who have left clear directives for medical management. Although reluctant to criticize the appeal to autonomy, Stoltzfus and Stamatos nevertheless rightly point out that heeding its dictates not only requires more time by the health care professional (who is often hard-pressed by time, conflicting views of family members, and other constraints related to the pain management unit in the hospital), but also that with the increased complexity of new techniques and technologies, it is likely if also unfortunate that increased complexity probably correlates inversely with patient autonomy.[14]

The assurance that the patient's autonomy is respected requires that the time spent with the patient by the physician be devoted to conversations with them[29]—both talking and, perhaps more importantly, listening and interpreting what is conveyed.[30] It has become more widely recognized, specifically concerning obtaining informed consent for withholding and withdrawal of life supports, that the ability to communicate effectively with patients and families or legal surrogates is one of the most vital professional skills in appropriate decision making.[31] In these terms, "the spoken language is the most important . . . diagnostic and therapeutic tool" that the physician possesses.[30] Reiser emphasizes that, although the "patient's role as narrator in the drama of illness has declined in the twentieth century, there are few tasks more important for contemporary medicine" than the careful cultivation and enhancement of "our communication skills" to seek the needed balance "between understanding general biologic processes that make us ill and understanding the illness as experienced . . . by the patient."[30] Katz also recognized that clinically conducted conversations or dialogues are essential for every medical consideration, not merely for patient compliance or consent.[32]

To be effective and sensitive in communication, physicians must learn to be as precise as the physician who auscultates a heart or palpates a spleen and as careful as is a surgeon with a scalpel,[30] both in providing information and in listening to their concerns (most of all about pain). Nevertheless, Kleinman emphasizes that physicians are currently not trained to be self-reflective interpreters of distinctive systems of meaning. They are rarely taught that biological processes are known only through socially constructed categories that constrain experience as much as does disordered physiology.[33]

Notwithstanding the significance of autonomy, it must be recognized that compliance with autonomy is fraught with real difficulties in clinical settings, and not merely due to experience of acute pain and understanding the complexities of new methods of pain management. Before addressing these issues, it is necessary to review the problems associated with the approach that Truog et al. recommend.

The appeal to "double effect"—employed specifically to determine whether the administration of barbiturates can ever be justified for terminally ill cancer patients—also presents serious difficulties. Acknowledging that their recommendation rests entirely on the concept of "intent," Truog et al. also recognize that it ineluctably courts the accusation of causing death (euthanasia) and not merely relieving pain or acting with a patient's competent request, which is assisted suicide. Justification based on the principle of double effect requires that the clinician intend only to relieve the patient's suffering and not to cause death. A problem arises, however, precisely because, for terminally ill patients, both effects are often seen as desirable. The justification of double effect may therefore function as a "fig leaf" for euthanasia, for in such cases "the true intent . . . would be the death of the patient"—a practice that is not permissible in traditional ethics.[2] Justification clearly rests on widespread approval of euthanasia, which, of course, does not in the least require the concept of intent.

"Double effect" relies on accepting the idea of "foreseen but unintended" effects, but in the very cases that give rise to its consideration, that idea is both unnecessary and possibly unacceptable (if any "traditional" ethic is invoked). At most, this approach might prove reasonable only for a narrowly defined set of cases, in which barbiturates are used strictly to relieve the burden of severe pain and suffering when every reasonable alternative has failed. Even in these cases, however, it should be noted that reliance on the distinction between intended and unintended (but foreseen) effects of an action harbors a well-recognized and potentially decisive difficulty: How can a physician's intent be determined? Barbiturates have often been used to kill patients intentionally[2] as well as to manage pain, but there is no obvious way to distinguish between an intention merely to relieve pain ("intended") and an intention to kill ("unintended but foreseen").

The Physician–Patient Relationship

It has taken many years to secure the recognition of the rights of self-determination and informed consent (autonomy) in health care[34] and thus should not be lightly impugned or dismissed. Autonomy has been often contrasted with medical paternalism—the idea that physicians are in a better position than patients or families to know the patient's best interests, and must therefore be the sole, or least the primary decision makers. This has contrasted with the increasingly accepted idea that the patient is the true source of authority for decisions, or, if not competent, a family member or legal surrogate, since either party has the right to control what happens.[31] Instead of acting paternalistically, physicians are enjoined to acknowledge autonomy and to act according to the standard of beneficence: the obligation to benefit the patient where the patient's best interests are determined (in whatever form) by the patient or legal surrogate.

Nevertheless, the difficulties mentioned previously require that these notions be looked at again. Although it is true that respect for persons is central to the concept of autonomy,[15] these concepts are not equivalent. Autonomy, even if restricted to the right of self-determination, presupposes the capacity for making one's own decisions; respect does not. To the contrary, patients should be respected *whether or not* they still have the capacity for making decisions—whether due to mental illness, incapacitating illness or pain, or the effects of medications. Beneficence also invokes the concept of respect.

Despite its frequent mention in the literature, the idea of respect seems ambiguous, since what it means exactly in any concrete situation may not be specifically clear, especially when the person is a patient in acute pain. Even so, to invoke respect for a patient is to affirm him or her as intrinsically valuable and worthwhile, and thus is to set up a *mutual relationship* with that person, a reflexive orientation that is quite complex.[35] In simple terms, the physician experiences and interprets the patient; likewise, the patient experiences and interprets himself or herself while also experiencing and interpreting the physician. In this relationship, both are aware of themselves as they relate to each another (although, to be sure, the patient's self-awareness may be muted or compromised, just as the physician's self-awareness may be suppressed, for whatever reason), and also of their relationship itself.

Several brief examples will help illustrate these points. Two persons are friends; each of them relates to, experiences, and values the other ("Joe is a good person"); likewise, each relates to, experiences, and values himself or herself within the relationship to each other ("I'm a better person when I'm with Joe"); and, each relates reflexively to, experiences, and values the relationship itself ("We have a solid friendship"). Similarly, within the physician's relationship with a patient, the patient relates to the physician ("She seems to understand what's wrong with me"); and both experience one another as well as the relationship itself ("I'd recommend her to anybody"; "It was a joy treating him").

This mutual and reflexive relationship is also asymmetric, with power, in the form of knowledge, skills, access to resources, social legitimization and legal authorization, on the side of the physician. In addition to being compromised by illness, pain, and fear, the patient is disadvantaged by the very relationship brought about by the illness. For that reason, physicians bear the responsibility not merely for attempting to communicate, but also for ensuring that effective communication occurs.[33] Accordingly, to respect the patient (whether or not he or she is alert or capable of making decisions) is to be oriented toward the patient in a specifically moral relationship. Negatively, as was already patent in the Hippocratic Oath, the physician must never take advantage of the multiply disadvantaged patient,[36] which, I suggest, is part of the core meaning of respect in health care situations. Positively, the concept of respect is central to that of beneficence as well: The responsibility to benefit a patient implies the active attempt to understand the patient.

In making medical recommendations, therefore, the clinician must focus on the patient's life, values, experience, and self-interpretation. When we speak of illness, we must include the patient's judgments about

how best to cope with the distress and with the practical problems in daily living it creates[32]: judgments that are expressed in the form of personal narratives. Frequently, however, neither the patient nor family is able to express the full narrative adequately or accurately, which is surely a requirement for judging whether she is truly informed, uncoerced, and capable of making decisions. Thus, another core clinical task

> is the empathetic interpretation of a life story that makes over the illness into the subject matter of a biography . . . [that] highlights core life themes—for example, injustice, courage, personal victory against the odds—for whose prosecution the details of illness supply evidence . . . [To do this,] the clinician must first piece together the illness narrative as it emerges from the patient's and the family's complaints and explanatory models; then he or she must interpret it in light of the different modes of illness meanings—symptom symbols, culturally salient illnesses, personal and social contexts.[33]

Respecting the patient does not necessarily presume decision-making capacity by the patient, nor does attempting to benefit the patient merely mean providing what the physician believes is the best treatment. Respect is a moral concept that indicates not only autonomy, beneficence, and nonmaleficence but also a complex clinical relationship between patient and physician that is mutual, reflexive, and asymmetric. This relationship is characterized precisely by the need for time and conversation—talking and listening so as to enrich mutual understanding so far as circumstances permit—that has, as noted, been too little appreciated.[29, 37]

The physician, in different terms, must not only try to understand the patient, but must also *be understanding* on behalf of the patient, a quality exhibited primarily through thoughtful and continuous conversation. This requires, however, that the physician develop an existential commitment to be with the sick person and to facilitate his or her building of an illness narrative that will make sense of and give value to the experience.[33] The doctor has to place himself in the lived experience of the patient's illness, so as to understand the situation as the patient understands, perceives, and feels it.[33]

Ethics of Pain Management

Morris et al. point out that pain is a personal experience, and because it is, attempts to objectively measure pain according to a single standard are intrinsically paradoxical.[1] Because of the intensely personal nature of pain, that paradox uniquely highlights both the clinical need and the difficulty of understanding and being understanding in managing the cancer patient's greatest fear and experience, which is pain and suffering.

Before proceeding, however, it will be helpful to introduce a crucial distinction, emphasized by Cassell, between these two frequently associated terms.[38] While patients may, and frequently do, suffer from pain, they also suffer when pain is not present. Cassell briefly recounts one of his patients—a 25-year-old sculptress with metastatic disease of the breast—who was treated by competent, caring physicians using the most advanced techniques and therapies. The treatments as well as the disease were both sources of pain and suffering. Her future had a brittle quality[39] marked by uncertainty and fear, but she could get little information from her doctors. She had no idea that her irradiated breast would become so disfigured, or that she would become hirsute, obese, and devoid of libido. Because of the tumor in the supraclavicular fossa, she lost strength in the hand and arm she used in sculpting, and grew increasingly depressed. When she fractured her femur, treatment was delayed while her physicians openly disagreed about placing pins in her hip. With each medical response to her disease or associated problems, she would become hopeful again, only to be confronted with still other problems. When a new course of chemotherapy was initiated, for instance, she felt the acute dilemma of being torn between a desire to live and work, and the all-too-familiar fear of allowing hope again when it only exposed her to misery if the treatment failed, as happened so often before. In addition to the inevitable side effects—nausea, vomiting, hair loss, etc.—her already brittle future contracted, causing increased pain and disability and the likelihood of death.

Distinct from the acute and continuing pain—or, rather, deeply texturing it—were several forms of suffering: about how she appeared to others, especially family and friends; about her sense of her own disfigured body; about her ability to understand the source of her pain and being abandoned; about what the future would bring; and ultimately about loss and death. Her suffering was thus not restricted to physical symptoms, but extended to re-

lationships and work, to her sense of her body and herself, as well as her prospects. She suffered from her disease and the pain (not fully understanding either), but also from the treatments and the pain and side effects they brought (not fully understanding these, either). Cassell emphasizes that one could not anticipate, but rather had to ask, what she would herself describe as reasons for her suffering.[38] Unfortunately, she was never asked.

Accordingly, it is manifestly inappropriate to treat sickness as something that happens merely to a person's body; ignoring the person who is sick only contributes to the suffering, especially the sense of being ignored and abandoned. Furthermore, like pain, suffering is intensely personal, for it is ultimately the threat of impending personal disaster, a "state of severe distress associated with events that threaten the intactness of the person."[38] Neither pain nor suffering can be understood and appropriately treated without ongoing, sensitive conversations with patients about their experiences and self-interpretations (especially about matters that are confusing and disturbing).

Pain and suffering may be, but are not always, closely connected. Some pains can be experienced as rewarding (childbirth, for instance), and there are pains that, although severe, are not sources of suffering (that experienced during the healing of a wound, for example). People report keen suffering from pain when they feel out of control, the pain is overwhelming, the source of the pain is unknown, the meaning of the pain is dire, or the pain is chronic.[38] Thus, patients may suffer from pain, but also over lost capacities, compromises to personal traits and abilities, disruptions in personal and familial life, and constrictions to the person's future (short or long term). Appropriate pain management clearly requires careful conversational probing to understand and exhibit understanding in treating patients.

Another patient, a 46-year-old barber, experienced pain in his upper leg and buttocks so severe that, as he put it, "it became a mental trauma." Visits with several doctors, each of whom diagnosed different problems (from hemorrhoids to prostate cancer) and prescribed different medications, proved unhelpful; the pain continued unabated. At one point, he got an infected toe from clipping his nails too short, and the pain in his foot brought a recommendation that he lose weight. He did, but all his pains continued; eventually, he experienced difficulties walking, standing, and even sitting. While he was cutting the hair of a friend (who happened also to be a physician) and relating his woes, his friend suggested that he see a podiatrist. When he did, it was determined that he had a fallen arch; the podiatrist then explained that this was the reason for his pains. He also got the first relief he had experienced in more than 2 years. As the patient reported, "I had no idea I had a foot problem because when your rear end hurts you don't think of your foot."[40]

Physicians and other providers need to establish good communication with patients, and in order to do this they must pay close attention to what patients relate about their illnesses. Two themes seem well established: (1) Sick people want to know what's wrong with them (their providers understand), and (2) they want to know that the people taking care of them also really care for them (their providers are understanding). Many patients, however, find it hard to talk about themselves; they may also experience compelling difficulties trying to find out what's wrong with them. Some patients may fear being regarded as too pushy; others may be apprehensive about appearing insulting; a few are more insistent. In any case, hospitals are rarely places that encourage persistent questions or conversations. They are busy places and patients often realize that their questions interrupt physicians and nurses, and that their questions may even make them appear selfish and presumptuous. Patients are rarely in a good position, moreover, to question physicians: They cannot evaluate precisely what is wrong, what is being done and why, nor can they judge whether treatments or procedures are appropriate or effective or whether there are available alternatives that might be better for them. Open and direct communication, difficult enough in hospitals anyway, can be compromised for other reasons. Some patients do not know how to talk with physicians; others may not want to do so (at a particular time, or at all); and some are content simply to act out the sick role they believe is expected of them by physicians and hospital staff. Most patients realize the premium placed on being a good patient: compliant, cooperative, and quiet.

These difficulties are enhanced when the patient experiences intense and continuing pain. When the pain is, or is thought to be, due to some form of cancer, the situation is often full of strong emotions,

fear in particular, and may be ripe for serious conflicts that affect decision making. It is important that physicians not only initiate conversations with patients early on (and sustain them over time), but also be patiently attentive to what is said. Pain is a quality of the patient's experience; managing it, therefore, requires careful listening to the patient's words, accompanied by sensitive assistance to help the patient discuss the experience.

It should be remembered, finally, that, as one patient emphasized, "if you can't communicate and you can't understand your disease, then you don't have any confidence in the medical help you are getting . . . there are lots of feelings that are hard to put into words, especially if you've never had the feeling before. I had to explain things to my doctor which were a brand new experience to me, and I had nothing to compare it to. So if you can't communicate back and forth, and explain to him what's bothering you, how can he help you?"[40]

Concluding Remarks

The typical emphasis given to autonomy, beneficence, nonmaleficence, and justice is not so much ethically incorrect as it is critically defective. What is defective about the received view is that, on the one hand, its focus on the competent patient with decision-making capacity does not provide guidance on how to manage most patients, especially cancer patients experiencing severe and prolonged fear, pain, and suffering. On the other hand, the idea of autonomy cannot stand by itself, because it invokes the closely connected but distinct idea of respect; indeed, the latter may be the key part of the former. The idea that autonomy, or the right of self-determination, is primary in health care (or in other contexts) risks ignoring the complex, asymmetric, and mutual relationship between provider and patient (family, associates, and legal surrogate) that is the core of autonomy, beneficence, nonmaleficence, and justice. In urging recognition of these, it has too often been forgotten that recognition is itself a basic moral orientation that has vitally important implications for the clinical management of patients. In a word, to say that the physician should acknowledge the autonomy of patients is inherently to urge that the provider should adopt a specific moral attitude toward all patients, and not merely those who are alert and capable of making decisions. That orientation or attitude is the core of the provider–patient relationship; it is what Pellegrino terms the "architectonic" of clinical medicine.[41]

The proposal that another principle ("double effect") might be appealed to in justifying the management of pain while avoiding the risk of open euthanasia is inadequate and highly problematic. It not only involves unacceptable risks and questionable assumptions about "intent," but in the end it presupposes and does not replace the terms of the standard approach.

There is a common flaw in both approaches. It is not enough to argue for certain norms as guides for action or merely to appeal to rational principles, of whatever sort and in whichever situation. Moral action requires not only that we understand the nature and implications of what we do, but also that we recognize and accept responsibility for our actions—perhaps as important, if not more so, it requires that we are *moved to act* in the first place. A physician may understand, for instance, that a patient's condition is so compromised and intractable that the time has come to withdraw life supports and allow the patient to die, yet, the physician may be unable to do that. A patient or family member may likewise understand that the time has come to withdraw supports, but may not yet be ready to accept that. It's one thing, if you will, to know what's right; it's quite another to be prepared to act in accord with that knowledge. Ethical understanding and theory must be based on a vital arch of feeling: We must not only understand but also be moved to act in light of that understanding, including recognizing the responsibility that our actions ineluctably carry with them. The idea of respect and its implications for ongoing dialogue between intimately interrelated participants, I believe, is directly responsive to that requirement of moral life.

There is, as Albert Schweitzer once noted, a "special league among those who have known anxiety and physical suffering . . . They know the terrible things man can undergo; they know the longing to be free of pain."[42] Each of us has in some way or other felt and vitally known the vulnerability that is so much a part of the experience of illness and pain. For the most part, our sundry ailments, abrasions, breaks, cuts, and fevers pass away or heal, leaving us with a sense of profound relief at their passing. With the relief, that sense of vulnerability and urgency, fear and apprehension, also usually pass away; the memory thankfully also dims.

Thus, Schweitzer continued, it may be that we need to be reminded of that inner, intimate experience, so as to appreciate anew that it is a veritable "special occasion" appealing for and compellingly evoking a moral sense that is, however, usually dormant. Illness, pain especially, diminishes our capacities and awareness, our abilities to choose and to feel, our self-image, and bodily integrity. It increases our reliance on other people and places us in an imbalanced, asymmetric relationship with them. To encounter another person going through severe illness and pain can, but need not, evoke those memories; it may, indeed, form us into a "fraternity of those marked by pain"[42]; it may function as one of those "special occasions" that may awaken our usually dormant moral sensibility and precisely thereby serve to move us to want to help, especially if we were fortunate enough ourselves to have been helped.

That awakening of a moral sense, I believe, is too frequently muted and overlooked in the usual discussions of ethics in clinical situations; it is also what must be accomplished if we would be appropriately attentive to those in pain and suffering brought on by debilitating forms of cancer.

References

1. Morris JN, Mor V, Goldberg RJ, et al. The effect of treatment setting and patient characteristics on pain in terminal cancer patients: A report from the National Hospice Study. J Chronic Dis 1986;39:27.
2. Truog RD, Berde CB, Mitchell C, Grier HE. Barbiturates in the care of the terminally ill. N Engl J Med 1992;327:1678.
3. Krant MJ. The hospice movement. N Engl J Med 1978;299:546.
4. Bonica JJ. The Management of Pain. Philadelphia: Lea & Febiger, 1990.
5. Hardy TK, Pritchard RI. Physical distress suffered by terminal cancer patients in hospital. Anaesthiology 1977;32:647.
6. Exton-Smith AN. Terminal illness in the aged. Lancet 1961;ii:305.
7. Goldberg IK, Kutscher AH, Schoenberg B, et al. Psychopharmacologic and Analgesic Agents Employed in Terminal Care of 100 Cancer Patients. In IK Goldberg, S Malitz, AH Kutscher (eds), Psychopharmacologic Agents for the Terminally Ill and Bereaved. New York: Columbia University, 1973.

8. Wilkes E. Some problems in cancer management. Proc R Soc Med 1974;67:100.

9. Twycross RG. The use of narcotic analgesics in terminal illness. J Med Ethics 1975;1:10.

10. Oster MW, Vizel M, Trugeon L. Pain of terminal cancer patients. Arch Intern Med 1978;138:1801.

11. Foley KM. The Management of Pain of Malignant Origin. In HR Tyler, D Dawson (eds), Current Neurology. Boston: Houghton Mifflin, 1979.

12. Foley KM. Clinical assessment of cancer pain. Acta Anaesth Scand 1982;74:91.

13. McKegney FP, Bailey L, Yates J. Prediction and management of pain in patients with advanced cancer. Gen Hosp Psychiatry 1981;3:95.

14. Stoltzfus DP, Stamatos JM. An appraisal of the ethical issues involved in high-technology cancer pain relief. J Clin Ethics 1992;2:113.

15. Ferrell BR, Rhiner M. High-tech comfort: Ethical issues in cancer pain management for the 1990s. J Clin Ethics 1992;2:108.

16. Edwards RB. Pain and the ethics of pain management. Soc Sci Med 1984;18:515.

17. Twycross RG. Ethical and clinical aspects of pain management in cancer patients. J Anaesth Scand 1982;74:83.

18. Pellegrino ED. The clinical ethics of pain management in the terminally ill. Hosp Forum 1982;25:1493.

19. Engelhardt HT. Ethical Issues in Pain Management. In HW Kosterlitz, LY Terenius (eds), Pain and Society: Report of the Dahlem Workshop on Pain and Society. Florida Verlag Chemie, 1980;461.

20. McCullough LB. Pain, Suffering and Life Extending Technologies. In RM Veatch (ed), Life span: Values and Life Extending Technologies. New York: Harper & Row, 1979;118.

21. Lisson EL. Ethical issues related to pain control. Nurs Clin North Am 1987;22:649.

22. Thomasma DC. Ethics and professional practice in oncology. Semin Oncol Nurs 1989;5:89.

23. Beauchamp T, Childress J. Principles of Biomedical Ethics. New York: Oxford, 1983.

24. LaPuma J. Consultations in clinical ethics—Issues and questions in 27 cases. West J Med 1987;6:633.

25. LaPuma J, Stocking CB, Silverstein MD. An ethics consultation service in a teaching hospital. JAMA 1988;260:808.

26. Schiedermayer DL, LaPuma J, Miles SH. Ethics consultations masking economic dilemmas in patient care. Arch Intern Med 1989;149:1303.

27. Agich CF. A role theoretic look. Soc Sci Med 1990;30:389.

28. Glover JJ, Ozar DT, Thomasma DC. Teaching ethics on rounds: The ethicist as teacher, consultant and decision-maker. Theor Med 1986;7:13.

29. Zaner RM. Voices and time: The venture of clinical ethics. J Med Phil 1993;18:9.

30. Cassell EJ. Talking with Patients. Boston: MIT Press, 1985.

31. Ruark JE, Raffin TA, and the Stanford University Medical Center Committee on Ethics. Initiating and withdrawing life support. N Engl J Med 1988;381:25.

32. Katz J. The Silent World of Doctor and Patient. New York: The Free Press, 1988.

33. Kleinman A. The Illness Narratives: Suffering, Healing and the Human Condition. New York: Basic Books, 1988.

34. Beauchamp T, Faden R. A History and Theory of Informed Consent. New York: Oxford, 1986.

35. Zaner RM. Illness and the Other. In GP McKenny, JR Sande (eds), Theological Analyses of the Clinical Encounter. Boston: Kluwer, 1994.

36. Zaner RM. Ethics and the Clinical Encounter. Englewood Cliffs, NJ: Prentice Hall, 1988.

37. Zaner RM. Medicine and dialogue. J Med Phil 1990;15:303.

38. Cassell EJ. The nature of suffering and the goals of medicine. N Engl J Med 1982;306:639.

39. Rawlinson M. Medicine's Discourse and the Practice of Medicine. In V Kestenbaum (ed), The Humanity of the Ill: Phenomenological Perspectives. Knoxville, TN: University of Tennessee Press, 1982;69.

40. Hardy RC. Sick: How People Feel about Being Sick and What They Think of Those Who Care for Them. Chicago: Teach'Em, 1978.

41. Pellegrino ED. The Healing Relationship: The Architectonics of Clinical Medicine. In EE Shelp (ed), The Clinical Encounter: The Moral Fabric of the Patient–Physician Relationship. Dordrecht: D. Reidel, 1983;153.

42. Speilgelberg H. Good fortune obligates: Albert Schweitzer's second ethical principle. Ethics 1975;85:227.

Chapter 43

Governmental Guidelines

Daniel B. Carr, Ada Jacox, and Richard Payne

Pain Control: A Patient-Centered Health Care Outcome

Debates about health care are becoming more widespread and more urgent. Economic pressure to find a way to pay for the rising costs of care has driven much of this debate; however, in many nations, sociopolitical concerns have had equal or greater prominence. Many current proposals to reformulate governments' role in health care emphasize the need to improve "health outcomes," the actual results (some would say the purpose) of medical therapy.[1] Proposed outcomes to be assessed are explicitly "patient-centered" in that they extend beyond physiologic measures or physical symptoms to encompass patient satisfaction with care, social and functional well-being, and quality of life (Table 43-1).[2] Objective, statistically oriented studies of health outcomes promise "rigorous determination of what works in medical care and what does not . . . Outcomes research, by informing the content of policy positions, payment rules, and practice guidelines, presumably both solves the problems of quality and cost that beset the health care system and does so by scientific rather than political means."[3]

Health professionals concerned with pain control have been worldwide leaders in clinical and health services research to delineate those therapies that benefit the multiple dimensions of patients' quality of life (Table 43-2).[4] For example, the Cancer and Palliative Care Unit of the World Health Organization (WHO)[5] has stated that "Nothing would have more immediate effect on quality of life and relief from suffering, not only for the cancer patients but also for their families, than implementing the knowledge accumulated in the field of palliative care." The WHO[6] has also urged that resources begin to shift from biologically focused antitumor treatment to analgesia and palliative care relatively soon after diagnosis. Pioneering studies on the undertreatment of acute and cancer pain[7–13] motivated organizations such as the International Association for the Study of Pain, and national and international agencies including the WHO, the Canadian Council on Health Facilities Accreditation, and the U.S. Agency for Health Care Policy and Research (AHCPR), to prepare and distribute standards or guidelines for management of acute[14] or cancer-related pain (Table 43-3).[15]

This chapter complements other chapters in this volume by describing the context in which the AHCPR clinical practice guideline on management of cancer pain was drafted, and in particular by contrasting its genesis and approach with those of the earlier and enormously influential WHO method for cancer pain relief. To do so, this chapter outlines the key features of the WHO method for relief of cancer pain, describes "the guideline movement" that has given rise to the WHO, AHCPR, and many other documents, and presents the corresponding policy and treatment contexts for the AHCPR guidelines—the recommendations of which will also be described.

Table 43-1. Sample Outcomes and Intermediate Process Variables

Outcomes
    Death
    Able to work
    Functioning socially
    Experiencing somatic complaints
    Patient satisfied
    Consuming health care resources
    Cost
    Health perceptions
Intermediate process variables
    Taking medication
    Disease
    Graft survival
    Transplant rejection
    Myocardial infarction
    Stroke
    Exercising
    Dieting

Source: Adapted from WB Brose. Health outcomes. Clin J Pain 1994;10:89.

Table 43-2. Commonly Identified Dimensions of Quality of Life

Physical concerns (symptoms; pain)
Treatment satisfaction (including financial concerns)
Functional ability (activity)
Family well-being
Emotional well-being
Social functioning
Occupational functioning
Spirituality
Sexuality/intimacy (including body image)
Future orientation (planning; hope)

Source: Adapted from JJ Clinch, H Schipper. Quality of Life Assessment in Palliative Care. In D Doyle, GWC Hanks, N McDonald (eds), Oxford Textbook of Palliative Medicine. New York: Oxford University Press, 1993;63.

Cancer Pain Relief and Public Health: The World Health Organization Initiative

Cancer has a profound impact on public health throughout the world. American Cancer Society estimates show that there are 520,000 deaths due to cancer and 1,130,000 new cases diagnosed each year in the United States alone.[16] Without proper symptom control, severe pain will afflict most advanced cases.[11, 17, 18] For these reasons, in 1980, the WHO began a three-step effort to prevent cancers with known causes, to improve detection and cure rates of cancer, and to relieve cancer pain.[19] The third component began in 1981 with surveys in five countries (Brazil, India, Israel, Japan, and Sri Lanka), which confirmed widespread prevalence of inadequate cancer pain relief. In 1982, a working group consisting of the 1981 survey participants, as well as six experts on the treatment of pain, met in Milan, Italy to draft a guideline on which the "Method for Cancer Pain Relief," Annex 1 in the initial WHO document, ultimately was based.[20] Further field testing and consultation were carried out prior to the first edition of *Cancer Pain Relief* in 1986. Postrelease validation studies have documented the effectiveness of the WHO method for cancer pain relief. The WHO approach is a "low-tech" one in which pharmacotherapy is delivered:

- By mouth
- By the clock
- By the ladder (see Figure 6-1)
- For the individual
- With attention to detail

As described in Chapters 20, 30 and 35, this approach also allows for nonpharmacologic therapies such as palliative radiotherapy or neurosurgical procedures, but these are hardly emphasized. If clinicians follow this method, only about 10% of patients with terminal cancer will experience severe pain that is only controllable by invasive means; most will have minimal-to-moderate pain.[21–25] From a policy perspective, the WHO approach may be viewed as having five dimensions as well:

1. Very broad geographic, professional, and institutional targeting: worldwide, for different types of practitioners, both medical and nonmedical (e.g., nursing), in developed and undeveloped countries, and different types of settings (hospice, clinic, university hospital).

2. Scant details as to how the different roles of varied types of clinicians involved in multidisciplinary care can be best fitted together on a day-to-day level (e.g., social service or discharge planning in developed countries).

Table 43-3. Representative Guidelines on Pain Management

Year	Organization	Publication
1986	World Health Organization	*Cancer Pain Relief*
1986	American Cancer Society	*The Treatment of Pain in the Patient with Cancer*
1988	Australian National Health and Medical Research Council	*Management of Severe Pain*
1989	American Pain Society	*Principles of Analgesic Use in the Treatment of Acute Pain and Chronic Cancer Pain*
1989	American Cancer Society	*Pain Control in the Patient with Cancer*
1989	Canadian Council of Health Facilities Accreditation	*Palliative Care Program Standards*
1990	Oncology Nursing Society	*Position Paper on Cancer Pain*
1990	Wisconsin Cancer Pain Initiative	*Handbook of Cancer Pain Management*
1990	Royal College of Surgeons of England/College of Anaesthetists	*Report of the Working Party on Pain After Surgery*
1990	American Academy of Pediatrics	*Report of the Consensus Conference on the Management of Pain in Childhood Cancer*
1991	World Health Organization	*Cancer Pain Relief, 2nd ed*
1991	American Pain Society	*Quality Assurance Standards for Relief of Acute Pain and Cancer Pain*
1992	United States Agency for Health Care Policy and Research	*Acute Pain Management: Operative or Medical Procedures and Trauma*
1992	American Society of Clinical Oncology	*Cancer Pain Assessment and Treatment Curriculum Guidelines*
1992	International Association for the Study of Pain	*Management of Acute Pain: A Practical Guide*
1994	United States Agency for Health Care Policy and Research	*Management of Cancer Pain*

3. Little guidance as to how to ensure that this method for pain control is implemented within any particular socioeconomic framework (e.g., quality assurance or total quality management in developed countries); only general statements (e.g., "Governments should encourage health care workers to report to the appropriate authorities any instance in which oral opioids are not available for cancer patients who need them").

4. No documentation of the relationship between the scientific and clinical literature and the formulation of the recommendations, i.e., did the expert panel come to a consensus first, then cite references to support its view, or exhaustively review and synthesize the literature according to explicit search criteria, and on that basis develop recommendations?

5. A deliberate and appropriate focus on a small number of standard oral medications, and away from invasive (e.g., neurosurgical) or technologically based approaches to pain relief (e.g., in-

traspinal catheters), even though improving economic conditions in many regions (Eastern Europe, Latin America, and Asia) foster the increased use of these modalities in selected cases.

Far overshadowing the previously mentioned critique is the overwhelming strength of the document's simplicity of approach, its wise emphasis on therapeutic (oral or rectal) routes that are nearly universally available, and its well-documented success at relieving cancer-related pain in approximately 90% of patients treated according to its recommendations.

How might one go about attempting to retain the successful aspects of the WHO document, while also addressing the shortcomings? Because there are not yet outcome-oriented studies to assess the end result on patient care and satisfaction of implementing one or another system of guideline development and to assess the effect of disseminating or otherwise adopting the resultant products, these remarks must be heuristic and not based on specific data. First, it is perhaps too general a target to aim for worldwide implementation of a treatment plan, given the vast differences in economic, social, and governmental conditions worldwide. Even a single region, such as Europe, embodies different languages and diagnostic categories, systems of medical practice, professional and governmental organizations, and their associated regulations and economics. Hence, a guideline effort might best be targeted to one nation, until it becomes clear that it is feasible to merge such guidelines among nations. Second, within a narrower geographical or social context, day-to-day and longer term treatment goals could be defined explicitly (e.g., reduction of pain intensity by a certain percentage or worst pain intensity no higher than a certain limit). This definition allows these performance standards to be measured through institutional quality assurance and review procedures, in order to sustain their effectiveness independent from the variations of individual practice and motivation levels. Third, clear specification of individual or institutional responsibility for surveying and attaining explicit pain treatment outcomes must be part of the guideline. Fourth, extensive peer review and field testing should be accomplished prior to releasing the guidelines, rather than leaving it to self-motivated centers and interested individuals to perform validation studies in the postrelease phase. Fifth, an a priori decision should be made concerning the specific approach to synthesize scientific evidence relevant to the guideline, and clear procedures should be established for gathering and analyzing this information. Finally, careful country- and context-specific plans must be implemented to disseminate guidelines through educational, medical review, and other channels, coupled with monitoring to assess their impact on clinical practice.

United States Agency for Health Care Policy and Research Guidelines

Background

The previously mentioned concerns, as well as others relating to guideline development in general, were part of an ongoing debate that followed the passage of the U.S. Omnibus Budget Reconciliation

Act of 1989, in which clinical practice guideline development was mandated through the AHCPR. Practice guidelines have been defined by an expert committee convened by the Institute of Medicine (IOM) of the U.S. National Academy of Sciences as "systematically developed statements to assist practitioner and patient decisions about appropriate health care for specific clinical circumstances."[26] Findings and conclusions of the same expert group included the following statement concerning the state of the art of guideline development:

> The process of systemic development, implementation, and evaluation of practice guidelines based on rigorous clinical research and soundly generated professional consensus, although progressing, has deficiencies in method, scope, and substance. Conflicts in terminology and technique characterize the field; they are notable for the confusion they create and for what they reflect about differences in values, experiences, and interests among different parties. Public and private development activities are multiplying, but the means for coordinating these efforts to resolve inconsistencies, fill in gaps, track applications and results, and assess the soundness of particular guidelines are limited. Disproportionately more attention is paid to developing guidelines than to implementing or evaluating them. Moreover, efforts to develop guidelines are necessarily constrained by inadequacies in the quality and quantity of scientific evidence on the effectiveness of many services.[26]

As the IOM points out, guidelines for clinical practice have, for thousands of years, formed a cornerstone of organized medical education and certification. Egyptian papyri, the writings of Hippocrates, Avicenna, and Galen, and numerous other manuscripts would no doubt have been considered by their authors to be "systematically developed," even though they fall short of present-day standards for evidence and documentation of the process by which clinical recommendations are distilled from clinical evidence.[27] Medical texts are also, in essence, guidelines.

At present, given the insistence of health insurers, managers, regulators, and consumers in reviewing care on a prospective or concurrent basis, the process of guideline development is a rapidly maturing and increasingly rigorous discipline. Guideline development is now a field of medical social science populated by economists, sociologists, political scientists, and "methodologists." For many years, medical societies have been leaders in guideline development. In the United States, medical groups such as the American Academy of Family Physicians, the American College of Cardiology, the American College of Physicians, the American Pain Society, and the American Society of Anesthesiologists, health maintenance organizations such as the Harvard Community Health Plan, and consultative organizations such as the RAND Corporation have all helped develop practice guidelines, treatment algorithms, and practice parameters. Newer initiatives are underway through the activities of the American Board of Medical Specialties, the American Medical Association, and the Council of Medical Specialty Societies, among other academic and health services research entities.

Which clinical circumstances are guidelines warranted for? This question has been approached by a variety of professional, third-party, and regulatory groups. An aggregate overview table has been prepared by the Priority Setting Group, Council on Health Care Technology, of the IOM.[26] The primary and secondary criteria decided on by the Priority Setting Group itself are also presented in Table 43-4. As an illustration of the results of topic selection, the other six AHCPR clinical practice guideline topics initially chosen besides pain are listed here:

- Visual impairment due to cataracts in the eyes of aging patients
- Diagnosis and treatment of benign prostatic hyperplasia
- Diagnosis and treatment of depressed outpatients in primary care settings
- Delivery of comprehensive care in sickle cell disease
- Prediction, prevention, and early treatment of pressure sores in adults
- Urinary incontinence in the adult

A guideline is successful if it improves practice; the guideline's educational content is only one part of this larger process.[28] Other parts include guideline dissemination and adoption of guideline recommendations into the realm of quality assurance and other review procedures. To foster successful dissemination and adoption of guidelines, based on IOM recommendations, the AHCPR has set forth eight guideline attributes to be achieved.[26]

1. *Validity.* Practice guidelines are valid if, when followed, they lead to the health and cost outcomes projected for them, other things being equal. A prospective assessment of validity will consider the projected health outcomes and costs of alternative courses of action, the relationship between the evidence and recommendations, the substance and quality of the scientific and clinical evidence cited, and the means used to evaluate the evidence.

2. *Reliability and Reproducibility.* Practice guidelines are reliable and reproducible (1) if, given the same evidence and methods for guidelines development, another set of experts would produce essentially the same statements, and (2) if, given the same circumstances, the guidelines are interpreted and applied consistently by practitioners or other appropriate parties. A prospective assessment of reliability may consider the results of independent external reviews and pretests of the guidelines.

3. *Clinical Applicability.* Practice guidelines should be as inclusive of appropriately defined patient populations as scientific and clinical evidence and expert judgment permit, and they should explicitly state the populations to which statements apply.

4. *Clinical Flexibility.* Practice guidelines should identify the specifically known or generally expected exceptions to their recommendations.

5. *Clarity.* Practice guidelines should use unambiguous language, define terms precisely, and use logical, easy-to-follow modes of presentation.

6. *Multidisciplinary Process.* Practice guidelines should be developed by a process that includes participation by representatives of key affected groups. Participation may include serving on panels that develop guidelines, providing evidence and viewpoints to the panels, and reviewing draft guidelines.

7. *Scheduled Review.* Practice guidelines should include statements about when they should be reviewed to determine whether revisions are warranted, given new clinical evidence or changing professional consensus.

8. *Documentation.* The procedures followed in developing guidelines, the participants involved, the evidence used, the assumptions and the rationales accepted, and the analytic methods employed should be meticulously documented and described.

By 1989 when AHCPR was created, more than 1,000 guidelines, practice parameters, consensus documents, and other codified recommendations had already been introduced in the United States to deal

Table 43-4. Representative Criteria for Guideline Topic Selection

Source	Criteria Listed	Relation to Council on Health Care Technology Criteria	
		Primary	**Secondary**
IOM/HCFA	1. Burden of the illness 2. High prevalence of the illness in the Medicare population 3. High costs to the Medicare program 4. Substantial variation across geographic areas 5. High level of controversy regarding the alternative strategies for managing the condition 6. Availability of data to address the effectiveness questions	Individual patient outcome: explicit Patient population: explicit Cost: explicit Variations: explicit	Social/ethical: not included Medical knowledge: implied Policy impact: implied Assessment capacity: not included Feasibility: explicit
NCHSR/ POARP	1. Benefits and risks to the patient 2. Amount of unexplained variation in medical practice 3. Volumes of cases and treatments 4. Cost/charge per treatment 5. Sufficient data for analysis 6. Importance of the problem to the population	Individual patient outcome: explicit Patient population: explicit Cost: explicit Variations: explicit	Social/ethical: not included Medical knowledge: not included Policy impact: implied Assessment capacity: not included Feasibility: explicit
NIH/OMAR	1. Subject should have public health importance 2. Topic should affect a significant number of people 3. There should be a scientific controversy that would be clarified 4. Topic must have an adequately defined and available base of scientific information 5. The topic should be amenable to clarification on technical grounds 6. Health care cost impact 7. Preventive impact 8. Public interest 9. Timing of the conference should be such that it is likely to have a meaningful impact	Individual patient outcome: implied Patient population: explicit Cost: explicit Variations: not included	Social/ethical: not included Medical knowledge: explicit Policy impact: explicit Assessment capacity: not included Feasibility: explicit

IOM/HCFA = Institute of Medicine Committee on Health Care Financing Administration; NCHSR/POARP = Patient Outcome Assessment Research Program (National Center for Health Services Research); NIH/OMAR = National Institutes of Health, Office of Medical Applications Research.
Source: Adapted from MJ Field, KN Lohr (eds). Institute of Medicine, Committee to Advise the Public Health Service on Clinical Practice Guidelines. Clinical Practice Guidelines. Directions for a New Program. Washington, D.C.: National Academy Press, 1990.

with numerous issues of clinical practice, and the "guideline movement" as well as the process of guideline development were receiving increasing attention within health services and health policy research. Considering that the organized development of guidelines according to explicit and rigorous methods is a recent phenomenon, it is not surprising that prior guidelines (not all of which have been named such) have been prepared according to different methods, by different types of committees using different methods, and issued to meet distinct needs of varied constituencies. If one excludes textbooks on cancer pain or textbook chapters dealing with this topic, examples of existing quasi-guidelines relevant to cancer pain are presented in Table 43-3.

In order to meet the mandate by Congress that AHCPR work to improve the quality, appropriatenesss, and effectiveness of health care in the United States, and to improve access to health care services, AHCPR allocated significant resources to the development of clinical practice guidelines. AHCPR guidelines, developed by multidisciplinary panels of health professionals and consumers, are based on systematic review of relevant scientific evidence as well as professional judgment. The "pain panel" whose chairs were selected by AHCPR in May 1990, held its first meeting on July 11, 1990. The panel considered that the extremely broad and pervasive topic of pain would best be split into at least three guidelines dealing (1) with acute pain (which, in many respects, was the easiest to synthesize from a relatively straightforward literature), (2) with cancer pain, and (3) with various aspects of chronic pain. Accordingly, the first guideline released by AHCPR in March 1992, dealt with the management of acute pain from operative or medical procedures and trauma.[14] That guideline, which was heavily influenced by earlier work from the American Pain Society,[29] recommended routine assessment of pain as a "vital sign," offering analgesic therapies consistent with available resources and expertise in each setting, using timed or patient-controlled delivery schedules in place of "as needed" (often delayed and inadequate) dosing, using patient education and relaxation techniques, and titrating ongoing treatment according to the individual patient's needs rather than standard orders—principles that equally apply to the management of cancer pain. Since then, approximately a dozen more guidelines have been released and a similar number are presently being developed.

view of current needs, therapeutic practices and principles, and emerging technologies. This process included review of all pertinent guidelines and standards, receipt of information and opinions from external consultants, commissioned papers on ethical, legal, and economic aspects of cancer pain management, an open forum to receive input from concerned parties, and extensive discussion among panel members.

The second process was a comprehensive review of published research on assessment and management of pain associated with cancer, including procedure-induced and treatment-related pain. The review included research related to both pharmacologic and nonpharmacologic treatments, with particular attention given to the effects of interventions on pain intensity, complications, patient satisfaction, length of inpatient hospitalization, and treatment cost.

The third process was peer review of drafts of the *Guideline* and pilot review by intended users in clinical sites. Physicians, nurses, pharmacists, psychologists, and other experts in various aspects of pain management reviewed complete drafts or sections of the *Guideline,* using as a framework the attributes of clinical practice guidelines described by the IOM (see previous discussion). Drafts were reviewed by approximately 470 physicians, nurses, and others involved in pain management for accuracy, clarity, and relevance, and tested for clarity and usefulness at 15 clinical sites. Consumer versions were developed and tested in clinical sites with patients, nurses, and physicians.

The entire process was anchored by an interdisciplinary panel of experts who used an integrated approach to synthesize scientific evidence and current clinical practice. Versions of the *Guideline* include the full *Guideline* (approximately 250 pages), two *Quick Reference Guides for Clinicians* (one focused on adults and the other on children), and brief consumer guides for children and adult patients and their families published in English and Spanish versions.

The Process

The guideline on cancer pain management was released on March 5, 1994. Three processes were used to develop this and earlier *guidelines.* The first one was an extensive interdisciplinary clinical re-

Content

The *AHCPR Guideline on Cancer Pain* is designed to help any clinician who works with any oncology patient in any setting understand the assessment and treatment of pain and associated symptoms. It also discusses briefly the management of pain in patients with human immunodeficiency virus and the acquired immunodeficiency syndrome (AIDS), because many principles of pain assessment and treatment are common to both cancer and AIDS.

The *Guideline* calls for (1) a collaborative interdisciplinary approach to the patient with cancer pain, (2) an individualized pain control plan developed and agreed on by patients, their families, and practitioners, (3) ongoing assessment and reassessment of the patient's pain, (4) the use of both drug and nondrug therapies to prevent and control pain, and (5) explicit institutional policies on the management of cancer pain, with clear lines of responsibility for pain management and for monitoring the quality of pain management.

Pain Assessment

Patients with cancer often have multiple pain problems from various sources, but in up to 90% of patients, the pain can be controlled through relatively simple means. Nevertheless, undertreatment of cancer pain is common owing to widespread inadequacy of clinicians' knowledge about effective assessment and management, negative attitudes of patients and clinicians toward the use of drugs for pain relief, and a variety of problems related to the costs of and reimbursement for effective pain management.[30]

Assessment of pain in the cancer patient is imperative because failure to do so is recognized to be a critical factor leading to its undertreatment. Patients with cancer can experience transient or long-term pain related to its diagnosis or treatment, or from unrelated preexisting painful conditions. Because of the multiple possible etiologies for pain, each time a clinician assesses a patient with cancer, evaluation of pain is required.

The initial evaluation of pain should include a detailed history, a physical examination with particular emphasis on the neurologic examination, a psychosocial assessment, and, when appropriate, a diagnostic plan to determine the cause of new or increasing pain.

Subsequent assessments should evaluate the effectiveness of the management plan and, if pain is unrelieved, determine whether the cause is related to the progression of disease, a new cause of pain, or to the cancer treatment.

Health professionals should ask about pain regularly because recent studies have shown that patients are reluctant to volunteer pain complaints.[31] The patient's self-report should be the primary source of assessment because it is more accurate than others' observations. Neither behavior nor vital signs should be used in lieu of a self-report.[32] Assessment of the patient's pain and the efficacy of the treatment plan should be ongoing, and the pain report should be documented.

Some causes of pain in the patient with cancer are relatively easy to diagnose and treat, such as pathologic fractures of the femur. However, clinicians treating patients with cancer should also be able to recognize common cancer pain syndromes that may cause intractable pain and that may signal disease recurrence. Prompt recognition of these syndromes may facilitate better cancer therapy as well as minimize the morbidity associated with unrelieved pain. Common pain syndromes are bone metastases, epidural metastases and spinal cord compression, plexopathies, peripheral neuropathies, abdominal pain, and mucositis.

Pharmacologic Management

Of the many modalities available to manage cancer pain, drug therapy is the cornerstone because it is relatively low-risk, usually inexpensive, and as a rule works quickly. An essential principle in using medications in managing cancer pain is to individualize the regimen to the patient.[12, 29]

Three major classes of drugs are used alone or, more commonly, in combination to manage pain: (1) nonsteroidal anti-inflammatory drugs (NSAIDs) and acetaminophen, (2) opioid analgesics, and (3) adjuvant analgesics.

When choosing drugs to manage pain or related symptoms, the simplest dosage schedules and least invasive routes of administration should be used first. In the case of opioid analgesics, if pain relief is inadequate, the dose should be increased until pain relief is achieved or unacceptable side effects occur. In the case of NSAIDs and adjuvant analgesic drugs, which have ceiling effects to their analgesic efficacy, if the upper limit of the recommended dose is reached and pain relief is not achieved, then that particular drug should be discontinued and other drugs in that same class tried.

Most cancer pain can be managed by oral administration of drugs. However, difficulty in swallowing, gastrointestinal dysfunction that renders drug absorption unreliable, the need to use large quantities of tablets, and many other factors may require other routes of administration to be used. The simple, well-validated, and effective method for ensuring rational titration of therapy for cancer pain advocated by the WHO[20] (see previous discussion) has as its first step the use of aspirin, acetaminophen, or other NSAIDs for mild-to-moderate pain. Adjuvant drugs to enhance analgesic efficacy, treat concurrent symptoms that exacerbate pain, and provide independent analgesic activity for specific types of pain are used at any step. When pain persists or increases, an opioid such as codeine or hydrocodone should be added to the NSAIDs and adjuvant drugs (second step of the WHO analgesic ladder). At this step, opioids are often administered in fixed-dose combinations with acetaminophen or aspirin because this combination provides added analgesia. When higher doses of opioid are necessary, separate dosage forms of opioid and nonopioid analgesics should be used to avoid exceeding maximally recommended doses of the NSAIDs.

Treatment of persistent or moderate-to-severe pain should be based on increasing opioid potency or dosage. This is the third step of the analgesic ladder. Drugs such as codeine or hydrocodone are replaced with more potent opioids, usually morphine, hydromorphone, methadone, fentanyl, or levorphanol. Medications for persistent cancer-related pain should be administered on an around-the-clock basis, with additional "as needed" doses, since regularly scheduled dosing maintains a constant level of drug in the body and helps prevent recurrence of pain. Patients who have moderate-to-severe pain when first seen by the clinician should be started at the second or third step of the ladder.

Morphine is the most commonly used opioid for moderate-to-severe pain due to its availability in a wide variety of dosage forms, well-characterized pharmacokinetics and pharmacodynamics, and relatively low cost. For use in meeting baseline analgesic needs that are stable, controlled-release tablets of morphine are commercially available, as are transdermal fentanyl "patches." Meperidine may be useful for brief courses (e.g., a few days) to treat acute pain, but generally should be avoided in patients with cancer due to its short duration of action (2.5–3.5 hours) and toxic metabolite, normeperidine. This metabolite accumulates during continued use, particularly when renal function is impaired, and causes dysphoria, agitation, or seizures.[33]

Tolerance and physical dependence are common and predictable consequences of long-term opioid administration. These terms are often confused with psychological dependence (addiction), manifested as drug abuse behavior. Misunderstanding of these terms related to opioid use leads to ineffective practices in requesting, prescribing, administering, and dispensing opioids for cancer pain and contributes to the problem of undertreatment.

Tolerance is defined as the increase in dose amounts over time that are necessary to maintain pain relief. For most cancer patients, the first indication of tolerance is a decrease in duration of analgesia for a given dose. Increasing dose requirements often herald disease progression or recurrence; patients with stable disease do not usually require increasing doses.[12]

Opioid doses should be adjusted to achieve pain relief with an acceptable level of adverse effects for each patient. There is no ceiling or maximum recommended dose for full opioid agonists: Very large doses of morphine, e.g., several hundred milligrams every 4 hours, may be needed for some patients with severe pain.[14] Effective pain relief can be accomplished by anticipating pain, such as with increases in activity, and averting this through preemptive breakthrough dosing.

It is usually advisable to try, sequentially, more than one opioid before switching routes of administration or trying an anesthetic, neurosurgery, or some other invasive approach to relieve persistent pain.[34] For example, patients who experience dose-limiting sedation, nausea, or mental clouding on oral morphine may be well managed with an equianalgesic dose of hydromorphone or fentanyl.

The oral route is the preferred route of administration because it is the most convenient for patients and the most cost-effective. When patients cannot take medications orally, noninvasive routes such as rectal or transdermal should be tried. Parenteral routes should be used only when simpler, less demanding, and less costly methods are inappropriate or ineffective.

Patient-controlled analgesia is designed to allow patients to control the amount of analgesia they receive.[35] It can be accomplished orally or by using a programmable pump to deliver the drug intravenously, subcutaneously, or epidurally. Patient-administered bolus doses are required to treat breakthrough pain and to provide a basis for more accurate and rapid upward titration of the daily infusion dose.

While constipation and sedation are the most common side effects associated with opioids, other potential side effects include confusion, nausea and vomiting, respiratory depression, dry mouth, urinary retention, pruritus, myoclonus, altered cognitive function, dysphoria, euphoria, sleep disturbances, sexual dysfunction, physiologic dependence, tolerance, and inappropriate secretion of antidiuretic hormone. Due to great individual variation in the development of opioid-induced side effects, clinicians should monitor for these potential side effects and prophylactically treat some inevitable ones, such as constipation.

Adjuvant drugs are used to enhance the analgesic efficacy of opioids, to treat concurrent symptoms that exacerbate pain, and to provide independent analgesic activity for specific types of pain. They may be used in all stages of the analgesic ladder. The most commonly used agents include corticosteroids, anticonvulsants, antidepressants, neuroleptics, and hydroxyzine.

Nonpharmacologic Management

Physical and Psychosocial Modalities

Physical and psychosocial modalities can be applied by families and clinicians concurrently with drugs or by themselves (Figure 19-2). Physical modalities include cutaneous stimulation such as application of heat, cold, or electrical stimuli, exercise, immobilization, and acupuncture. The use of these modalities may reduce the need for drugs but they should not be used as substitutes. These modalities should be introduced early to treat generalized weakness and deconditioning as well as myofascial pain associated with periods of inactivity and immobility related to cancer diagnosis and therapy.

Psychosocial interventions are an important part of a multimodal approach to pain management and commonly are used in conjunction with analgesics. One goal of psychosocial intervention is to help the patient gain a sense of control over the pain. Cognitive techniques are designed to influence how one interprets events and bodily sensations. Giving patients information about pain and its management and helping them to think differently about their pain can increase their sense of control. When psychosocial interventions are successful in relieving pain, one should never conclude that the pain was not real.

Invasive Therapies

With rare exceptions, noninvasive analgesic approaches should precede invasive palliative approaches, such as anesthetic techniques, neurosurgery, and surgery. In an estimated 1–15% of patients, use of these invasive therapies is necessary.

More than one-third of the practice of radiation therapy is designed to relieve pain quickly and maintain symptom control for the duration of the patient's life.[36] Radiation therapy can be useful in relieving pain due to bone metastases, plexopathies, and in general, to any location of symptomatic primary or metastatic disease. The literature is divided regarding optimal radiation protocols to achieve tumor regression and disease palliation—at either primary or metastatic sites. A balance is required between the killing of tumor cells and the adverse radiation effects on normal tissues. To promote patient comfort and convenience, the desired dosage should be administered in the fewest fractions possible.

Intractable pain can be controlled transiently by applying a local anesthetic or for a longer period with the use of a neurolytic (destructive) agent for neural blockade. Benefits from nerve blocks for cancer pain may be seen in approximately 50–80% of patients.[37] Patient selection and timing of nerve division or destruction for pain relief are based on exhaustion of more conservative modalities, lack of availability of clinically superior options, and access to capable physician and support systems after the procedure.

Neurosurgical procedures for relief of pain are classified into three categories: neuroablation, implantation of drug infusion systems, and neuroaugmentation. The choice of a neurosurgical procedure is based on the location and type of pain (somatic, visceral, deafferentation), the general condition of the patient, the patient's life expectancy, and the expertise available.

With regard to surgical operations, pain control is usually a secondary goal when curative tumor excision is performed. In contrast, when surgery is palliative because the tumor is unresectable, pain control is frequently the operative indication. The oncologic surgeon should be familiar with the interactions of chemotherapy, radiation therapy, and surgical interventions so that iatrogenic complications may be avoided or anticipated (e.g., multiple fistulas resulting from bowel resection performed after radiation).

Table 43-5. Clinical Approach to Cancer Pain: A Mnemonic

A   Ask about pain regularly
    Assess pain systematically
B   Believe the patient and family in their reports of pain and what relieves it
C   Choose pain control options appropriate for the patient, family, and setting
D   Deliver interventions in a timely, logical, and coordinated fashion
E   Empower patients and their families
    Enable patients to control their course to the greatest extent possible

Continuity of Pain Management

Most cancer patients are treated for pain in outpatient and home care settings. Patients should be taught to report changes in their pain or any new pain so that appropriate reassessment and changes to the treatment plan can be initiated.

Patients and their families may have difficulty understanding and remembering the details of the plan for managing pain. Therefore, patients should be given a written pain management plan whenever possible. Discharge planners should advise patients and clinicians to communicate the pain management plan to other clinicians when the patient is being transferred from one health care facility to another, such as from an acute care facility to a hospice.

Other Aspects of Pain Management Included in the Guideline

In addition to more extensive discussion of the pharmacologic and nonpharmacologic interventions described previously, the Guideline focuses attention on several other areas, including procedure-related pain in adults and children. Pain in several special populations is addressed, including neonates, children, and adolescents, elderly patients, patients with psychiatric problems associated with cancer pain, substance abusers, minority populations, and patients with AIDS.

A final section of the Guideline recommends that formal means for evaluating pain management practices be developed and used within each institution. The Guideline suggests how such processes may be carried out in settings where patients with cancer receive care. In summary, the clinical approach recommended in the Guideline can be schematized by the flowchart presented in Figure 19-1 or the mnemonic "ABCDE" presented in Table 43-5.

The Guideline includes tables showing type, strength, and consistency of the evidence for the various interventions, sample pain assessment instruments for adults and children, drug dosage tables for NSAIDs and opioids, sample relaxation exercises, and sites where the guidelines were tested. Copies are available on request by calling 1-800-358-9295.

This discussion of the content and context of the AHCPR guideline for cancer pain management is presented with the goal of evoking discussion to refine planning for, management of, and adaptation of evolving versions of this uniquely influential document. As of early 1994, more than 2.5 million copies of AHCPR guidelines on acute and chronic pain had been distributed. As prophesied by the IOM, however, there have been hardly any studies on the impact of the guideline on cancer pain management. As co-chairs of the panel that labored to prepare this document, we acknowledge our bias in believing that our efforts will indeed have impact on pain management. Nonetheless, the sheer numbers of copies requested and distributed, the wide attention received in the lay press, and the impressions by clinicians that patients are asking more about options for pain relief cannot be dismissed. We believe strongly that the next step in the evolution of this guideline will be to assess its impact and shortcomings systematically, and to enlarge its scope to reflect changes in therapeutic options, so that when the second edition is issued it will have benefited from "quality improvement" as it was being modified from the first edition. Possibly, those around the world will have sufficient interest and optimism in its utility that translations for use in other countries will be prepared and disseminated. If this does occur, then the cost-effectiveness of the AHCPR guideline in improving the quality of life of patients suffering from cancer pain can be compared with the impact of the simpler and less expensive WHO guideline effort.[20, 38]

References

1. Miaskowski C, Nichols R, Brody R, Synold T. Assessment of patient satisfaction utilizing the American Pain Society's quality assurance standards on acute and cancer-related pain. J Pain Symptom Manage 1994;9:5.
2. Brose WB. Health outcomes. Clin J Pain 1994;10:89.
3. Tanenbaum SJ. What physicians know. N Engl J Med 1993;329:1268.
4. Calman KC, Hanks GWC. Clinical and Health Services Research in Palliative Care. In D Doyle, GWC Hanks, N Macdonald (eds), Oxford Textbook of Palliative Medicine. Oxford: Oxford University Press, 1993;73.
5. World Health Organization Cancer Control Program. Policies for cancer pain control. Geneva: WHO, 1992.
6. World Health Organization Cancer Control Program. How to set up national cancer control programmes. Geneva: WHO, 1992.
7. Marks RM, Sachar EJ. Undertreatment of medical inpatients with narcotic analgesics. Ann Intern Med 1973;78:173.
8. Sriwatanakul K, Kelvie W, Lasagna L, et al. Analysis of narcotic usage in the treatment of postoperative pain. JAMA 1983;250:926.
9. Donovan M, Dillon P, McGuire L. Incidence and characteristics of pain in a sample of medical-surgical inpatients. Pain 1987;30:69.
10. Melzack R, Ofeish JG, Mount BM. The Brompton mixture: Effects on pain in the cancer patient. Can Med Assoc J 1976;115:125.
11. Bonica JJ. Treatment of Cancer Pain: Current Status and Future Needs. In HL Fields, R Dubner, F Cervero (eds), Advances in Pain Research and Therapy (Vol. 9). Proceedings of the IV World Congress on Pain. New York: Raven Press, 1985;589.
12. Foley KM. The treatment of cancer pain. N Engl J Med 1985;313:84.
13. Saunders C. Terminal patient care. Geriatrics 1966;21:70.
14. Carr DB, Jacox AK, Chapman CR, et al. Acute Pain Management: Operative or Medical Procedures and Trauma. Clinical Practice Guideline. AHCPR Publication No. 92–0032. Rockville, MD: Agency for Health Care Policy and Research, Public Health Service, Department of Health and Human Services, February 1992.
15. Jacox A, Carr DB, Payne R, et al. Management of Cancer Pain. Clinical Practice Guideline No 9. AHCPR Publication No. 94–0592. Rockville, MD: Agency for Health Care Policy and Research, U.S. Department of Health and Human Services, March 1994.
16. American Cancer Society. Cancer Facts and Figures, 1992. Atlanta, GA: American Cancer Society, 1992;2.
17. Twycross RG. Clinical experience with diamorphine in advanced malignant disease. Int J Clin Pharmacol 1974;9:184.
18. Daut RL, Cleeland CS. The prevalence and severity of pain in cancer. Cancer 1982;50:1913.
19. Swerdlow M. The WHO concept of cancer pain relief. Schmerz Pain Douleur 1989;10:130.
20. World Health Organization. Cancer Pain Relief. Geneva: WHO, 1986.
21. Takeda F. Results of field-testing in Japan of the WHO draft interim guidelines on relief of cancer pain. Pain Clin 1986;1:83.
22. Ventafridda V, Tamburini M, Caraceni A, et al. A validation study of the WHO method for cancer pain relief. Cancer 1987;59:850.
23. Walker VA, Hoskin PJ, Hanks GW, White ID. Evaluation of WHO analgesic guidelines for cancer pain in a hospital-based palliative care unit. J Pain Symptom Manage 1988;3:145.
24. Schug SA, Zech D, Dörr U. Cancer pain management according to WHO analgesic guidelines. J Pain Symptom Manage 1990;5:27.
25. Grond S, Zech D, Schug SA, et al. Validation of World Health Organization guidelines for cancer pain relief during the last days and hours of life. J Pain Symptom Manage 1991;6:411.
26. Field MJ, Lohr KN (eds). Institute of Medicine, Committee to Advise the Public Health Service on Clinical Practice Guidelines. Clinical Practice Guidelines. Directions for a New Program. Washington, D.C.: National Academy Press, 1990.
27. Siraisi NG. Medieval & Early Renaissance Medicine. Chicago: University of Chicago Press, 1990.
28. Max MB. Improving outcomes of analgesic treatments: Is education enough? Ann Intern Med 1990;113:885.
29. Max MB, Donovan M, Portenoy RK, et al. American Pain Society Quality Assurance Standards for Relief of Acute Pain and Cancer Pain. In MR Bond, JE Charlton, CJ Woolf (eds), Proceedings of the VIth World Congress on Pain. New York: Elsevier, 1991;185.
30. Cleeland CS. Barriers to the management of cancer pain. Oncology 1987;1(Suppl. 2):19.
31. Von Roenn JH, Cleeland CS, Gonin R, et al. Physician attitudes and practice in cancer pain management: A survey from the Eastern Cooperative Oncology Group. Ann Intern Med 1993;119:121.
32. Grossman SA, Sheidler VR, Swedeen K, et al. Correlation of patient and caregiver ratings of cancer pain. J Pain Symptom Manage 1991;6:53.

33. Kaiko RF, Foley KM, Grabinski PY, et al. Central nervous system excitatory effects of meperidine in cancer patients. Ann Neurol 1983;13:180.

34. Galer BS, Coyle N, Pasternak GW, Portenoy RK. Individual variability in the response to different opioids: Report of five cases. Pain 1992;49:87.

35. Ferrante FM, Ostheimer GW, Covino BG. Patient Controlled Analgesia. Boston: Blackwell Scientific, 1990.

36. Arcangeli G, Micheli A, Arcangeli G, et al. The responsiveness of bone metastases to radiotherapy: The effect of site, histology and radiation dose on pain relief. Radiother Oncol 1989;14:95.

37. Patt RB. Cancer Pain. Philadelphia: Lippincott, 1993.

38. Carr DB. The WHO Concept of Cancer Pain Treatment: A Guideline Prototype and Its Context. In J Chrubasik, M Cousins, E Martin (eds), Advances in Pain Therapy (Vol. I). Berlin: Springer, 1992;8.

Chapter 44

The Changing Face of Cancer Pain

Hugh Raftery

It is not the fear of death, but the fear of pain and of dying alone and in pain, that haunts the mind of the patient with a diagnosis of cancer. It reflects badly on our profession that so many families have the experience of caring for a relative whose worst fears are realized, and whose pain is inadequately relieved. Despite the improvement in the cure rate of some malignant conditions, cancer continues to be one of the major causes of death, with more than five million deaths annually throughout the world. Without appropriate treatment, most of these patients will die in severe pain; but with proper care, most of them may be kept pain free until death. This requires the expertise of doctors, nurses, and other health care providers with special education and training in pain management.

The problem is as real today as it was in the early 1950s, but back then, there were very few doctors with the knowledge and commitment to offer comprehensive pain relief to their patients. The mode of action of pain-killing drugs was not well understood, and there was widespread fear of the problems of overdosage, tolerance, and addiction. The natural progression of cancer was predictable: from diagnosis to death in less than 1 year. Within that timeframe, the period of very severe pain was about 3 months.

My introduction to cancer pain relief (in the early 1950s) was to perform nerve-blocking procedures for pain relief. These were very effective most of the time, provided the patient did not live too long. When I reviewed my results, I found that although most of my patients died within 3 months of

nerve block therapy, some achieved satisfactory pain relief until death. However, a significant minority, who survived longer, developed pain syndromes that were much more difficult to treat, and for whom repeat nerve block was not helpful.

Since 1950, new and more effective techniques of radiotherapy and anticancer chemotherapy have been developed, as well as the combination of these treatments with surgery. Many patients survive to enjoy a normal life span, and many, for whom cure is not an option, survive for years with their cancer. This has led to a changed pattern in cancer pain and pain syndromes that was not seen in the 1950s.

These problems arise from a variety of causes, but are all related to the improved direct anticancer treatments. The patient may have an enhanced expectation of cure that is not realized. If a treatment has a success rate of 75%, it must be used; however, for the 25% failure group, the disappointment is devastating. These patients need skillful comprehensive help from their doctors to treat the pain and other symptoms that may follow from the treatment itself, notwithstanding its failure. The progress of their tumor may be slowed but not halted, and they may develop pain mechanisms related to nerve injury or destruction of weight-bearing structures.

Some very important contributions to the understanding and management of cancer pain were made by Dame Dr. Cecily Saunders of St. Christopher's Hospice in London.[1] Dr. Saunders brought a rational view to the role of morphine in cancer pain relief and also introduced the concept of "total pain." By this concept, she meant the sum of the distress caused by the tumor, pain, sense of impending death, and side effects of the drugs. There are some problems that are tolerable in the short-term, or in isolation, but in the overall context of cancer-related death, they are too much to bear.

The hair loss following chemotherapy may be acceptable to some patients but horrifying to others, so we must be sensitive to this. To patients with lung cancer, persistent smoking by their spouse, friends, or family is a cause of great distress and a constant reminder of their own condition. A simple request by the perceptive doctor may help much more than a sedative. Where there is a sexual relationship, cancer of the genital tract is bound to create tensions that may express themselves as pain, when actually they are really a cry for help of a different nature. Although learning of breast cancer is always traumatic for a woman, the disfigurement following surgery may be an even greater distress than the cancer diagnosis. These are a few examples of how factors, other than pain, may lead to distress, that is articulated by the patient as pain. The absence of specific pain mechanisms does not make the suffering less real, but it does mean that several alternative options in addition to narcotic analgesics should be explored.

Modern anticancer drugs are very powerful, and have various unpleasant side effects. In addition to hair loss, there may be pyrexia, itching, nausea, and vomiting. The hope of cure will support a patient through this, but there is an ethical imperative on doctors not to put their patients through this misery, if cure is not an option. Pope Pius XII stated an ethical guideline for us: "Thou shalt not kill; but need not strive officiously to keep alive."[2] We should keep this in mind as we stand back and assess the result of our treatment, and if we decide that the treatment is only to prolong suffering, then it is not justified. It is important to attempt to maintain satisfactory quality of life.

Many tumors do respond to palliative treatment, and extra months or even years of life may be achieved, but there may be a price to pay. A pain syndrome may develop that is much more difficult to treat. When a tumor presses on a nerve it causes a referred pain that is easily controlled by analgesics. As time passes and the tumor eventually causes nerve destruction, a different and more recalcitrant pain problem arises.[3] A deafferentation pattern may develop with symptoms of sympathetic overactiv-

ity and this, of course, is resistant to simple medication and will require more invasive therapeutic options including hospital care and direct intraspinal drug delivery. Widely disseminated metastatic bone tumors may develop from primary breast or prostatic cancer. Initially, these tumors are sensitive to radiotherapy, but eventually the loss of bone structure may give rise to severe pain associated with movement. Treatment of mobility pain poses particular problems, as adequate analgesia may lead to oversedation at rest. Neurodestructive procedures may help alleviate these conditions, even though many of these procedures are infrequently used.

Cancers of the lymphatic and hemopoietic systems have a much more optimistic prognosis than in the 1950s. The potential for cure from conditions such as leukemia or lymphoma is good, and this assurance will support the patient through the rigors and trials of treatment. Unfortunately, while many patients survive to enjoy a normal life span, others must be supported through a long and losing battle with their disease, and their pain problems may be greater because of the disappointment and despair following treatment failure. With the decision to confine treatment to palliative symptom (pain) control, it is best that a new team take over in whom the patient may have renewed confidence. Similar problems arise with failure of treatment for cancer of the uterus. The local recurrent tumor invades and destroys pelvic nerves, bones, and blood vessels, but does not affect any vital organs. Pain control and patient support will demand a high degree of skill, and are best delivered by a team, rather than by an individual.

The past 10 years have seen great developments in the care of patients dying of cancer. The World Health Organization guidelines[4] on the use of drugs and the identification of symptoms have brought the whole problem into focus. Most of the patients may be cared for at home by family and a team of specially trained nurses, using analgesics and other drugs, according to the philosophy of the right drug at the right dose at the right time. The nursing team must be trained to recognize the situations where a simple increase in approach is required. It is a paradox that the more sophisticated the oncology service, the more difficult the pain problems. The doctors who assume this work must understand how cancer kills and how cancer pain is caused. They must also understand how other treatments affect the natural history of tumors and how all this affects the individual patients and their families.

The communication of a diagnosis of cancer to a patient and family is never an easy task for a doctor, and there is no standard approach. A conspiracy of silence, where the family is informed and the patient is kept in ignorance, is no longer acceptable. Tact and sensitivity are essential, with due regard given to the patient's right to know and ability to cope. The conversation may take several visits before the patient fully understands his or her condition. Palliative cancer care and pain control were a neglected area in medicine, but in the light of modern understanding of cancer pain syndromes, the mode of action of analgesics, and the impact of pain on dying patients, it is now possible to offer comprehensive pain relief, which was not previsouly available. More educational programs of cancer pain management need to be organized to continue this positive trend.

The past 25 years have seen a lot of progress in oncology centers, pain clinics, and hospices. Despite this, the World Health Organization predicts that 12,000,000 people will die of cancer by the year 2000.[4] Because we now know how to care for these patients and how to relieve their pain and ease their other symptoms, I hope that the fear of a lonely, painful death will become a thing of the past.

References

1. Saunders CMS. The care of the dying patient and his family. Contact 1972;38(Suppl.):12.
2. Flatt B. Some stages of grief. Journal of Religion and Health 1987;26:143.
3. Payne R. Cancer pain, anatomy, physiology and pharmacology. Cancer 1989;63:2266.
4. Cancer Pain Relief and Palliative Care. Technical Report Series 804. Geneva: World Health Organization, 1990.

Chapter 45

Cancer Pain: A Japanese Perspective

Tsutom Oyama

This chapter introduces the state of cancer pain management in Japan based on the recent survey of 39,971 cancer patients hospitalized in large hospitals. The primary region of cancer was gastric (14.3%), followed by hepato-biliary-pancreatic (13.9%) and lung (11.7%). Pretreatment patients represented 11.3%, patients under radical treatment represented 63%, conservative therapy patients represented 13%, and the terminal patients represented 12.7%. Of these patients, 30.4% underwent pain therapy. Forty-four percent of the patients who underwent conservative cancer therapy had experienced pain, whereas 73.5% of terminal cancer patients complained of pain. As a whole, adequate pain relief was obtained in 46.9% of the patients and moderate relief was observed in 50.2% of the patients who had not experienced satisfactory relief of pain. No pain relief was seen in 2.9% of patients. Adequate pain relief was obtained in 38.4% of the terminal cancer patients and in 45.8% of the conservative cancer therapy patients (Table 45-1).

The possible factors that contribute to the difficulty of pain management in cancer patients include:

1. *Patients and families.* Hesitation to complain of pain to doctors; incorrect knowledge about pain; variable relationships in family; traditional value of tolerating pain
2. *Doctors and nurses.* Too busy to take care of pain; inadequate understanding of pain; lack of team work
3. *Hospital.* Inadequate number of hospices and special care wards

4. *Society.* Unwillingness to communicate the diagnosis of cancer to the patients; only about 54% of the doctors tell the truth; difficulty managing pain at home; inconvenient and rigid regulation of narcotic use in Japan

We tend to focus on narcotics as being the main method of pain management in cancer patients. Of course, no one doubts their role in pain management. However, they also have several side effects including nausea, vomiting, constipation, loss of appetite, physical and psychic dependency, drowsiness, itching, and many others. We must weigh the tradeoffs between pain management and the quality of life of the cancer patients.

What Is Kampo?

Traditional herbal medicine has been used for more than 3,000 years in China, while its use has been documented for more than 1,000 years in Japan, albeit with some changes to the original Chinese formulations. Recently, for many reasons, there has been a revival of interest in herbal medicines in Japan. One of these reasons is that the population of the elderly has increased. The population of people older than 65 years old was 7% in 1970, but it jumped to 14% in 1994, and is projected by the year 2040 to be approximately 28%. Therefore, due to the older population, Japan has seen an increase in the number of patients who suffer from chronic diseases including cancer, arteriosclerotic diseases, and

Table 45-1. Effect of Analgesics in Cancer Patients*

Analgesics	Application (%)	Adequate Analgesia (%)	Moderate	None
NSAIDs (PO, PR)				
Conservative	56.8	37.3	59.3	3.3
Terminal	41.1	24.5	69.2	6.3
NSAIDS (IM, IV)				
Conservative	29.0	45.8	51.6	2.5
Terminal	35.5	35.8	60.0	4.2
Morphine (PO, PR)				
Conservative	31.1	49.1	48.4	2.5
Terminal	36.7	43.6	52.5	4.0
Narcotics and anesthetics (injection)				
Conservative	5.7	54.2	42.7	3.1
Terminal	18.9	54.5	43.4	2.1

* Survey in Japan in 1990.
Conservative = patients under conservative therapy; Terminal = terminal cancer patients.
Source: Modified from K Hiraga, T Mizuguchi, F Takeda. The incidence of cancer pain and improvement of pain management in Japan. Postgrad Med 1991;67(Suppl. 2):S14.

autoimmune and allergic disorders. It has become evident from a steady increase in Kampo use by physicians and numerous clinical reports that traditional Oriental herbal medicines can help manage chronic pain. One main drawback of modern Western medicine is the frequency and severity of side effects related to treatment modalities.

Kampo medicines are extracts of several unrefined herbal drugs. They are always taken orally, never parenterally. In Japan, there are 131 Kampo drugs available and approved by the Government and the National Insurance Plan. Each Kampo compound has many ingredients, and the effect of Kampo is not necessarily attributable to just one component. The onset of the effect is slow compared with Western medicine. However, there are far fewer side effects compared with Western medicines. Kampo compounds typically influence the whole body and not any specific organ. Kampo medicines improve the metabolism, peripheral circulation, and endocrine and immunologic systems.

The Analgesic Effect of Processed Aconiti Tuber and Its Alkaloids

Aconiti tuber has been used for many years in Japan and China as an indispensable traditional Oriental medicine for analgesia and improvement in hypometabolism. Aconiti tuber termed *Shuchi-bushi-matsu* (TJ-3021) in Japanese, is produced by autoclaving the raw aconiti root to decrease its toxicity. The oral administration of TJ-3021 produces antinociception in rats and mice using several nociceptive tests.[1] Mesaconitine (MA), one of the main aconitine alkaloids contained in TJ-3021, has a potent analgesic effect (Figure 45-1; Table 45-2).

Intrathecal and intraperitoneal administration of selective alpha$_2$-adrenoreceptor antagonists—idazoxan and methylsergide—a serotonin receptor antagonist, reduced significantly the analgesic effect of TJ-3021 in repeated cold stress (RCS) rats. RCS is defined as repeated exposure to cold temperature over a few days and is a unique model for long-lasting hyperalgesia without any inflammation in the periphery. In RCS-induced hyperalgesia, TJ-3021 had clear analgesic activity.[1]

Intraperitoneal administration of the opioid-receptor antagonist, naloxone, provided the slight effect to analgesia that was produced by TJ-3021. Both oral and intracisternal administration of MA, which is one of the main potent aconitine alkaloids in TJ-3021, produced remarkable analgesic effect in non-RCS rats. These effects were significantly reduced by either intraperitoneal administration of idazoxan or methylsergide. These results suggest that

Table 45-2. Analgesic Activity and Acute Toxicity

	ED50* (SC mg/kg)	LD50 (SC mg/kg)	LD50/ED50
Aconitine	0.06	0.55	9.2
Mesaconitine	0.039	0.25	6.4
Jesaconitine	0.032	0.26	8.1
Morphine	0.38	531	1397

* By the acetic acid-induced writhing method.
ED50 = 50% effective dose; LD50 = 50% lethal dose.

the activation of descending inhibitory alpha$_2$-adrenergic and serotonergic systems, but not the opioid system, contribute to the antinociceptive mechanism of TJ-3021 and MA. The important contribution of the descending pain inhibitory system on the antinociceptive mechanism is well known (Figure 45-2). This pathway has important brain stem components that include periaqueductal gray, the nucleus reticularis paragigantocellularis, the nucleus raphe magnus, the rostral ventral medulla, and projections to the spinal dorsal horn. The analgesia produced by morphine has been a demonstration of the descending stimulation of opioid and monoaminergic systems, especially with noradrenergic and serotonergic systems, as well as inhibited effect on the ascending nociceptive mechanism.

We explored the possible role of the specific regions in the brain stem on the antinociceptive actions of MA by microinjecting it into nucleus reticularis paragigantocellularis, nucleus raphe magnus, and periaqueductal gray. Microinjection into these regions elicited dose-dependent antinociceptive action.[2] These results suggest that the analgesic effect of TJ-3021 would depend in part on MA, which acts at the brain stem, mediated by both alpha$_2$-adrenergic and serotonergic systems.

The analgesic effect of TJ-3021 depends partly on the actions of MA on the brain stem, mediated by both alpha$_2$-adrenergic and serotonergic systems, but probably not through opioid receptors.[3] Furthermore, we reported that the effects of TJ-3021 on the cerebral cortex appeared to be mini-

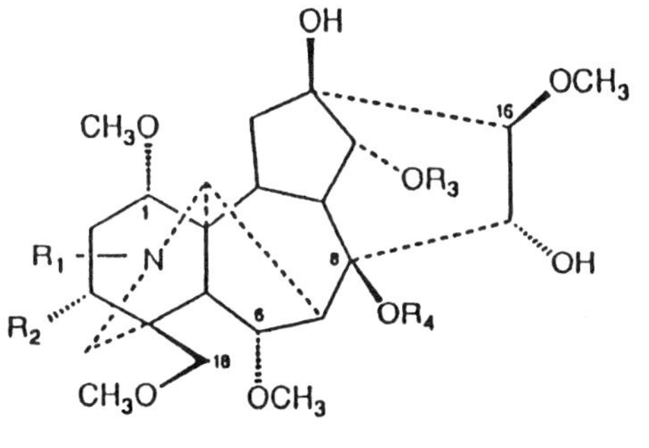

Figure 45-1. Chemical structures of Aconitum alkaloids. (Ac = COCH3; Bz = Benzoyl; As = Anisoylo.)

	R$_1$	R$_2$	R$_3$	R$_4$
aconitine	C$_2$H$_5$	OH	Bz	Ac
mesaconitine	CH$_3$	OH	Bz	Ac
hypaconitine	CH$_3$	H	Bz	Ac
jesaconitine	C$_2$H$_5$	OH	As	Ac
benzoylaconine	C$_2$H$_5$	OH	Bz	H
benzoylmesaconine	CH$_3$	OH	Bz	H
benzoylhypaconine	CH$_3$	H	Bz	H

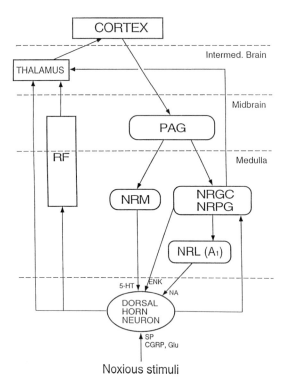

Figure 45-2. Hypothesis concerning the pain transmission and regulation in the spinal dorsal horn. (RF = reticular formation; PAG = periaqueductal gray; NRM = nucleus raphe magnus; NRGC = nucleus reticularis gigantocellularis; NRPG = nucleus reticularis paragigantocellularis; NRL = nucleus reticularis lateralis; 5-HT = serotonin; ENK = enkephalin; NA = noradrenaline; SP = substance P; CGRP = calcitonin gene-related peptide; Glu = glutamate.)

mal.[4] We suggest that the antinociceptive effects of TJ-3021 may be mediated by an action on the descending pain inhibitory system in the brain stem.[2]

The Possible Application of Kampo to Cancer Patients

Preliminary study in mice in our laboratory showed that the combined use of TJ-3021 and morphine for 2 weeks prolonged the antinociceptive effects of morphine and also reduced constipation and loss of appetite. Therefore, this combination could contribute not only to reduce the necessary dose of morphine but may also increase the quality of life for cancer patients.

Yamamoto et al.[5] reported on one of the Kampo medicines, Toki-shakuyakusan (TJ-23), tested on morphine-tolerant rats. Components of TJ-23 are paeoniae radix, atractyloids lanceae rhizoma, alismatis rhizoma, angelicae radix, hoelen, and cnidii rhizoma. This formula has been used for dymenorrhea, amenorrhea, and perimenstrual abdominal pain.

Yamamoto et al. found that TJ-23 potentiates morphine analgesia in morphine-tolerant rats and may therefore promote recovery from morphine tolerance. Although they observed that single and repeated doses of TJ-23 had no effect on morphine analgesia in development of tolerance to morphine analgesia in normal rats. On the other hand, the repeated doses of TJ-23 potentiated morphine analgesia dose dependently in morphine-tolerant rats.

References

1. Oyama T, Isono T, Suzuki Y, Hayakawa Y. Anti-nociceptive effects of Aconiti tuber and its alkaloids. Am J Chinese Med 1994;22:175.
2. Suzuki Y, Oyama T, Ishige A, et al. Antinociceptive mechanism of Aconitine alkaloids. Planta Med 1994;60:391.
3. Isono T, Oyama T, Suzuki Y, et al. The analgesic mechanism of processed Aconiti tuber (TJ-3021): The involvement in descending inhibitory system. Am J Chinese Med 1994;22:83.
4. Oyama T, Isono T, Suzuki Y, et al. The Analgesic Effect and Mechanism of Processed Aconiti Tuber and Its Alkaloid. In T Oyama, G Smith (eds), Pain and Kampo. Berlin: Springer-Verlag, 1994;16.
5. Yamamoto H, Kishioka S, Ozaki M, et al. TJ-23 (Toki-shakuyaku-san) potentiates the actions of morphine in morphine-tolerant rats. Report of an International Scientific Workshop, Bergen, Norway, May 31, 1991.

Chapter 46

Cancer Pain: A South African Perspective

Gordon Irving, C.W. Allwood, V. Levin, and E. Shipton

Cancer Treatment in Southern Africa

The Southern African region comprises 10 independent nations with a combined population of more than 100 million (Figure 46-1). Oncology services in most of these nations are rudimentary or nonexistent. South Africa has the most advanced treatment centers, with seven academic hospitals (Figure 46-2). In South Africa, which has a population of 42.9 million, there are about 70 specialized radiation therapists and medical oncologists and 200 therapy radiographers. There are approximately 40 megavoltage and 24 orthovoltage machines in use.[1, 2] The only other country in Southern Africa with functional radiation facilities is Zimbabwe, which has a population of 9.8 million. Cost is major stumbling block for effective oncology services in these countries. This limits the use of chemotherapy as well as effective pain medications. In fact, only two countries have per capita gross national products in excess of $2,000: South Africa ($2,200) and Botswana ($2,040) (1990 figures). Strife-torn Angola and Mozambique have gross national products of about $100.

There are no reliable statistics of the incidence of carcinoma in the Southern African countries. The only statistics are from South Africa where the Cancer Registry,[3] which is based on pathologically verified tumors, indicates an incidence of one case of cancer per 1,000 population per year. Adjustments for unreported cases, clinical diagnoses, and the youthful population suggest that about 25% of the total population of South Africa will develop some form of cancer. This is similar to First World statistics.

The prevalence of most types of cancer is unknown. In South Africa, however, cervical cancer has an age-specific incidence rate that is similar to the incidence of breast cancer (28.3 versus 27.6). Endometrial cancer has a relatively low incidence. Esophageal cancer is common in men and is equal in prevalence with head and neck, bronchial, and prostatic carcinoma. In other regions of Southern Africa, hepatocellular carcinoma (east coast) and Kaposi's sarcoma (central region) are common.

Southern Africa has a predominantly black population. The population is composed of many different tribes: the Tswana in Botswana; the Zulus and Xhosa in South Africa; Tonkas in Zambia; Mashona and Matabele in Zimbabwe; Swazis in Swaziland; Ovambos and Hereros in Namibia and Southern Angola; and Basotho in Lesotho. It is important that the health care giver recognizes and addresses the emotional aspects of each culture, with special reference given to tribal origin.

Those individuals who live near the major academic or larger regional hospitals may have access to First World medicine and, consequently, will receive pain management on a level comparable to that offered in North America or Western Europe. However, even in these urban centers, many tribes maintain their strong traditional beliefs and seek witch doctor or "Sangoma" treatment as first-line therapy.

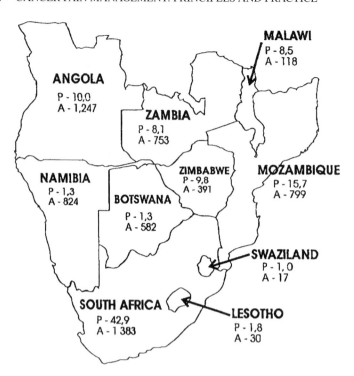

Figure 46-1. Countries that make up the Southern African group of nations. (P = population in millions; A = area in thousand square kilometers.)

Cultural Attitudes

It is important to recognize some generalizations about the attitudes of Southern African black patients toward pain and illness. African peoples in the south and east of South Africa have languages and traditions that are broadly related. The following description relates to the Nguni people of the eastern seaboard of South Africa and the vernacular used will be Zulu. Most of the concepts have close parallels in the other South African black tribes and have been modified but not eliminated by powerful forces including education, contact with other religions, relocation, urbanization, and contact with the Western medical system.[4]

The traditional African person lives within a theistic cosmology. The spiritual world is part of the present reality. Spiritual forces of good and evil have always been and continue to be present. The spirits of the forefathers, the Ancestral Spirits, are the recently deceased—usually three generations or less—who reside in or near the home and who are generally benign and protective. The family keeps in contact with the ancestral spirits through rites and rituals of varying regularity and importance, ac-

knowledging the presence and protection of the spirits through offerings of food and drink, and the sacrifices of different animals. If neglected or deliberately offended, the Ancestral Spirits may become angry and may then be punitive toward the family in general or toward individual members. This punishment may be inflicted in the form of bad luck, illness, or calamity. Usually, the influence of the Ancestral Spirits is limited to the family or members of the immediate clan.

A further possible cause of illness or ill fortune may be evil perpetrated by a witch ("witchcraft"). Being bewitched is a theory of causation: It does not deny natural or empirical causes but seeks supernatural reasons for them.[5] This may extend beyond the family to the clan or tribe, even to such things as national disasters. A witch is believed to carry out his or her art in secret, especially at night. This practice is, however, socially proscribed in almost all African tribes. Anyone discovered practicing witchcraft is punished, ostracized, or even killed. Spells are cast by people of evil intent. A witch may cause evil that is unbeknown to them, because the evil deeds may be done in unconscious states. Evil spells are usually cast on the victim in

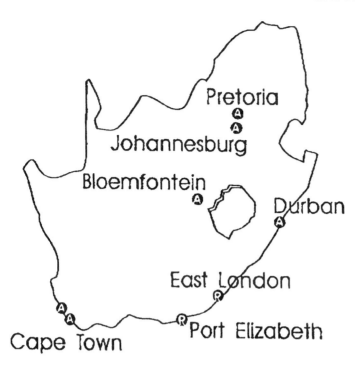

the form of something to be inhaled or ingested, stepped on or over, or may be introduced through sexual intercourse. Some spells may have their effect without any physical contact at all.

When illness or calamity befall a person it is a problem for the family and the next of kin, and possibly for the clan. Individuals rarely suffer alone. The sharing of good and bad, even beyond the family, is part of the concept of *ubuntu,* which means literally, but not very accurately, *personhood.* (To appreciate this concept, the following saying gives some indication of the depth of the underlying meaning: "Umuntu ungumuntu ngabantu"—a person is only a person through others.)

To the African patient, illness or calamity may have many explanations, including a Western medical explanation, that are all held together without apparent contradiction (so-called "syncretism"). Ultimately, however, the most important question to be answered by the person, family, or clan is, why has this person become ill at this time? This is a spiritual or cosmological question and the answer will be sought by the patient in conjunction with the family. The person to be consulted is the Sangoma or diviner healer.

The Sangoma is a venerated member of the community who has been especially called by his or her Ancestral Spirits to a vocation of divination and healing. The power to divine is given to the Sangoma by an Ancestral Spirit(s).

The patient who comes for Western medical treatment has probably already consulted a Sangoma. Many of these patients have scarifications from the Sangoma on their bodies at the site of pain. This is almost certain to be so if it has been a long illness. The Sangoma will tell the patient and the family why the illness has happened and who is responsible for the illness, and then what needs to be done. The treatment may include several different possibilities, ranging from the placatory sacrifice of a cow, goat, or sheep, to a prolonged stay with the Sangoma for repeated treatments, which may be both physical and ritual. The treatments are usually very costly and may have to be postponed until the family has raised the money. At sometime in this process, it is likely that the patient will probably have come, or been brought, for Western medical attention. It is usually only after delays of months or even years and because of intractable pain or obviously advancing disease.

However, Sangomas are not the only traditional healers. "Inyangas" are healers who have specialist knowledge of traditional healing methods, mainly of herbal and animal origin. Other compounds (e.g., potassium permanganate, or household disinfectants and detergents) may also be used.

The relationship among the patient, the family, traditional healing systems, and the medical profession is complex and extremely variable. There are an infinite number of possible permutations. Some traditional healers are knowledgeable about medicine and thus will refer patients early for medical treatment and will work closely with the medical profession. This scenario is probably more true of those healers that practice in the urban areas. Unfortunately, in rural areas, the opposite is often the norm and the patient may be trapped between two healing systems that conflict in their respective recommendations. This will frequently result in a lack of cooperation with Western medical treatment programs with noncompliance and eventual dropout.

Another factor that is very important to a black patient relates to the spirit returning home after death. The belief is that the body has to return home, and it must be buried in the ancestral burial place. The black patient will often want to be discharged to go home if he or she thinks that death is imminent. If one openly discusses these matters with the patient, it demonstrates an understanding of these important matters and will do much to gain the patient's trust.

For the medical profession to provide the best service for cancer pain management, it must take the belief system of the patient seriously. This not only is true of African patients but also of all patients. The ultimate outcome of any medical intervention will be decided on how well Western science can be merged with the attitudes and belief system of the patient. While the patient does not expect the doctor to subscribe to a belief system, the patient can demand that his or her world view be respected and taken seriously by the doctor. Ultimately, the patient will decide either by decision or default and may have the last say. Although the medical staff may find it difficult to understand the patient and his or her traditional and spiritual needs, the time and effort invested will usually greatly benefit the patient. Understanding brings reality into the therapeutic relationship.

Practical Management of Cancer Pain

Many rural Africans are reluctant to take oral medication on a regular basis. Follow-up is also often erratic, perhaps because of expense, transportation difficulties, long waits for treatment, or cultural beliefs. Because of these factors and the fact that many patients request injections for their pain, neurolytic blockade, where appropriate, often becomes the treatment of choice at an earlier stage than in more Westernized cultures.

Neurolytic Blockade

Ideally, neurolytic destructive procedures are best suited for patients whose fragility, debility, or short life expectancy make them unsuitable for neurosurgery. The major drawback of most of these procedures is limited duration of pain relief, which lasts from 2 weeks to several months (with an average of 2–4 months), after which sensation and pain often return.[6] In the author's (G.I.) experience, repeat neurolytic blockade may not be as effective.

Agents Used

Neurolytic agents include alcohol, phenol, and chlorocresol. With alcohol, a concentration of 95% reliably lyses sympathetic, sensory, and motor components.[7] Phenol has an initial local anesthetic effect that decreases after 24 hours to reveal its neurolytic effect. It has been reportedly shown to spare motor function at a concentration of 3%. This makes it useful for neurolysis of structures such as the stellate ganglion. For intrathecal neurolysis, all the previously mentioned neurolytic agents can be used, with each having its own particular indication.

Patient Selection

Patients should have localized pain. Ideally, diagnostic blocks with local anesthetics should always precede the use of neurolytic agents by a few days in order to assess effects. In Southern Africa, however, whereas local anesthetic blocks may be used to assess the potential effect, it is usually followed immediately by the neurolytic agent. This is to optimize the use of the medical personnel and to ensure the patient gets the appropriate treatment without having to wait for long periods or risking the patient not returning for follow-up.

Complications

Neurolytic blocks that use chemical agents unfortunately have an inability to precisely control the spread of destructive agents. Postinjection neuritis of a peripheral nerve may occur. In the lumbar intrathecal space, neurolytics should be deposited as peripherally as possible to avoid spillover onto the sacral roots destined for the bladder or rectum. Loss of motor function or inability to control bowel or bladder function will greatly impair quality of life. However, in many cancer pain patients who require intrathecal neurolysis, bladder and bowel function are often already compromised.

Cryoanalgesia

The clinical application of cold to produce analgesia was introduced in 1976. The term *cryoanalgesia* describes the destruction of peripheral nerves by extreme cold in order to relieve pain that required somatic blockade.[8]

The advantages of this technique are its simplicity, relatively low cost, and the reversibility of the lesion. It also has apparently few side effects. Less fibrous tissue may be produced than with other forms of peripheral nerve destruction. Unsubstantiated claims have been made that the incidence of postlesion neuritis is less with cryoanalgesia than with neurolytic agents.

The cost of the cryotherapy equipment and the need to renew the gases (either nitrous oxide or carbon dioxide) that are used to generate a temperature drop at the end of a probe may prove to be unaffordable in many poorly funded hospitals. The duration of pain relief depends on the completeness of nerve destruction. The median duration of pain relief varies from about 2 days to about 6 months, but usually with a minimum of about 3 weeks.

Radiofrequency Neural Ablation

Radiofrequency current can be used to produce neurolytic heat lesions in the peripheral or central nervous systems. The indications for use in the periphery are similar to those for cryotherapy. Central lesioning or cordotomies usually require the expertise of a neurosurgeon, of whom there are few in the Southern African countries. Again, cost is a major factor that limits its more widespread use. Radiofrequencies lesioning, however, produces pain relief that is likely to be longer lasting than other neurolytic procedures.

Conclusion

The treatment of cancer in patients of differing cultures should integrate not only the patient's viewpoint, but also the viewpoint of the therapist. A detailed inquiry into the patient's past, which is not seen by the patient to be pertinent, should be avoided. Ideally, the language used by the therapist should include concepts, myths, and ideas that are congruent to those of the patient. The content of dreams may be inquired into and can be used to increase a patient's morale. Traditional healers such as Sangomas and Inyangas have to be recognized as playing an important role in the well-being of certain population groups and should be incorporated, where possible, into the treatment plan. The fact that death itself has different connotations in different populations must also be respected. Even though the patient may wish to do something contrary to Western medical philosophies, the physician must respect the patient's right to do so. As in other parts of the world, education is fundamental in all aspects of oncology care. Cigarette consumption is rapidly increasing in the poorer populations, which will undoubtedly increase the number of cancer victims in years to come. Populations are becoming more urbanized, and pollution, unsanitary living conditions, and malnutrition are commonplace. Over the last decade there has been a marked increase in the number of cases of tuberculosis, sexually transmitted diseases, and human immunodeficiency virus in Southern Africa. All of these factors provide an immunologic assault that will increase the number of new neoplasms. The challenge is to educate and to provide better living conditions, as well as to offer better health care. Doctors and medical students need to be taught practical ways of treating cancer that may be different from their European or westernized counterparts. Traditional healers need to be taught to both recognize and to teach patients to recognize cancer early, so that a timely referral to a treatment center can be made. The epidemic of human immunodeficiency virus has already encouraged practical, innovative ways of providing effective education to the underdeveloped rural areas in Southern Africa. These have included the use of radio, traveling movie theaters, and traveling puppet shows. Some of these educational methods may be appropriate for other medical issues such as cancer recognition, prevention, and the control of pain in cancer patients.

Efforts are currently underway in South Africa to integrate cancer prevention, early diagnosis, treatment, and palliative care into more accessible regional hospitals. This was in part stimulated by a National Cancer Control Program Congress held in 1993. The leaders of all communities are being encouraged to work together to create practical solutions for the management of cancer pain in rural societies where there are few medical facilities. The models being developed in South Africa should have relevance to neighboring countries in the Southern African continent.

References

1. Levin CV, Sitas F, Odes RA. Radiation therapy services in South Africa. S Afr Med J (in press).
2. Durosinmietti FA, Nofal M, Mahfouz MM. Radiotherapy in Africa: Current needs and prospects. IAEA Bulletin 1991;4:24.
3. Sitas F. Incidence of Histologically Diagnosed Cancer in South Africa in 1988. Johannesburg: South African Institute of Medical Research, 1992.
4. Wessels WH. Understanding culture-specific syndromes in South Africa: The Western dilemma. Modern Medicine 1985;10:51.
5. Neki JS, Joinet B, Ndosi N, et al. Witchcraft and psychotherapy. Br J Psychiatry 1986;149:145.
6. Charlton JE. Common pain syndromes and their management. Can J Anaesth 1989;36:S9.
7. Budd K. The Pain Clinic: Chronic Pain. In JF Nunn, JE Utting, BR Brown (eds), General Anaesthesia (5th ed). London: Butterworth, 1989;1349.
8. Lloyd JW, Barnard JDW, Glynn CJ. Cryoanalgesia: A new approach to pain relief. Lancet 1976;2:932.

Chapter 47

Cancer Pain: An Indian Perspective

Dipankar Das Gupta, M.V.L. Kothari, and Lopa A. Mehta

Pain is a more terrible lord of mankind than even Death Himself. The fellowship of those who bear the Mark of Pain. Who are the members of this Fellowship? Those who have learnt by experience what physical pain and bodily anguish mean, belong together all the world over; they are united by a secret bond.

Albert Schweitzer[1]

All of the literature regarding *pain* and *cancer* seems to weld the two into a synonymy, whereby *pain in cancer* has acquired a clinical status of its own. It is little wonder that a *pain clinic* has come to form an integral part of any modern cancer hospital.

The Tata Memorial Hospital, regarded as the pioneer cancer hospital and cancer research center in India, was established in 1941. It is fully equipped for comprehensive cancer care. Under the aegis of the department of anesthesiology, it runs a regular pain clinic, that offers both outdoor and indoor service. The Tata Memorial Hospital Registry joined the National Cancer Registry Programme network in 1984. From 1984–1991, 179,330 new patients from all over India and the neighboring countries were seen at the Tata Hospital. Of these, 109,356 cases (56% male and 44% female patients) were diagnosed with cancer. In 1984, 10,615 new cancer cases were diagnosed; in 1991 the figure rose to 15,719, showing an increase of more than 48%. Of these, 30,674 (28%) were head and neck cancer, 15,385 (14%) gastrointestinal tract cancer, 13,750 (12.6%) cervical and uterine cancer, 10,875 (9.9%) breast cancer, 11,682 (10.7%) lymphomas and leukemias, and 4,814 (4.4%) lung cancer.

The patients attending the pain clinic are mainly those having head and neck cancer, gastrointestinal tract, bones and soft tissue in the men and breast and uterine malignancies in the women.

The clinical overview of cancer, as described at the Tata Memorial Hospital, is representative of the approach to cancer seen in India, except in regard to the pain clinic. The need for a pain clinic as an integral part of cancer management has yet to be widely recognized. This chapter presents a wider, Indian perspective on pain in cancer, both in retrospect and in prospect, as an attempt to give cancer dolorology a status of its own in India and in other Third World countries.

Ancient Indian History of Pain in Cancer

The description of cancer, in Indian Vedic texts, is traceable to pre-Buddha times, nearly 4,000 years ago. The vedic equivalent of cancer was *arbuda,* which means a swelling or tumor. A benign arbuda was classified as *saumya* (gentle) and the malignant one as *ghatak* (fatal). The clinical description of saumya versus ghatak arbuda compares well with the modern description of benign versus malignant tumor. A tissue-wise classification of arbuda was made with the nomenclature having modern ring-tissue type suffixed by arbuda. Hence, for example asthyarbuda, medaburda, and dentarbuda, respectively, meant bone tumor, marrow tumor (myeloma), and dental tumor.

The allusion to cancer pain, in the Vedic texts, is scarce. The chief reason for this omission resides probably in the continual forbidding of any treatment of ghatak or malignant tumors. There is a categoric declaration that states that treating the malignant tumors creates more trouble than the disease itself.

Pain in Cancer from an Indian Perspective

Genesis and Incidence of Pain in Cancer

"Pain is a protective mechanism for the body; it occurs whenever any tissues are being damaged, and it causes the individual to react to remove the pain stimulus."[2] "Pain," declared Paul Brand, the missionary reconstructive surgeon for leprosy patients at Christian Medical Center, Vellore, South India, "is our license to survive." The foregoing generalizations, the first by an eminent physiologist and the second by a surgeon of rich experience, give to pain some credit, some purpose long overdue. Pain, prior to cancer diagnosis, guides the patient to seek a clinician, and the clinician to assess the cancer. Pain, following treatment, declares the inevitably iatrogenic nature of pain in cancer—a realization that teaches rational restraint in cancer therapy and compassionate persistence and innovation in the alleviation of pain.

An autochthonous cancer's dogged refusal to cytobiologically and immunologically differ from other tissues renders radical surgery mutilative, and radiotherapy or chemotherapy cytotoxic, vasculotoxic, neurotoxic, and myelotoxic. All such necessary side effects of cancer therapy should alert oncologists all over India to the need for an up-to-date pain clinic wherever cancer is being treated by modern methods.

We do not know for certain the exact figures regarding the incidence in India of the presence of pain associated with cancer. But a statement on this from a leading American oncology text is revealing:

Although large-scale national epidemiologic studies on the incidence and severity of cancer pain are lacking, existing studies suggest that moderate to severe pain is experienced by one-third of cancer patients receiving active therapy and by 60% of patients with advanced cancer. These data have been generated from several surveys of small groups of patients in specific medical care settings. The dates are very consistent in cross-cultural studies. Data from India, Thailand, Vietnam and the Philippines report a similar prevalence of pain in cancer in patients in active therapy and advanced disease.[3]

Psychopathology of Pain in Cancer

A toast to Allah? Yes, I shall propose it: For giving pain, but not the knowledge why!

Goethe[4]

Pain is comprehended only through theories that unfortunately change with changing neurophysiology. So, instead of beating round the theoretical bush, we shall adhere to the "pattern theory" of pain, quite relevant from the Indian context.

The pattern theory proposes that most pain perception depends on stimulus intensity, with central summation as the critical determinant. Some investigators have suggested that central summation mechanisms are more important than excessive peripheral stimulation in determining the occurrence and severity of pain. Regardless, it is important that the patient and the pain therapist attend to both the peripheral site of injury, and the central side of the patient's psyche. Another name for central summation is affective dimension.

Foley reported that "Several studies that have focused on both patient and physician attitudes toward cancer pain suggest that cancer pain is perceived as the most feared consequence of cancer. Sixty-nine percent of patients interviewed reported that they would consider suicide if their cancer pain became intolerable."[3] The media-marketed cancerophobia perpetuated by modern society helps promote a central summative mechanism that is prepared to send more facilitatory impulses than inhibitory impulses toward the final experience of pain.

Why has it not been emphasized to the cancerophobic lay that the cliché-worn "seven danger signals" that herald a cancer do not have pain as a party to them? In fact, only 15% of the patients with nonmetastatic cancer present with pain. Pain and cancer need to be treated as separate entities.

The Eastern, particularly the Indian psyche, tends to view the occurrence of cancer and the subsequent suffering as a consequence of faulty actions or *Karma* in the past and hence a phenomenon to be borne stoically, willingly, even smilingly. Such a lofty approach is not exercisable by an average Indian patient, yet paying attention to the patient's psychological fortitude can help minimize not only the medication and procedures needed but also the pain itself. Any kind of pain is relieved by pleasurable distraction, joyful environment, a mood of relaxation, or words of cheer. If a cancer therapist is himself not afraid of cancer, he will be able to change the affective state of the patient into a therapeutic gain.

Philosophy of Pain Management

Not only degrees of pain,
But its existence, in any
degree, must be taken upon
the testimony of the patient.

Peter Mere Latham[5]

The utter subjectivity of pain, the total abstractness of any affective state joyful or sorrowful, and the hopeless immeasurability of any human emotion render it imperative that dolorologists believe and trust the patient in pain. The patient actually experiences the pain and the pain reliever presumably knows about the patient's pain. This is an epistemologic equation that places the patient superior to the physician vis-à-vis the reality of pain. Thus, one could aphorize: Pain can be imagined more easily than expressed and, pain exists more truly than imagined.

A set of unwritten rules have been globally arrived at to guide a dolorologist to adopt a modus operandi while attempting to relieve a cancer patient's pain:

1. Trust the patient's complaint.
2. Elicit carefully the relevant history.
3. Evaluate the patient psychologically.
4. Do a thorough medical and neurologic examination.
5. Ask for and scrutinize appropriate investigations.
6. Strive to provide total, immediate, protracted relief from pain.
7. Periodically reassess the patient's response to therapy.

8. Treat the patient as an individual and not as part of some protocol.
9. Brief the patient and family on future eventualities and the remedial measures to be taken thereof.
10. Be constructively compassionate. A judicious combination of philosophy and religion are the best adjuvants to measures to relieve pain. It pays to accept Buddhism's refrain that all existence is painful. The acceptance of pain as an integral part of being, growing, and dying greatly assuages the pain itself and the hurt feelings of being a victim of inscrutable fate.
11. Pain in cancer is the presenting facade of a curious personal and sociocultural mix of physiopathology, psychopathology, aversion, fear, "why me?" syndrome, and existential ennui. The verbal and nonverbal communication of the dolorologist can help elevate and fortify the morale of the patient. In the remote parts of the country, patients have to take recourse to naturopathy, biopathy, homeopathy, home remedies, wheat-grass therapy, hydrotherapy electroenergizers (ultrasound in place of acupuncture needles), acupuncture, acupressure, reflexology (acupressure sandals), magnetotherapy, autourine therapy, osteopathy, and Vipasana. The most well-placed and well-cared cancer patient in a metropolis may have to take recourse to one or more of the previously mentioned options, when the best of allopathy fails to provide pain relief. This real-life fact is well portrayed by Gunther in *Death Be Not Proud*, the valiant struggle of the family against a son's brain tumor.[6]
12. The pain therapist must constantly keep in mind the palliative nature of cancer therapy as also pain therapy. He or she should always be fully aware of the adverse effects of both of these.
13. Treatment of pain in cancer in a Third World nation such as India may be neither easy nor rewarding. An ever expanding population coupled with poverty of resources make the appropriate therapy unavailable to many cancer patients.
14. Remember what Dr. Vaidya,[7] a general practitioner of Bandra, Bombay said: "All pathies are good when mixed with enough sympathy."

Of the directives outlined previously, the top priority has been assigned, worldwide, to the need to believe the complaint of pain from the cancer patient. The Consensus Development Conference of the National Institutes of Health held in 1986 issued a report appropriately titled "The Integrated Approach to the Management of Pain."[8] The thrust was twofold: (1) to raise the pain awareness among practicing physicians, and (2) to offer an integrated approach to the art and science of pain relief.

This report discussed and detailed three types of pain:

1. Acute pain associated with surgery, radiation, chemotherapy, tumor invasion, pathologic fracture, and so on
2. Chronic pain of malignant origin
3. Chronic pain of nonmalignant origin, i.e., pain arising from ischemia, deafferentation, fibrosis, etc.

Pain Management

Pain management is a subject that is best summarized in the form of four paradigms that help take care of the soma, psyche, and spirit of a cancer patient nursing an unbearable pain. Figures 47-1, 47-2, and 47-3 are paradigms for cancer pain management.

Both central and peripheral mechanisms related to pain are too complex, nebulous, and multiple to be detailed here. It is enough to say that therapy modulates them to make the cancer patient feel better through pain relief.[9]

General Measures

1. Much of pain relief is empirical.
2. All measures have their side effects.
3. As disease mounts, one is forced to be painfully aggressive against cancer pain.
4. The step-up begins with common, simple, harmless measures to uncommon, complex, noxious measures—from medicative to modulative to mutilative.
5. Pain relief is not the end, but a means to a better quality of life.[10]

Specific Measures

Oral Medication

The three-step ladder approach recommended by the World Health Organization is simple, easy, and inexpensive to implement.

1. Nonopioids and adjuvants
2. Weak opioids, nonopioids, and adjuvants
3. Strong opioids and adjuvants

Although there is no reason why the three-step ladder approach cannot be applied globally, the limiting factor is that simple drugs such as oral morphine are not freely available in many developing countries.[11] This obstacle needs to be overcome through pressure applied on governmental agencies. The responsibility for bringing about this change lies with physicians. In the United Kingdom, the Royal College of Physicians has recently recognized palliative medicine as a new subspecialty of general internal medicine; however, in developing countries, where most of the future deaths from cancer are likely to occur, there is little progress in this direction.

Reversible Neurolysis

Reversible neurolysis is the most common procedure to achieve pain relief.[12] Its forte resides in its ability to provide dramatic immediate relief and the certainty of restricting the neurolysis to a well-defined area. The following modes of reversible neurolysis are practiced at the Tata Pain Clinic.

Regional Analgesia Using Local Anesthetics. These include three types of blocks: (1) diagnostic, (2) prognostic, and (3) therapeutic. *Diagnostic blocks* help determine specific nociceptive pathways, define the mechanism of pain, and define the differential diagnosis of the nociceptive input.[13] *Prognostic blocks* help predict the efficacy of analgesics and also the side effects of neurolytic block or neurosurgical procedures. They can let the doctor and the patient know what to contend with just in case irreversible neurolysis is necessary. *Therapeutic blocks* with local anesthetics provide quick relief from excruciating cancer pain for short or long peri-

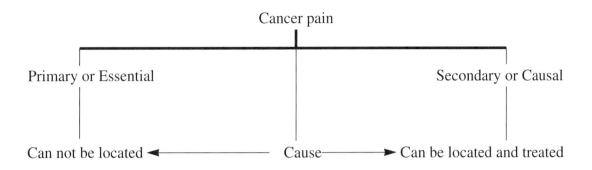

Figure 47-1. Paradigm 1 for cancer pain management. Always carefully determine and eliminate causal cancer pain before starting a pain relief program.

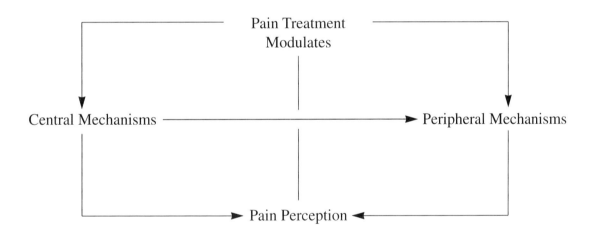

Figure 47-2. Paradigm 2 for cancer pain management.

ods.[14] They provide long-term relief by blocking the sensory input that bombards the spinal transmission cells, thus interrupting the vicious self-sustaining cycle of neuronal loops that are responsible for chronic pain.[15] They also allow patients to return to normal motor activity, which in turn closes the gate mechanism and prevents recurrence of pain.

Intraspinal Narcotics. Epidural or subarachnoid injection of small quantities of opiates can provide sustained pain relief without blocking other sensory inputs. These can be given as a single-shot or repeatedly through a catheter retained in place. Side effects include nausea, vomiting, pruritis, urinary retention, and tolerance.

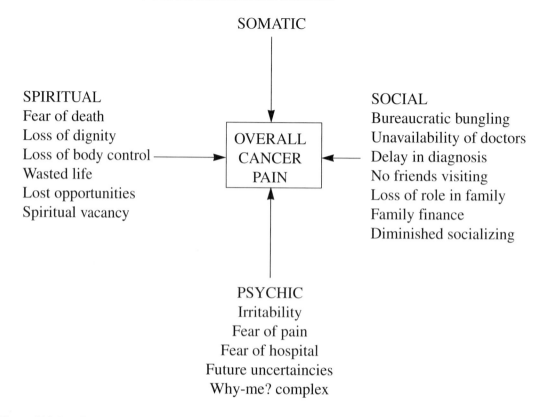

Figure 47-3. Paradigm 3 shows the components of pain in cancer management.

Regional Analgesia Using Neurolytic Agents.
Epidural or subarachnoid injection of hypertonic saline, alcohol, or phenol gives sustained relief for weeks and months. As described by Hitchcock,[16] a large volume (15 ml) of chilled (5–7°C) hypertonic (5.0–7.5%) saline under light general anesthesia produces reversible chemical rhizotomy without attendant motor loss. The site of injection is selected from cisterna magna (in patients with head and neck cancer) to lumbar levels, depending on the primary location of cancer.

Neurolysis of trigeminal ganglion or sensory root by alcohol or phenol effectively relieves pain in cancer in patients with head and neck cancer.

Celiac plexus block using alcohol or phenol is effective for patients with advanced gastrointestinal malignancy.[17]

Neuroadenolysis of the pituitary gland can be effected by a transsphenoidal intrapituitary needle delivering absolute alcohol. The relief from severe, diffuse cancer pain is noticeable in more than 50% of patients.

Trigger Point Injections. A short-term, empirical measure is to inject small quantities of a local anesthetic and steroid in trigger spots. Trigger spots acquired their name because of the fact that localized pressure on them triggers pain over a wide musculoskeletal area.[18] Its chief value lies in its ease, inexpensiveness, and ubiquitousness of application. Even if it is mainly a placebo, it comes in handy when the patient is losing hope and wants something to be done urgently.

Physical Measures

These methods give a holistic appearance to the pain clinic and prove useful in being the least harmful to the patient. These measures are believed to increase blood flow to part of the body, thereby promoting removal of pain-producing substances and repair of damaged tissues. They also provide sensory inputs that inhibit pain signals by closing the gate. The physical measures are listed here:

1. Massage or manipulation
2. Traction or compression
3. Physiotherapeutic exercise
4. Short-wave diathermy, infra-red lamp, sonic waves
5. Ice massage or ice packs

Psychological Methods

With these methods, the patient's soma is paid less attention to, but the psyche is relaxed and restructured, through several psychological techniques such as operant conditioning, biofeedback, muscle relaxation, hypnosis, willed ignorance of pain, and determined attention to the positive aspects of being and becoming, e.g., an awareness of the bountiful and beautiful world, a flower, a sunset, a seashore. No setup is needed except an aware therapist and a willing patient.

Neurostimulatory Methods

Stimulation-produced analgesia comprises such measures as transcutaneous electrical neural stimulation, dorsal column stimulation, and percutaneously implanted spinal cord epidural stimulation. These techniques are used to relieve advanced cancer pain.

Neurosurgical Sections

This is the final recourse of the desperate; a willing sacrifice of the patient's neural tissues to make her or him forget pain. Some of the modalities are listed below, and are used occasionally in India.

1. Spinal sensory rhizotomy
2. Cranial sensory rhizotomy
3. Differential rhizotomy[19]
4. Spinothalamic tractotomy
5. Stereotactic ablations

We end this section in due humility, with the sense that one is forced to hurt a patient so that he or she can forget a greater hurt—his or her cancer pain.

Cancer Pain Paradigm 4

All pain is relieved to some extent by distraction and a pleasurable environment and exacerbated by anxiety or psychological stress.

Foley[20]

My final word before I am done
Is cancer can be rather fun
Provided one confronts the tumor
With a sufficient sense of humour.
I know that cancer often kills,
But so do cars and sleeping pills;
And it can hurt till one sweats,
So can bad teeth and unpaid debts.

J.B.S. Haldane[21]

Obstacles in Pain Management

In India, the major reasons for unsatisfactory management of pain can be briefly stated as follows:

1. Lack of recognition by various health professionals to the established methods of pain relief.
2. Governmental apathy at both federal and state levels.
3. Lack of availability of drugs.
4. Fear of addiction, which is a phobia that is allowed to have its sway even when the patient has not much time left to develop an addiction.
5. Curricular lack of systematic education regarding pain relief to health professionals, nurses, medical students, and doctors.
6. The inordinate regard that most practicing oncologists have for the "latest" in the "multidisciplinary" treatment of cancer is coupled with poor regard for the phenomenon of pain in cancer, much less so for its scientific management.

The news on relief from cancer pain in First World countries is not necessarily encouraging:

Several barriers interfere with the appropriate management of patients with pain and cancer. Although pain can be controlled in most patients, an analysis of 11 published reports of cancer pain treatment covering nearly

2000 patients in nonhospice settings estimated that 50–80% did not have adequate control.[22]

In hopes of explaining the gross chasm between expectation and fulfillment, the following possible reasons have been advanced (ranked in order of decreasing priority):

1. Inadequate assessment of pain and relief
2. Reluctance by patient to report pain
3. Reluctance by patient to take opiates
4. Reluctance by doctor to give opiates
5. Poor equipment skills
6. Reluctance by nursing staff to administer opiates
7. Excessive governmental regulation on narcotic prescription
8. Poor psychological support service
9. Paucity of neurodestructive methods
10. Limited range of analgesics
11. Scarcity of pain therapists

"Among the remedies which it has pleased Almighty God to give to man to relieve his sufferings, none is so universal and so efficacious as opium."[23] This monumental opiophilic generalization by the "English Hippocrates" Thomas Sydenham, made in 1680, has not lost its flavor nor its worth. The global drug wars, drug trafficking, and all the fear thereof have pushed regulating bodies into irrationally clamping a common physician's access to the gift of *Poppy somniferum* from the Almighty.

Maybe those who ban opium as a blanket measure have not experienced excruciating, dehumanizing pain. They ought to keep in mind that De Quincey who wrote *Confessions of an English Opium-Eater,* conquered by sheer will, his addiction which as its zenith meant 8,000 drops of laudanum a day.[24] So let us not be afraid of opium and opiates, and let there be a global awakening, blessed by the World Health Organization, toward the wider, rational use of opium products.

References

1. Schweitzer A. In MB Strauss (ed), Familiar Medical Quotations. Boston: Little, Brown, 1968.
2. Guyton AC. Textbook of Medical Physiology (8th ed). Philadelphia: Saunders, 1993;520.
3. Foley KM. Management of Cancer Pain. In VT De Vita, S Hellman, RA Rosenberg (eds), Cancer Principles and Practice of Oncology. Philadelphia: Lippincott, 1993;2417.
4. Goethe. In MB Strauss (ed), Familiar Medical Quotations. Boston: Little, Brown, 1968.
5. Peter Mere Latham. In MB Strauss (ed), Familiar Medical Quotations. Boston: Little, Brown, 1968.
6. Gunther J. Death Be Not Proud. A Memoir. New York, Harper & Row, 1965.
7. Vaidya B. Personal communication, 1994.
8. Lipman AG. Reassessment of pain management. Clin Pharmacol Ther 1986;5:825.
9. Lipman AG. Drug therapy in cancer pain. Cancer Nurs 1980;3:39.
10. Twycriss RG, Fairfield S. Pain in far advanced cancer. Pain 1982;14:303.
11. Bonica JJ. Pain. In J Walton, P Beason, SR Bodley (eds), The Oxford Companion to Medicine. Oxford: Oxford University Press, 1986;984.
12. Foley KM. The treatment of cancer pain. N Engl J Med 1985;313:84.
13. Bonica JJ. Basic principles in managing chronic pain. Arch Surg 1977;112:783.
14. Amer S. The role of nerve blocks in treatment of cancer pain. Acta Anaesthesiol Scand 1982;74(Suppl.):104.
15. Ashburn MA, Fine PG. Evaluation and treatment of chronic pain syndromes. Compr Ther 1990;16:37.
16. Hitchcock E. Hypothermic subarachnoid irrigation for intractable pain. Lancet 1967;1:1133.
17. Brown DL, Bulley CK, Quiel EL. Neurolytic celiac plexus block for pancreatic cancer pain. Anesth Analg 1987;66;869.
18. Foley KM, Posner JB. Pain and Its Management. In JB Wyngaarden, LH Smith (eds), Cecil Textbook of Medicine (18th ed). Philadelphia: Saunders, 1989;104.
19. Arbit E, Gelicich JH, Burt M, Mallya K. Modified open thoracic rhizotomy for treatment of intractable chest wall pain of malignant etiology. Ann Thorac Surg 1989;48;820.
20. Foley KM. Pain syndromes in patients with cancer. Med Clin North Am 1987;71:169.
21. Haldane JBS. In MB Strauss (ed), Familiar Medical Quotations. Boston: Little, Brown, 1968.
22. Ventafridda V, Caraceni A. Cancer pain classification: A controversial issue. Pain 1991;46:1.
23. Singhal GD, Patterson TJS. Synopsis of Ayurveda (Based on a translation of Sysruta Samhita). Delhi: Oxford University Press, 1993.
24. Lanman CR. Atharva veda Samhita. Delhi: Motilal Banarasidass, 1984.

Chapter 48

Recent Advances and Future Challenges

Winston C. V. Parris

Since the publication of "Pain Mechanisms: A New Theory," by Melzack and Wall[1] in 1965, there has been a flurry of research activity in the area of pain medicine. This activity intensified as the pharmacology of the opioids[2] became better understood and the recognition of the role of neuropeptides,[3] endorphins,[4] enkephalins, and other vasoactive amino acids in pain mechanisms became clearer. Thus, in 1995, 30 years after Melzack and Wall's publication on the gate-control hypothesis, the intensity of research activity in pain medicine in general and cancer pain management in particular continues to increase. This activity implies that new therapeutic modalities are constantly being proposed for cancer pain management along with new mechanisms hypothesized as important in the treatment and understanding of cancer pain. Although some publications are of questionable quality, many papers are of high quality and make meaningful contributions toward solving the puzzle of cancer pain. It is hoped that with time, the quality and quantity of both basic science and clinical papers will increase and, in fact, become more useful in practical terms and easier to evaluate in clinical practice. This chapter reviews some of the recent advances in cancer pain management and speculates on the implications of those advances in light of future challenges for cancer pain management.

The recent advances made in cancer pain management are closely linked with the progress made in the treatment of cancer itself. In fact, as aggressive therapies are introduced to treat cancer, minor and major complications of those therapies may de-velop. Some of those complications may be associated with pain and may have unique presentations requiring specific therapeutic regimens for management. The current modalities for managing cancer include radical and palliative surgery,[5] radiotherapy[6] including brachytherapy, chemotherapy,[7] and biological therapy.[8] The complications of these therapeutic modalities have been discussed in Chapters 19, 20, 23, 30, 34, and 35; however, it is important to stress that as more advances are made in cancer therapy, it may be anticipated that more complications including pain may develop as a result of these advances.

It is important to make sure that pain-related complications of cancer therapy are adequately controlled for three primary reasons. First, uncontrolled pain in cancer patients may produce undesirable pathophysiologic effects including tachycardia, hypertension, myocardial hypoperfusion, immunologic dysfunction, and an enhanced catabolic phase of metabolic activity. Second, when cancer pain is unrelieved, inevitable suffering and anguish results. This suffering and anguish are totally unnecessary and usually avoidable. Third, if the cancer has been controlled or cured, but pain is unrelieved, the quality of life[9] may become unacceptable and activities of daily life including recreation, eating, communication with others, and sexual activity are all compromised to the patient's ultimate detriment. For these reasons, one must strive to achieve adequate pain control, while at the same time maintaining a satisfactory quality of life. An important principle of providing pain control is to determine the delicate balance of providing optimal pain relief with minimal side effects. It is important to keep this principle in mind as new concepts are introduced and new regimens investigated.

A major advance in cancer pain management (March 1994) has been the publication of the Clinical Practice Guideline on "The Management of Cancer Pain."[10] That guideline published by the Agency for Health Care Policy and Research (an agency of the U.S. Department of Health and Human Services) was universally acclaimed as a positive step in sensitizing physicians (specialists and generalists alike) and other health care providers to the need to improve pain management for cancer patients. This publication was well received, widely distributed, and has apparently made a positive impact on physicians and other health care providers who treat cancer patients.

In 1990, the World Health Organization (WHO)[11] reaffirmed the implementation of the "analgesic ladder" in managing cancer pain patients. A major prerequisite of that ladder was the need for comprehensive assessment of the patient including meticulous assessment of pain and its characteristics. It also emphasized that following initial assessment, regular subsequent reassessments of the patient's physical status and pain be made to optimize appropriate therapy for managing cancer pain. The general principles behind WHO recommendations were that following patient assessment if pain was deemed to be due to cancer that it would be appropriate to initiate the analgesic ladder. The analgesic ladder has three arbitrary steps based on pain intensity and the response of that pain to treatment. For patients with mild pain, the use of a nonopioid with or without analgesic adjuvant is recommended; this is the first step of the ladder. If this mild pain does not improve or if it progresses to moderate pain, then a mild opioid (e.g., oxycodone) is introduced; this is the second step of the ladder. If the moderate pain becomes severe or does not respond to treatment, then a strong opioid may be added to the pre-existing pharmacologic regimen; this is the third step of the ladder. The gold standard for strong opioids is morphine sulfate and most patients usually respond to adequate doses of oral morphine.

A significant development in morphine pharmacology is the manufacture of controlled-release morphine preparations. MS Contin,[12] Oxycontin, and Roxanol-SR are representative of controlled-release morphine. MS Contin has a unique matrix within the capsule that allows morphine to be slowly released over approximately 12 hours. This characteristic gives the patient much greater freedom from having to take repetitive medications, thus providing longer-lasting analgesia. It lets the patient have a good night's sleep rather than having to wake up to take pain medications. Several trials have shown these preparations to be safe and efficacious and that they are not associated with any more side effects than regular morphine. While titrating patients on these controlled-release morphine preparations, it is important to provide oral immediate-release morphine if and when breakthrough pain occurs. At the next dosing schedule, it is appropriate to increase the dose of the controlled-release morphine preparation if necessary and to evaluate the efficacy of that increase for both side effects and the presence of breakthrough pain. Thus, whenever MS Contin, Oxycontin, or Roxanol-SR is prescribed, it is important to give additional doses of immediate-release oral morphine in order to deal with breakthrough pain. It is also important to provide the patient with stool-softening medication to deal with constipation that is commonly associated with the administration of opioid drugs.

The search for new drugs continues along with new applications of old drugs. It is hoped that new pharmacologic developments will occur that will add to the armamentarium of the physician managing cancer pain. One such drug is tramadol (Ultram).[13] Tramadol, which was recently approved by the Food and Drug Administration and officially released in the United States in April 1995, represents a new class of analgesic. It is a centrally acting binary analgesic that has been shown to produce antinociception in both animals and humans. It is thought to have two mechanisms of action. The first is that of a partial mu-agonist with a weak affinity for mu-opioid receptors. This mechanism of action makes it similar to morphine except that the affinity for mu-opioid receptors is approximately 6,000 times less than morphine. The other mechanism of action is related to its ability to inhibit the neuronal reuptake of 5-hydroxy tryptamine (serotonin) and norepinephrine.[14] It is thought that these two mechanisms of action interact in a synergistic way to produce enhanced antinoiception. Further, tramadol is metabolized to an active metabolite O-desmethyl tramadol. This compound binds with greater affinity to the mu-receptor than the parent compound and probably contributes to the overall analgesic efficacy. Tramadol is believed to have a low abuse potential and appears to have fewer side effects than morphine. However, some adverse effects have been reported in long-term trials and these include nausea, dizziness, vomiting, and headache. The most troublesome of all these adverse effects is nausea.[15] It is opined from the European experience with tramadol that a slow titration regimen reduces the incidence of side effects. The recommended dose in adults is 50–100 mg every 4–6 hours. It is recommended that a total dose should not exceed 400 mg in patients with normal hepatic and renal function. Prior to its use in the United States, Tramadol had been used extensively in Latin America, the Philippines, South Africa, and several European countries. It appears to be a satisfactory substitute for those patients who have developed severe adverse effects to the commonly prescribed narcotic analgesics. Because of its efficacy, safety, and low potential for abuse, tramadol appears to have a role in the management of some cancer pain syndromes. More scientifically conducted clinical studies investigating its efficacy in that patient population are needed to justify this claim.

As previously discussed, morphine represents the prototype for opioid management of cancer pain. However, some patients are unable to take oral medication and some develop adverse effects or tolerance to morphine. For that patient population, alternative drugs or alternative routes of administration need to be developed. Transdermal fentanyl[16] has been a significant advance in providing for that need. Transdermal fentanyl formulation is available in systems that deliver 25, 50, 75, and 100 µg per hour. This system consists of a drug reservoir separated from the patient's skin by a rate-limiting membrane that controls the rate of drug delivery in such a manner that fentanyl is released at a nearly constant rate per unit time. In most situations, the dosing interval of each system is approximately 72 hours. However, individual pharmocokinetic variabilities do occur and the dosing interval may vary from 48–96 hours in a small but distinct group of patients. Thus, it is important to assess the efficacy of the transdermal delivery system, especially after initial application. Its limitations in normal circumstances include the relative high cost and the need to use an alternative short-acting opioid when necessary for breakthrough pain. Clinical trials with other opioids using the same transdermal technology may produce beneficial applications of cancer pain management in the future. Other routes of administration of opioids include sublingual, subcutaneous, epidural, intrathecal, rectal, transnasal (inhalational), intraventricular, and intravenous. These routes should be considered when patients have problems with the oral route of administration. The intramuscular route should be discouraged because it is unpredictable both in its delivery and metabolism and is associated with unnecessary pain on administration.

In the practical management of cancer pain, adequate pain control may be satisfactorily attained using oral opioids. However, side effects may be discomforting and, occasionally, intolerable. The most common and unacceptable adverse effects include severe constipation, nausea, vomiting, and sedation. Other adverse effects include delirium, pruritus, myoclonus, and respiratory depression. These adverse effects are usually dose limiting and may be controlled by altering the dose of the opioid. The management of side effects of opioid administration is just as important as the management of the cancer pain. Constipation is usually managed by the prophylactic administration of a combination of a stool-softening agent and a cathartic agent. The doses of those drugs may be increased if prophylactic administration is ineffective. In exceptional circumstances, the constipation may be intractable and extreme measures like the use of the oral bowel preparation (e.g., polyethylene glycol 3350 [GoLYTELY]) may be necessary to alleviate this uncomfortable symptom. Sykes[17] and Culpepper-Morgan et al.[18] have described the use of oral naloxone for the treatment of refractory constipation. Oral naloxone has a bioavailability of less than 3% and possibly acts selectively on opioid receptors in the bowel. The initial dose may be from 0.8–1.2 mg once or twice a day, and this dose may be slowly increased until the constipation is alleviated or until unacceptable adverse effects (i.e., abdominal cramps and diarrhea) develop. This therapeutic approach represents a recent advancement in the management of the side effects of opioids and warrants further investigation, since the risk of systemic withdrawal from oral naloxone has not been thoroughly studied.

Recent studies have demonstrated that more Americans are either losing confidence in established medicine or are resorting to alternative therapies while continuing to use conventional medical therapy.[19] This trend is even more alarming in cancer pain patients. The intense interest in Laetrile as a cure for cancer and, more recently, the use of shark cartilage as an alternative therapy for cancer has created widespread public interest in exploring unconventional therapies. This increase in public interest has had its political implications. In 1991, the United States government created the Office of Alternative Medicine (OAM) within the National Institutes of Health structure. The primary purpose of the OAM is to act as a clearinghouse for research ideas relating to alternative medicine and to fund appropriate studies and investigate alternative modalities and drugs using established research procedures. Most alternative modalities have been alleged to be effective following anecdotal reports.[20] Very few randomized, placebo-controlled, double-blind studies have been performed to validate the efficacy of these modalities. Thus, it is hoped that the OAM will facilitate the scientific investigation of those modalities that have been purported to be therapeutically effective. Recently, the OAM has funded studies for investigating the use of intercessionary prayer, music therapy,[21] biofeedback,[22] selective herbal medicine,[23] and others for use in cancer pain patients.

This approach is productive in that several papers have been published on the efficacy of alternative modalities in cancer pain management. Fishman[24] showed that cognitive behavioral therapy may be effective in alleviating pain-related suffering in patients with advanced malignancy. This modality is noninvasive and teaches patients to practice relaxation and develop active coping skills so as to increase pain tolerance. It also teaches patients to modify thoughts and attitudes that increase perception of personal disintegration. Although this modality is not dramatic and is not associated with "high-tech" equipment, it may be very effective in appropriate patients. Rhiner et al.[25] examined the use of a structured nondrug interventional program for cancer pain. Their study consisted of three parts including an overview of pain, pharmacologic management of pain, and nondrug interventions for pain. The nondrug component of the program consisted of using heat, cold, massage, vibration, distraction, and relaxation techniques. This study showed that these noninvasive modalities may be effective in selected patients with advanced malig-

nancy. These observations have been validated by other studies. Beck[26] has demonstrated that music may help manage cancer pain. Whereas, it is not appropriate to discontinue established medications and introduce music therapy as the sole modality for managing pain, it is appropriate to use music therapy as an adjunct to other modalities in patients for whom music therapy may be of tremendous therapeutic value. The same approach is being adopted to investigate low-power laser therapy, acupuncture, magnetic field therapy, and other modalities that are anecdotally reported to be effective in cancer pain management.

From a radiotherapeutic standpoint, many techniques have been shown to be effective in cancer pain management. This is particularly true in cancer patients who have multiple bony metastases.[27] The techniques for administering radiotherapy include those in the following list:

1. External beams
   A. Megavoltage using linear accelerators, cobalt, or cyclotron machine
   B. Kilovoltage using an x-ray machine with photon beams
   C. Superficial beam using an x-ray machine with lower voltage photon beams
2. Radioisotopes
   A. Intracavitary sealed applicators using radium, cesium, or iridium needles
   B. Unsealed oral preparations (e.g., iodine [I-131])
   C. Injected unsealed radioisotopes (e.g., strontium 89 [Sr-89] or phosphorus 32 [P-32])

Some of these applications have already been discussed in Chapter 30 and new applications of those techniques are currently being proposed as new technology is developed. Strontium 89 has been successfully used to treat metastatic bone pain,[28] while phosphorus has been used effectively to treat polycythemia rubra vera. Intracavitary and interstitial implanted needles are commonly used for cancers of the cervix and uterus and head and neck tumors. They have also been used to treat skin tumors. The external beams are effective in treating superficial lesions while the megavoltage external beams have greater tissue penetrative characteristics. However, although the megavoltage external beams may minimize significant trauma to the skin, they may also cause major neurologic complications that in themselves may be associated with pain. Thus, radiation neuritis[29] is a common complication of radiotherapy using external beams. As that technology improves, it is hoped that interventional radiotherapeutic principles will have an expanded and important role in palliation and cancer pain management.

Preemptive analgesia is currently advanced as a technique that may significantly decrease postoperative pain. Surgery is an important therapeutic modality for some forms of cancer. It is clear that removal of limb, breast, and any appendage in the body may be associated with phantom sensation or phantom pain. The treatment of phantom phenomena is generally unsatisfactory. Thus, prevention of phantom pain is an effective technique for dealing with that complication. As early as 1910, George Crile[30] indicated that "General anesthesia does not anesthetize the spinal cord." Surgical manipulation and plasticity of the central nervous system[31] contribute to creating an afferent barrage of the spinal cord, which ultimately produces a hypersensitivity state in the spinal cord. This afferent barrage and hypersensitivity state may not cease after surgery but may continue long afterward and be manifest as severe postoperative pain or as phantom limb pain in patients following amputations. Bach et al.[32] showed that preoperative lumbar epidural blockade prior to limb amputation prevents the development of phantom phenomena. This excellent example of preemptive analgesia highlights the need for preoperative neural blockade of the affected appendage area prior to its amputation or excision. This represents a progressive form of preemptive analgesia.

Pain education in general, and cancer pain education in particular, are deficient in the training and education of medical and nursing students. The same situation exists for physicians undergoing postgraduate training. Many reasons exist for this continuing deficiency in spite of the strides being made in pain medicine. The directors of medical and nursing curricula (with a few exceptions) are still resistant to acknowledging pain medicine as a legitimate specialty or subspecialty in medicine. Fortunately, the American Medical Association has recognized this deficiency and has granted pain medicine a seat in its House of Delegates. Further, pain management is recognized by the American Board of Medical Specialties by permitting the American Board of Anesthesiology to offer an examination for a certificate of added qualifications in pain management. This and other related certification activity notably by the American Board of Pain Medicine (formerly, the American College of Pain Medicine) may help authenticate the importance of chronic pain management and cancer pain management in the United States.

It is imperative that directors of medical and nursing programs, directors of relevant residency programs (i.e., anesthesiology, neurosurgery, general surgery, family medicine, internal medicine, oncologic medicine, and pediatric oncology) and other appropriate groups focus their attention on sensitizing their respective trainees to the need for improved pain management of cancer patients and, also provision of the clinical experience necessary to provide competency of their trainees in cancer pain management. In order to accomplish these two objectives, it is important that the leaders of the different specialties put aside petty parochial differences of opinion and be prepared to be receptive to new ideas and not to be rigidly adherent to old ones. These leaders should also take a fresh look at the pain patient from a different perspective that includes not just the treatment of a tumor but the management of the consequences produced by the treatment of that tumor and to address ultimately the patient's quality of life after treatment. This process will not be easy because change is never easy. However, in the light of the health care reform initiatives (i.e., managed care, managed costs, and managed competition), there ought to be no "sacred cows." An honest effort at reviewing old approaches and an openness to new ideas may be a modest first step in an attempt to introduce new educational material into medical and nursing school curricula and to possibly eliminate or diminish those areas that are not as relevant as cancer pain management. It may be legitimately argued that cancer pain management is more appropriately addressed in postgraduate training programs. However, just as neurosurgery is a postgraduate discipline, some limited exposure to neurosurgical principles at an undergraduate level prepares the would-be trainee for an appreciation of the scope of the discipline prior to actually deciding on a career specialty. Correspondingly, with cancer pain management and chronic pain, it would be desirable if a limited but well-organized exposure of cancer pain and chronic pain management be introduced at the undergraduate level to medical students. Thus, most students would become familiar with the concepts and principles of pain management by the time it is necessary to make choices about a specialty. Even if a prospective trainee does not choose to be trained in cancer pain management or in pain management, the awareness of the functions of the cancer pain specialist would be better understood and appropriate referrals initiated when necessary. The net effect of all this proposed activity is that patient care would be enhanced and patient quality of life significantly improved.

The need for continued and expanded research on pain mechanisms and on the treatment of specific pain syndromes will require more funding. As the research dollars continue to diminish, funding of these endeavors may become increasingly difficult. New strategies for research grant applications may have to be undertaken and clear objectives and priorities may have to be established prior to application. A fundamental principle that should not be understated is that any cancer research project that does not address quality of life issues is almost irrelevant since it is important to determine not only pharmacologic, medical, or surgical therapeutic efficacy but the impact of that modality on the patient's activities of day-to-day living and other factors that would make a difference in lifestyle. Because government inclination to and capability of funding most major cancer research projects is decreasing, it is important to increase the involvement of private industry, foundations, or other philanthropic organizations in funding cancer pain research. In pursuit of that support, it is important to maintain high objectivity, sound ethics, and good science in proposing research objectives. It is also important to describe clearly the role and participation of the sponsor in the particular research and to establish appropriate review boards to scrutinize proposed studies and research protocols when applicable. An area of medicine that has gone unattended is pediatric cancer pain management. In fact, the whole issue of pediatric pain[33] has only been seriously addressed in the past 4–6 years. Infants and young children do develop cancer and these cancers are frequently associated with pain. Thus, pain management of that population needs to be addressed as vigorously as the adult population. Important strides have been made in the assessment of pain in pediatric patients. A determination of pain intensity and

periodic changes in intensity would help determine the need to treat and the vigor with which that treatment should be implemented. There are many procedures, which in both pediatric cancer patients and adult cancer patients, produce pain or are associated with pain. These procedures include bone marrow biopsy, vascular access procedures, lumbar puncture, radiation therapy, some chemotherapeutic protocols and, of course, most surgical procedures. Patient management should be individualized; pain intensity should be assessed and a particular strategy for pain management should be developed for each patient's individual needs.

The use of intravenous analgesics and sedatives, nerve blocks, and oral medication have been used to provide periprocedure analgesia. The advent of patient-controlled analgesia (PCA)[34] represents a major advance in postoperative analgesia. PCA has been used via the intravenous route and has been used effectively in pediatric patients. Currently, PCA is being used in children via the epidural route but it is too early to assess the efficacy of that route of administration. Notwithstanding, newer techniques need to be evaluated in order to determine which procedures are most effective in the pediatric cancer pain patient.

There are some patients whose pain may not be adequately controlled with any routine modality. For those patients who have a long life expectancy, it is quite appropriate to attempt a variety of alternative medical interventions with or without the modalities that have been used previously. These noninvasive interventions include alternative pharmacologic approaches, the use of psychological interventions,[35] neurostimulatory techniques[36] (including transcutaneous electrical nerve stimulation and dorsal column stimulation), rehabilitative interventions, and physiatric techniques[37] depending on the physical status of the patient. Some patients may even request the introduction of a holistic approach, whereas others may opt for spiritual interactions. An open mind should be maintained without necessarily condemning or condoning a particular option. No attempts should be made to interfere with or change a patient's personal belief unless that belief may produce harm to the patient. The expanded use of hospice services may better help care for terminally ill cancer patients in the future. With the exception of the contribution of diverse hospice groups, it is unfortunate, but true, that comprehensive medical care of the dying patient has long been neglected and may be greatly improved. This situation is in need of urgent redress.

Certain physiatric techniques have been used to manage some states in cancer patients that are associated with pain. For example, lymphedema may be a source of tremendous pain and is best managed using a variety of physiatric techniques. These techniques include electrical stimulation, cryotherapy, heat, and orthotic devices. Brennan[38] recently described the use of pressure stockings and pneumatic pump devices to decrease pain and improve function in patients with lymphedema. These measures were very effective in some situations when other standard modalities had failed.

There is a small but select group of patients who have intractable cancer pain and who have not responded to routine conservative therapeutic options for cancer pain management. These patients may be considered ideal candidates for intraspinal opioid therapy.[39] The criteria that influence the implantation of catheters delivering intraspinal opioids should be carefully discussed and agreed on by all members of the pain team. Those criteria may vary from institution to institution but the general principles should be the same, irrespective of the institution. In some cancer pain patients, intraspinal opioids have been very effective and, in fact, their efficacy has led to a decrease in the neuroablative procedures that were performed previously to palliate intractable cancer pain. The side effects associated with the use of intraspinal opioids include respiratory depression, gastrointestinal dysfunction including constipation, nausea and vomiting, urinary retention, pruritus, catheter malfunction including breakage, dislodgement, blockage, anaphylactic reactions, infectious complications including meningitis, myelitis, encephalitis, and inadvertent injection of neurotoxic compounds other than the prescribed opioids. The challenge for the future is to continue research in determining the ideal opioid or the ideal opioid and local anesthetic combination most suitable for intrathecal or epidural injection. The search for improved catheter material, which would minimize catheter-related complications, is currently ongoing and evaluation of new delivery systems and pump devices may ultimately produce better patient care. These new devices may be more efficient and less expensive than current ones. Criteria for the ideal opioid would include determining the hy-

drophilicity and lipophilicity of the agent, the presence or absence of preservatives, consideration of the baricity of the agent, the need to use synthetic beta-endorphins or other neuropeptides and considerations of the use of agonists-antagonists analgesic agents.

The future may introduce improvements in PCA technology as other agents or combinations of agents are used, thereby producing improved efficacy in pain management of cancer patients. Opioids have been administered via intraventricular routes or, more specifically, via intracerebroventricular routes; preliminary results of these techniques are encouraging. It is hoped that more research will be continued in an attempt to improve existing modalities and technology.

The 11-amino-acid neuropeptide, somatostatin[40] is a potent analgesic. It has been reported to be effective when administered intrathecally in patients with advanced cancer. This finding is encouraging and should be explored further, particularly if the side effects and complications of intrathecal somatostatin are minimal. Research into alternative routes of administration (e.g., epidural somatostatin administration) may be investigated and possibly implemented. Further, the use of other neuropeptides including substance P antagonists, calcitonin gene-related peptide, and related compounds may be evaluated for possible use in treating terminal cancer pain patients. It is important to stress that some of the previously mentioned modalities, although effective, may be very expensive. In addition to determining the risk–benefit ratio of the treatment or modality, it is also relevant to determine the cost-effectiveness of the treatment. It is almost counterproductive to install a $10,000 device and all its appendages in a patient for 1 week when $100 worth of oral narcotic analgesic therapy may have kept that patient just as comfortable. The "high-tech" treatment that is offered should be administered with sensitivity toward patient selection and observation of the criteria necessary for appropriate use of a particular treatment modality. In fact, the Agency for Health Care Policy and Research, the WHO, the National Cancer Pain Institute, and the American Pain Society have attempted to address those difficult socioeconomic and philosophical issues that affect the delivery of health care in cancer pain management. Some of the difficult areas include the cost of treating cancer pain, the regulatory perspectives affecting the use of opioids for cancer pain, access of nonaffluent patients to adequate and competent care for pain management, and the ethical and legal issues affecting pain management. These previously neglected areas are just beginning to be recognized and it is hoped that in the future, more discussion, investigation, and analyses of those issues may lead to more efficient and compassionate delivery of health care to all cancer patients in pain.

The task of prevention, early detection, and aggressive treatment of cancer still remains a cornerstone of cancer management. If the disease may be prevented and if it may be treated early, many of the complications and treatment of the disease may be prevented or minimized. For example, there appears to be a general recognition at many levels of government and in society that smoking is definitely harmful to health. If this trend continues and if smoking does in fact decrease, then it is quite clear that the resulting cancer complications of smoking would be decreased and pain associated with some of those complications would also decrease. Furthermore, early treatment of pain, before it becomes intractable, may make treatment easier to implement and decrease the likelihood of the development of addiction, pseudoaddiction, tolerance, and those other difficult complications that may occur as a result of treating a patient aggressively and too late in the course of the disease process.

As cancer treatment improves, patients may inevitably live longer; however, in living longer they still have the threat that there could be a recurrence or sudden deterioration in their clinical condition. This uncertain situation and also the reaction of the patient's spouse and family to the pain is always difficult to deal with and to understand. Thus, these issues are best dealt with using support groups.[41] These support groups are very important in teaching patients coping mechanisms to help them reduce emotional stress, promote increasing physical activity, and continue with the activities of normal daily living. It is sometimes more effective when a patient receives some information regarding cancer and its effect on everyday activities and on family interactions from another patient rather than to hear it from a doctor. A well-managed support group with some limited medical and nursing interaction goes a long way toward helping patients deal with trivial but very important personal issues from the patient's perspective. It is hoped that support groups would develop and increase their scope and provide enhancing support for appropriate patients.

Recently, physician-assisted suicide has been the subject of medical, legal, religious, social, political, and ethical discussions. The debate has intensified as to whether euthanasia or mercy killing is acceptable and, in fact, desirable. As of this writing, Oregon is the only state in the United States where it is legal to obtain physician-assisted suicide. The obligations of physicians in Oregon toward a patient who requests that service are not clear. It is hoped that no law forcing a physician to render a treatment that he or she may be unwilling or unable to perform would ever be initiated or enforced. Irrespective of the individual predisposition for or against physician-assisted suicide, it is quite clear that most patients requesting that service are patients in whom pain management has been less than adequate. It appears that when patients with terminal cancer or other terminal conditions associated with pain are able to function satisfactorily and if adequate pain control is accomplished, the number of patients requesting physician-assisted suicide decreases significantly. It is important to stress that doctors are in the business of life and assisting to maintain life; it would be unfortunate if doctors become involved in the business of ending lives, e.g., as in execution or the use of physician-assisted suicide. It is hoped that in the future as more information becomes available on the use of palliative care, the hospice movement, and in particular cancer pain management, physicians caring for cancer patients will have a much greater understanding of the issues and enhanced knowledge so as to make sound scientific choices for the ultimate good and comfort of the cancer pain patient.

References

1. Melzack R, Wall PD. Pain mechanisms: A new theory. Science 1965;150:971.
2. Kosterlitz HW. Opioid Peptides and Pain: An Update. In JJ Bonica, U Lindblom, A Iggo (eds), Advances in Pain Research and Therapy. New York: Raven, 1983.
3. Hughes J, Smith TW, Kosterlitz HW, et al. Identification of two related pentapeptides from the brain with potent opiate agonist activity. Nature 1975;258:5779.
4. Hughes J. Biogenesis release and inactivation of enkephalins and dynorphins. Br Med Bull 1983;39:17.
5. Bedard J, Dionne A, Dionne L. The experience of La Maison Michael Sarrazin (1985–1990): Profile analy-

sis of 952 terminal-phase cancer patients. J Palliat Care 1991;7:42.

6. Bates T. Radiotherapy for bone metastases. Clin Oncol 1989;1:57.

7. Hellmann K, Carter SK (eds). Fundamentals of Cancer Chemotherapy. New York: McGraw-Hill, 1987.

8. Le J, Vilcek J. Tumor necrosis factor and interleukin-1: Cytokines with multiple overlapping biological activities. Lab Invest 1987;56:234.

9. Walsh TD. Symptom control in patients with advanced cancer. Am J Hospice Palliat Care 1990;7:60.

10. Jacox A, Carr DB, Payne R, et al. Management of cancer pain. Clinical Practice Guideline No. 9. U.S. Department of Health and Human Services. AHCPR Publication No. 94-0592. Agency for Health Care Policy and Research, March 1994.

11. World Health Organization. Cancer pain relief and palliative care. Report of a WHO expert committee (World Health Organization Technical Report Series, 804). Geneva, Switzerland: World Health Organization, 1990;1.

12. Kaiko RF, Wallenstein SL, Rogers AG, et al. Narcotics in the elderly. Med Clin North Am 1982;66:1079.

13. Vickers MD, O'Flaherty D, Szekely SM, et al. Tramadol: Pain relief by an opioid without depression of respiration. Anesthesia 1992;47:291.

14. Raffa B, Friedrichs E, Reimann W, et al. Opioid and non-opioid components independently contribute to mechanism of action of tramadol. J Pharmacol Exp Ther 1992;260:275.

15. Canlo NB, Cordova S. A comparative study of tramadol 100mg versus tramadol 50mg. Curr Ther Res 1992;51:112.

16. Miser AW, Narang PK, Dothage JA, et al. Transdermal fentanyl for pain control in patients with cancer. Pain 1989;37:15.

17. Sykes NP. Oral naloxone in opioid associated constipation. Lancet 1991;337;475.

18. Culpepper-Morgan JA, Inturrisi CE, Portenoy RK, et al. Treatment of opioid-induced constipation with oral naloxone: A pilot study. Clin Pharmacol Ther 1992;52:90.

19. Eisenberg DM, Kessler RC, Foster C, et al. Unconventional medicine in the United States: Prevalence, costs and patterns of use. N Engl J Med 1993;326:266.

20. McGinnis LS. Alternative therapies 190. An overview (review). Cancer 1991;67(Suppl. 6):1788.

21. Lee MHM, Itoh M, Yang GW, Eason AL. Physical Therapy and Rehabilitation Medicine. In JJ Bonica (ed), The Management of Pain (2nd ed, Vol. 2). Philadelphia: Lea & Febiger, 1990;1769.

22. Fotopoulos SS, Graham C, Cook MR. Psychophysiologic Control of Cancer Pain. In JJ Bonica, V Ventafridda (eds), Advances in Pain Research and Therapy (Vol. 2). New York: Raven, 1979.

23. Kenner DJ. Pain forum. A total approach to pain management. Conceptual overview (review). Aust Fam Physician 1994;23:1267.

24. Fishman B. The cognitive behavioral perspective on pain management in terminal illness. Hospice J 1992;8:73.

25. Rhimer M, Ferrell BR, Ferrell BA, Grant MM. A structured non-drug intervention program for cancer pain. Cancer Pract 1993;1:137.

26. Beck SL. The therapeutic use of music. Oncol Nurs Forum 1991;18:1327.

27. Poulsen HS, Nielsen OS, Klee M, et al. Palliative irradiation of bone metastases. Cancer Treat Rev 1989;16:41.

28. Silberstein EB, Williams C. Strontium-89 therapy for the pain of osseous metastases. J Nucl Med 1985;26:345.

29. Berger PS. Neurological Complications of Radiotherapy. In A Silverstein (ed), Neurological Complications of Therapy: Selected Topics. Mount Kisco, NY: Futura, 1982.

30. Crile GW. Phylogenetic association in relation to certain medical problems. Boston Med Surg J 1910;163:893.

31. Woolf CJ. Evidence for a central component of post-injury pain hypersensitivity. Nature 1983;306:686.

32. Bach S, Noreng MF, Tjéllden NU. Phantom limb pain in amputees during the first 12 months following limb amputation, after preoperative lumbar epidural blockade. Pain 1988;33:297.

33. McGrath PJ. Paediatric pain: A good start. Pain 1990;41:253.

34. Bruera E, Brenneis C, Michaud M, et al. Patient-controlled subcutaneous hydromorphone versus continuous subcutaneous infusion for the treatment of cancer pain. J Natl Cancer Inst 1988;80:152.

35. Turk DC, Fernandez E. On the putative uniqueness of cancer pain: Do psychological principles apply? Behav Res Ther 1990;28:1.

36. Young RF, Brechner T. Electrical stimulation of the brain for relief of intractable pain due to cancer. Cancer 1986;57:1266.

37. Linton SL, Melin L. Applied relaxation in the management of cancer pain. Behav Psychother 1983;11:337.

38. Brennan MJ. Lymphedema following the surgical treatment of breast cancer: A review of pathophysiology and treatment. J Pain Symptom Manage 1992;7:110.

39. Benedetti C. Intraspinal analgesia. An historical overview. Acta Anaesthesiol Scand 1987;85:17.

40. Chrubasik J, Meynadier J, Blond S, et al. Somatostatin, an important analgesic. Lancet 1984;2:1208.

41. Yalom I, Greaves C. Group therapy with the terminally ill. Am J Psychiatry 1977;134:396.

Index